Modern Trends in Vascular Surgery

The Ischemic Extremity
New Findings and Treatment

Heron E. Rodriguez, M.D.
Assistant Professor of Surgery
Division of Vascular Surgery
Department of Surgery
Northwestern University
Feinberg School of Medicine
Chicago, IL

William H. Pearce, M.D.
Violet R. and Charles A. Baldwin
Professor of Vascular Surgery
Chief, Division of Vascular Surgery
Department of Surgery
Northwestern University
Feinberg School of Medicine
Chicago, IL

James S. T. Yao, M.D., Ph.D.
Professor Emeritus
Division of Vascular Surgery
Department of Surgery
Northwestern University
Feinberg School of Medicine
Chicago, IL

2010
PEOPLE'S MEDICAL PUBLISHING HOUSE—USA
SHELTON, CONNECTICUT

People's Medical Publishing House—USA
2 Enterprise Drive, Suite 509
Shelton, CT 06484
Tel: 203-402-0646
Fax: 203-402-0854
E-mail: info@pmph-usa.com

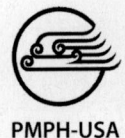

PMPH-USA

© 2010 PMPH–USA, Ltd.

09 10 11 12 13/PMPH/9 8 7 6 5 4 3 2 1

13-digit ISBN 13: 978-1-60795-050-9
10-digit ISBN 10: 1-60795-050-2

Printed in China by People's Medical Publishing House of China
Copyeditor/Typesetter: Spearhead Global, Inc.; Cover Designer: Mary McKeon

Library of Congress Cataloging-in-Publication Data on File

Notice: The authors and publisher have made every effort to ensure that the patient care recommended herein, including choice of drugs and drug dosages, is in accord with the accepted standard and practice at the time of publication. However, since research and regulation constantly change clinical standards, the reader is urged to check the product information sheet included in the package of each drug, which includes recommended doses, warnings, and contraindications. This is particularly important with new or infrequently used drugs. Any treatment regimen, particularly one involving medication, involves inherent risks that must be weighed on a case-by-case basis against the benefits anticipated. The reader is cautioned that the purpose of this book is to inform and enlighten; the information contained herein is not intended as, and should not be employed as, a substitute for individual diagnosis and treatment.

Sales and Distribution

Canada
McGraw-Hill Ryerson Education
Customer Care
300 Water Street
Whitby, Ontario L1N 9B6
Canada
Tel: 1-800-565-5758
Fax: 1-800-463-5885
www.mcgrawhill.ca

Foreign Rights
John Scott & Company
International Publisher's Agency
P.O. Box 878
Kimberton, PA 19442
USA
Tel: 610-827-1640
Fax: 610-827-1671

Japan
United Publishers Services Limited
1-32-5 Higashi-Shinagawa
Shinagawa-ku, Tokyo 140-0002
Japan
Tel: 03-5479-7251
Fax: 03-5479-7307
Email: kakimoto@ups.co.jp

United Kingdom, Europe, Middle East, Africa
McGraw Hill Education
Shoppenhangers Road
Maidenhead
Berkshire, SL6 2QL
England
Tel: 44-0-1628-502500
Fax: 44-0-1628-635895
www.mcgraw-hill.co.uk

*Singapore, Thailand, Philippines, Indonesia,
Vietnam, Pacific Rim, Korea*
McGraw-Hill Education
60 Tuas Basin Link
Singapore 638775
Tel: 65-6863-1580
Fax: 65-6862-3354
www.mcgraw-hill.com.sg

Australia, New Zealand
Elsevier Australia
Locked Bag 7500
Chatswood DC NSW 2067
Australia
Tel: +61 (2) 9422-8500
Fax: +61 (2) 9422-8562
www.elsevier.com.au

Brazil
Tecmedd Importadora e Distribuidora
de Livros Ltda.
Avenida Maurilio Biagi 2850
City Ribeirao, Rebeirao, Preto SP
Brazil
CEP: 14021-000
Tel: 0800-992236
Fax: 16-3993-9000
Email: tecmedd@tecmedd.com.br

India, Bangladesh, Pakistan, Sri Lanka, Malaysia
CBS Publishers
4819/X1 Prahlad Street 24
Ansari Road, Darya Ganj, New Delhi-110002
India
Tel: 91-11-23266861/67
Fax: 91-11-23266818
Email:cbspubs@vsnl.com

People's Republic of China
PMPH
Bldg 3, 3rd District
Fangqunyuan, Fangzhuang
Beijing 100078
P.R. China
Tel: 8610-67653342
Fax: 8610-67691034
www.pmph.com

Contents

SECTION IV Advances in Wound Care and Amputation   241

40 The Management of Upper Extremity Arterial Trauma   463

David L. Gillespie, M.D., F.A.C.S.

SECTION VIII Upper Extremity Ischemia   477

41 Quality Measures in Thoracic Outlet Syndrome   479

Julie Ann Freischlag, M.D.

42 Arterial Injuries in Thoracic Outlet Compression   489

William H. Pearce, M.D., Jon S. Matsumura, M.D.,
and James S.T. Yao, M.D., Ph.D.

Preface

For the last 31 years the Northwestern Vascular Symposium in Chicago has been a premier forum for the dissemination of knowledge in the field of vascular surgery. Every year, we invite a select group of recognized experts from all over the country and abroad to discuss a wide variety of topics related to our profession. From traditional open surgery, to endovascular techniques, regulatory issues, economic aspects, training related topics, emerging technology and many others, these state-of-the art dissertations have been recorded in a book that is published every year. This collection of books represents a major contribution to the surgical literature. Unfortunately, for the last several years, only those who attend the Vascular Symposium have had access to this series of great textbooks.

In another one of our educational efforts, a compilation of the most relevant chapters contained in the five most recent symposium books has been prepared. This collection of books will allow readers all across the globe to gain access to the invaluable contributions of the amazing group of renowned leaders in vascular surgery that have formed the faculty of the Northwestern Vascular Symposium from 2005 to 2009.

This book–the fourth in this collection–is devoted to topics related to the management of ischemia affecting the extremities. Divided in eight sections, it is a comprehensive review of the most current understanding of limb ischemia and its management. The first section deals with the perioperative management of patients suffering from limb ischemia. It touches on the natural history of limb ischemia, the different strategies for its management and also discusses non-invasive approaches and the different pharmacological adjunctive therapies used in the treatment of this group of disorders. The second and third sections are excellent compilations of the most updated techniques in the endovascular and open surgical armamentarium. The fourth section reviews wound management and advances in amputation and prosthesis. The presentation and management of complications after both open and endovascular interventions are reviewed in section V. In section VI, cutting edge technologies such as stem cell therapy, bioengineered and modified conduits and molecular therapy are discussed. The last two sections are devoted to arterial trauma and upper extremity disorders.

It has been a privilege for us to be able to put together in this book the many great contributions of the Northwestern Vascular Symposium faculty. We are proud to present "Ischemic Extremities" and to make it available to the public, hoping that it will become a useful reference tool for the practicing vascular surgeon in his or her continuous efforts to adapt to the ever-changing world of vascular surgery.

Acknowledgments

We thank the administrative staff of the Division of Vascular Surgery—Sara Minton and Jan Goldstein—for their support. Special thanks to Susan Parmentier of Greenwood Academic for reprocessing chapters of the last five Northwestern Symposia. We would also like to thank W.L. Gore & Associates for a generous education grant to support the Northwestern Vascular Symposium over the years. Finally, we thank Mr. Jason Malley of People's Medical Publishing House-USA and Mr. Harjeet Singh from Spearhead Global, Inc. for their expert assistance.

Heron E. Rodriguez
William H. Pearce
James S.T. Yao

Contributors

Samuel S. Ahn, M.D.
University Vascular Associates-Westwood
Los Angeles, CA

David G. Armstrong, D.P.M., Ph.D.
Professor of Surgery
Director, Southern Arizona Limb Salvage
Alliance (SALSA)
Arizona Health Science Center
Department of Surgery
Tucson, AZ

Marvin D. Atkins, M.D.
Texas A&M HSC
Scott & White Hospital and Clinic
Temple, TX

Christopher Attinger, M.D.
Departments of Surgery and Sections
    of Plastic Surgery
VA Medical Center and Georgetown
    University Medical Center
Washington, DC

Michael Belkin, M.D.
Harvard University Medical School
Department of Vascular Surgery
Brigham & Women's Hospital
Boston, MA

Marshall E. Benjamin, M.D.
Associate Professor of Surgery
Division of Vascular Surgery
University of Maryland School of
    Medicine
Baltimore, MD

Ana Silvia Bonilla, M.D.
Department of Cardiovascular-Thoracic
    Surgery
Rush University Medical Center
Chicago, IL

David C. Brewster, M.D.
Professor of Surgery
Vascular and Endovascular Surgery
Massachusetts General Hospital
Boston, MA

Richard K. Burt, M.D.
Associate Professor of Immunotherapy for
    Autoimmune Diseases
Northwestern University
Feinberg School of Medicine
Chicago, IL

Keith D. Calligaro, M.D.
Clinical Associate Professor of Surgery
Chief, Section of Vascular Surgery
Pennsylvania Hospital
Philadelphia, PA

Christopher G. Carsten, III, M.D.
Academic Department of Surgery
Section of Vascular Surgery
Greenville Hospital System
Greenville, SC

Mary Ella Carter, M.D.
Departments of Surgery and Sections
    of Plastic Surgery
VA Medical Center and Georgetown
    University Medical Center
Washington, DC

Jeffrey A. Caves, Ph.D.
Department of Surgery
Emory University School of Medicine
Atlanta, GA

Elliot L. Chaikof, M.D., Ph.D.
Professor of Surgery
Division of Vascular Surgery and
    Endovascular Therapy
Department of Surgery
Emory University School of Medicine
Atlanta, GA

Benjamin B. Chang, M.D.
Associate Professor of Surgery
Institute for Vascular Health and Disease
Albany Medical College
Albany, NY

Kenneth J. Cherry, M.D.
Department of Surgery
University of Virginia
Charlottesville, VA

Dolores F. Cikrit, M.D.
Indiana University School of Medicine
Indianapolis, IN

Ryan Crews, M.S.
Dr. William M. Scholl College of
    Podiatric Medicine
Rosalind Franklin University of
    Medicine and Surgery
North Chicago, IL

Michael C. Dalsing, M.D.
The E. Dale and Susan E. Habegger
    Professor of Surgery
Director of Vascular Surgery
Indiana University School of Medicine
Indianapolis, IN

R. Clement Darling, III, M.D.
Professor of Surgery
Albany Medical College
Albany Medical Center Hospital
The Institute for Vascular Health and
    Disease
The Vascular Group, PLLC
Albany, NY

Ricardo Deleon, M.D.
Department of Surgery
Johns Hopkins Medical Institutions
Baltimore, MD

Matthew J. Dougherty, M.D.
Clinical Associate Professor of Surgery
Chief, Section of Endovascular Surgery
Pennsylvania Hospital
Philadelphia, PA

Gregory A. Dumanian, M.D.
Professor of Surgery
Division of Plastic Surgery
Northwestern University
Feinberg School of Medicine
Chicago, IL

Mark L. Edwards, M.H.P.E., C.P.
Department of Physical Medicine and
    Rehabilitation
Northwestern University
Chicago, IL

Karen F. Kim Evans, M.D.
Departments of Surgery and Sections of
    Plastic Surgery
VA Medical Center and Georgetown
    University Medical Center
Washington, DC

William R. Flinn, M.D.
Professor of Surgery
Chief, Division of Vascular Surgery
Division of Vascular Surgery
Univ of Maryland Med Systems
Baltimore, MD

Julie A. Freischlag, M.D.
Professor of Surgery
Johns Hopkins School of Medicine
Chair, Department of Surgery
Surgeon-in-Chief
Johns Hopkins Medical Institutions
Baltimore, MD

David L. Gillespie, M.D., R.V.T., F.A.C.S.
Professor of Surgery
School of Medicine and Dentistry
University of Rochester
Rochester, NY

Rao Gutta, M.D.
Division of Vascular Surgery
University of Maryland Medical Systems

Peter K. Henke, M.D.
Section of Vascular Surgery
University of Michigan Medical School
Ann Arbor, MI

Karen J. Ho, M.D.
Harvard University Medical School
Department of Vascular Surgery
Brigham & Women's Hospital
Boston, MA

Melissa E. Hogg, M.D.
Division of Vascular Surgery
Northwestern University's Feinberg
  School of Medicine
Northwestern Memorial Hospital
Chicago, IL

Chad E. Jacobs, M.D.
Department of Cardiovascular-
  Thoracic Surgery
Rush University Medical Center
Chicago, IL

Muneera R. Kapadia, M.D.
Department of Surgery
University of Minnesota
Minneapolis, MN

Melina R. Kibbe, M.D.
Associate Professor
Division of Vascular Surgery
Northwestern University's Feinberg
  School of Medicine
Northwestern Memorial Hospital
Chicago, IL

Robert Kim, M.D.
The Polyclinic
Seattle, WA

Paul B. Kreienberg, M.D.
Associate Professor of Surgery
Institute for Vascular Health and
  Disease
Albany Medical College
Albany, NY

Toshifumi Kudo, M.D., Ph.D.
Tokyo Medical and Dental University,
  Graduate School
Dept. of Vascular and Applied Surgery
Yushima, Bunkyo-ku

Todd A. Kuiken, M.D., Ph.D.
Associate Professor
Department of Physical Medicine and
  Rehabilitation
Northwestern University
Feinberg School of Medicine
The Rehabilitation Institute of Chicago
Chicago, IL

Woo-Hyung Kwun, M.D., Ph.D.
Endovascular Research Fellow
University of California at Los Angeles
Gonda Vascular Center
Los Angeles, CA

Glenn M. Lamuraglia, M.D.
Associate Professor of Surgery
Harvard Medical School
Massachusetts General Hospital
Boston, MA

Gregory J. Landry, M.D.
Associate Professor
Division of Vascular Surgery
Oregon Health Sciences University
Dotter Interventional Institute
Portland, OR

Eugene M. Langan III, M.D.
Program Director of Vascular
  Surgery
Academic Department of Surgery,
  Section of Vascular Surgery
Greenville Hospital System
Greenville, SC

Frank W. LoGerfo, M.D.
William V. McDermott Distinguished
  Professor of Surgery
Division of Vascular and
  Endovascular Surgery
Beth Israel Deaconess Medical Center
Boston, MA

John D. Martin, M.D.
Cardiology Associates PC
Annapolis, MD

Jon S. Matsumura, M.D.
University of Wisconsin
Madison, Wl

Walter J. McCarthy, M.D.
Department of Cardiovascular-Thoracic
  Surgery and the College of Health
  Sciences
Department of Vascular Ultrasound
Rush University Medical Center
Chicago, IL

Mary McGrae McDermott, M.D.
Professor Dept of Medicine
Northwestern University Feinberg School
  of Medicine
Northwestern Medical Faculty Foundation
Chicago, IL

James F. Mckinsey, M.D.
Interim Chief of Vascular Surgery
Columbia University College of Physicians
  and Surgeons
Weill Medical College of Cornell University
New York Presbyterian Hospital
New York NY

Manish Mehta, M.D., M.P.H.
Institute for Vascular Health and Disease
Albany Medical College
Albany, NY

Spencer J. Melby, M.D.
Senior Resident in General Surgery
Department of Surgery
Barnes-Jewish Hospital and Washington
  University School of Medicine
St. Louis, MO

Joseph L. Mills, Sr., M.D.
Professor of Surgery
Chief, Division of Vascular Surgery
University of Arizona Health Sciences
  Center
Tucson, AZ

Laura A. Miller, Ph.D., C.P
Department of Physical Medicine and
  Rehabilitation
Northwestern University, Feinberg School
  of Medicine
The Rehabilitation Institute of Chicago
Chicago, IL

Thomas S. Monahan, M.D.
UCSF
San Francisco, CA

Gregory L. Moneta, M.D.
Professor and Chief
Vascular Surgery
Oregon Health & Science University
Portland, OR

Raghunandan Motaganahalli, M.D.
Indiana-Purdue University,
  Indianapolis
Indianapolis, IN

Michael Murphy, M.D.
Indiana University School of Medicine
Indianapolis, IN

Ryan Nachreiner, M.D.
Inland Vascular Institute
Spokane, WA

Samer F. Najjar, M.D.
Vascular Surgery & Associates
Arlington Heights, IL

Patrick O'Hara, M.D., F.A.C.S.
Professor of Surgery
Cleveland Clinic Lerner College of
  Medicine of Case Western Reserve
  University
Department of Vascular Surgery
Cleveland Clinic Foundation
Cleveland, OH

Kenneth Ouriel, M.D.
New York-Presbyterian Hospital
New York, NY

Kathleen J. Ozsvath, M.D.
Assistant Professor of Surgery
Institute for Vascular Health and Disease
Albany Medical College
Albany, NY

Jean M. Panneton, M.D.
Vascular Surgery Chief and Program
  Director
Eastern Virginia Medical School
Norfolk, VA

Frederico E. Parodi, M.D.
Tampa, FL

Juan C. Parodi, M.D.
University of Miami
Miami, FL

Sheela T. Patel, M.D.
Assistant Professor of Surgery
Miami, Florida

Philip S.K. Paty, M.D.
Associate Professor of Surgery
Albany Medical College
Albany Medical Center Hospital
The Institute for Vascular Health and
  Disease
The Vascular Group
PLLC
Albany, NY

William H. Pearce, M.D.
Violet R. and Charles A. Baldwin
Professor of Vascular Surgery
Chief, Division of Vascular Surgery
Department of Surgery
Northwestern University
Feinberg School of Medicine
Chicago, IL

Brian G. Peterson, M.D.
Assistant Professor of Surgery
Division of Vascular Surgery
St. Louis University
St. Louis, MO

Richard H. Pin, M.D.
Grant Medical Center
Columbus, OH

Daniel A. Popowich, M.D.
General Surgery Resident
Northwestern University Feinberg School
  of Medicine
Chicago, IL

C. Steven Powell, M.D.
Section of Vascular Surgery
Department of Cardiovascular
  Sciences
East Carolina University
Greenville, NC

Soo J. Rhee, M.D.
Division of Vascular Surgery
Columbia University College of
  Physicians and Surgeons
Weill Medical College of Cornell
  University
New York Presbyterian Hospital
New York NY

John J. Ricotta, M.D.
Chair, Department of Surgery
Washington Hospital Center
Washington, DC

Sean P. Roddy, M.D.
Professor of Surgery, Albany Medical
  College/Albany Medical Center
The Institute for Vascular Disease
Albany, NY

David Rosenthal, M.D.
Atlanta Medical Center
Atlanta, GA

Alan P. Sawchuk, M.D.
Indiana University School of Medicine
Indianapolis, IN

Andres Schanzer, M.D.
University of Massachusetts
  Medical School
Div. of Vasc. and Endovascular Surg.
Worcester, MA

Peter J. Schubart, M.D.
O'Connor Hospital
San Jose, CA

Eric C. Scott, M.D.
Vascular Surgery Fellow
Eastern Virginia Medical School
Norfolk, VA

Shoab Shafique, M.D.
Oklahoma City, OK

Dhiraj M. Shah, M.D.
Professor of Surgery
Albany Medical College
Albany Medical Center Hospital
The Institute for Vascular Health and
    Disease
The Vascular Group
PLLC, Albany, NY

Anton N. Sidawy, M.D., M.P.H.
Chief, Surgical Services
VA Medical Center
Professor of Surgery
Georgetown and George Washington
    Universities
Washington, DC

Michelle E. Sohn, M.D.
St Joseph Hospital
Peace Health Medical Group
Bellingham, WA

Michael C. Stoner, M.D.
Assistant Professor
Section of Vascular Surgery
Department of Cardiovascular
    Sciences
East Carolina University
Greenville, NC

Gale L. Tang, M.D.
Puget Sound VA Health Care System
Surgical Services
Seattle, WA

Lloyd M. Taylor, Jr., M.D.
Professor of Surgery
Division of Vascular Surgery
Portland, OR

Robert W. Thompson, M.D.
Professor of Surgery (Section of Vascular
    Surgery),
Radiology, and Cell Biology and Physiology
Vice-Chariman for Research
Department of Surgery
Washington University School of Medicine
St. Louis, MO

Jonathan B. Towne, M.D.
Professor Emeritus
Medical College of Wisconsin
Milwaukee, WI

Maria G. Uberti, M.D.
University of Miami, Miami, FL

Vinit N. Varu, M.D.
Department of Surgery
University of Illinois at Chicago
Chicago, IL

Daniel B. Walsh, M.D.
Professor of Surgery
Vice Chair
Department of Surgery
Dartmouth-Hitchcock Medical Center
Lebanon, NH

Eric D. Wellons, M.D.
Department of Vascular Surgery
Atlanta Medical Center
Atlanta, GA

Nicole M. Wheeler, M.D.
Department of Surgery
Division of Vascular Surgery
Oregon Health & Science University
Portland, OR

Stephanie C. Wu, D.P.M., M.S
Dr. William M. Scholl College of Podiatric
    Medicine
Rosalind Franklin University of Medicine
    and Surgery
North Chicago, IL

James S.T. Yao, M.D., Ph.D.
Emeritus Professor of Surgery
Division of Vascular Surgery
Northwestern University
Feinberg School of Medicine
Chicago, IL

New Strategies in Perioperative Care

1

Critical Limb Ischemia

Vinit N. Varu, M.D. Melissa E. Hogg, M.D.
Melina R. Kibbe, M.D.

The international consensus on the definition of critical limb ischemia (CLI) is the following: any patient with chronic ischemic rest pain, ulcers, or gangrene attributable to objectively proven arterial occlusive disease.[1] Traditionally, given that CLI is a severe manifestation of peripheral arterial disease (PAD), these patients would be classified as stage III–IV in the Fontaine classification or Grades 4–6 in the Rutherford classification (Table 1–1). However, recent evidence shows CLI does not progress though the various stages of these classification systems.[2] In fact, a multicenter prospective study looking at amputations in patients with ischemia found that over half of their cohort did not have any PAD symptoms six months prior to onset of CLI.[3] Moreover, rigid guidelines on the proper surgical management of these patients are currently unavailable, due, in part, to the relatively small incidence and prevalence of

TABLE 1-1. CLASSIFICATION SCHEMES OF PERIFERAL ARTERIAL DISEASE

Classification	Stage	Clinical Description
Fontaine	I	Asymptomatic
	IIa	Mild claudication
	IIb	Moderate-to-severe claudication
	III	Rest pain
	IV	Ulceration or gangrene
Rutherford	0	Asymptomatic
	1	Mild claudication
	2	Moderate claudication
	3	Severe claudication
	4	Rest pain
	5	Minor tissue loss
	6	Severe tissue loss or gangrene

CLI. Additionally, large numbers of patients with CLI are lost to follow-up or die from other causes in these study populations.

Patients with CLI experience significant morbidity with cardiovascular event rates surpassing those seen in patients with symptomatic coronary artery disease.[4] Amputations continue to be performed despite recent advances in revascularization, partly because patients with CLI are referred to vascular surgeons late in their course, but perhaps more importantly, because there is no agreed upon definition of a nonsalvageable limb.[5] Possibly even more concerning, of the little data that exist, most of it focuses on a physician-oriented view of success: graft patency, limb salvage, and survival.[6] Only in the past few years has patient-oriented outcomes research begun to gather attention. Between the vascular exam, the ankle-brachial index (ABI), and a number of imaging modalities, diagnosing this disease is straightforward, but vascular surgeons as a united group have yet to understand how to optimally manage patients with CLI, whether surgically or medically. Further, it is unclear what the ultimate treatment goal is for patients with CLI. This review serves to explore these issues and examine what challenges the vascular surgeon will continue to face in managing patients with CLI. The epidemiology and natural history of CLI will be discussed, along with the pathophysiology of the disease process. A review of the literature in regards to the different treatment modalities will be presented to help the vascular surgeon optimize the type of therapy for the CLI patient, as well as new scoring systems to help predict surgical outcomes in CLI patients undergoing revascularization procedures. Next, an overview of the current status of patient-oriented outcomes will be given, and how this may potentially alter how patients with CLI may be treated. Finally, we will look at emerging therapies in the treatment of CLI as an alternative to medical and surgical management of this devastating disease.

EPIDEMIOLOGY AND NATURAL HISTORY

PAD affects eight to 10 million Americans, and is associated with a three- to six-fold increased risk of cardiovascular morbidity and mortality compared to individuals without PAD.[7] Patients with CLI represent about 1% of the total number of patients with PAD.[8] CLI is the devastating end-manifestation of PAD, with overall mortality in these patients approaching 50% over five years.[9] The one-year mortality in patients wih CLI is approximately 20%, mainly as a result of cardiac events, while 35% will require amputation; the remainder will enter a more chronic state.[10,11] Following surgical intervention, data from the Veterans Affairs National Surgery Quality Improvement Plan (NSQIP) revealed a 30-day mortality rate of 2.1%, 6.3%, and 13.3% for femoral-distal bypass, below-knee amputation (BKA), and above-knee amputation (AKA), respectively.[12,13] Immediate postoperative mortality and major limb amputation is also considerable with recent series ranging from 1–3% and 1–5%, respectively.[14,15] The economic burden is considerable as well. The estimated cost of clinical care alone of patients with CLI has been estimated at $43,000 per patient-year in 1990.[16] Further, the median cost of managing a patient after amputation is estimated to be almost twice that of successful limb salvage.[17] Clearly, CLI represents a challenging disease state with a lot of room for improvement in the approach toward management of these patients. To fully understand how to accomplish this, the vascular surgeon must first recognize the inherent problems that cause CLI.

PATHOPHYSIOLOGY

The pathophysiology of CLI is a chronic and complex process that affects the macro-vascular systems and microvascular systems, as well as surrounding tissues. CLI starts with atherogenesis, which leads to arterial stenosis. From here, multiple processes occur in no defined order including inadequate tissue oxygen extraction, microvascular dysfunction, and impaired vasomotor control (Table 1–2). However, it is not fully known why the physiologic mechanisms that regulate structure and function of the vasculature breakdown lead to circulatory failure. Atherosclerotic vascular disease is responsible for the majority of cases of cardiovascular disease in both developing and developed countries, including PAD.[18] And as such, their risk factors are the same. Major modifiable risk factors include hypertension, dyslipidemia, smoking, obesity, and diabetes mellitus.[19] Emerging risk factors are also being discovered including C-reactive protein, lipoprotein A, fibrinogen, and homocysteine.[18]

Atherosclerosis

Initiation of the lesion is largely an inflammatory process. First, leukocytes chemotax and adhere to the endothelium with the help of selectins and adhesion molecules,

TABLE 1-2. PATHOPHYSIOLOGY OF CRITICAL LIMB ISCHEMIA

Atherosclerosis	Leukocyte chemotaxis
	Increased adhesion molecule expression
	Foam cell formation
	Fatty streaks
	VSMC proliferation, calcification, and increased matrix deposition
Arterial Stenosis	Angiogenesis
	Arteriogenesis
	Increased VEGF, stromal cell-derived factor-1, and CXCR4 expression
	Demand greater than supply
	Inadequate tissue perfusion
Inadequate Tissue Oxygen Extraction	Redistribution of blood flow
	Change in mitochondrial density and distribution in tissue
	Impaired myogenic control
	Decreased cross-sectional area of muscle fibers
	Altered expression of myosin heavy chain isoforms
Microvascular Dysfunction	Increased reactive oxygen species production
	Decreased nitric oxide production
	Increased peroxynitrite production
	Increased platelet activation
	Microvascular thrombosis
	Precapillary arteriole collapse
	Impaired oxygen exchange
Impaired Vasomotor Control	Vasomotor paralysis
	Arterial remodeling with decreased wall thickness
	Increased skin perfusion

P-selectin, and vascular cell adhesion molecule (VCAM-1).[20] Diapedesis occurs, which allows deposition of leukocytes into the intimal layer.[20] Monocytes acquire morphologic characteristics of macrophages, and these macrophages become lipid-laden and lead to foam cell formation. Foam cells form the fatty streak and characterize the early atherosclerotic lesion.[20] These early stages are reversible.[20]

Progression to plaque formation occurs when further foam cells and vascular smooth muscle cells (VSMC) accumulate within the lesion. With more VSMC, the plaque becomes more fibrous and a cellular matrix is formed.[20] VSMC also express proteins involved in osteogenesis and this leads to accumulation of calcium. Through these processes, the lesion grows and starts to impede blood flow.

Arterial Stenosis

Inadequate blood flow is the hallmark of occlusive arterial disease. The disease can either be functional or critical. Functional ischemia is when blood flow is normal at rest but insufficient during exercise.[21] This leads to intermittent claudication. "Critical Limb Ischemia" occurs when blood flow supplied to the distal extremity is insufficient to provide the basal oxygen demand. Critical ischemia is a result of a perfusion deficit at rest causing rest pain or trophic lesions of the legs.[21] Gangrene occurs when arterial perfusion is so inadequate that spontaneous necrosis occurs in the most poorly perfused areas.[22] Arterial occlusion results in development of collateral supply vessels through a process called angiogenesis or arteriogenesis.[21] These are physiologic responses to increased demand for blood supply, and are stimulated by factors such as tissue hypoxia and alterations in blood flow.[23] Angiogenesis, or capillary sprouting, involves coordinated migration, proliferation, assembly, and maturation of endothelial cells and VSMC.[22,23] This results in formation of major collateral feeder vessels in addition to nutritive blood vessels. The extent of development of these vessels is dependent on the degree of stenosis within the native vessel. Arteriogenesis is the process that promotes the enlargement of preexisting collaterals.[22,23] Both angiogenesis and arteriogenesis have been shown to occur in experimental models of hind-limb ischemia.[22] Several factors, including vascular endothelial growth factor (VEGF), stromal cell-derived factor-1, and chemokine receptor 4 (CXCR4), have been identified that enhance angiogenesis or arteriogenesis, but randomized human clinical trials have not yielded successful results when delivering some of these agents to patients.[24,25]

Inadequate Tissue Oxygen Extraction

Many earlier studies have shown that exercise improves muscle function in claudicants, not only due to increased collateralization, but also to peripheral change within the muscle.[25] Muscle adaptations include redistribution of flow to better perfused active fibers, increased oxygen exchange capacity due to change in mitochondrial density and distribution within the fiber, and enhanced capillary networks surrounding the fibers.[25,26] In a rat model of peripheral arterial insufficiency, Yang et al. showed that a treadmill trained rat had increased exercise tolerance, a better ability to maintain muscle tension, increased peak oxygen consumption, increased oxygen extraction, and a greater capillary-to-fiber ratio.[26] Furthermore, muscle ischemia, as a result of peripheral vascular disease, is a factor that causes adaptations in the contractile apparatus of muscle. McGuigan et al. biopsied the gastrocnemius muscle of subjects with PAD and controls, and found that subjects with PAD had altered expression of myosin heavy chain isoforms, a significant decrease in the cross-sectional area of the muscle fibers, and an enhanced capillary density.[27]

Microvascular Dysfunction

The endothelium protects the integrity of the blood vessel by modulating vascular tone, controlling vascular permeability, and acting as an antithrombogenic barrier. Chronic ischemia from macroscopic disease leads to alterations in structure and function of endothelial cells, and alterations in pressure unloading, which results in microcirculatory adaptations. This endothelial dysfunction leads to hemostasis and microthrombosis within the capillaries, as well as edema formation in the extremity.[23] Furthermore, endothelial trauma results in increased free radical production, inappropriate platelet activation, and leukocyte adhesion, all of which lead to microthrombi formation.[23] The increase in reactive oxygen species also leads to decreased bioavailability of nitric oxide through a direct reaction between superoxide and nitric oxide, and also through diminished production of nitric oxide from endothelial nitric oxide synthase.[28] Furthermore, as superoxide reacts with nitric oxide, peroxynitrite is produced, which has deleterious effects in tissue.[28] Also, due to the inflammatory response produced locally as a result of atherosclerosis and systemically as a result of ongoing tissue damage, severe microvascular dysfunction occurs. Tissue oxygen exchange at the capillary level is impeded and less effective. The ultimate timeline leading to diminished capillary perfusion is not clearly established, and microthrombosis is one theory. Others include collapse of precapillary arterioles because of low transmural pressure, arteriolar vasospasm, and abnormal vasomotion.[29] Immune system activation locally and capillary occlusion caused by endothelial cell swelling, rigid adhesive leukocytes, platelet aggregation, and rigid red blood cells are also factors believed to further lead to diminished blood delivery.[29] Edema is a major concern in these patients. Most patients with CLI have edema due to a combination of impaired vasomotor control leading to maximal vasodilation along with holding their limb in a dependent position to alleviate ischemic rest pain. This increases the hydrostatic pressure within the distal portion of the limb. Edema is harmful because an increase in interstitial pressure compresses already compromised capillaries and impairs diffusion of nutrients to the tissue.[23] This pathologic process occurs in arteries, arterioles, capillaries, and the tissue surrounding these structures. These processes occurring simultaneously are what make critical limb ischemia such a difficult disease to treat. Simply reinstating blood flow on a macrovascular level alone will not reverse this derangement. In fact, doing so initiates reactive hyperemia and a cascade of events that may further exacerbate an already complex problem.[23]

Impaired Vasomotor Control

Arterioles in patients with critical limb ischemia are already maximally vasodilated. Arteriolar vasodilation and consequent reduction of peripheral vascular resistance is a primary compensatory response to ischemia.[23] It has been shown that, compared to controls, peripheral arterioles in CLI patients are insensitive to provasodilatory stimuli.[23] This phenomenon has been called "vasomotor paralysis," which is thought to be the result of chronic exposure to vasorelaxing factors in patients with diseased vessels.[23] It has been shown that CLI patients have increased circulating inflammatory mediators.[18] These inflammatory mediators have also been found to correlate with endothelial dysfunction.[23] This appears to have systemic consequences as well as local implications. A study performed on patients with lower extremity PAD showed that flow-mediated vasodilation of the brachial artery was reduced compared to matched controls.[23] Also, blood vessels in patients with CLI are associated with decreased wall thickness, decreased cross-sectional area, and decreased wall-to-lumen ratio compared to controls.[23] These are responses to relative hypotension and hypoperfusion in the limb.[23] Microvascular vasodilation maintains nutritive flow in the presence of proximal arterial occlusion. Paradoxically, some patients with CLI have increased total skin blood flow in the ischemic foot, probably because of maximal vasodilation in the neighboring tissue. This maldistribution of skin microcirculation contributes to the sequelae of CLI in addition to the reduction in total blood flow.[29] Clinically, we see implications of this phenomenon with "dependent rubor" or reddening of an extremity when in the dependent position as a result of increased perfusion. Conversely, lifting the leg results in a pallor from capillary collapse.

MODIFIABLE RISK FACTORS

Risk factors for CLI certainly parallel those for PAD: diabetes, hypercholesterolemia, hypertension, and smoking, among others. In theory, if the root cause of the disease process could be modified or controlled, then the consequences of CLI should not manifest. While this is an overly simplified means of analysis, the following studies were conducted to determine if controlling these risk factors does indeed show benefit.

Progression of CLI to gangrene occurs in 40% of diabetic patients compared to 9% of nondiabetic patients.[30] Further, limb-salvage rates in diabetic patients with CLI have been reported to be lower versus nondiabetic patients, and diabetes is an independent risk factor for postoperative amputation and complications in CLI.[31] In Type II diabetic patients with established macrovascular disease, pioglitazone treatment has recently been shown to reduce composite of all-cause mortality, nonfatal myocardial infarction, and stroke, whereas no significant effect was observed with leg revascularization or amputation.[32] Yet it is unclear if similar glycemic control influences prognosis for CLI patients specifically.

It is known that plasma levels of total and low-density lipoprotein cholesterol are important risk factors for coronary heart disease. While patients with elevated lipoprotein levels have been associated with higher mortality in patients with CLI, it has been shown that hypertryglyceridemia independently increases the risk for progression of intermittent claudication to CLI.[33] While data is sparse in regard to the effect of lipid reduction in CLI, statin use is associated with improved survival in CLI patients one year after infrainguinal bypass graft surgery (*see* Treatment, Nonsurgical Management, below).

Current recommendations for antihypertensive treatment in high-risk subjects, including PAD, propose target blood pressure of <140/90 in subjects without diabetes and <130/80 in subjects with diabetes.[34] While some advocate that the blood pressure target in CLI patients should be set above recommended levels to increase perfusion to the ischemic limb, this has yet to be examined scientifically. Randomized trials have shown a reduction in vascular death, myocardial infarction, and stroke in PAD patients receiving angiotensin-converting enzyme (ACE)-inhibitors for four to six years, regardless of ABI.[35] Moreover, ACE-inhibitors are associated with lower mortality after infrainguinal bypass surgery.[36] Still, no specific studies have been conducted with these agents in patients with CLI. A meta-analysis showed that β-blockers do not adversely effect walking capacity or symptoms of intermittent claudication in patients with mild to moderate PAD.[37] However, potentially unfavorable effects in the more severely ischemic patients with CLI cannot be excluded since this has not been extensively studied.

No individual randomized trials have demonstrated the efficacy of aspirin for reduction of cardiovascular events in PAD, but meta-analyses have shown antiplatelet medications reduce the risk of vascular death, myocardial infarction (MI), and stroke by approximately 25%.[38] Moreover, the CAPRIE study showed clopidogrel conferred an 8.7% further relative risk reduction for stroke, MI, or vascular death compared to aspirin among patients with myocardial infarction, ischemic stroke, or PAD.[39] Still, aspirin is considered first-line therapy for patients with PAD,[40] but no studies have been conducted specifically for CLI patients.

Smoking is a major risk factor for both the occurrence and progression of CLI, and continued smoking in PAD patients increases the risk for progression to CLI, amputation, and the need for invasive intervention.[41] Cessation of smoking leads to improved graft patency after surgery and decreased risk for fatal vascular complications in PAD.[42] Even though the effect of tobacco has yet to be studied in the CLI population, it is prudent to say all patients with CLI should be advised to quit smoking and be given access to nicotine replacement therapy to increase the odds of successfully quitting smoking.

TREATMENT

The diagnosis of CLI cannot be stressed enough, given the high morbidity and mortality associated with the disease process. In fact, observational studies of patients with CLI who are not candidates for revascularization suggest that one year after onset of CLI, only 50% of the patients will remain amputation-free, though may still be symptomatic, while 25% will require a major amputation. The remaining 25% will have died.[1] Therefore, even though CLI is a clinical diagnosis, it should be confirmed objectively and early in the disease process through ABI, toe systolic pressures, or transcutaneous oxygen tension (TcPO$_2$). Once diagnosis is confirmed, the goals of treating CLI are to relieve ischemic pain, heal ischemic ulcers, prevent limb loss, improve patient function and quality of life (QOL), and prolong survival. While revascularization, in theory, could optimally achieve these goals, the severity of comorbidities along with durability of the reconstruction in patients with CLI demands a risk-benefit analysis to determine the optimal therapy for these patients.

Nonsurgical Management

CLI confers a poor prognosis in medically treated patients, as conservative management is associated with a major amputation rate at one year of 70–95%, while surgical revascularization may decrease this risk to 24–28%.[43] Revascularization may not always be an option. Patients present to vascular surgeons who are poor candidates for surgical or endovascular procedures due to medical comorbidities, institutionalized nonambulatory status, or poor outflow vessels in the limb. Furthermore, data is currently lacking to determine which patients should definitively be treated with early amputation. Marston et al. reported on a subset of patients that satisfied the TransAtlantic

Intersociety Consensus (TASC) criteria for CLI who presented with extensive but uncomplicated and stable tissue loss. These patients were managed nonoperatively and were treated with a dedicated wound management plan. The primary outcome revealed that most patients did not require amputation (38%) at one year; however, ulcer healing was slow, with only 25% healed at six months and just over 50% healed at one year.[11] The group also looked at the ability of noninvasive diagnostic tools to predict the probability of limb loss, and found that an ABI < 0.5 was a significant predictor of limb loss, although ABIs were obtainable in only half the limbs studied. Neither ankle nor toe pressures were predictive of limb loss or wound closure.

The natural history of patients with CLI treated with pharmacological means has also been studied. Placebo-controlled studies have evaluated the use of iloprost, a prostacyclin analogue, for CLI. Norgen et al. reported an average incidence of limb loss of 39% in the placebo group with no significant difference in the iloprost group.[44] Similarly, Brass et al. showed lipo-ecraprost failed to modify the six-month amputation rate in patients with CLI who were not candidates for revascularization.[45]

Prevent III was a prospective, randomized, double-blinded multicenter trial designed to determine the efficacy of edifoligide, a molecule that inhibits the expression of genes that stimulate VSMC proliferation and thus hypothesized to reduce neointimal hyperplasia, in preventing autogenous vein graft failure in CLI patients undergoing infrainguinal bypass grafting.[15] The primary study endpoint was the time to occurrence of nontechnical index graft failure resulting in graft revision or major amputation within 12 months. Secondary endpoints included all-cause graft failure, clinically significant graft stenosis, amputation/reintervention-free survival, and nontechnical primary graft patency. Results of the study showed no significant difference between the treatment groups in the primary or secondary trial endpoints, primary graft patency, or limb salvage.

Various reports have demonstrated that cardioprotective medications such as statins, antihypertensive medications, and antiplatelet agents are associated with a decreased cardiovascular event rate in patients with PAD.[46] However, little is known about the effectiveness of these drugs in the patient population at greatest risk—patients with CLI—as these studies have been performed in heterogenous populations. Schanzer et al. utilized the Prevent III cohort to shed light on this.[47] In this cohort, 45% were taking statins, 59% were taking β-blockers, and 80% were taking antiplatelet therapy. It was found that only statin use was associated with improved survival in CLI patients one year after revascularization, while β-blockers and antiplatelet medication had no impact on survival. The group also reported that significant predictors of mortality in patients with CLI undergoing infrainguinal bypass graft surgery were age >75 years, coronary artery disease, chronic kidney disease stages 4 and 5, and tissue loss.

Spinal cord stimulation has been proposed as an alternative to amputation in patients with CLI and severe pain. It involves the implantation of stimulation electrodes at the level of L3–L4, as well as a pulse generator subcutaneously. While a recent meta-analysis of randomized, controlled studies showed a modest positive effect of spinal cord stimulation in CLI patients in terms of pain relief, spinal cord stimulation compared to the best medical treatment does not prevent amputations in CLI.[48]

Surgical Management: Revascularization or Primary Amputation

Surgical therapy should only be offered if the benefit-to-risk ratio is high and if anatomical characteristics suggest a favorable and durable result. Revascularization strategies include bypass surgery, with or without thromboendarterectomy, as well as endovascular techniques. Overall, in CLI patients undergoing infrainguinal bypass, the one-year primary graft patency is 61%, secondary patency is 80%, and limb salvage is 88%.15 However, these data reflect only a subgroup of vascular centers specializing in the management of CLI and, therefore, these results may lack generalizability.[49] This is further evidenced by Chung et al. who showed a 25% wound complication rate in CLI patients undergoing infrainguinal bypass with reversed saphenous vein, with primary patency rates of 63% and 50%, and limb salvage rates at 85% and 79%, at one and three years, respectively.[50] While there is debate whether emerging endovascular treatment is preferable over open surgery, there is a general consensus that bypass surgery is preferable to angioplasty in patients with a TASC Type D lesion.[51] Further, those who favor surgery usually emphasize good long-term anatomical patency and clinical durability. However, this preference could come at the cost of high morbidity and mortality, as well as substantial resource use.[49] The bypass versus angioplasty in severe ischemia of the leg (BASIL) study was a multicenter, randomized controlled trial that set out to compare the outcomes of a bypass-surgery-first strategy versus an angioplasty-first strategy in patients presenting with CLI due to infrainguinal disease.[52] When examined in the medium term, the amputation-free survival, all-cause mortality, and health-related quality of life were similar in both groups, though in the surgery-first group, more morbidity was incurred and hospital costs were one-third higher within the first year. Yet it was found for those patients that remained alive with an intact limb for more than two years, surgery prolonged their subsequent life more so than the angioplasty group. Vessel or graft patency rates were not reported for this trial.

While advances in open and endovascular techniques continue to be made, amputation rates are rising, with nearly 25 major amputations per 100,000 people performed annually in the United States.[53] In fact, TASC has identified indications for those patients with CLI who would benefit from primary amputation: unreconstructable arterial occlusive disease, necrosis of significant areas of the weight-bearing portion of the foot, a fixed and irremediable flexion contracture of the leg, a terminal illness, or a very limited life expectancy because of comorbid conditions.[8] Further, amputation may offer an expedient return to a useful QOL. While not specific to CLI, it bears mentioning that PAD patients who are ambulatory preoperatively and are capable of healing a BKA, the likelihood of ambulation with a prosthesis ranges from 66–81% in most studies. For similar patients with AKA, the likelihood of ambulation falls below 50%.[54] However, it can be conjectured that these rates would be lower for patients with CLI given their increased comorbidities.

A recent prospective study by Abou-Zamzam et al. examined factors leading to primary amputation versus revascularization.[55] Over a four-year period, 224 patients underwent surgery for critical limb ischemia, with 43% receiving primary amputation and 57% undergoing revascularization. On univariate analysis, nonwhite ethnicity, diabetes mellitus, end-stage renal disease, major tissue loss, dependent living situation, and non-ambulatory status were independent predictors of amputation versus revascularization. Moreover, the group examined system-related factors such as time to vascular surgery evaluation, and found these factors did not influence treatment. The authors implied limb salvage could be improved by aggressive treatment of medical comorbidities to prevent late complications of CLI along with earlier recognition of tissue loss. It should be noted that most series comparing perioperative mortality or long-term survival in CLI have favored revascularization over amputation overall.[56] Yet, these are not randomized trials, and given the increased comorbidities in patients receiving primary amputations, if patients were to be randomized to revascularization or amputation, the mortality and long-term survival rates would likely be improved in the amputation groups.

To reiterate, patients with CLI undergoing revascularization procedures suffer less mortality versus patients receiving a BKA or AKA, but this is due to the fact that patients undergoing amputation are generally more debilitated and at higher preoperative risk. In terms of morbidity, healing incisions below the knee is difficult regardless of the surgical procedure. Approximately 25% of infrainguinal bypass patients suffer some type of incisional wound complication postoperativley.[57] For those CLI patients undergoing primary amputation, failure of BKA requiring re-amputation or conversion to AKA occurs in 10–20% of cases.[9] The revascularization group also incurs a 1% graft infection rate secondary to wound breakdown with a 15% mortality rate and a 40% incidence of major limb loss.[58] While there are circumstances in which revascularization is favored over amputation, or vice-versa, it cannot be stated with confidence which is the superior course of action in a patient until more randomized data are available.

Predictive Indices

Although lower limb revascularization for CLI is advocated if there is a reasonable chance of patient survival and limb salvage at one year, a risk assessment method to predict poor outcome in patients with CLI undergoing surgical revascularization could more accurately stratify which patients are most at risk for postoperative mortality and/or major limb amputation. Biancari et al. developed a risk-scoring method to better predict immediate postoperative outcome following femoral endarterectomy, femorpopliteal bypass, or infrapopliteal bypass surgery in CLI patients.[59] The group used a registry that included data on 3,925 infrainguinal surgical revascularization procedures, and found in the overall series that 30-day postoperative mortality and major amputation rates were 3.1% and 6.3%, respectively. The 30-day postoperative mortality and/or limb loss rate was 9.2%. Numerous risk factors were included in the analysis (i.e., coronary artery disease [CAD], cerebrovascular accident [CVA], renal disease, and so on), but multivariate analysis showed that only diabetes, CAD, foot gangrene, and urgent operation were independent risk factors of mortality and/or limb loss. Thus, a risk score was developed by assigning 1 point each to these risk factors (Table 1–3). In the derivitization set, the 30-day post-operative mortality or amputation rates in patients with scores of 0, 1, 2, 3, and 4 were 7.7%, 6.4%, 11.1%, 20.4%, and 27.3%, respectively (p<.0001); mortality rates were 1.3%, 2.3%, 4.1%, 7.7%, and 12.1%, respectively, (P < 0.0001); and major amputation rates were 6.4%, 4.3%, 7.1%, 12.7%, and 18.2%, respectively, (P < 0.0001). In the validation data set, the 30-day postoperative mortality or amputation rates in patients with scores of 0, 1, 2, 3, and 4 were 4.8%, 7.5%, 10.1%, 15.9%, and 22.2%, respectively, (P < 0.0001); mortality rates were 0.7%, 2.3%, 4.2%, 5.5%, and 14.8%, respectively, (P < 0.0001); and major amputation rates were 4.6%, 5.3%, 6.4%, 11.0%, and 14.0%, respectively (P = 0.011). Thus, while in its infancy, this bedside risk-scoring system appears to provide meaningful information to the clinician that may aid in the decision process when contemplating surgical revasularization in a patient with CLI.

PATIENT-ORIENTED OUTCOMES

While there is a moderate amount of data on the physician-oriented view of success in patients with CLI (i.e., graft patency, limb salvage, and survival), patient-oriented out-

TABLE 1-3. RISK STRATIFICATION METHOD OF BIANCARI ET AL. FOR PREDICTING
POSTOPERATIVE OUTCOME AFTER SURGICAL REVASULARIZATION IN PATIENTS WITH CLI.[59]

Risk Factor	Points
Diabetes mellitus	1
Coronary artery disease	1
Foot gangrene	1
Urgent operation	1

Overall Score	30-day Mortality Rate	30-day Amputation Rate
0	0.7%	4.6%
1	2.3%	5.3%
2	4.2%	6.4%
3	5.5%	11.0%
4	14.8%	14.0%

comes are only now beginning to come to light. In fact, the TASC consortium has stated there are no QOL instruments that have been standardized in a large population of patients with CLI, and has identified this as a "critical issue".[8] This may be because patients are often not clinically stable, the treatments offered this patient population involve significant morbidity, or the outcomes for this "end-of-life" population are complex.[9] If the vascular surgeon approaches the treatment of CLI in a more patient-focused manner as opposed to the current lesion-focused manner, subgroups of the CLI population undergoing extensive limb salvage may be better off with primary amputation or nonoperative management.

Abou-Zamzam et al. evaluated patient-oriented outcomes in a retrospective study evaluating pre- and postoperative living situation and ambulatory status in CLI patients undergoing lower extremity bypass.[60] At six months, 99% of patients who were living independently and 97% of patients who were ambulatory preoperatively maintained these outcomes. Yet, only 4% of patients who were in a dependent living situation preoperatively went on to live independently at six months, while 21% who did not ambulate preoperatively were independently ambulatory six months following surgery. Multivariate analysis confirmed preoperative living situation and ambulatory status as predictors of outcome at six months postoperatively. A subsequent study by Nicoloff et al. followed similar patients for 42 months and found that with longer follow-up, there is greater decline in independent ambulation and living status.[61] Further, only 14% of patients had an uncomplicated operation, relief of symptoms, complete wound healing, no need for reoperation, and maintenance of functional status. The remaining 86% spent a major portion of their remaining life undergoing treatment for CLI. Taylor et al. evaluated functional outcomes at five years for surgical revascularization procedures.[62] In this retrospective analysis, ambulatory and living status were assessed, as well as traditional outcomes measures. The five-year overall graft patency rates and limb salvage were 72.4% and 72.1%, respectively, with a five-year survival of 41.9%. Independent ambulatory and living status were 70.6% and 81.3%, respectively, with impaired ambulatory status at presentation and dementia as predictors of poor functional outcomes, while location or type of reconstruction, as well as comorbidities, did not predict functional outcomes.

Even with the paucity of retrospective data for functional outcomes in patients with CLI, the amount of prospective data in terms of QOL is lacking even further, and data that is available involve mainly patient questionnaires. The Short Form 36 (SF36) and Nottingham Health Profile (NHP) have been most widely used in patients with PAD, but to date, there is no consensus on the ideal questionnaire in evaluating patients with CLI.[63] The largest study performed to date that prospectively analyzed patient QOL after surgical revascularization was the PREVENT III trial[15] (*see* Treatment, Nonsurgical Management, above). Significant improvements in QOL were identified in patients undergoing surgical revascularization at three and 12 months compared to baseline, and factors associated with failure of QOL improvement included diabetes and graft-related events. Of note, questionnaires were completed by 92% at baseline, 61% at three months, and 52% at 12 months, and analysis showed that patients not completing the QOL assessment were more likely to have had an adverse event. The BASIL trial evaluated heath-related QOL in patients with CLI undergoing lower extremity bypass versus angioplasty[52] (*see* Treatment, Surgical Management, above). The health-related QOL were similarly improved in both treatment arms, and with longer follow-up, there was a trend for improved health-related QOL in the surgery group, although this difference was not significant.

FUTURE DIRECTION

Exploring new strategies for revascularization in patients with CLI is of the utmost importance given the large number of patients with CLI not eligible for revascularization procedures, coupled with the fact that amputation confers an even worse prognosis, and that medical management at this time is suboptimal. Currently, the ultimate goal of increasing or stimulating angiogenesis is being evaluated through clinical trials in patients with PAD and CLI. A phase I clinical trial utilizing a naked human plasmid encoding an isoform of VEGF165 was injected in 10 limbs of nine CLI patients with nonhealing ischemic ulcers or rest pain.[64] The ABI improved significantly from 0.33 to 0.48, along with newly seen collateral blood vessels documented by contrast angiography. Ischemic ulcers healed or markedly improved in four of seven limbs, including successful limb salvage in three patients initially planned for BKA. Rajagopalan et al. performed a phase II, randomized, double-blinded, placebo-controlled trial in patients with severe intermittent claudication using an adenovirus carrying the VEGF121 gene, but found no difference in peak walking time, ABI, claudication onset time, and QOL after 12 weeks time.[65] Powell et al. examined hepatocyte growth factor (HGF) plasmid injection in a double-blind, placebo-controlled, dose-escalating, multicenter HGF-STAT trial in 104 CLI patients with rest pain or tissue loss. Increase of $TcPO_2$ in the high-dose group was shown, though rate of amputation, wound healing, and ABI did not reveal a difference between treatment groups.[66] A similar trial evaluated intramuscular administration of NV1FGF, a plasmid-based angiogenic gene delivery system for local expression of fibroblast growth factor 1 (FGF-1) in patients with CLI. Improvements in ulcer healing were similar for all treatment groups, yet the use of NV1FGF significantly reduced the risk two-fold of all amputations and major amputations. Moreover, the adverse event incidence was similar between the groups, but there was a trend for reduced risk of death with the use of NV1FGF.[67] Gene therapy offers a potential efficacious therapy for patients with CLI, especially given that in the more than

1,000 individuals treated with gene therapy for therapeutic angiogenesis in phase I/II trials, adverse events have been similar between treatment and control groups. Long-term safety data must be gathered before widespread use of these treatments, given the potential for angiogenesis-triggered malignancies and the impact of angiogenesis on physiological and pathological processes such as retinopathy and atherosclerotic plaque destabilization.[68]

Endothelial progenitor cells (EPC) derived from bone marrow or peripheral blood are implicated in the regeneration of injured endothelium and neoangiogensis after tissue ischemia, and thus have been identified as a new potential therapeutic target in CLI. The first human trial of cell therapy in CLI consisted of a pilot study in which patients with unilateral ischemia received intramuscular implantation of bone marrow-mononuclear cells (BM-MNCs) in the ischemic leg and saline in the contralateral leg. The procedure was deemed safe and significantly improved ABI, TcPO$_2$, rest pain, and increased pain-free walking time at four and 24 weeks.[69] The group then randomly injected patients with bilateral CLI with BM-MNCs in one leg and peripheral blood-mononuclear cells (PB-MNCs) in the contralateral leg. The ABI, TcPO$_2$, and rest pain significantly improved in the BM-MNC group, but much smaller, nonsignificant, increases were seen in the PB-MNC group.[69] Granulocyte colony stimulating factor is known to stimulate production of hematopoetic stem cells and EPCs from the BM to the circulation.[70] In a randomized controlled trial, Huang et al. studied diabetic patients with CLI who received subcutaneous injections of granulocyte colony stimulating factor for five days prior to collection of PB-MNCs. Improvements were seen in pain-free walking distance, diabetic foot ulcers, ABI, and angiographic scores.[71]

While both gene and cell therapy studies in CLI seem promising in a subset of patients, all of these studies, to date, lack adequate power as well as double-blinded controls. Also, other endpoints need to be examined in greater detail (i.e., amputation rates, QOL, etc) before a definite conclusion can be reached in regard to safety and efficacy of this novel therapy.

CONCLUSION

As proposed by Nehler et al., a possible approach is to look at the problem of CLI from three sides: technical issues of revascularization, foot wound healing issues, and co-morbidity.[49] Patients with marginal outlook in more than one category would not be considered revascularization candidates. Yet the group states that even more important may be the need for more prospective and randomized trials that focus on CLI patients and patient-oriented outcomes as the guide to optimal therapy. For instance, in selected high-risk patients, early amputation may improve QOL, in which these patients may spend the remainder of their lives at home instead of being hospitalized for multiple failed revascularization procedures. Moreover, patients with extensive co-morbidities who may undergo a successful operation may still be unable to ambulate due to these comorbidites, further signaling the need to look into patient-focused outcomes in more detail. It must be kept in mind that high-risk patients are victims of the limitations of surgical and medical management, and potential for increased morbidity. As such, newer techniques with promise, such as cell and gene therapy in patients with CLI, need prospective and randomized studies to continue. The vascular surgeon is armed with a repertoire of skills and modalities to confront a patient with CLI, but much work lies ahead in what the appropriate outcomes to measure should be so that the appropriate therapy can be optimally directed toward patient well-being.

REFERENCES

1. Norgren L, Hiatt WR, Dormandy JA, Nehler MR, Harris KA, Fowkes FGR. Inter-society consensus for the management of peripheral arterial disease (TASC II). *Eur J Vasc Endovas Surg*. 2007;33:S5–S75.
2. White JV, Rutherford RB, Ryjewski C. Chronic subcritical limb ischemia: A poorly recognized stage of critical limb ischemia. *Semin Vasc Surg*. 2007 Mar;20(1):62–7.
3. Dormandy J, Belcher G, Broos P, Eikelboom B, Laszlo G, Konrad P, et al. Prospective-Study of 713 Below-Knee Amputations for Ischemia and the Effect of A Prostacyclin Analog on Healing. *Br J Surg*. 1994 Jan;81(1):33–7.
4. Caro J, Migliaccio-Walle K, Ishak KJ, Proskorovsky I. The morbidity and mortality following a diagnosis of peripheral arterial disease: long-term follow-up of a large database. *BMC Cardiovasc Disord*. 2005;5–14.
5. Connelly J, Airey M, Chell S. Variation in clinical decision making is a partial explanation for geographical variation in lower extremity amputation rates. *Br J Surg*. 2001 Apr;88(4): 529–35.
6. Rutherford RB, Baker JD, Ernst C, Johnston KW, Porter JM, Ahn S, et al. Recommended standards for reports dealing with lower extremity ischemia: Revised version. *J Vasc Surg*. 1997 Sep;26(3):517–38.
7. Criqui MH, Langer RD, Fronek A, Feigelson HS, Klauber MR, Mccann TJ, et al. Mortality Over A Period of 10 Years in Patients with Peripheral Arterial-Disease. *N Engl J Med*. 1992 Feb 6;326(6):381–6.
8. Dormandy JA RRB. Management of peripheral arterial disease (PAD). TASC Working Group. *TransAtlantic Inter-Society Consensus (TASC)*. (1 Pt 2):S1-S296 ed. 2000.
9. Nehler MR, Peyton BD. Is revascularization and limb salvage always the treatment for critical limb ischemia? *J Cardiovasc Surg*. 2004 Jun;45(3):177–84.
10. Gottsater A. Managing risk factors for atherosclerosis in critical limb ischaemia. *Eur J Vasc Endovas Surg*. 2006 Nov;32(5):478–83.
11. Marston WA, Davies SW, Armstrong B, Farber MA, Mendes RC, Fulton JJ, et al. Natural history of limbs with arterial insufficiency and chronic ulceration treated without revascularization. *J Vasc Surg*. 2006 Jul;44(1):108–14.
12. Feinglass J, Pearce WH, Martin GJ, Gibbs J, Cowper D, Sorensen M, et al. Postoperative and amputation-free survival outcomes after femorodistal bypass grafting surgery: Findings from the department of veterans affairs national surgical quality improvement program. *J Vasc Surg*. 2001 Aug;34(2):283–90.
13. Feinglass J, Pearce WH, Martin GJ, Gibbs J, Cowper D, Sorensen M, et al. Postoperative and late survival outcomes after major amputation: Findings from the Department of Veterans Affairs National Surgical Quality Improvement Program. *Surgery*. 2001 Jul;130(1):21–9.
14. Albers M, Romiti M, Brochado-Neto FC, De Luccia N, Pereira CAB. Meta-analysis of popliteal-to-distal vein bypass grafts for critical ischemia. *J Vasc Surg*. 2006 Mar;43(3): 498–503.
15. Conte MS, Bandyk DF, Clowes AW, Moneta GL, Seely L, Lorenz TJ, et al. Results of PREVENT III: A multicenter, randomized trial of edifoligide for the prevention of vein graft failure in lower extremity bypass surgery. *J Vasc Surg*. 2006 Apr;43(4):742–50.
16. Hunink MGM, Wong JB, Donaldson MC, Meyerovitz MF, Devries J, Harrington DP. Revascularization for Femoropopliteal Disease - A Decision and Cost-Effectiveness Analysis. *JAMA*. 1995 Jul 12;274(2):165–71.
17. Singh S, Evens L, Datta D, Gaines P, Beard JD. The costs of managing lower limb-threatening ischaemia. *Eur J Vasc Endovas Surg*. 1996 Oct;12(3):359–62.

18. Hackam DG, Anand SS. Emerging risk factors for atherosclerotic vascular disease - A critical review of the evidence. *JAMA*. 2003 Aug 20;290(7):932–40.
19. Shammas NW. Epidemiology, classification, and modifiable risk factors of peripheral arterial disease. *Vasc Health Risk Manag*. 2007;3(2):229–34.
20. Ouriel K. Peripheral arterial disease. *Lancet*. 2001 Oct 13;358(9289):1257–64.
21. Hernando FJS, Conejero AM. Peripheral artery disease: Pathophysiology, diagnosis and treatment. *Revista Espanola de Cardiologia*. 2007 Sep;60(9):969–82.
22. Tang GL, Chang DS, Sarkar R, Wang R, Messina LM. The effect of gradual or acute arterial occlusion on skeletal muscle blood flow, artcriogenesis, and inflammation in rat hindlimb ischemia. *J Vasc Surg*. 2005 Feb;41(2):312–20.
23. Coats P, Wadsworth R. Marriage of resistance and conduit arteries breeds critical limb ischemia. *Am J Physiol-Heart Circ Physiol*. 2005 Mar;288(3):H1044–H1050.
24. van Weel V, Seghers L, de Vries MR, Kuiper EJ, Schlingemann RO, Bajema IM, et al. Expression of vascular endothelial growth factor, stromal cell-derived factor-1, and CXCR4 in human limb muscle with acute and chronic ischemia. *Arterioscl Thromb Vasc Biol*. 2007 Jun;27(6):1426–32.
25. Yang HT, Ogilvie RW, Terjung RL. Peripheral Adaptations in Trained Aged Rats with Femoral-Artery Stenosis. *Circ Res*. 1994 Feb;74(2):235–43.
26. Yang HT, Ogilvie RW, Terjung RL. Low-Intensity Training Produces Muscle Adaptations in Rats with Femoral-Artery Stenosis. *J Appl Physiol*. 1991 Nov;71(5):1822–9.
27. McGuigan MRM, Bronks R, Newton RU, Sharman MJ, Graham JC, Cody DV, et al. Muscle fiber characteristics in patients with peripheral arterial disease. *Med Sci Sports Exerc*. 2001 Dec;33(12):2016–21.
28. Griendling KK, FitzGerald GA. Oxidative stress and cardiovascular injury - Part I: Basic mechanisms and in vivo monitoring of ROS. *Circulation*. 2003 Oct 21;108(16):1912–6.
29. Kempczinski RF. The Chronically Ischemic Leg: An Overview. In: Rutherford RB. ed. *Vascular Surgery. 5th ed*. Philadelphia; WB Saunders. 2000:91 7–927.
30. Kannel WB. Risk factors for atherosclerotic cardiovascular outcomes in different arterial territories. *J Cardiovasc Risk*. 1994 Dec;1(4):333–9.
31. Virkkunen J, Heikkinen M, Lepantalo M, Metsanoja R, Salenius JP. Diabetes as an independent risk factor for early postoperative complications in critical limb ischemia. *J Vasc Surg*. 2004 Oct;40(4):761–7.
32. Dormandy JA, Charbonnel B, Eckland DJA, Erdmann E, Massi-Benedetti M, Kmoules IK, et al. Secondary prevention of macrovascular events in patients with type 2 diabetes in the PROactive Study (PROspective pioglitAzone Clinical Trial In MacroVascular Events): a randomised controlled trial. *Lancet*. 2005 Oct 8;366(9493):1279–89.
33. Smith I, Franks PJ, Greenhalgh RM, Poulter NR, Powell JT. The influence of smoking cessation and hypertriglyceridaemia on the progression of peripheral arterial disease and the onset of critical ischaemia. *Eur J Vasc Endovasc Surg*. 1996 May;11(4):402–8.
34. De Backer G, Ambrosioni E, Borch-Johnsen K, Brotons C, Cifkova R, Dallongeville J, et al. European guidelines on cardiovascular disease prevention in clinical practice - Third Joint Task Force of European and other Societies on Cardiovascular Disease Prevention in Clinical Practice. *Eur Heart J*. 2003 Sep;24(17):1601–10.
35. Ostergren J, Sleight P, Dagenais G, Danisa K, Bosch J, Yi QL, et al. Impact of ramipril in patients with evidence of clinical or subclinical peripheral arterial disease. *Eur Heart J*. 2004 Jan;25(1):17–24.
36. Henke PK, Blackburn S, Proctor MC, Stevens J, Mukherjee D, Rajagopalin S, et al. Patients undergoing infrainguinal bypass to treat atherosclerotic vascular disease are underprescribed cardioprotective medications: Effect on graft patency, limb salvage, and mortality. *J Vasc Surg*. 2004 Feb;39(2):357–64.
37. Radack K, Deck C. Beta-Adrenergic Blocker Therapy Does Not Worsen Intermittent Claudication in Subjects with Peripheral Arterial-Disease - A Metaanalysis of Randomized Controlled Trials. *Arch Inter Med*. 1991 Sep;151(9):1769–76.

38. Baigent C, Sudlow C, Collins R, Peto R. Collaborative meta-analysis of randomised trials of antiplatelet therapy for prevention of death, myocardial infarction, and stroke in high risk patients. *Br Med J.* 2002 Jan 12;324(7329):71–86.

39. Gent M, Beaumont D, Blanchard J, Bousser MG, Coffman J, Easton JD, et al. A randomised, blinded, trial of clopidogrel versus aspirin in patients at risk of ischaemic events (CAPRIE). *Lancet.* 1996 Nov 16;348(9038):1329–39.

40. Clagett GP, Sobel M, Jackson MR, Lip GYH, Tangelder M, Verhaeghe R. Antithrombotic therapy in peripheral arterial occlusive disease. *Chest.* 2004 Sep;126(3):609S–26S.

41. Jonason T, Ringqvist I. Factors of Prognostic Importance for Subsequent Rest Pain in Patients with Intermittent Claudication. *Acta Medica Scandinavica* 1985;218(1):27–33.

42. Jonason T, Bergstrom R. Cessation of Smoking in Patients with Intermittent Claudication - Effects on the Risk of Peripheral Vascular Complications, Myocardial-Infarction and Mortality. *Acta Medica Scandinavia.* 1987;221(3):253–60.

43. Wolfe JHN, Wyatt MG. Critical and subcritical ischaemia. *Eur J Vasc Endovas Surg.* 1997 Jun;13(6):578–82.

44. Norgren L. Non-surgical treatment of critical limb ischaemia; *Eur J Vasc Surg.* 1990 Oct. 4(5):449–54 ed.

45. Brass EP, Anthony R, Dormandy J, Hiatt WR, Jiao J, Nakanishi A, et al. Parenteral therapy with lipo-ecraprost, a lipid-based formulation of a PGE1 analog, does not alter six-month outcomes in patients with critical leg ischemia. *J Vasc Surg.* 2006 Apr;43(4):752–9.

46. Hankey GJ, Norman PE, Eikelboom JW. Medical treatment of peripheral arterial disease. *JAMA.* 2006 Feb 1;295(5):547–53.

47. Schanzer A, Hevelone N, Owens CD, Beckman JA, Belkin M, Conte MS. Statins are independently associated with reduced mortality in patients undergoing infrainguinal bypass graft surgery for critical limb ischemia. *J Vasc Surg.* 2008 Apr;47(4):774–81.

48. Ubbink DT, Vermeulen H. Spinal cord stimulation for non-reconstructable chronic critical leg ischaemia. *Cochrane Database of Systematic Reviews.* 2005;(3).

49. Nehler MR, Hiatt WR, Taylor LM. Is revascularization and limb salvage always the best treatment for critical limb ischemia? *J Vasc Surg.* 2003 Mar;37(3):704–8.

50. Chung J, Bartelson BB, Hiatt WR, Peyton BD, McLafferty RB, Hopley CW, et al. Wound healing and functional outcomes after infrainguinal bypass with reversed saphenous vein for critical limb ischemia. *J Vasc Surg.* 2006 Jun;43(6):1183–90.

51. Ballard JL MJS. Surgical management of critical limb ischemia. *Tech Vasc Intervent Radiol.* 2005 Dec;8(4):169–74.

52. Bradbury AW, Ruckley CV, Fowkes FGR, Forbes JF, Gillespie I, Adam DJ, et al. Bypass versus angioplasty in severe ischaemia of the leg (BASIL): multicentre, randomised controlled trial. *Lancet.* 2005 Dec 3;366(9501):1925–34.

53. Feinglass J, Brown JL, LaSasso A, Sohn MW, Manheim LM, Shah SJ, et al. Rates of lower-extremity amputation and arterial reconstruction in the United States, 1979 to 1996. *Am J Pub Health.* 1999 Aug;89(8):1222–7.

54. Aulivola B, Hile CN, Hamdan AD, Sheahan MG, Veraldi JR, Skillman JJ, et al. Major lower extremity amputation - Outcome of a modern series. *Arch Surg.* 2004 Apr;139(4):395–9.

55. Abou-Zamzam AM, Gomez NR, Molkara A, Banta JE, Teruya TH, Killeen JD, et al. A prospective analysis of critical limb ischemia: Factors leading to major primary amputation versus Revascularization. *Ann VascSurg.* 2007 Jul;21(4):458–63.

56. Taylor LM, Hamre D, Dalman RL, Porter JM. Limb Salvage Vs Amputation for Critical Ischemia - the Role of Vascular-Surgery. *Arch Surg.* 1991 Oct;126(10):1251–8.

57. Treiman GS, Copland S, Yellin AE, Lawrence PF, McNamara RM, Treiman RL. Wound infections involving infrainguinal autogenous vein grafts: A current evaluation of factors determining successful graft preservation. *J Vasc Surg.* 2001 May;33(5):948–54.

58. Kikta MJ, Goodson SF, Bishara RA, Meyer JP, Schuler JJ, Flanigan DP. Mortality and Limb Loss with Infected Infrainguinal Bypass Grafts. *J Vasc Surg.* 1987 Apr;5(4):566–71.

59. Biancari F, Salenius JP, Heikkinen M, Luther M, Ylonen K, Lepantalo M. Risk-scoring method for prediction of 30-day postoperative outcome after infrainguinal surgical revascu-

larization for critical lower-limb ischemia: a Finnvasc registry study. *World J Surg.* 2007 Jan;31(1):217–27.

60. AbouZamzam AM, Lee RW, Moneta GL, Taylor LM, Porter JM. Functional outcome after infrainguinal bypass for limb salvage. *J Vasc Surg.* 1997 Feb;25(2):287–95.

61. Nicoloff AD, Taylor LM, McLafferty RB, Moneta GL, Porter JM. Patient recovery after infrainguinal bypass grafting for limb salvage. *J Vasc Surg.* 1998 Feb;27(2):256–63.

62. Taylor SM, Kalbaugh CA, Blackhurst DW, Cass AL, Trent EA, Langan EM, et al. Determinants of functional outcome after revascularization for critical limb ischemia: An analysis of 1000 consecutive vascular interventions. *J Vasc Surg.* 2006 Oct;44(4):747–55.

63. Landry GJ. Functional outcome of critical limb ischemia. *J Vasc Surg.* 2007 Jun;45:141A–8A.

64. Baumgartner I, Pieczek A, Manor O, Blair R, Kearney M, Walsh K, et al. Constitutive expression of phVEGF(165) after intramuscular gene transfer promotes collateral vessel development in patients with critical limb ischemia. *Circulation.* 1998 Mar 31;97(12):1114–23.

65. Rajagopalan S, Mohler ER, Lederman RJ, Mendelsohn FO, Saucedo JF, Goldman CK, et al. Regional angiogenesis with vascular endothelial growth factor in peripheral arterial disease - A phase II randomized, double-blind, controlled study of adenoviral delivery of vascular endothelial growth factor 121 in patients with disabling intermittent claudication. *Circulation.* 2003 Oct 21;108(16):1933–8.

66. Powell RJ, Simons M, Mendelsohn FO, Daniel G, Henry TD, Koga M, et al. Results of a double-blind, placebo-controlled Study to Assess the Safety of Intramuscular Injection of Hepatocyte Growth Factor Plasmid to Improve Limb Perfusion in Patients with Critical Limb Ischemia. *Circulation.* 2008 Jul 1;118(1):58–65.

67. Nikol S, Baumgartner I, Van Belle E, Diehm C, Visona A, Capogrossi MC, et al. Therapeutic angiogenesis with intramuscular NV1FGF improves amputation-free survival in patients with critical limb ischemia. *Mol Ther.* 2008 May;16(5):972–8.

68. Tongers J, Roncalli JG, Losordo DW. Therapeutic angiogenesis for critical limb ischemia - Microvascular therapies coming of age. *Circulation.* 2008 Jul 1;118(1):9–16.

69. Tateishi-Yuyama E, Matsubara H, Murohara T, Ikeda U, Shintani S, Masaki H, et al. Therapeutic angiogenesis for patients with limb ischaemia by autologous transplantation of bone-marrow cells: a pilot study and a randomised controlled trial. *Lancet.* 2002 Aug 10; 360(9331):427–35.

70. Honold J, Lehmann R, Heeschen C, Walter DH, Assmus B, Sasaki K, et al. Effects of granulocyte colony simulating factor on functional activities of endothelial progenitor cells in patients with chronic ischemic heart disease. *Arterioscler Thromb Vasc Biol.* 2006 Oct;26(10): 2238–43.

71. Huang PP, Li SZ, Han MZ, Xiao ZJ, Yang RC, Han ZC. Autologous transplantation of granulocyte colony-stimulating factor-mobilized peripheral blood mononuclear cells improves critical limb ischemia in diabetes. *Diabetes Care.* 2005 Sep;28(9):2155–60.

2

Exercise Training Programs for Patients with Intermittent Claudication

Mary McGrae McDermott, M.D.

Lower extremity peripheral arterial disease (PAD) affects 8 to 12 million men and women in the United States. Persons with PAD have increased functional impairment and increased rates of functional decline compared to persons without PAD.[1-3] Patients with intermittent claudication (IC) have slower walking speed, poorer walking endurance, lower physical activity, and more impaired quality of life compared to individuals without PAD.[1,2] The functional limitations associated with PAD have been linked to increased rates of health care utilization and institutionalization. The social and economic costs associated with PAD-related functional limitations are substantial. Identifying therapies to improve lower extremity functioning and prevent functional decline are important to prevent mobility loss, poor quality of life, and other adverse outcomes in patients with PAD. This review summarizes data regarding exercise treatments that have been demonstrated to be effective for patients with PAD. Gaps in knowledge regarding optimal exercise therapies for PAD patients are also outlined.

Only 20% to 30% of persons with PAD have classic symptoms of intermittent claudication. Many patients with PAD are asymptomatic (i.e., have no exertional leg symptoms) or have exertional leg symptoms that are not typical of classic intermittent claudication.[1,2] Although significant functional impairment has been documented in PAD patients who are asymptomatic or who do not have classic symptoms of intermittent claudication, most clinical trials of exercise interventions in patients with PAD have been limited to patients with intermittent claudication.[1-4] Thus, this review summarizes data on effective exercise therapies for patients with PAD and intermittent claudication.

BENEFITS OF SUPERVISED TREADMILL EXERCISE PROGRAMS IN PATIENTS WITH PAD

Supervised exercise training has been well studied in patients with intermittent claudication. Multiple randomized controlled clinical trials of supervised walking exercise have been conducted for PAD patients with intermittent claudication. To quantify the benefit associated with supervised exercise and identify features of the most effective exercise programs for patients with intermittent claudication, Gardner et al. analyzed 21 clinical trials in a meta-analysis of exercise training for patients with intermittent claudication.[5] In their meta-analysis, Gardner et al. included any clinical trials that used treadmill testing to assess walking-related intermittent claudication pain before and after a supervised exercise program. Of the 21 studies included in the meta-analysis, three were randomized controlled trials, four were nonrandomized, and 14 were uncontrolled. Seventeen of the studies included 25 or fewer participants. Results of the meta-analysis demonstrated an overall 179% increase in treadmill-measured pain-free walking distance and a 122% increase in treadmill-measured maximal walking distance.[5] In addition, Gardner et al. identified three characteristics of the exercise training interventions that accounted for nearly 90% of the variation in results across the 21 studies.[5] These three characteristics, in descending order of importance, were 1) the claudication pain endpoint employed during exercise training, 2) total duration of the exercise training program, and 3) mode of exercise. For claudication pain endpoint, exercise training programs in which participants exercised to *maximal severity* of claudication pain were more effective than training programs in which participants exercised to the *onset* of claudication symptoms. With regard to length of training, exercise training programs lasting 26 weeks or more were more effective than those lasting less than 26 weeks. Finally, clinical trials that employed walking exercise were more effective than training programs that either combined walking exercise with other forms of exercise or did not include walking exercise at all. In the meta-analysis, Gardner et al. also found that older patients experienced greater improvement from exercise training than younger patients. Claudication patients with lower average ankle brachial index (ABI) levels benefited to a greater degree than claudication patients with higher ABI values. Finally, claudication patients with a longer duration of symptoms on entry into the exercise program benefited more than patients with shorter symptom duration (Table 2–1). Based on the findings of Gardner et al., the most effective supervised exercise training program for patients with intermittent claudication is one that incorporates walking to near-maximal claudication symptoms during training, lasts a minimum of six months, and uses walking exercise as the primary mode of exercise.[5] Although less important than the other characteristics, exercise training programs that take place at least three times per week were more effective than exercise training programs with

TABLE 2-1. CHARACTERISTICS OF PAD PATIENTS WITH INTERMITTENT CLAUDICATION WHO ARE MOST SENSITIVE TO THE BENEFITS OF SUPERVISED TREADMILL WALKING EXERCISE.

The following patient characteristics are associated with better response to supervised walking exercise rehabilitation programs.

Older age
Lower ankle-brachial index values
Longer leg symptom duration

TABLE 2-2. CHARACTERISTICS OF THE OPTIMAL WALKING EXERCISE TRAINING PROGRAM FOR INTERMITTENT CLAUDICATION.

- Exercise sessions are supervised by a nurse or exercise physiologist
- Exercise sessions occur at least three times weekly
- Begin with 15 minutes of walking exercise and increase duration of exercise by five minutes per session each week to attain 40 to 50 minutes of walking exercise each session .
- Patients walk to maximal claudication pain before resting
- On reaching maximal claudication pain, the patient rests and resumes walking as soon as he or she is able
- Exercise training lasts a minimum of six months

less frequent sessions.[5] Table 2–2 delineates desirable characteristics of an exercise program for patients with intermittent claudication, based on results of Gardner et al.'s meta-analysis and other available literature.

Prescribing an Effective Supervised Exercise Program

Supervised exercise rehabilitation programs for patients with intermittent claudication should be held at least three times weekly. Sessions typically begin with a five-minute warm-up period and conclude with a five-minute cool-down period to help minimize injuries. Prior to beginning a supervised exercise training program, absolute and initial claudication distances are determined using a baseline graded exercise treadmill protocol. In the initial training session, the intensity of the workload is the same as that at which claudication symptoms first develop during the baseline graded treadmill test. During the active exercise period, treadmill walking is interspersed with periods of rest, as determined by the onset of near-maximal claudication pain. Near-maximal claudication is defined by a claudication severity score of 3 or 4 on a 1–5 pain scale (5 = most severe pain). In the first session, the goal is to achieve a total of 10 to 15 minutes of walking exercise on the treadmill, exclusive of the warm-up and cool-down periods, and exclusive of the periods of rest necessitated by claudication symptoms. After the initial training session, the goal is to increase the amount of time spent walking on the treadmill by five minutes each session until the total time spent exercising is 40 to 50 minutes. After the initial training session, either the treadmill speed or grade is increased if the patient is able to walk for at least 10 minutes continuously at the lower workload without achieving moderate to near-maximal claudication pain. Either treadmill speed or grade can be increased, but increasing the grade is recommended if the patient is able to walk at least two miles per hour.[6]

Baseline Exercise Stress Testing

Prior to beginning an exercise program, it is advisable to have patients with PAD perform an exercise stress test with continuous 12-lead electrocardiography. The baseline exercise stress test serves two purposes. First, the exercise stress test helps identify PAD patients whose walking exercise performance is associated with coronary ischemia. These PAD patients should undergo additional coronary evaluation prior to beginning a new exercise program. Second, performance on the baseline stress test helps guide the starting intensity of treadmill walking exercise. The initial exercise intensity (i.e., treadmill speed and grade) is determined based on the treadmill speed and grade at which the patient first developed leg symptoms during treadmill testing.

Constant Load vs. Graded Exercise Stress Testing.   Older studies frequently used constant-load treadmill testing to measure baseline treadmill walking performance in patients with intermittent claudication. In constant-load treadmill testing, patients walk at a speed of approximately 1.5–2.0 miles per hour at a fixed grade of 8% to 12%. However, constant-load treadmill testing has a high coefficient of variability (30% to 45%) for initial and absolute claudication distance. Another limitation of constant-load treadmill testing is that some patients who experience large improvements in walking performance following an exercise intervention are able to walk indefinitely on the constant-load treadmill testing at follow-up. For these reasons, constant-load treadmill testing, although previously used in many clinical trials involving patients with intermittent claudication, has been more recently replaced with graded treadmill exercise testing.

In graded treadmill testing, treadmill grade is increased at specified intervals, while treadmill speed is held stable at 2.0 miles per hour and the treadmill grade is increased at specified intervals. Two commonly used treadmill protocols increase the treadmill grade by 3.5% every three minutes and by 2.0% every two minutes, while maintaining treadmill speed at 2.0 miles per hour.[6] Graded treadmill protocols have a low coefficient of variability (12% to 13% for maximal treadmill distance) and, therefore, provide much more reproducible results than constant-load treadmill testing. Because the grade increases at specified intervals, a maximum treadmill walking distance can be obtained for virtually all claudication patients using the graded protocol. Patients who are unable to begin walking at 2.0 miles per hour can begin at 0.50 miles per hour. For these patients, treadmill speed is increased at 0.50 miles per hour in increments every two minutes until 2.0 miles per hour is achieved. Subsequently, treadmill grade is increased using one of the methods described above. Because of their low variability and superior ability to measure changes in treadmill performance, graded treadmill tests should be used rather than constant-load treadmill tests for patients with PAD.

EXERCISE REHABILITATION AND FUNCTIONAL OUTCOMES IN PERSONS WITH PERIPHERAL ARTERIAL DISEASE AND INTERMITTENT CLAUDICATION

Most studies evaluating the benefits of exercise in patients with intermittent claudication have used treadmill performance as the primary study outcome. While treadmill walking is a rigorous, well-accepted, standardized outcome measure for patients with intermittent claudication, treadmill testing may not simulate walking ability in the community, particularly among older patients.[7-9] For example, older patients may be intimidated or uncomfortable with treadmill walking as compared to corridor or other forms of walking that are more directly applicable to walking during daily life. Another limitation associated with using treadmill walking performance as the primary outcome measure is a "learning" effect associated with the treadmill test. Patients in the supervised treadmill walking group have the advantage of "practicing" treadmill walking during their exercise sessions.

To determine whether exercise rehabilitation programs are associated with improvements in functional outcome measures other than treadmill walking that may be more relevant to functioning in daily life, Gardner et al. measured change in six-minute walk performance and free living physical activity levels in PAD patients randomized to six months of walking exercise rehabilitation versus no exercise.[10] Participants were 61 PAD patients with intermittent claudication. Six months after randomization, participants in the intervention arm had significantly improved their six-minute walk performance by 12% (388 meters ± 16 to 433 meters ± 16, p <0.001), while the usual care group experienced no change (406 ± 18 to 388 ± 23, p = NS). Physical activity, measured over two days with a vertical accelerometer, increased by 38% in the exercise rehabilitation group (366 Kcal ± 39 to 504 Kcal ± 49), while the control group experienced no change in accelerometer-measured physical activity (472 Kcal ± 9 to 311 Kcal ± 72, p = NS). These results indicate that supervised walking exercise increases physical activity levels and functional performance in patients with PAD. These outcomes may be more relevant to walking performance in the community than treadmill walking.

SAFETY OF EXERCISE REHABILITATION

Exercise rehabilitation programs are safe for patients with intermittent claudication. No increased cardiovascular morbidity or mortality has been reported as a result of exercise rehabilitation programs.[6,7] As described above, a baseline treadmill test helps identify PAD patients with unstable or significant coronary ischemia for whom initiation of an exercise program might be inadvisable. In addition, preliminary evidence suggests that supervised walking exercise may improve atherosclerotic risk factors in patients with PAD and intermittent claudication,[11] thereby potentially reducing long-term cardiovascular morbidity and mortality in patients with PAD.

INTENSITY VERSUS DURATION OF EXERCISE AS PREDICTORS OF OUTCOMES IN SUPERVISED EXERCISE REHABILITATION PROGRAMS

In non-PAD populations, more intensive exercise (i.e., faster speed of walking exercise) is associated with greater benefits. However, available data suggest that intensity of exercise may be less important for patients with PAD. Gardner et al. compared the gains in treadmill walking performance between a high- versus low-intensity treadmill exercise rehabilitation program in 33 patients with PAD and intermittent claudication.[12] Participants were randomized to either a high- versus low-intensity walking exercise rehabilitation program. For both groups, the exercise program consisted of six months of walking exercise three times weekly at 2.0 miles per hour. The low exercise intensity group exercised at 40% of the grade achieved during the baseline treadmill exercise test. The low-intensity group exercised for 15 minutes for the first month and increased treadmill exercise duration by five minutes per session each month to 40 minutes of exercise during the final month of the intervention. The high-intensity exercise group exercised at 80% of the grade achieved during the baseline treadmill test. Duration of exercise in the high-intensity group was shorter to achieve the same work load (i.e., Kcals expended) as the low-intensity group.[12] At six-month follow-up, gains in treadmill walking performance were nearly identical between the two groups. Time to onset of claudication symptoms on the treadmill increased by 109% in each group. Maximal treadmill walking distance increased by 61% in the low-intensity group versus 63% in the high-intensity group. These data suggest that low-intensity treadmill exercise rehabilitation in PAD patients can achieve gains that are comparable to higher intensity treadmill exercise rehabilitation, as long as walking duration in the low-intensity group is increased to achieve a comparable workload to that of higher intensity exercise.[12]

MAINTENANCE OF GAINS ACHIEVED DURING EXERCISE REHABILITATION IN PAD

Benefits of exercise rehabilitation do not persist once exercise rehabilitation stops.[5] However, a recent study by Gardner et al. demonstrated that gains made during a 26-week, three times weekly walking exercise rehabilitation program can be largely maintained for an additional 12 months when the frequency of walking exercise rehabilitation is reduced to twice weekly.[13] Participants in the study by Gardner et al. were 31 patients with PAD randomized to exercise rehabilitation versus usual care. During the first six months of walking exercise rehabilitation, participants attended exercise sessions three times weekly. After six months, exercise rehabilitation continued with twice weekly sessions. These twice weekly sessions employed the same intensity and duration of exercise achieved at the end of the first six months of exercise.[13] Eighteen months after baseline testing, the exercise group had increased maximal treadmill walking distance by 80% as compared to baseline. Time to onset of leg symptoms on the treadmill had increased by 189%. Six-minute walk performance and physical activity (measured by vertical accelerometer) had increased by 10% and 31%, respectively, compared to baseline. Furthermore, these 18-month improvements were comparable to those attained after six-month follow-up. Improvements in the exercise group at both six- and 18-month follow-up were significantly greater than gains in the control group. This study suggests that gains made during a six-month walking exercise rehabilitation program can be successfully maintained for an additional year with less frequent (twice weekly) exercise rehabilitation sessions.[13]

SUPERVISED VERSUS UNSUPERVISED WALKING EXERCISE PROGRAMS

Although supervised treadmill exercise rehabilitation programs improve treadmill walking performance in patients with PAD, most patients with PAD do not participate in these programs.[7] Barriers to participation in exercise rehabilitation programs include lack of medical insurance coverage for many patients, and the requirement for regular travel back and forth to the exercise facility. Home-based (unsupervised) walking exercise programs are potentially attractive for patients with PAD, since they are less costly and eliminate the requirement for regular transportation. However, home-based walking exercise programs may be less effective than supervised exercise rehabilitation programs for patients with PAD and intermittent claudication.

The Cochrane Collaboration summarized data from eight clinical trials that compared supervised exercise rehabilitation programs with home-based (unsupervised) exercise programs for patients with PAD. The eight studies included 319 participants ranging in age from 40 to 86 years (mean age = 67 years). The clinical trials lasted from three to 12 months duration.[14] The home-based unsupervised exercise programs typically involved advice at baseline to walk for exercise at home at least three times weekly, for at least 30 minutes each exercise session.[14] Most of the studies included telephone calls to participants in the home-based exercise programs. These telephone contacts varied in frequency from once per week to once per month. At three-month follow-up, collective data from the eight clinical trials demonstrated greater benefit in maximal treadmill walking performance in the supervised treadmill exercise groups compared to the home-based exercise groups. Participants in the supervised exercise programs increased their walking distance by approximately 150 meters as compared to the home-based exercise groups. Baseline maximal walking distance was approximately 300 meters among participants in these trials. The benefits favoring the supervised exercise group were maintained at six-month and 12-month follow-up assessments of treadmill walking performance. However, only two of the eight trials measured treadmill walking performance at 12-month follow-up. It is important to point out that most of the eight trials incorporated treadmill walking exercise in the supervised exercise rehabilitation study arms and that the primary outcome measure was treadmill walking performance. Since there is a learning effect associated with treadmill walking performance in persons with PAD, it is conceivable that some of the greater treadmill gains in the supervised exercise groups were related to the extensive "practice" associated with frequent treadmill walking during the supervised exercise sessions. Two studies included in this critical review did not include treadmill walking in the supervised exercise rehabilitation arm of the study.[14] One of these showed no improvement in the supervised exercise rehabilitation arm as compared to the home-based exercise group. It is conceivable that at least some of the greater gains in treadmill performance in the supervised exercise rehabilitation groups may be related to greater "practice" with treadmill walking. Table 2–3 summarizes outcomes that have been demonstrated to improve in response to walking exercise programs in patients with PAD.

SELF-DIRECTED WALKING EXERCISE AND RATES OF FUNCTIONAL DECLINE IN PERIPHERAL ARTERIAL DISEASE

The Cochrane Collaboration critical review compared home-based walking exercise to supervised treadmill exercise programs and suggested comparatively little benefit from home-based exercise. However, observational data support a benefit of home-based

TABLE 2-3. DOCUMENTED BENEFITS OF WALKING EXERCISE REHABILITATION IN PATIENTS WITH INTERMITTENT CLAUDICATION.

- Increased pain-free and maximal walking distance on treadmill testing
- Improved cardiovascular risk factor profiles
- Improved Walking Impairment Questionnaire and Medical Outcomes Study scores
- Increased physical activity levels
- Improved oxygen uptake during exercise
- Improved six-minute walk performance

walking exercise compared to *no* walking exercise in patients with PAD.[15] In a study of 417 patients with PAD who were followed annually for three years, PAD participants who went walking for exercise three or more times per week (34%) had significantly less decline in six-minute walk performance and walking speed over four meters, compared to those who went walking for exercise one to two times per week or not at all.[15] Similar associations were observed between the amount of time engaged in walking exercise and decline in six-minute walk performance or walking speed.[15] These associations were independent of the ankle-brachial index, age, sex, comorbidities, and other potential confounders. Similar associations between more frequent walking exercise and less functional decline were observed among PAD participants who were asymptomatic (i.e., had no exertional leg symptoms) and those with exertional leg symptoms other than intermittent claudication (i.e., atypical exertional leg symptoms). These observational data suggest that self-directed regular walking exercise may be beneficial to patients with PAD compared to the alternative of no exercise.

MECHANISMS BY WHICH WALKING EXERCISE INCREASES PAIN-FREE AND MAXIMAL WALKING DISTANCE IN INTERMITTENT CLAUDICATION

Mechanisms by which walking exercise increases pain-free and maximal walking distance are not well understood. However, a number of hypotheses have been proposed.[16] These include favorable changes in distribution of arterial perfusion to the legs, improved blood rheology (reduced blood viscosity), improved oxidative metabolism of lower extremity muscles, increased pain tolerance, and increased gait efficiency (Table 2–4). Exercise may also have favorable effects on inflammation, which may, in turn, favorably affect functioning over time.

Walking Exercise Training and the ABI

Many studies of exercise training in intermittent claudication have shown that the ABI does not undergo meaningful change in response to exercise training. However, other changes in the microcirculation may improve arterial perfusion of lower extremity skeletal muscle independently of the ABI. These changes may include an increase in capillary surface area, improved endothelial function, or favorable change in the distribution of arterial perfusion (without changing total perfusion).

Muscle biopsies of patients with intermittent claudication indicate that metabolic efficiency of lower extremity muscles improves in response to walking exercise train-

---

TABLE 2-4. POTENTIAL MECHANISMS BY WHICH WALKING EXERCISE REHABILITATION MIGHT INCREASE WALKING PERFORMANCE IN INTERMITTENT CLAUDIATION.

- Favorable changes in the distribution of arterial perfusion to the legs*
- Increased pain tolerance and/or improved gait efficiency
- Improved efficiency of oxidative metabolism of lower extremity muscles
- Improved blood rheology (reduced blood viscosity)
- Improved endothelial function

*While available data indicate that the ankle-brachial index does not undergo meaningful change in response to exercise training, other microcirculatory changes may improve in response to exercise.

ing. In the claudicating lower extremity muscle, impairment in normal mitochondrial oxidative metabolism is reflected by an increase in intracellular acyl carnitine.[17] Exercise training lowers muscle concentration of acylcarnitine. In one study of 19 men with disabling claudication randomized to a 12-week supervised treadmill exercise program versus a control (no exercise) group, exercising subjects increased maximal treadmill walking time by 123% while their acylcarnitine concentration decreased by 26%.[18] Subjects in the exercise training group with the greatest improvement in walking had the greatest reduction in acylcarnitine concentration. Maximal treadmill walking time and acylcarnitine concentration were highly correlated (correlation coefficient = -0.78 [$p<0.05$] in the treated group). This study suggests that exercise training may improve oxidative metabolism in claudicating muscle.

UPPER AND LOWER LIMB AEROBIC EXERCISE IN PERIPHERAL ARTERIAL DISEASE

Relatively few data are available on the benefits of modes of exercise other than walking. However, a barrier to walking exercise in patients with intermittent claudication is exertional leg pain associated with walking exercise. Identifying effective modes of exercise, other than walking, may improve adherence to exercise programs in patients with PAD and intermittent claudication. Table 2–5 summarizes data on modes of exercise that have been studied in randomized controlled clinical trials for their ability to improve walking performance in PAD patients with intermittent claudication.

A large clinical trial recently demonstrated the benefits of upper and lower limb aerobic exercise, using upper and lower limb cranking, in patients with PAD. The study included 104 participants with PAD and intermittent claudication (median age = 69 years). Participants were randomized to upper limb aerobic exercise, lower limb aerobic exercise, and usual care (i.e., no exercise). The upper and lower limb aerobic

TABLE 2-5. EXERCISE MODALITIES IN PATIENTS WITH PERIPHERAL ARTERIAL DISEASE AND INTERMITTENT CLAUDICATION.

Mode of Exercise	Demonstrated Efficacy in Clinical Trials	Comments
Supervised treadmill walking exercise.	Yes	Demonstrated to be efficacious in multiple randomized controlled clinical trials.
Upper arm exercise with an arm crank	Yes	Demonstrated to be efficacious in at least one randomized controlled clinical trial.
Lower extremity exercise with a leg crank	Yes	Demonstrated to be efficacious in at least one randomized controlled clinical trial.
Unsupervised walking exercise	No	Not effective as compared to supervised treadmill walking exercise programs. Observational data suggest a potential benefit.
Lower extremity resistance training	Both positive and negative findings.	Improves treadmill walking performance, but to a lesser degree than supervised treadmill walking exercise. Associated with greater benefits in Walking Impairment Questionnaire scores than treadmill walking. Associated with favorable changes on muscle biopsy.

exercises consisted of arm and leg cranks, respectively, rotated at 50 revolutions per minute throughout exercise.

Baseline Measurements

At baseline, peak upper and lower limb aerobic power were measured with a calibrated, electronically braked, cycle ergometer. Participants performed incremental arm and leg cranking on the ergometer to maximal exercise tolerance. For both the upper and lower limbs, participants cranked at 50 revolutions per minute for two-minute intervals, each separated by three minutes rest. Initial intensity of the crank was nine watts for both the upper and lower limbs. Power was incrementally increased at each two-minute interval by seven watts in the upper limb and by 14 watts in the lower limb.

Initial exercise intensity for the upper and lower limb exercise groups was based on the penultimate power output for the upper and lower limb crank test outcomes, respectively. Participants exercised for two-minute intervals at 50 revolutions per minute, with two minutes rest between each exercise interval for a total of 20 minutes of exercise in each 40-minute exercise session. Maximal power, using the crank test described above, was remeasured at six-week intervals. Within the exercise groups, the intensity of exercise was adjusted according to the maximal power results.

The primary outcome measure during this study was maximal walking distance and time to onset of claudication symptoms during a shuttle walk test. The shuttle walk test is performed in a hall corridor between two cones that are placed 10 meters apart. Walking is paced by an audiotape that beeps to indicate the desired walking pace. At 24-week follow-up, maximal walking distance had increased significantly by 29% in the upper arm aerobic exercise group and by 31% in the lower limb aerobic exercise group. Time to onset of claudication pain during the shuttle walk test increased by 51% in the upper extremity exercise group and by 57% in the lower extremity exercise group. There were no changes in maximal walking distance or time to onset of claudication pain in the control group.

This study indicates that exercise with upper and lower limb cranking benefits patients with intermittent claudication. Improved cardiovascular fitness may be a mechanism of improved walking performance in the arm cranking group. The exercise groups also demonstrated improved leg pain tolerance during the shuttle test. Peak oxygen uptake during the crank test measurements were also significantly increased in the both the upper and lower arm exercise groups, while the control group did not change. The ankle-brachial index did not change in any of the three study groups. This study is important in part because exercise modalities other than walking exercise may be more acceptable to patients with intermittent claudication who wish to avoid leg symptoms associated with walking exercise.

LOWER EXTREMITY STRENGTH TRAINING IN PERIPHERAL ARTERIAL DISEASE

Two prior studies have assessed the ability of lower extremity resistance training to improve lower extremity functioning in participants with PAD and IC.[20,21] There is reason to believe that strength training may be beneficial for patients with PAD. Men and women with PAD have reduced leg strength compared to persons without PAD.[22]

In addition, poorer knee extension strength is associated significantly with poorer lower extremity functional performance in patients with PAD.[22] In older frail populations and in patients with coronary heart disease, leg strengthening programs improve functional performance and treadmill walking performance.

Hiatt et al. compared a 12-week treadmill training program to a 12-week leg strengthening program and a control group in 29 men with peripheral arterial disease and intermittent claudication (average age = 67 years).[20] The primary outcome measure was maximal walking distance on the treadmill. At 12-week follow-up, both exercise groups had significantly increased their treadmill walking times (9.6 ± 5.7 minutes to 14.7 ± 7.3 minutes for the treadmill trained group [$p<0.05$], and 6.5 ± 2.9 minutes to 8.5 ± 5.2 minutes in the strength trained group [$p<0.05$]). In contrast, the control group experienced no significant change in treadmill walking performance. Improvement in treadmill walking performance was greater in the treadmill exercise rehabilitation group compared to the resistance trained group. The strength trained group had a significant increase in gastrocnemius strength, but the treadmill-trained group had no change in leg strength after treadmill training. While the authors concluded that the results indicated lack of benefit of lower extremity strength training in patients with PAD, it is important to point out that *both* exercise groups significantly improved their treadmill walking performance. Possibly, patients randomized to the treadmill exercise rehabilitation group, who participated in treadmill walking exercise three times weekly, may have "learned" how to walk further on a treadmill. This may be one reason for the greater improvement in the treadmill training group as compared to the strength trained group. At 12-week follow-up, the treadmill exercise group had no change in their Walking Impairment Questionnaire (WIQ) scores for walking distance, walking speed, or stair climbing. In contrast, the strength trained group had significant improvement in WIQ scores for both walking speed and stair climbing.

In a second randomized controlled clinical trial of strength training in patients with PAD and claudication, 20 subjects (nine men) with symptomatic PAD were randomized to either 24 weeks of progressive resistance training of the lower extremities versus usual care.[21] Muscle biopsies from the medial gastrocnemius were taken before and after the intervention. Participants were average age 70 ± 6 years (intervention group) and average age 66 ± 5 years (control group). After 24-weeks of resistance training, subjects in the intervention group had significant increases in leg strength. Muscle biopsies showed significant increases in type I muscle fibers, type II muscle fibers, and capillary density in the strength trained group. Control subjects had no change in the amounts of muscle fiber, capillary density, or leg strength. These two studies suggest that leg strengthening may be of some benefit to patients with PAD. However, sample sizes were small and further study is needed.

POTENTIAL BARRIERS TO PARTICIPATION IN EXERCISE TRAINING PROGRAMS

Many intermittent claudication patients have comorbid diseases that may interfere with exercise training programs including arthritis and significant atherosclerosis in other vascular beds. Additionally, insurance companies frequently do not pay for supervised exercise programs, despite the demonstrated benefits of supervised treadmill exercise programs. However, a study of patients with intermittent claudication in the United States found that only 9% of claudication patients referred for an exercise program were ineligible.[23] All 9% were ineligible because severe cardiac ischemia was identified on their initial treadmill test. Of those enrolled, 73% completed the exercise program successfully. An additional barrier to enrollment in an exercise program may be lack of physician recommendation.[24]

CONCLUSION

Supervised treadmill walking exercise programs benefit patients with PAD who have intermittent claudication symptoms. The most effective supervised exercise programs are those that include walking exercise at least three times weekly for at least 30 minutes per session and continue for a minimum of six months. Unfortunately, barriers limit participation in supervised walking exercise programs by patients with PAD. These barriers include lack of medical insurance coverage and the requirement for frequent transportation to and from the exercise center. Observational data suggest that PAD patients who engage in self-directed walking exercise three or more times weekly have less functional decline than PAD patients who do not engage in self-directed walking exercise. Further study is needed to identify optimal exercise regimens for the large number of PAD patients who do not have classical symptoms of intermittent claudication. Further study is also necessary to further examine potential benefits of lower extremity resistance training for patients with PAD.

REFERENCES

1. McDermott MM, Greenland P, Liu K, Guralnik JM, Celic L, Criqui MH, Chan C, Martin GJ, Schneider J, Pearce WH, Taylor L, Clark ET. The ankle brachial index as a measure of leg functioning and physical activity in peripheral arterial disease: The Walking and Leg Circulation Study. *Ann Intern Med* 2002;136(12);873–883.
2. McDermott MM, Liu K, Greenland P, Guralnik JM, Criqui MH, Chan C, Pearce WH, Schneider JR, Ferrucci L, Celic L, Taylor LM, Vonesh E, Martin GJ, Clark E. Functional decline in peripheral arterial disease: associations with the ankle brachial index and leg symptoms. *JAMA* 2004;292:453–461.
3. McDermott MM, Mehta S, Liu K, Guralnik JM, Martin GJ, Criqui MH, Greenland P. Leg symptoms, the ankle brachial index, and walking ability in peripheral arterial disease. *J Gen Intern Med* 1999;14:173–181.
4. McDermott MM, Fried L, Simonsick E, Ling S, Guralnik JM. Asymptomatic peripheral arterial disease is independently associated with impaired lower extremity functioning: The Women's Health and Aging Study. *Circulation* 2000;101:1007–1012.
5. Gardner AW, Poehlman ET. Exercise rehabilitation programs for the treatment of claudication pain. *JAMA* 1995;274:975–980.
6. Regensteiner JG, Gardner A, Hiatt WR. Exercise testing and exercise rehabilitation for patients with peripheral arterial disease: status in 1997. *Vasc Med* 1997;2:147–155.
7. Falcone RA, Hirsch AT, Regensteiner JG, et al. Peripheral arterial disease rehabilitation: A review. *J Cardiopulm Rehabil.* 2003;23:170–5.
8. Swerts PMJ, Mostert R, Wouters EFM. Comparison of corridor and treadmill walking in patients with severe chronic obstructive pulmonary disease. *Phys Ther* 1990;70;439–442.
9. Greig C, Butler F, Skelton D, Mahmud S, Young A. Treadmill walking in old age may not reproduce the real life situation. *J Am Geriatr Soc* 1993;41:15–18.

10. Gardner AW, Katzel LI, Sorkin JD, et al. Exercise rehabilitation improves functional outcomes and peripheral circulation in patients with intermittent claudication: A randomized controlled trial. *J Am Geriatr Soc* 2001;49:755–62.
11. Izquierdo-Porrera AM, Gardner AW, Powell CC, Katzel LI. Effects of exercise rehabilitation on cardiovascular risk factors in older patients with peripheral arterial occlusive disease. *J Vasc Surg* 2000;31:670–7.
12. Gardner AW, Montgomery PS, Flinn WR, KIatzel LI. The effect of exercise intensity on the response to exercise rehabilitation in patients with intermittent claudication. *J Vasc Surg* 2005;42:702–9.
13. Gardner AW, Katzel LI, Sorkin JD, Goldberg AP. Effects of long-term exercise rehabilitation on claudication distances in patients with peripheral arterial disease: A randomized controlled trial. *J Cardiopulm Rehabil* 2002;22:192–198.
14. Bendermacher BLW, Willigendael EM, Teiink JAW, Prins MH. Supervised exercise therapy versus non-supervised exercise therapy for intermittent claudication. *The Cochrane Database of Systemic Reviews* 2006, Issue 2. Art. No.: CD005263.pub2. DOI: 10.1002/14651858. CD005263.pub2.
15. McDermott MM, Liu K, Ferrucci L, Criqui MH, Greenland P, Guralnik JM, Tian L, Pearce WH, Tan J, Martin GJ. Physical performance in peripheral arterial disease: A slower rate of decline in patients who walk more. *Ann Intern Med* 2006;144:10–20.
16. Stewart KJ, Hiatt WR, Regensteiner JG, Hirsch AT. Exercise training for claudication. *N Engl J Med* 2002;12:1941–1951.
17. Hiatt WR, Wolfel EE, Regensteiner JG, Brass EP. Skeletal muscle carnitine metabolism in patients with unilateral peripheral arterial disease. *J Appl Physiol* 1992;53:346–353.
18. Hiatt WR, Regensteiner JG, Gargarten ME, Wolfel EE, Brass EP. Benefit of exercise conditioning for patients with peripheral arterial disease. *Circulation* 1990;81:602–609.
19. Zwierska I, Walker R, Choksy SA, Male JS, Pckley AG, Saxton JM. Upper vs lower limb aerobic exercise rehabilitation in patients with symptomatic peripheral arterial disease: A randomized controlled trial. *J Vasc Surg* 2005;42:1122–30.
20. Hiatt WR, Wolfel EE, Meier RH, Regensteiner JG. Superiority of treadmill walking exercise versus strength training for patients with peripheral arterial disease. *Circulation.* 1994;90:1866–1874.
21. McGuigan MR, Bronks R, Newton RU, Sharman MJ, Graham JC, Cody DV, Kramer WJ. Resistance training in patients with peripheral arterial disease: Effects on myosin isoforms, fiber type distribution, and capillary supply to skeletal muscle. *J Gerontol A Biol Sci Med Sci* 2001;56(7):B302–310.
22. McDermott MM, Criqui MH, Greenland P, Guralnik JM, Liu K, Pearce WH, Taylor L, Chan C, Celic L, Woolley C, Schneider JR. Leg strength in peripheral arterial disease: Associations with disease severity, revascularization, and lower extremity performance. *J Vasc Surg* 2004;39:523–30.
23. Williams LR, Ekers MA, Collins PS, Lee JF. Vascular rehabilitation: benefits of a structured exercise/risk modification program. *J Vasc Surg* 1991; 14:320–326.
24. McDermott MM, Mehta S, Ahn H, Greenland P. Atherosclerotic risk factors are less intensively modified in peripheral arterial disease than in coronary artery disease. *Journ Gen Intern Med* 1997;12:209–215.

10. Gardner AW, Katzel LI, Sorkin JD, et al. Exercise rehabilitation improves functional outcome and peripheral circulation in patients with intermittent claudication: A randomized controlled trial. J Am Geriatr Soc 2001;49:755–62.

11. Izquierdo-Porrera AM, Gardner AW, Powell CC, Katzel LI. Effects of exercise rehabilitation on cardiovascular risk factors in older patients with peripheral arterial occlusive disease. J Vasc Surg 2000;31:670–7.

12. Gardner AW, Montgomery PS, Flinn WR, Katzel LI. The effect of exercise intensity on the response to exercise rehabilitation in patients with intermittent claudication. J Vasc Surg 2005;42:702–9.

13. Gardner AW, Katzel LI, Sorkin JD, Goldberg AP. Effects of long-term exercise rehabilitation on claudication distances in patients with peripheral arterial disease: A randomized controlled trial. J Cardiopulm Rehabil 2002;22:192–8.

14. Bendermacher BLW, Willigendael EM, Teijink JAW, Prins MH. Supervised exercise therapy versus non-supervised exercise therapy for intermittent claudication. The Cochrane Database of Systematic Reviews 2006, Issue 2. Art. No.: CD005263. DOI: 10.1002/14651858. CD005263.pub2.

15. McDermott MM, Liu K, Ferrucci L, Criqui MH, Greenland P, Guralnik JM, Tian L, Pearce WH, Tan J, Martin GJ. Physical performance in peripheral arterial disease: A slower rate of decline in patients who walk more. Ann Intern Med 2006;144:10–20.

16. Stewart KJ, Hiatt WR, Regensteiner JG, Hirsch AT. Exercise training for claudication. N Engl J Med 2002;347:1941–51.

17. Hiatt WR, Wolfel EE, Regensteiner JG, Brass EP. Skeletal muscle carnitine metabolism in patients with unilateral peripheral arterial disease. J Appl Physiol 1992;73:346–53.

18. Hiatt WR, Regensteiner JG, Hargarten ME, Wolfel EE, Brass EP. Benefit of exercise training for peripheral arterial disease. Circulation 1990;81:602–9.

19. Greenhalgh RM, Belch JJF, Brown LC, et al. Preferential benefit of angioplasty over supervised exercise in patients with intermittent claudication on quality of life at 24 months of follow-up. Circulation 2008;118:2296.

20. Walters R, Clarke J, Greenhalgh RM. Cilostazol and peripheral arterial disease. Expert Opin Pharmacother 2009;10:2009.

21. Mehler PS, Coll JR, Estacio R, Esler A, Schrier RW, Hiatt WR. Intensive blood pressure control reduces the risk of cardiovascular events in patients with peripheral arterial disease and type 2 diabetes. Circulation 2003;107:753–6.

22. McDermott MM, Criqui MH, Greenland P, Guralnik JM, Liu K, Pearce WH, Taylor L, Chan C, Celic L, Woolley C. Leg strength in peripheral arterial disease. J Am Coll Cardiol 2004;44:1158–62.

23. Williams PT, Monteith KE, Mitchell GS. Effect of insoles for the treatment of plantar fasciitis. Am J Sports Med 2009;37:1819–28.

3

Value of Preoperative Duplex Scanning in Planning Infrainguinal Bypass

Daniel B. Walsh, M.D.

In the most recent edition of Rutherford's *Vascular Surgery*, the section on preoperative evaluation for infrainguinal bypass states that "duplex mapping of saphenous or alternative veins . . . may be desirable to establish the presence of adequate vein and place incisions accurately." The chapter goes on to say that "duplex examination . . . does not provide anatomic resolution to the degree necessary for accurate preoperative planning."[1] Data forthcoming in this chapter should convince an open-minded reader that this statement, which represents the belief of a majority of vascular surgeons, is either patently wrong or, at least, out of date.

In order to perform successful lower revascularization three elements are required: an adequate inflow artery, an adequate outflow or target artery, and a useable conduit. Even the traditional experts in Rutherford's text agree that preoperative vein mapping to establish the presence and location of a usable venous conduit is a useful adjunct to a lower extremity revascularization. The utility of duplex vein mapping prior to lower extremity bypass, thus, is an accepted standard.

The traditional method for determining the adequacy of the inflow and target arteries for bypass has been contrast arteriography. Yet, in 1985 and again in 1987, Jager and Moneta from the University of Washington reported and confirmed that duplex ultrasound scanning from the infrarenal aorta to the popliteal arteries was as accurate in identifying significant arterial stenosis as independently read contrast arteriograms.[2,3] Furthermore, in 1992, Moneta went on to demonstrate duplex arterial mapping of the tibial and peroneal arteries was accurate in predicting occlusion in 90% and 82%, respectively, when compared with contrast arteriography.[4] These findings have since been confirmed by multiple authors.[5-8]

The true "gold standard" for testing the value of duplex arterial mapping in planning lower extremity revascularization, however, is not contrast arteriography. The standard must be the actual artery used at surgery. In 2003, we blinded vascular surgeons to the actual operation performed.[9] These surgeons then reviewed either the contrast or the duplex arteriograms and selected the target tibial or peroneal artery best suited for bypass. This selection was then compared with the artery actually used at bypass surgery and chosen by the operating surgeon who had full knowledge of all available duplex and contrast arteriography images. Data for this study was obtained from 40 lower extremities in 38 patients. This provided 110 arteries for comparison. Duplex arteriography failed to identify ten infragenicular arteries, eight peroneal, and two anterior tibial arteries. Contrast arteriography failed to identify one anterior tibial artery (Table 3–1). Duplex and contrast arteriograms agreed on the condition of the tibial and peroneal vessels in 81% (Table 3–2). Four arteries selected as targets by duplex arteriogram were seen as occluded at contrast arteriography; one of these was used as the actual bypass recipient. Three arteries seen as occluded at duplex were selected as target arteries by contrast arteriography. These three arteries were all peroneal arteries and were all used as actual bypass graft recipients. Surgeons using duplex arteriograms and surgeons using only contrast arteriograms concurred in their selection of target artery for bypass grafting in 85% of targets selected.

Duplex arteriography correctly predicted the actual bypass recipient artery in 88% of patients (35 over 40 patients) (Table 3–3). Contrast arteriography correctly predicted the actual bypass graft recipient artery in 93% of patients (37 over 40 patients). There was no significant statistical difference in ability of duplex or contrast arteriograms to correctly predict target arteries. However, contrast arteriography was clearly more effective for correct identification of peroneal arteries that were chosen as bypass graft recipients.

TABLE 3-1. AGREEMENT BETWEEN DU AND CA IN VISUALIZATION OF TIBIAL AND PERONEAL ARTERIES

	DU		CA	
Artery	Seen	Not Seen	Seen	Not Seen
Anterior tibal (%)	38	2	39	1
Peroneal (%)	32	8	40	0
Posterior tibial (%)	40	0	40	0
Total (%)	110	10	119	1

Arteries not seen with one technique were seen with the other.
DU, Duplex ultrasound scanning; CA, contrast-enhanced arteriography.
From: *J Vasc Surg.* 2003;37(6):1186–1190. With permission from: The Society for Vascular Surgery and the American Association for Vascular Surgery.

TABLE 3-2. AGREEMENT BETWEEN DU AND CA IN EVALUATION OF TIBIAL AND PERONEAL ARTERIES

DU	Occluded	CA patent, not target	CA target
Occluded	36	3	3
Patent, not target	8	18	3
DU target	4	1	34

Total arteries = 110; agreement, 81%; 95% CI, 73% -87%.
DU, Duplex ultrasound scanning; CA, contract-enhanced arteriography.
From: *J Vasc Surg.* 2003;37(6):1186–1190. With permission from: The Society for Vascular Surgery and the American Association for Vascular Surgery.

TABLE 3-3. ACCURACY OF DU AND CA IN SELECTION OF ACTUAL BYPASS GRAFT RECIPIENT ARTERY.

Artery	Actual bypass artery	No. of DU targets chosen	No. correct	% correct	No. of targets chosen	No. correct	% correct
Anterior tibial	11	12	11	92	9	9	100
Peroneal	10	5	5	50.	10	9	88
Posterior tibial	19	23	19	83	21	19	91
Total	40	40	35	88	40	37	93

From: *J Vasc Surg.* 2003;37(6):1186–1190. With permission from: The Society for Vascular Surgery and the American Association for Vascular Surgery.

Only five of 10 peroneal arteries used as bypass graft recipients at operation were selected by duplex. In one patient both the peroneal and posterior tibial arteries were seen as patent by duplex arteriography. The posterior tibial artery was chosen by the duplex reviewer because of its better run-off vessels. The operating surgeon selected the peroneal artery as the actual recipient of the bypass graft. In one patient, duplex failed to visualize the distal peroneal artery and determined it was occluded. Contrast arteriography demonstrated this peroneal artery is patent and it was selected as the bypass recipient at surgery.

In two patients, contrast arteriography failed to select the actual artery used for bypass grafting. In one, an anterior tibial artery selected at surgery as the bypass graft recipient was not visualized at contrast arteriography. In the other, the operating surgeon using both the duplex and contrast arteriograms believed the anterior tibial artery was the superior choice for bypass grafting over a patent posterior tibial artery selected by the reviewer using contrast arteriography.

In one patient, both duplex and contrast arteriogram reviewers believed the posterior tibial artery was the better target for bypass grafting, compared with the patent peroneal artery. The surgeon at operation chose the peroneal artery as the bypass graft recipient, thereby demonstrating that in some patients, there may be more than one quality target artery.

In one patient, the anterior tibial artery chosen with duplex was used 24 hours after the peroneal artery selected by the operating surgeon and the contrast arteriogram reviewer failed. No technical flaws were found at repeat exploration. This anterior tibial arterial graft remains patent. If arteries without adequate visualization are eliminated, the surgeon reviewer using duplex arteriography successfully chose 28 of 30 target vessels actually used, a 93% success rate, virtually the same as the success rate with contrast arteriography.

The final standard for comparison of duplex arteriography with contrast arteriography rests on the performance of infrainguinal bypass performed using each technique. Ascher, et al. have successfully performed infrapopliteal bypass graft based on duplex alone in 89% of a series of patients presenting with critical lower limb ischemia.[10] In 2002, Mazzariol reported a series of 57 patients who had infrapopiteal bypass grafts based on duplex arteriography alone. These patients achieved one and three month patency rates of 90% and 83% respectively.[11]

In 2001, we published our initial experience with duplex arteriography as the sole preoperative imaging study used for planning infragenicular bypass. To determine if duplex guided bypass gives acceptable results, we compared patency and limb salvage rates with the demographically matched historical control group who underwent similar procedures based on contrast arteriography alone.[12]

The study cohort was comprised of 23 consecutive patients who underwent infragenicular vein bypass graft based duplex arteriography alone in a 20-month period from 1998 through 2000. The comparison group included 50 consecutive patients who underwent infragenicular vein graft for critical ischemia based on contrast arteriography alone in the two-year period from 1996 through 1998. Surgical procedures were performed with similar standard techniques that did not change over the study period.

Preoperative duplex was performed with the ATL 3000 or ATL 5000 duplex ultrasound machine (Philips ATL, Bothall, Washington). Patients undergoing duplex arteriograms had duplex interrogation of the full length of all arteries in the ischemic lower extremity. Significant stenoses were identified by two-fold or greater increase in peak systolic velocity whereas an occlusion was defined as a well-seen artery with absent blood flow. Peak systolic velocity and endostic velocity were determined with spectral wave forms obtained from each arterial segment as viewed during the B-mode imaging. The operating surgeon chose proximal and distal anastomotic findings based on duplex findings. Along with criteria such as vessel diameter, amount of calcification, and condition of the vessels distally, velocity data were used by the primary surgeon to help select the optimal target. In general, higher duplex arteriogram target artery velocities in nondiseased arterial segments were thought to represent more optimal targets.

All patients, in both the study and the comparison groups, had duplex vein mapping to determine the length and quality of conduit available for bypass grafting. In situ saphenous vein was used preferentially for conduit with reverse saphenous vein composite vein or arm vein use when in situ saphenous vein was not available. All grafts were assessed intraoperatively for technical adequacy with completion duplex or contrast arteriography.[13] Grafts surveillance was performed with duplex ultrasound and limb pressure measurements at one, four, six, and 12 months, and every six months thereafter.

There was no statistical difference in conduit or target artery between the two groups. A larger number of grafts in the contrast arteriography group had more distal inflow origins than grafts in the duplex arteriogram group. Of the 23 operations performed based on duplex, one anastomostic site was abandoned due to dense calcification. This change in target artery required lengthening the original incision so that a more distal sight on the same artery could be used.

The 12-month primary graft patency rates for the duplex and contrast arteriography groups were 78% and 70%, respectively (Figure 3–1). The difference in patency was not significant. Primary assisted and secondary patency rates were also similar.

The 12-month limb cell salvage rates were comparable between the two groups (Duplex 70%, contrast 81%) (Figure 3–2). These trends continued at two years, but the number of patients followed was insufficient for meaningful statistical comparison. Seven grafts in the duplex group failed. In two patients, overwhelming sepsis led to amputation despite patent bypass graft. In three patients, intimal hyperplasia caused graft thrombosis, and in two patients, poor quality veins were thought to cause graft failure. The above mentioned data establishes that results achieved in lower extremity bypasses when duplex arteriography is used in planning are equivalent to those achieved when contrast arteriography is used for operative planning. This is particularly true if the peroneal artery is visualized by duplex.

The final method for establishing the value of duplex ultrasound in planning lower extremity revascularization is comparison of the cost and efficacy of the two

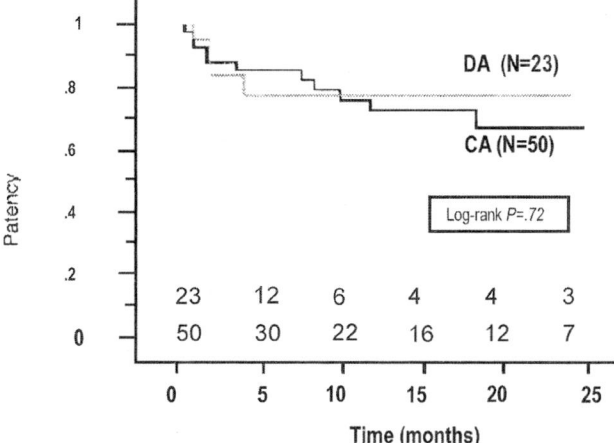

Figure 3-1. Kaplan-Meier life table comparing primary graft patency of duplex arteriography *(DA)* group versus conventional arteriography *(CA)* group. Numbers at the bottom of graph represent number of patients at risk to fail in each group at beginning of each time interval. Statistical analysis performed with Mantel-Cox log-rank test. From: *J Vasc Surg.* 2001;33(6):1165–1170. With permission from: The Society for Vascular Surgery and the American Association for Vascular Surgery.

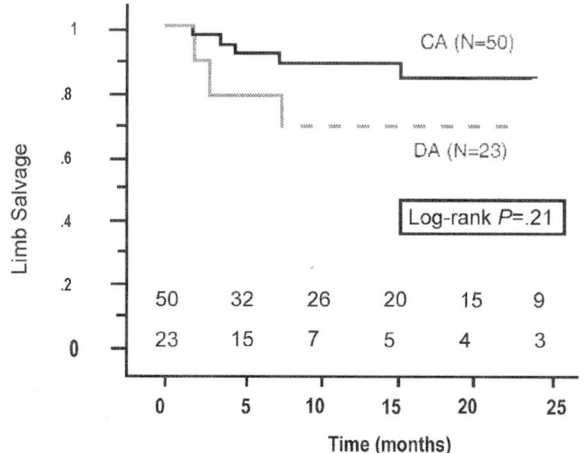

Figure 3-2. Kaplan-Meier life table comparing limb salvage rates of duplex arteriography *(DA)* group with conventional arteriography *(CA)* group. Numbers at the bottom of graph represent number of limbs at risk in each group at beginning of each time period. SE>10% when graph is *dashed*. Statistical analysis performed with Mantel-Cox log-rank test. From: *J Vasc Surg.* 2001;33(6):1165–1170. With permission from: The Society for Vascular Surgery and the American Association for Vascular Surgery.

technologies. It must be pointed out at the outset of this analysis that duplex arteriography has no associated complications, whereas contrast arteriography does have a low but measurable rate of associated complications, the worst being renal failure.[14-16]

If we ignore the complication rate, however, value can be considered to be a calculable figure. To illustrate this, we can arbitrarily set Value = 1/cost × efficacy. The larger the number obtained, the higher the value of the technology. For example, the value of a technology that has an accuracy of 99% and a cost of $100 per test would be Value = 1/.99 × 100 = .01. For contrast arteriography, the pertinent CPT codes are

36200, 75625, and 75710. These produce a professional component reimbursement of $157.92, $59.16, and $59.49, respectively, for a total of $276.59. Therefore, if we use the data from Grassbaugh, et al, Value (CA) = 1/.93 × 276.57 = .004. In contrast, for duplex arteriography, the relative codes are 93978, 93931, 93926, and 93971. The typical combination for one ischemic lower extremity duplex arteriogram from aorta to foot plus a vein mapping would use the codes 93979, 93931, and 93971. For 2004, the professional reimbursement for these three codes totals $75.05. Therefore, Value (DA) = 1/.88 × 75.05 = .015. This number is higher than that achieved by either contrast arteriography or our nearly perfect test with a cost of $100.

Because of the above data, we advocate a so called "duplex first" strategy. At the time of initial operative planning, if adequate tibial level targets and venous conduit are available, particularly if the peroneal artery is seen, revascularization may proceed without need for contrast arteriography with the expectation of patency and limb salvage results equivalent to those obtained with more traditional contrast arteriography. If the tibial arteries targets identified are suboptimal or the peroneal artery is inadequately visualized, a focused contrast arteriogram should be performed. This strategy would have eliminated the need for contrast arteriography in 32 of the 40 patients in our study. Avanerious et al. concluded in their own study that perhaps as few as 10% of revascularization procedures would benefit from contrast arteriograms.[17]

The benefits of the use of a "duplex first" approach would be significant. The cost associated with duplex arteriography would be significantly lower than those incurred with contrast arteriography. An additional benefit would be the lack of associated morbidity.

One concern of surgeons reluctant to adopt duplex as a first-line technique for tibial/peroneal arterial imaging is the issue of vascular technologists' accuracy. Duplex ultrasound arteriography is operator dependent. Validation of the vascular laboratory use in a "duplex first" revascularization program is a necessary part of implementing this algorithm for pre-operative planning. However, the techniques and training at our facility are similar to other vascular laboratories certified by the Intrasocietal Commission for the Accreditation of Vascular Laboratories (ICAVL). Furthermore, all registered Vascular Technologists at DHMC perform tibal imaging, demonstrating that the arterial mapping technique is not limited to an elite group of specifically selected or trained technicians.

In conclusion, we believe that duplex arteriography can accurately identify the target for bypass grafting for infragenicular bypasses in most patients. Particularly if the peroneal artery is seen, contrast arteriography is unlikely to provide additional information that would alter the execution of the operation. Tibial level bypasses can be performed with the same patency results as are achieved with contrast arteriography. Due to a lower cost in complications and dollars, duplex arteriography is a higher value approach to lower extremity revascularization. We believe that duplex arteriography should be the primary pre-operative technique for planning tibial level revascularization.

REFERENCES

1. Whittemore A, Belkin, M. Infraguinal Bypass. In: Rutherford RB. *Vascular Surgery*. (5ed), Vol. 1, 2000:998–1018.
2. Jager KA, Phillips DJ, Martin RL, et al. Noninvasive mapping of lower limb arterial lesions. *Ultrasound Med Biol*. 1985;11(3):515–21.

3. Kohler TR, Nance DR, Cramer MM, et al. Duplex scanning for diagnosis of aortoiliac and femoropopliteal disease: a prospective study. *Circulation*. 1987;76(5):1074–1080.

4. Moneta GL, Yeager RA, Antonovic R, et al. Accuracy of lower extremity arterial duplex mapping. *J Vasc Surg*. 1992;15(2):275-283; discussion 283–284.

5. Sensier Y, Hartshorne T, Thrush A, et al. A prospective comparison of lower limb colour-coded Duplex scanning with arteriography. *Eur J Vasc Endovasc Surg*. 1996;11(2):170–175.

6. Sensier Y, Fishwick G, Owen R, et al. A comparison between colour duplex ultrasonography and arteriography for imaging infrapopliteal arterial lesions. *Eur J Vasc Endovasc Surg*. 1998;15(1):44–50.

7. Wilson YG, George JK, Wilkins DC, Ashley S. Duplex assessment of run-off before femoro-crural reconstruction. *Br J Surg*. 1997;84(10):1360–1363.

8. Karacagil S, Lofberg AM, Granbo A, et al. Value of duplex scanning in evaluation of crural and foot arteries in limbs with severe lower limb ischaemia—a prospective comparison with angiography. *Eur J Vasc Endovasc Surg*. 1996;12(3):300–303.

9. Grassbaugh JA, Nelson PR, Rzucidlo EM, et al. Blinded comparison of preoperative duplex ultrasound scanning and contrast arteriography for planning revascularization at the level of the tibia. *J Vasc Surg*. 2003;37(6):1186–1190.

10. Ascher E, Mazzariol F, Hingorani A, et al. The use of duplex ultrasound arterial mapping as an alternative to conventional arteriography for primary and secondary infrapopliteal by-passes. *Am J Surg*. 1999;178(2):162–165.

11. Mazzariol F, Ascher E, Hingorani A, et al. Lower-extremity revascularisation without pre-operative contrast arteriography in 185 cases: lessons learned with duplex ultrasound arterial mapping. *Eur J Vasc Endovasc Surg*. 2000;19(5):509–515.

12. Proia RR, Walsh DB, Nelson PR, et al. Early results of infragenicular revascularization based solely on duplex arteriography. *J Vasc Surg*. 2001;33(6):1165–1170.

13. Rzucidlo EM, Walsh DB, Powell RJ, et al. Prediction of early graft failure with intraoperative completion duplex ultrasound scan. *J Vasc Surg*. 2002;36(5):975–981.

14. Johnson BL, Bandyk DF, Back MR, et al. Intraoperative duplex monitoring of infrainguinal vein bypass procedures. *J Vasc Surg*. 2000;31(4):678–690.

15. Hessel SJ, Adams DF, Abrams HL. Complications of angiography. *Radiology*. 1981;138(2):273–281.

16. Waugh JR, Sacharias N. Arteriographic complications in the DSA era. *Radiology*. 1992;182(1):243–246.

17. Avenarius JK, Breek JC, Lampmann LE et al. The additional value of angiography after colour-coded duplex on decision making in patients with critical limb ischaemia. A prospective study. *Eur J Vasc Endovasc Surg*. 2002;23(5):393–7.

4

Infrainguinal Graft Duplex Surveillance: Detection and Treatment of Graft-Threatening Lesions

Joseph L. Mills Sr., M.D. and Sheela T. Patel, M.D.

Duplex-based surveillance is the current standard of care for the serial postoperative follow-up of every patient following infrainguinal vein graft reconstruction. Although clinical history, physical examination, and Doppler-derived ankle brachial index determinations are important components of patient aftercare, duplex scanning is the essential and most critical element of any graft surveillance program. Surveillance allows detection and grading of inflow, outflow, and most importantly, intrinsic vein graft lesions; such defects can be identified, categorized, and monitored for progression. Generally accepted criteria for lesions warranting intervention have been developed. While surgical revision is generally the most durable treatment for intrinsic graft lesions, many inflow and outflow lesions, as well as selected intrinsic graft lesions, respond well to less invasive percutaneous interventions. Recent improvements in angioplasty technology may lead to more widespread use of percutaneous treatment of threatened-vein grafts in the near future. These newly evolving techniques will be addressed as part of the present review.

Postoperative duplex surveillance should be routine, but some clinicians begin surveillance in the operating room at the time of the initial vein graft reconstruction. Intraoperative duplex may be especially appropriate in reoperative settings when using spliced or arm vein conduits, or when using techniques requiring valve lysis.

INTRAOPERATIVE DUPLEX SCANNING

Intraoperative duplex scanning provides both an anatomic assessment of the vein bypass and hemodynamic information of potential clinical utility in the rational application of adjunctive procedures designed to improve graft patency such as distal arteriovenous fistulae, postoperative anticoagulation, and graft surveillance. The major downsides of intraoperative duplex scanning include scanner expense and availability, increased operative time, and the requisite for acquiring the expertise to correctly perform and interpret the intraoperative study. Papanicolau et al reported a series of 81 vein grafts. They compared the use of color-flow duplex to angiography for completion study of infrainguinal bypass. Among 49 such studies, duplex detected abnormalities in 17 cases (34.7%), 9 (18.4%) of which were immediately revised.[1] Specific criteria for revision included a focal peak systolic velocity (PSV) > 200 cm/s or a low graft flow velocity < 45 cm/s. Unrepaired duplex-detected defects were followed to determine their contribution to the need for early or late graft revision. All of the grafts with unrepaired abnormalities required revision in the postoperative period. None of the grafts with normal intraoperative scans developed lesions requiring revision during a mean follow-up interval of 16.1 months. Bandyk et al, in a prospective study of 275 infrainguinal vein graft bypasses undergoing intraoperative color-duplex evaluation, identified abnormalities requiring immediate operative intervention in 16% of grafts.[2] Criteria for intraoperative graft revision were a focal PSV > 180 cm/sec associated with a velocity ratio (Vr) > 2.5. Reversed vein grafts exhibited the lowest scan abnormality and revision requirement rates (7%) while translocated, in-situ, and arm vein grafts harbored significant duplex-detectable flow abnormalities in 15–23% of cases. A normal intraoperative scan was associated with a 90-day graft thrombosis rate of only 0.4%. In contrast, 40% of grafts harboring residual or unrepaired duplex defects thrombosed. These data suggest that a normal intraoperative duplex correlates highly with early and intermediate graft patency; that intraoperative duplex scanning has a higher yield when applied to translocated, in-situ, or arm vein conduits; and that significant unrepaired defects compromise graft patency.

Johnson et al proposed that vein grafts with low intraoperative PSV (<30–40 cm/s) and high outflow resistance (absent diastolic flow) should undergo adjunctive procedures to augment flow such as distal arteriovenous fistulae or sequential bypass grafting.[3] If such adjunctive procedures were not applicable, then postoperative antithrombotic therapy was initiated. Their group used intraoperative color-duplex scanning to assess vein graft patency and hemodynamics in 626 infrainguinal vein bypass grafts. Criteria for immediate intraoperative repair were PSV > 180 cm/s with spectral broadening and a Vr > 3. In their experience, duplex scanning prompted revision of 104 lesions in 96 (15%) bypass grafts. A normal intraoperative scan on initial imaging or after revision was associated with a 30-day thrombosis rate of 0.2% and a revision rate of only 0.8%. In contrast, 29% of the grafts with residual or unrepaired stenoses or a low flow state later required a re-intervention for graft thrombosis or stenosis. Although these data are fairly impressive, widespread application of intraoperative duplex scanning at the time of the initial reconstruction has been limited by skepticism concerning the yield of duplex when used routinely as well as by the practicalities of everyday surgical practice.

POSTOPERATIVE VEIN GRAFT EVALUATION

Serial vein graft attrition remains the most significant obstacle to long-term clinical success. Without re-intervention, only 50–70% of infrainguinal vein grafts will be patent five years after implantation; only 40–50% will be primarily patent after the first decade.[4] The ultimate goal of infrainguinal vein graft surveillance is to prevent graft occlusion through accurate identification and timely repair of graft-threatening lesions. Graft failure is a persistent threat and may result from anastomotic or conduit defects, myointimal hyperplasia, or progressive atherosclerotic disease in the inflow or outflow arteries, or even within the vein graft itself. The time courses over which these potentially deleterious lesions develop differ, but nearly all of them are identifiable and correctable by vigilant surveillance. Strategic re-intervention improves long-term graft patency and limb salvage rates. An improvement in one-year patency rate of approximately 15% has been reported in patients who were prospectively followed by duplex scanning.[5, 6] The primary goal of graft surveillance is to prevent the catastrophe of graft occlusion, an occurrence that is technically demanding for the surgeon, potentially disastrous for the patient, and generates significant health care costs.

RATIONALE FOR SURVEILLANCE

Failing infrainguinal autogenous venous conduits are most commonly preceded by the development of intrinsic graft stenoses. Such lesions may progress to hemodynamic significance, reduce graft flow below the thrombotic threshold velocity, and result in graft thrombosis. Szilagyi et al performed serial angiographic studies in 377 reversed lower extremity vein grafts and identified stenoses in 33% of grafts within five years of implantation.[7] Nearly all subsequent studies employing less-invasive duplex surveillance have borne out Szilagyi's seminal observation by confirming that 20 to 35% of grafts develop stenoses within the graft or in the native arterial inflow or outflow vessels.[6, 8-12] Numerous reports also suggest that 60–80% of graft-threatening lesions are focal, identifiable, and potentially correctable. Donaldson et al reported a detailed analysis of the causes of graft failure in a consecutive series of 440 in situ vein grafts.[13] Over 63% of failures were caused by intrinsic defects within the vein conduit itself or its anastomoses. Mills et al identified intrinsic graft lesions as the cause of failed or failing grafts in 60% of cases in a prospective duplex study of 227 consecutive reversed vein grafts.[14] Intrinsic graft stenosis is undeniably the most common cause of both in situ and reversed vein graft failure over time.

The incidence of stenotic lesions in vein grafts varies among reports, dependent on the screening technique and diagnostic criteria employed as well as the duration of follow-up. In patients monitored only by clinical means and simple ABI (ankle-brachial index) determinations, the incidence ranges from 5–21%. Duplex scanning is much more accurate and sensitive, reportedly detecting lesions in 20–37% of grafts.[6, 14, 15]

Clinical examination is important but limited in that it only detect the presence or absence of a pulse in a graft or run-off vessels. It provides no information concerning the potential likelihood of graft thrombosis. Pulses may be enhanced by reflected waves from a very high resistance peripheral bed and pulses may be difficult to palpate in obese or edematous patients. Pulse palpation has serious limitations since the graft may be located in a deep anatomic compartment and be inaccessible to direct palpation. Bandyk et al demonstrated that 68% of patients with pre-occlusive vein graft stenoses had no clinical symptoms whatsoever. Ankle-brachial index is likewise a poor predictor of long-term graft function.[16] Up to 40% of grafts fail without a premonitory drop in ABI. Symptom recurrence and a decreased ABI are more likely the result of a failed graft unsuitable for surgical or endovascular intervention than an indicator of a failing, potentially readily salvageable graft. Idu et al reported that clinical symptoms identified only 33% of stenotic grafts.[6] A significant drop in ABI (> 0.15) was observed in only 38% of grafts with significant duplex-detected stenoses. Although of limited utility when used alone, the ABI is useful prognostically when used in conjunction with duplex graft surveillance data. Green et al found that grafts harboring duplex surveillance-detected stenoses associated with an ABI decrease of 10% or greater had a 66% incidence of thrombosis within three months; if the ABI was normal but the duplex scan was abnormal, the corresponding risk of failure within three months was only 4%; no graft thrombosed if both scan and ABI were normal.[17]

The function of autogenous vein grafts implanted into the arterial circulation is best monitored by serial duplex surveillance because it is noninvasive, sensitive, accurate, reproducible, and economical. At least 80% of graft lesions develop within the first two postoperative years; the first six months (vein graft adolescence) is the interval of highest risk. Several reports have noted a high incidence of duplex-detected flow abnormalities in both in situ and reversed vein grafts studied within 30 days of implantation despite normal completion arteriograms. Such data suggest that maximizing the utility of graft surveillance would require increased surveillance intensity during this early, infancy period of particular graft vulnerability.

Vein graft stenoses developing during the first three to six postoperative months may behave in a particularly aggressive manner. Several investigators have suggested that such lesions are more prone to rapid progression and vein graft thrombosis than later, more slowly developing lesions.[10,18-20] Early and late-appearing graft lesions, therefore, exhibit differing biological behaviors. Early flow disturbances may be associated with platelet aggregation at sites of technical imperfection, areas of intimal injury, or at valve leaflet defects. During the period of adaptation to the arterial circulation, these early flow disturbances may be subjected to a more unfavorable milieu of growth factors and cytokines than lesions developing at later intervals. Nielsen et al reported that patients who developed stenoses within three months of surgery had a greater risk of graft thrombosis than patients who developed stenoses at a later stage (12 month patency 40% versus 83%, p = 0.01).[20] They proposed that early stenoses exceeding specific velocity parameters (Vr >2.5) should be revised even in the absence of ankle-brachial index reduction. Ihnat et al observed that grafts with early postoperative duplex-detected flow disturbances were associated with a nearly three-fold increase in subsequent development of graft-threatening stenosis and requirement for revision when compared to grafts with normal early scans.[21]

Vein grafts with serial normal duplex studies exhibit a remarkably low rate of graft occlusion during long-term follow-up. In contrast, the natural history of grafts harboring high-grade intrinsic stenoses, particularly those detected within the first three to six months of surgery, is sudden occlusion. Unrevised grafts with critical stenoses are associated with a short-term occlusion rate of almost 80%.[22] Prophylactic intervention for such high-grade lesions is justified because prophylactic revision of stenotic grafts is durable and the treatment outcome for graft occlusion is poor. Robinson and colleagues found that vein grafts requiring thrombectomy within 30 days of surgery had a two-fold risk of developing stenosis as well as reduced secondary patency rates.[23] Vein grafts that occlude in the intermediate and late postoperative periods also fare poorly. Long-term patency rates for grafts following thrombectomy and thrombolysis are unsatisfactory (range - 19–28%).[24-28] In contrast, surgical correction of a failing vein prior to thrombosis yields five-year assisted patency rates (80–85%) comparable to those for nonstenotic grafts, effectively restoring the life-table curve to normal.[24, 29, 30]

Graft Surveillance Algorithm

The purpose of a graft surveillance program is to maximize the detection of graft-threatening lesions and allow targeted intervention before the occurrence of graft thrombosis. The protocol design must consider both the progression rate and natural history of vein graft stenosis. Nearly 80% of graft stenoses develop within 12 months of graft implantation, the majority of which are detectable within the first six postoperative months. Early graft lesions (< three months) tend to progress more rapidly and are more threatening than lesions developing at later time intervals. Mills et al prospectively performed duplex surveillance, beginning in the intra- and early postoperative period, to determine the origin of vein graft lesions and delineate their propensity for progression.[31] They found that significant stenoses appeared to develop at sites of pre-existing or early-appearing conduit abnormalities or unrepaired technical defects; only 2% of stenoses developed de novo in graft segments that were entirely normal at the time of graft implantation. Of 42 grafts (32% of series) with abnormal scans within the first three months, 18 (43%) subsequently developed high-grade stenoses. In addition, 27 grafts (22% of series) demonstrated suspicious areas on the one-week scan and eight of them (30%) subsequently developed hemodynamically significant stenoses requiring revision.

We currently recommend early (one scan within four weeks of reconstruction, two scans within three months) postoperative scanning because it allows the surgeon to stratify grafts into high-, intermediate-, and low-risk categories for thrombosis. The criteria we use consist of low-flow and high-velocity thresholds and are summarized in Table 4–1. Grafts with early flow disturbances require more intensive surveillance. Although the risk of developing a graft stenosis greatly diminishes after one to two years, there persists an annual 2–4% incidence of late-appearing graft stenosis and a 5–10% lifetime risk of inflow/outflow disease progression requiring intervention.[21] Reifsnyder et al reported that more than 50% of venous conduits will develop significant lesions beyond five years.[32] Landry et al noted that while most vein bypass revisions were required in the first year, 34% of revisions were performed between the first and fifth year, and 11% after five years.[30] Long-term follow-up, albeit of diminished intensity, is thus still worthwhile.

We recommend a surveillance paradigm (Figure 4–1) that incorporates available natural history and disease progression data. The first postoperative scan is obtained

TABLE 4-1. STRATIFICATION OF RISK OF GRAFT THROMBOSIS BASED ON SURVEILLANCE DATA.

Category	High velocity criteria		Low velocity criteria		Drop in ABI
I (highest risk)	PSV > 300 cm/s or Vr > 3.5	and	GFV < 45 cm/s	or	> 0.15
II (high risk)	PSV > 300 cm/s or Vr > 3.5	and	GFV > 45 cm/s	and	< 0.15
III (intermediate risk)	180 < PSV < 300 cm/s or Vr > 2.0	and	GFV > 45 cm/s	and	< 0.15
IV (low risk)	PSV < 180 cm/s and Vr < 2.0	and	GFV > 45 cm/s	and	< 0.15

PSV = Duplex-derived peak systolic velocity at site of flow disturbance;
GFV – graft flow velocity (global or distal);
Vr = velocity ratio of stenosis to more proximal graft segment of same caliber;
ABI = Doppler-derived ankle-brachial index.

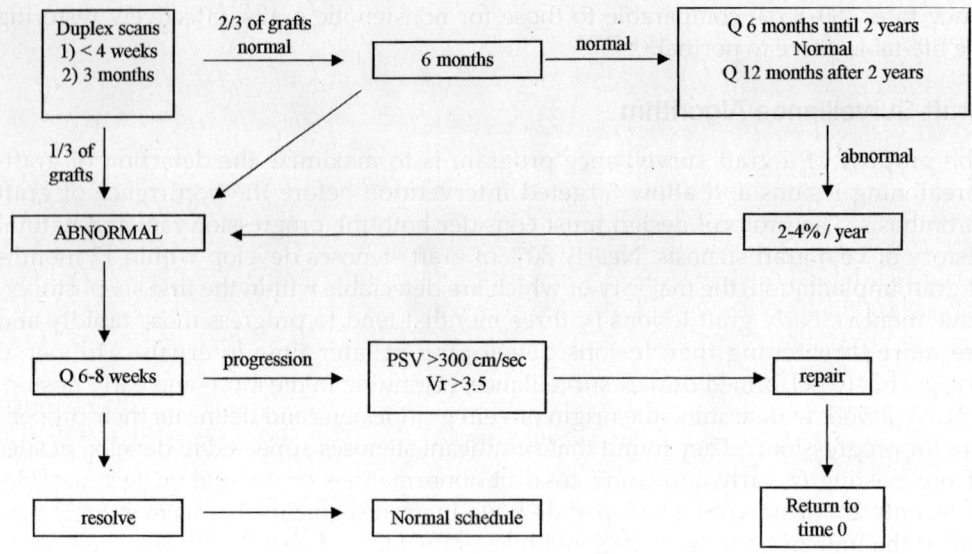

Figure 4-1. Vein Graft Surveillance Algorithm

prior to hospital discharge or at the time of the first postoperative clinic visit (within four weeks of graft implantation). A repeat study is performed three months after graft implantation. If these two studies are normal (about 2/3 of grafts), the surveillance visits are extended to every six months until two years after surgery. Annual studies are performed after two years for the lifetime of the patient. If lesions are detected during intermediate or late follow-up, scanning frequency is increased to identify grafts with progressive lesions. Grafts with low and intermediate-grade lesions are monitored for progression by performing surveillance studies every six to eight weeks until the lesion either resolves or becomes high grade. High-grade lesions are addressed.

A complete graft surveillance examination includes a physical examination (pulse palpation), ABI determination, and color-duplex interrogation of the adjacent inflow and outflow arteries, both proximal and distal anastomoses, and the entire venous conduit. If there is a significant drop in ABI or a low-flow graft is identified but duplex surveillance fails to detect the culprit lesion, conventional arteriography or MRA is performed.

The essential component of graft surveillance is thorough duplex interrogation of the bypass conduit. Surveillance is simpler if the graft has been subcutaneously tunneled and when color-flow imaging is utilized. Doppler imaging with either a 5.0 or 7.5 MHz linear-array probe is initiated in the native artery proximal to the origin of the reconstruction. Velocity spectra measurements should be made at a Doppler angle less than or equal to 60 degrees. Arterial waveforms and velocities are recorded from the inflow artery, proximal anastomosis, the proximal graft, the mid-graft, the distal graft, the distal anastomosis, and the outflow artery. Findings suggestive of a possible iliac artery stenosis include a rounded upstroke on the waveform tracing and a clearly prolonged upstroke acceleration time. If a focal, mosaic color-flow disturbance is noted, the peak systolic velocity (PSV) is measured and compared with a normal caliber, turbulence-free site in the graft proximal to the flow disturbance. The ratio of the PSV at the stenosis (V2) to normal proximal PSV (V1) is termed the velocity ratio (Vr). The advantage of employing a ratio is that changes in graft flow due to alterations in peripheral resistance or cardiac output are negated. The use of Vr is accurate and facilitates comparison of stenosis progression on serial studies. PSV and Vr determinations are the most useful duplex-derived surveillance measurements, but Vr is the single most accurate criterion for the determination of the presence and degree of graft stenosis. The mean PSV in a normal infrainguinal vein graft is generally 60–80 cm/s. A stenosis is defined as a PSV > 180 cm/s with a Vr > 1.5. A focal vein graft PSV > 300 cm/s and a Vr > 3.5 indicate a high-grade stenosis. Measurements of end-diastolic velocity (EDV) can also be readily performed. Although the EDV is less sensitive than PSV and Vr, an EDV exceeding 75 to 100 cm/s at the site of flow disturbance is a very specific finding for a stenosis exceeding 75% diameter-reduction.[33] We utilize both high- and low-flow/velocity criteria to guide intervention (Table 4–1). High-velocity criteria include a PSV > 300 cm/s at the site of stenosis and/or Vr > 3.5. Peak systolic graft flow velocity generally should exceed 45 cm/s in a normal caliber infrainguinal vein graft. If the graft flow velocity falls below this critical threshold, the probability of graft thrombosis increases. We also perform ABI determinations at each surveillance visit. Low-velocity criteria include a global graft PSV < 45 cm/s and/or a decrease in ABI > 0.15.

Two factors influence the flow characteristics of a vein graft: outflow resistance and graft diameter. Belkin and colleagues suggested that graft diameter be considered when analyzing PSV measurements.[34, 35] They noted a significant inverse correlation between PSV and diameter for tibial and popliteal grafts, but not for inframalleolar level grafts. Fillinger et al recommended calculation of shear stress during graft surveillance because it reflects both velocity and diameter.[36] This measurement may obviate the problem of detecting high or low velocities that are due to conduit diameter rather than focal stenosis. No single threshold for PSV is accurate in identifying all grafts at risk for failure. Serial measurements should be used to detect deterioration in graft function over time.

Four categories of thrombotic risk have been defined based on four hemodynamic parameters: PSV, Vr, GFV (distal or global flow velocity), and ABI (Table 4–1). The graft category at highest risk for thrombosis includes those grafts with PSV greater than 300 cm/s, Vr greater than 3.5, and a reduction in ABI exceeding 0.15. Such lesions are unlikely to regress; revision to prevent graft thrombosis is mandatory. Lesions of intermediate hemodynamic significance (PSV > 180 cm/s and Vr > 1.5) should be monitored by duplex every four to eight weeks until resolution or progression to threshold for intervention occurs. Normal graft surveillance studies are associated with a very low risk of graft thrombosis. Sladen et al[37] described nearly identical criteria. There are minor variations in the literature concerning the definition of high-grade stenosis. In general, a PSV > 250–300 cm/s or a Vr > 3–4 is felt by most clinicians to mandate either arteriography or intervention.

The surveillance program is most intense during the first one to 18 months, which is the period of greatest risk for graft stenosis and occlusion. Surveillance is continued for the lifetime of the patient to uncover hemodynamically significant atherosclerotic deteriorations in outflow and inflow arteries and late development of lesions within the graft conduit itself.

There have been minor inconsistencies in published reports with respect to the magnitude of stenosis mandating revision. An understanding of the natural history of vein graft stenosis is critical before one recommends intervention. Idu et al described the impact of a color-flow duplex surveillance program on infrainguinal vein graft patency.[6] Two patient groups were followed for a median of 21 months: 160 bypass grafts were monitored with clinical assessment and duplex scanning and compared to 41 bypass grafts followed by clinical assessment alone. Stenoses > 30% were identified in 29% of vein grafts (32% in surveillance group versus 7% in clinical assessment only group, p = 0.005). None of the grafts with stenoses between 30–49% diameter-reduction failed during follow-up. Occlusion occurred in 57% of the nonrevised versus only 9% of the revised grafts (p = .047) harboring stenoses in the 50–69% category. Stenoses with > 70% diameter-reduction were associated with graft failure in 100% of nonrevised bypasses versus 10% of revised grafts (p = 0.004). Mills et al reported that 7/9 grafts with unrepaired critical stenoses (PSV > 300 cm/s, or > 4) thrombosed within four months.[22]

Identification of subgroups of patients who might benefit from more intensive surveillance has been the subject of a number of clinical studies. However, clinical and technical variables appear to offer little prognostic value as to the risk of graft stenosis. The presence of severe comorbid illnesses such as coronary artery disease, diabetes mellitus, and end-stage nephropathy, do not appear to significantly influence the development of graft stenosis. Operative technique, specifically the controversy between reversed and in situ conduit configurations, has received considerable attention, but there has been no convincing evidence that either technique offers a significant patency advantage.[12, 38, 39] Tobacco smoking increases the risk of graft stenosis.[12] There are conflicting data as to whether female gender is a risk factor for graft stenosis.[40, 41] Alternative venous grafts (arm, lesser saphenous, spliced) are associated with an increased incidence of graft stenosis as well as poorer patencies, factors that mandate more aggressive surveillance.[21, 42, 43] Ihnat et al reported a 30-month 73% assisted primary patency rate of alternate vein conduits compared to 93% for greater saphenous grafts.[21] Interestingly, it also has been demonstrated that low-graft flow is a predictor of graft stenosis after infrainguinal bypass.[44, 45]

GRAFT REVISION

Not all stenoses are progressive and the criteria for bypass revision remain controversial. Patients with early stenoses, most often caused by myointimal hyperplasia, appear to benefit from revision even in the absence of ABI reduction.[20, 21] Stenoses reaching the threshold criteria in the early postoperative period represent rapidly progressing lesions, whereas stenoses identified later represent more slowly developing lesions. Recent reports have questioned the necessity of correcting proximal inflow lesions in the absence of clinical symptoms. Some investigators have reported that these lesions do not have a negative impact on graft patency and thus surveillance of these areas may be unnecessary.[46]

Preoperative arteriography prior to repair controversial and depends on how aggressive the surgeon is and what option for repair he chooses. Landry et al observed that arteriography significantly contributed to operative planning in 42% of open revision cases.[8] Duplex surveillance criteria for arteriography suggested by these authors include a PSV > 200 cm/s, Vr > 3.0, presence of a mid-graft velocity less than 45 cm/s, interval drop in ABI > 0.2, and/or change in clinical status. Arteriography was critical for identifying significant lesions when the proximal anastomosis was to the profunda femoris artery or in the presence of tandem graft lesions. The authors repaired lesions with > 50% angiographically confirmed stenosis which led to a five-year assisted primary patency rate of 91%. They concluded that preoperative arteriography was mandatory before revision of failing vein grafts. Idu et al recently published the results of a multicenter Dutch study assessing the role of angiography before graft revision.[47] A standardized postoperative vein graft surveillance protocol was performed in 300 patients, of whom 84 (28%) subsequently underwent vein graft revision. These authors found a Vr > 3 highly correlated with > 70% angiographic stenosis. According to their proposed algorithm, patients with a Vr < 2.5 underwent conservative treatment without angiography or revision, patients with a Vr > 4 underwent revision on the basis of duplex scan findings alone without angiography, and patients with a Vr between 2.5 and 4.0 underwent angiography before revision. This policy of selective arteriography resulted in a five-year assisted-primary patency of 74%. Mills et al suggested that intermediate graft stenoses (PSV< 300 cm/sec, Vr < 4) could be safely followed with close serial duplex surveillance, and that high-grade lesions (Vr > 4, PSV > 300) could be repaired based on duplex-findings alone.[22]

The anatomic distribution of vein graft stenoses has been examined by several investigators. Interestingly, lesion location may be dependent on the grafting technique. Mills et al prospectively studied 227 infrainguinal reversed vein grafts over a five-year period and found 33 intrinsic graft stenoses in 29 grafts, of which the majority (53%) were juxta-anastomotic and only 29% of the lesions were mid-graft.[14] Berkowitz et al reported anatomic data in a series of reversed saphenous vein graft stenoses in which the majority of lesions (40%) were just distal to the proximal anastomosis hood and 29% were juxta-anastomotic.[48] In contrast, Donaldson et al detailed the causes of primary failure of 85 in situ bypass grafts and found that 63% of graft thromboses were caused by intrinsic graft lesions, with the majority being in the mid-graft, while only 27% were juxta-anastomotic lesions.[13] Some authors have suggested that proximal lesions are more common in reversed grafts and distal lesions more frequent in in-situ grafts, but the available data do not support this assertion.

A patent graft does not necessarily guarantee limb preservation. Most authors have suggested that graft surveillance improves both graft patency and limb salvage rates.[6,49-51] The only prospective randomized study supporting an intensive surveillance program found an improvement of 25% in assisted primary patency rate compared with routine clinical follow-up in patients with autogenous infrainguinal bypass grafts. The authors did not report limb salvage rates.[52] A meta-analysis of graft surveillance by Golledge et al[51] concluded that although the patency of infrainguinal vein grafts was improved by surveillance, no improvement could be demonstrated with respect to limb salvage rates. The lack of level I evidence and differing interpretations of available duplex surveillance data resulted in the initiation of a prospective, randomized trial in the United Kingdom to determine the efficacy of duplex ultrasound graft surveillance.[53] The study is underway but the trial is incomplete and results are not yet available.

Economics of Graft Surveillance

Two studies, one in North America, and one in western Europe, have carefully evaluated the economics of vein graft surveillance. Wixon et al[54] analyzed 155 consecutive autogenous infrainguinal bypass grafts performed in 141 patients. Grafts revised for duplex-detected stenosis in comparison with those revised after thrombosis had improved one-year patency, required fewer amputations, and generated fewer expenses at 12 months ($17,688 versus $45,252). Visser et al[55] also concluded that duplex surveillance was cost effective in both claudicants and those with critical limb ischemia and reduced the risk of major limb amputation. Both studies suggest that the prevention of a small to moderate number of vein graft occlusions by judicious use of a duplex surveillance protocol makes clinical sense and yields substantial economic benefit.

INTERVENTION FOR GRAFT STENOSIS

There are three options following the detection of a graft-threatening lesion: continued observation, percutaneous endovascular repair, or open surgical revision. Continued observation without intervention is inappropriate for grafts harboring a severe stenosis as well as for those with marked hemodynamic deterioration due to inflow or outflow disease progression. Failure to intervene for vein graft stenoses exceeding 70% diameter reduction inevitably leads to graft thrombosis.

Once a hemodynamically significant graft stenosis has been confirmed and treatment deemed necessary, the decision then becomes one of selecting either endovascular intervention (PTA) or open surgical revision. Although no randomized prospective trials have been reported, available data suggest that conventional PTA is inferior to open repair.[56-59] Additionally, the indiscriminate use of PTA frequently results in an increased requirement for multiple re-interventions. Conventional PTA may be relatively effective compared to open repair if lesions are appropriately selected. Avino et al. noted that results of PTA were nearly equivalent to surgical revision when specifically applied to focal lesions (< 2cm in length), developing more than four months after the original bypass procedure, in good caliber veins (> 3.5 mm).[60]

Carlson et al recently reported the results of 45 PTA procedures in 36 failing infrainguinal vein grafts. While the initial angiographic success rate was 91.7%, one- and two-year primary patency rates were only 63% and 58%, respectively.[61] Complication rates were low, but conventional PTA results remain inferior to those reported for open revision. Recurrent stenosis develops in as many as 50% of vein grafts treated by conventional PTA (Figure 4–2).

Two recent technologic advances may improve the results of PTA for vein graft stenosis: cryoplasty and cutting balloon angioplasty (Figure 4–3). Cutting balloons

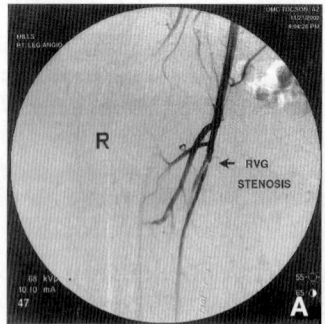
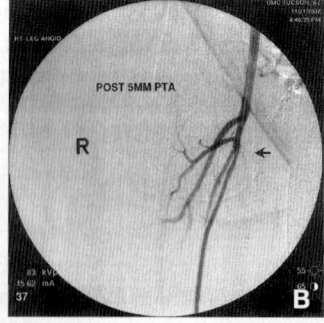
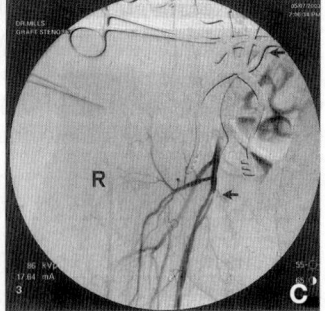

Figure 4-2. A. Severe focal, proximal, juxta-anastomotic vein graft lesion identified by duplex surveillance eight months following femoropopliteal bypass for critical limb ischemia. **B.** Excellent technical result following 5 mm conventional PTA. PSV at lesion fell from 450 cm/s to 211 cm/s and ankle-brachial index normalized. **C.** Lesion recurred at same site and with equivalent severity six months after PTA. It was repaired with open vein patch angioplasty and has not recurred during 13 months of follow-up.

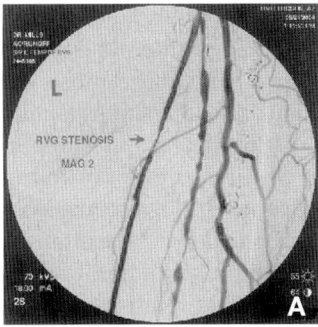 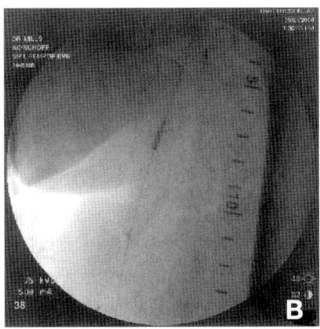 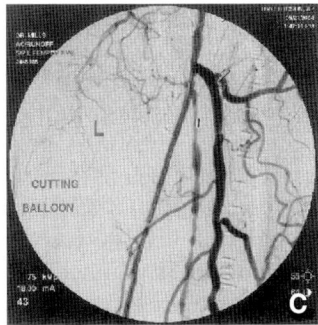

Figure 4-3. A. Recurrent femoropopliteal vein graft stenosis 10 months following basilic vein interposition graft to treat early restenosis in small caliber, spliced vein conduit. **B.** Treatment with 2.5 mm cutting balloon (CB) angioplasty. **C.** An excellent, early angiographic result was produced by CB angioplasty. Duplex-derived PSV at site of stenosis fell from 700 cm/s to 215 cm/s and the ABI doubled.

have been approved for treatment of stenoses in coronary artery bypass grafts. Results in the coronary circulation, however, may not represent an improvement over conventional PTA. Mauri et al randomized 1,238 patients with coronary arterial stenoses to cutting balloon (CB) or standard balloon (PTCA) angioplasty.[62] The primary endpoint, angiographic restenosis at six months, was 31.4% for CB and 30.4% for PTCA (p = NS). The authors recommended reserving CB for "difficult lesions." There are only two reports in the literature of the use of CB for lower extremity bypass grafts; both are small series with limited follow-up. Engelke et al used CB angioplasty in 15 consecutive lower extremity prosthetic or vein graft stenoses.[63] In six instances, CB was employed after failed or suboptimal results from conventional PTA. Procedural success rate was 94% and 12 month-patency rates were 67% (primary) and 83% (secondary). Kasirajan and Schneider have reported a 100% initial technical success rate in the treatment of nineteen focal (< 2 cm) vein graft stenoses.[64] Follow-up was too limited to permit life table analysis, but only one restenosis was observed over a mean follow-up interval of 11.4 months. We currently favor CB over conventional PTA for vein stenoses but realize that data are presently insufficient on which to make an evidence-based recommendation. The initial results (angiographic and duplex) of CB PTA appear superior to those obtained with conventional PTA (Figure 4–2). The maximal diameter of currently available cutting balloons is 4 mm and their use requires a 0.014-inch wire system.

A second new development is the Polarcath Balloon Catheter (Boston Scientific).[65] Available balloons range from 2.5 to 8 mm (0.014″ and 0.035″ systems available). The balloon is expanded with supercooled nitrous oxide (−10 degrees C) to perform "Cryoplasty." The cold is thought to reduce elastic recoil and also serves to induce apoptosis in the cells at the site of the myointimal lesion, thereby reducing further neoinitimal formation. Follow-up is extremely limited with company-provided IDE data showing a "94% procedural success rate" and an "18% target lesion revascularization rate at nine months."[65] We have just begun to employ this technique and available data are inadequate to recommend its widespread use.

Although PTA is useful in selected patients for short lesions, open surgical revision is still the most durable procedure to address the majority of severe vein graft stenoses. The specific technique of open repair is dictated by the location and etiology of the lesion. Mid-graft lesions are often the result of retained or sclerotic valve leaflets and are often correctable by partial excision of the valve leaflets and vein patch angio-plasty. Circumferential fibrotic lesions, however, will require total, segmental excision with interposition vein graft replacement. Stenoses occurring near the anastomosis are termed juxta-anastomotic lesions. Whether proximal or distal, these lesions usually occur on the venous side of the anastomosis and are the result of focal intimal hyper-plasia. Such lesions can sometimes be repaired by excision of the stenotic portion of the vein graft and translocation of the anastomosis to an adjacent arterial site, thus ob-viating the need to harvest additional conduit. Proximal graft lesions may often be treated in this manner if the original anastomosis was to the common femoral artery and the origin and proximal deep femoral artery is widely patent and relatively free of obstruction. If there is insufficient length to allow relocation of the vein graft, an inter-position vein graft can be used.

A variety of procedures such as interposition vein grafting, vein patch angio-plasty, or anastomotic translocation can be employed to repair focal juxta-anastomotic stenoses. The technique of anastomotic translocation is of specific utility when the stenosis is at the proximal anastomosis and when additional vein conduit is in short supply.

Occasionally, juxta-anastomotic stenoses may be too long to be amenable to either angioplasty or translocation. In such cases, vein graft interposition can be used to cor-rect the abnormality. Almost equal in frequency to proximal juxta-anastomotic stenoses are distal juxta-anastomotic lesions. These are most easily repaired using ei-ther vein patch angioplasty or by resection and interposition vein grafting.

Regardless of the technique selected for open repair, it is essential that the inter-vention minimize potential additional injury to the arterialized vein conduit during the revision and to document resolution of the lesion and restoration of normal graft hemodynamics at the conclusion of the procedure. The graft is especially subject to in-jury during dissection in a scarred field or by traumatic clamp placement directly on the vein. These injuries can be minimized by using distal exsanguination with an Esmarch bandage and proximal tourniquet control obviating the need for clamp place-ment. Revision of focal graft stenosis can often be performed under local anesthesia, especially if the graft has been subcutaneously tunneled. Since redo vein grafts and those employing alternate conduits such as arm vein are associated with an increased requirement for subsequent revision, we frequently tunnel such grafts subcutaneously. This approach renders graft surveillance studies easy and also simplifies open graft re-pair should the need arise.

ARTERIAL DISEASE PROGRESSION

Graft failures occurring more than three years after implantation are frequently the re-sult of progressive arterial occlusive disease in either the inflow or outflow tract. These lesions may be isolated to the native arterial tree or may develop in conjunction with juxta-anastomotic graft stenosis; all such lesions are readily identifiable by duplex sur-veillance. Less frequently seen are high-grade stenoses or occlusive lesions in outflow arteries below patent functioning grafts. When such lesions result in low graft flow ve-locities, there is an increased risk of graft thrombosis and recurrent foot ischemia. Occasionally, lesions of this type may be treated by translocating the distal anastomo-sis to an alternate runoff artery, if available, or if not, by extending the bypass to a more distal target artery.

Progressive atherosclerotic occlusive disease may also develop over time in the inflow arteries leading to stenosis or even occlusion of the inflow artery while the graft itself remains patent but in a low flow state. The patient may be asymptomatic or may notice return of claudication or rest pain; a key finding is a diminished or absent femoral pulse on physical examination. In addition, DUS will reveal low-flow velocities within the graft (<45cm/s, usually < 30 cm/s). While mature, arterialized vein grafts without intrinsic defects are remarkably tolerant to low flow states, such a situation will put the graft at increased risk for eventual failure, making it essential that the responsible lesion be corrected. Procedures commonly used to restore adequate inflow include percutaneous transluminal iliac angioplasty or local endarterectomy for focal lesions, and aortofemoral bypass, axillofemoral bypass or femorofemoral bypass for more diffuse disease. The appropriate procedure must be based on the anatomic distribution of disease and the patient's medical condition. PTA is an excellent choice for selected, focal inflow and outflow lesions. PTA is less satisfactory for intrinsic vein graft lesions than open repair, but appropriate lesion selection and improved PTA technology may lead to better results in the percutaneous treatment of vein graft stenosis. Surveillance is essential to identify offending lesions and allows intervention before the development of graft occlusion.

REFERENCES

1. Papanicolaou G, Aziz I, Yellin AE, et al. Intraoperative color duplex scanning for infrainguinal vein grafts. *Ann Vasc Surg*. 1996;10:347–355.
2. Bandyk DF, Johnson BL, Gupta AK, et al. Nature and management of duplex abnormalities encountered during infrainguinal vein bypass grafting. *J Vasc Surg*. 1996;24:430–438.
3. Johnson BL, Bandyk DF, Back MR et al. Intraoperative duplex monitoring of infrainguinal vein bypass procedures. *J Vasc Surg*. 2000;31:678–690.
4. Veith FJ, Gupta SK, Ascer E, et al. Six-year prospective multicenter randomized comparison of autologous saphenous vein and expanded polytetrafluoroethylene grafts in infrainguinal arterial reconstructions. *J Vasc Surg*. 1986;3:104–111,114.
5. Moody P, Gould DA, Harris PL. Vein graft surveillance improves patency in femoropopliteal bypass. *Eur J Vasc Surg*. 1990;4:117–121.
6. Idu MM, Blankstein JD, de Gier P, et al. Impact of a color-flow duplex surveillance program on infrainguinal vein graft patency: a five-year experience. *J Vasc Surg*. 1993;17:42–53.
7. Szilagyi DE, Elliot JP, Hageman J, et al. Biologic fate of autogenous vein implants as arterial substitutes: clinical, angiographic, and histo-pathologic observations in femoro-popliteal operations for atherosclerosis. *Ann Surg*. 1973;178:232–246.
8. Landry GJ, Moneta GL, Taylor LM Jr, et al. Duplex scanning alone is not sufficient imaging before secondary procedures after lower extremity reversed vein bypass graft. *J Vasc Surg*. 1999;29:270–281.
9. Nehler MR, Moneta GL, Yeager RA, et al. Surgical treatment of threatened reversed infrainguinal vein grafts. *J Vasc Surg*. 1994;20:558–565.
10. Caps MT, Cantwell-Gab K, Bergelin RO, et al. Vein graft lesions: time of onset and rate of progression. *J Vasc Surg*. 1995;22:466–475.
11. Erickson CA, Towne JB, Seabrook GR, et al. Ongoing vascular laboratory surveillance is essential to maximize long-term in situ saphenous vein bypass patency. *J Vasc Surg*. 1996;23:18–27.
12. Gentile AT, Mills JL, Gooden MA, et al. Identification of predictors for lower extremity vein graft stenosis. *Am J Surg*. 1997;174:218–221.
13. Donaldson MC, Mannick JA, Whittemore AD. Causes of primary graft failure after in situ saphenous vein bypass grafting. *J Vasc Surg*. 1992;15:113–120.

14. Mills Jl, Fujitani RM, Taylor SM. The characteristics and anatomic distribution of lesions that cause reversed vein graft failure: a five-year prospective study. *J Vasc Surg.* 1993;17:195–206.
15. Laborde AL, Synn AY, Worsey MJ, et al. A prospective comparison of ankle/brachial indices and color duplex imaging in surveillance of the in situ saphenous vein bypass. *J Cardiovasc Surg.* 1992;33:420–425.
16. Bandyk DF, Bergamini TM, Towne JB, et al. Durability of vein graft revision: the outcome of secondary procedures. *J Vasc Surg.* 1991;13:200–210.
17. Green RM, McNamara J, Ouriel K, et al. Comparison of infrainguinal graft surveillance techniques. *J Vasc Surg.* 1990;11:207–215.
18. Ferris BL, Mills JL Sr, Hughes JD, et al. Is early postoperative duplex scan surveillance of leg bypass grafts clinically important? *J Vasc Surg.* 2003;37:495–500.
19. Wilson YG, Davies AH, Currie IC, et al. Vein graft stenosis: incidence and intervention. Eur *J Vasc Endovasc Surg.* 1996;11:164–169.
20. Nielsen TG. Natural history of infrainguinal vein bypass stenoses: early lesions increase the risk of thrombosis. *Eur J Vasc Endovasc Surg.* 1996;12:60–64.
21. Ihnat DM, Mills JL, Dawson DL, et al. The correlation of early flow disturbances with the development of infrainguinal graft stenosis: a 10-year study of 341 autogenous vein grafts. *J Vasc Surg.* 1999;30:8–15.
22. Mills JL Sr, Wixon CL, James DC, et al. The natural history of intermediate and critical vein graft stenosis: recommendation for continued surveillance or repair. *J Vasc Surg.* 2001;33: 273–280.
23. Robinson KD, Sato DT, Gregory RT, et al. Long-term outcome after early infrainguinal graft failure. *J Vasc Surg.* 1997;26:425–438.
24. Belkin M, Conte MS, Donaldson MI, et al. Preferred strategies for secondary infrainguinal bypass: lessons learned from 300 consecutive reoperations. *J Vasc Surg.* 1995;21:282–295.
25. Belkin M, Donaldson MI, Whittemore AD, et al. Observations on the use of thrombolytic occlusion of infrainguinal vein grafts. *J Vasc Surg.* 1990;11:289–296.
26. Cohen JR, Mannick JA, Couch NP, et al. Recognition and management of impending vein-graft failure: importance for long-term patency. *Arch Surg.* 1986;121:758–759.
27. Graor RA, Risius B, Young JR, et al. Thrombolysis of peripheral arterial bypass grafts: surgical thrombectomy compared with thrombolysis: a preliminary report. *J Vasc Surg.* 1988;7: 347–355.
28. Ouriel K, Shortell CK, DeWeese JA, et al. A comparison of thrombolytic therapy with operative revascularization in the initial treatment of acute peripheral arterial ischemia. *J Vasc Surg.* 1994;19:1021–1030.
29. Bandyk DF, Schmitt DD, Seabrook GR, et al. Monitoring functional patency of in situ saphenous vein bypasses: the impact of a surveillance protocol and elective revision. *J Vasc Surg.* 1989;9:286–296.
30. Landry GJ, Moneta GL, Taylor LM Jr, et al. Long-term outcome of revised lower-extremity bypass grafts. *J Vasc Surg.* 2002;35:56–63.
31. Mills JL, Bandyk DF, Gahtan V, et al. The origin of infrainguinal vein graft stenosis: a prospective study based on duplex surveillance. *J Vasc Surg.* 1995;21:16–25.
32. Reifsnyder T, Towne JB, Seabrook GR, et al. Biologic characteristics of long-term autogenous vein grafts: a dynamic evolution. *J Vasc Surg.* 1993;17:207–217.
33. Buth J, Disselhoff B, Sommeling C, et al. Color-flow duplex criteria for grading stenosis in infrainguinal vein grafts. *J Vasc Surg.* 1991;14:716–728.
34. Belkin M, Mackey WC, McLaughlin R, et al. The variation in vein graft flow velocity with luminal diameter and outflow level. *J Vasc Surg.* 1992;15:991–999.
35. Belkin M, Raftery KB, Mackey WC, et al. A prospective study of the determinants of vein graft flow velocity: implications for graft surveillance. *J Vasc Surg.* 1994;19:259–267.
36. Fillinger MF, Cronenwett JL, Besso S, et al. Vein adaptation to the hemodynamic environment of infrainguinal vein grafts. *J Vasc Surg.* 1994;19:970–999.
37. Sladen JG, Reid JD, Cooperberg PL, et al. Color flow duplex screening of infrainguinal grafts combining low- and high-velocity criteria. *Am J Surg.* 1989;158:107–112.

38. Wengerter KR, Veith FJ, Gupta SK, et al. Prospective randomized multicenter comparison of in situ and reversed vein infrapopliteal bypasses. *J Vasc Surg.* 1991;13:189–199.
39. Moody AP, Edwards PR, Harris PL. In situ versus reversed femoropopliteal vein grafts: long-term follow-up of a prospective, randomized trial. *Br J Surg.* 1992;79:750–752.
40. Harris EJ Jr, Taylor LM Jr, Moneta GL, et al. Outcome of infrainguinal arterial reconstruction in women. *J Vasc Surg.* 1993;18:627–636.
41. Magnant JG, Cronenwett JL, Walsh DB, et al. Surgical treatment of infrainguinal arterial occlusive disease in women. *J Vasc Surg.* 1993;17:67–78.
42. Chang BB, Darling RC III, Bock DEM, et al. The use of spliced vein bypasses for infrainguinal arterial reconstruction. *J Vasc Surg.* 1995;21:403–412.
43. Chew DKW, Conte MS, Donaldson MC, et al. Autogenous composite vein bypass graft for infrainguinal arterial reconstruction. *J Vasc Surg.* 2001;33:259–264.
44. Ihlberg LHM, Alback NA, Lassila R, et al. Intraoperative flow predicts the development of stenosis in infrainguinal vein grafts. *J Vasc Surg.* 2001;34:269–276.
45. Lundell A, Bergqvist D. Prediction of early graft occlusion in femoropopliteal and femorodistal reconstruction by measurement of volume flow with a transit time flowmeter and calculation of peripheral resistance. *Eur J Vasc Surg.* 1993;7:704–708.
46. Treiman GS, Ashrafi A, Lawrence PF. Incidentally detected stenoses proximal to grafts originating below the common femoral artery: do they affect graft patency or warrant repair in asymptomatic patients? *J Vasc Surg.* 2000;32:1180–1189.
47. Idu MM, Buth J, Hop WCJ, et al. Vein graft surveillance: is graft revision without angiography justified and what criterial should be used? *J Vasc Surg.* 1998;27:399–413.
48. Berkowitz HD, Fox AD, Deaton DH. Reversed vein graft stenosis: early diagnosis and management. *J Vasc Surg.* 1992;15:130–141.
49. Mattos MA, van Bemmelen PS, Hodgson KJ, et al. Does correction of stenoses identified with color duplex scanning improve infrainguinal graft patency? *J Vasc Surg.* 1993;17:54–66.
50. Bergamini TM, George SM Sr, Massey HT, et al. Intensive surveillance of femoropopliteal-tibial autogenous vein bypasses improves long-term graft patency and limb salvage. *Ann Surg.* 1995;221:507–516.
51. Golledge J, Beattie DK, Greenhalgh RM, et al. Have the results of infrainguinal bypass improved with the widespread utilization of postoperative surveillance? *Eur J Vasc Endovasc Surg.* 1996;11:388–392.
52. Lundell A, Lindblad B, Bergqvist D, et al. Femoropopliteal-crural graft patency is improved by an intensive surveillance program. A prospective randomized study. *J Vasc Surg.* 1995;21:26–34.
53. Kirby PL, Brady AR, Thompson SG, et al. The Vein Graft Surveillance Trial: rationale, design, and methods. VGST participants. *Eur J Vasc Endovasc Surg.* 1999;18:469–474.
54. Wixon CL, Mills JL, Westerband A, et al. An economic appraisal of lower extremity bypass graft maintenance. *J Vasc Surg.* 2000;32:1–12.
55. Visser K, Idu MM, Buth J, et al. Duplex scan surveillance during the first year after infrainguinal autologous vein bypass grafting surgery: costs and clinical outcomes compared with other surveillance programs. *J Vasc Surg.* 2001;33:123–30.
56. Perler BA, Osterman FA, Mitchell SE, et al. Balloon dilatation versus surgical revision of infrainguinal autogenous vein graft stenosis: long-term follow-up. *J Cardiovasc Surg.* 1990;31:656–661.
57. Gahtan V, Weiss JP, Kerstein MD, et al. Percutaneous transluminal angioplasty in the treatment of vein graft stenosis. *Vasc Surg.* 1997;31:721–726.
58. Sanchez, LA, Suggs WD, Marin ML, et al. Is percutaneous balloon angioplasty appropriate in the treatment of graft and anastomotic lesions responsible for failing vein bypasses. *Am J Surg.* 1994;168:97–101.
59. Whittemore AD, Donaldson MC, Polak JF, et al. Limitations of balloon angioplasty for vein graft stenosis. *Vasc Surg.* 1991;14:340–345.
60. Avino AJ, Bandyk DF, Gonsalves AJ, et al. Surgical and endovascular intervention for infrainguinal vein graft stenosis. *J Vasc Surg.* 1999;29:60–71.

61. Carlson GA, Hoballah JJ, Sharo WJ. Balloon angioplasty as a treatment of failing infrainguinal autologous vein bypass grafts. *J Vasc Surg*. 2004;39(2):421–426.
62. Mauri L, Bonan R, Weiner BH et al. Cutting balloon angioplasty for the prevention of restenosis: results of the cutting balloon global randomized trial. *Am J Card*. 2002;90:1079–1083.
63. Engelke C, Morgan RA, Belli AM. Cutting balloon percutaneous transluminal angioplasty for salvage of lower limb arterial bypass grafts: Feasibility. *Radiology*. 2002;223(1):106–114.
64. Kasirajan K, Schneider PA. Early outcome of "cutting" balloon angioplasty for infrainguinal vein graft stenosis. *J Vasc Surg*. 2004;39(4):702–708.
65. PolarCath Peripheral Dilatation System. Available at: http://www.bostonscientific.com/med_specialty/deviceDetail.jhtml.

5

Statin Management for Vascular Surgery Patients

Walter J. McCarthy, M.D., Chad E. Jacobs, M.D., and Ana Silvia Bonilla, M.D.

Ample evidence exists that to provide quality care for vascular surgery patients with arterial disease, their comorbidities need to be managed.[1] Besides providing arterial bypass, endarterectomy, or angioplasty, other issues need to be considered. Once a patient is identified to have significant arterial disease, whether that person has an operation or intervention or not, he or she will require lifetime attention on several different fronts. Thus, competent management of diabetes, hypertension, and smoking cessation are priorities. Less intuitive, but now well established, are the benefits of several oral medical interventions for these patients. These include the use of ACE inhibitors, beta-blocking medications, antiplatelet medications, and cholesterol reducing formularies including statins. These medical interventions have been shown to have not only salutary effects at the time of arterial intervention, but also, for some, to provide improved long-term arterial patency and protection from myocardial mortality or even all-cause mortality.

While an analysis of all these different medications is intriguing, the focus of this presentation will be on the impact of statin medications for patients with peripheral arterial disease. The effects of statins on myocardial arterial disease has been known for many years, but specific benefit for peripheral arterial patients has become convincingly available in the last five years.[2,3] For example, a distinct patency benefit was demonstrated in a large group of patients from the Brigham and Women's Hospital with primary autogenous infrainguinal reconstruction.[4] In a similar paper reviewing all types of lower extremity bypass from the University of Michigan, long-term patency was also better.[5] Several papers from Rotterdam and Leiden in the Netherlands have demonstrated both better perioperative survival and better long-term survival for aortic aneurysm patients treated with statins.[6,7]

Many papers have shown that carotid artery intimal-medial thickness is decreased over time with statins[8-12] and, remarkably, a comprehensive paper from the Massachusetts General Hospital recently demonstrated a similar result after carotid endarterectomy.[13] They found improved long-term carotid patency in patients treated with chronic statin use. Besides reviewing these important papers, a consideration of the described effects of statins on arteries will be reviewed. A review of other cholesterol-lowering drugs as well as guidelines for statin use along with their risks, will be presented.

WHAT ARE STATINS?

There are three classes of medications used for first-line treatment of hyperlipidemia.[14] Statins, the third group, are considered the most effective and best tolerated of the three. The first group includes the bile acid-binding resins such as cholestyramine and colestipol. These drugs interrupt the reabsorption of bile acids in the intestine and thereby regulate LDL receptors in the liver. These medications are used for young people who have high LDL cholesterol and normal triglycerides, but are often poorly tolerated as there are gastrointestinal side effects such as constipation, gas, and bloating. These agents are safe and have been used for over 30 years. Niacin is the second group. Its mechanism is not fully understood. Niacin is also safe and has been used for over 30 years, but often results in unpleasant side effects such as cutaneous flushing. Liver enzymes may become elevated in 3% to 5% of patients using niacin.

Statin is a commonly used, shorter term for HMG- CoA reductase inhibitors.[15] Statins competitively inhibit 3-hydroxy 3-methylglutaryl coenzyme A reductase that is responsible for catalyzing a rate limiting step in cholesterol biosynthesis in the liver. The original statin came from the mold *Penicillium citrinium* and was shown to be an inhibitor of cholesterol synthesis in 1976. It subsequently was proved to be an inhibitor of HMG CoA reductase in 1978. Scientists at Merck developed the first statins to be approved in humans from *Aspergillus terreus*, and consequently lovastatin (Mevacor) was approved by the U.S. FDA in 1987. Since then at least five other statins have been approved. Pravastatin (Pravacol) and simvastatin (Vytorin, Zocor) are chemically modified from lovastatin. More recent compounds including atorva-statin (Caduet, Lipitor), fluvastatin (Lescol), and cerivastatin (recently withdrawn by the FDA) are synthetic.

Statins function by reducing LDL cholesterol but seem to have other effects in addition.[16] The observed reduction of cardiac and vascular endpoints may be achieved by a combination of biological effects. As outlined by Abbruzzese, these include improved endothelial function particularly related to nitric oxide.[4] There is reduced smooth muscle cell proliferation and migration, which results in an inhibition of neointimal hyperplasia and inflammation. There is a reduction in plaque smooth muscle cell content and collagen content, and there is a suppression of certain tissue factors and matrix metalloprotinases that may enhance plaque stability. These beneficial results may reduce recurrent stenosis by suppressing intimal hyperplasia, slow development of atherosclerosis, and stabilize existing plaque. The commonly described model of myocardial infarction after existing plaque rupture causing coronary artery occlusion and adjacent thrombosis may be modified by this plaque stabilization, and explain reduction in myocardial mortality.

DIRECT BENEFICIAL EFFECTS OF STATINS FOR VASCULAR PATIENTS

As mentioned above, there is considerable literature to support the use of statins in patients with lower extremity occlusive disease, aortic disease, and carotid disease. In addition to the cardioprotective benefits and improved mortality rates well documented with statins in this patient group, several authors have recently described improved bypass graft patency, increased limb salvage, and decreased rates of carotid restenosis after endarterectomy.

In 2003, Eagle reported on a large series of consecutive infrainguinal bypasses performed at the University of Michigan.[5] His group sought to evaluate if statin drugs and ACE inhibitors conferred on this cohort an improvement in graft patency, limb salvage, and operative mortality. All patients undergoing infrainguinal bypass at that institution from 1997 to 2002 were included in the analysis. Medication use was documented either during the preoperative, perioperative, or postoperative period to include beta-blockers, ACE inhibitors, statins, aspirin, clopidogrel, warfarin, and multivitamins.

The analysis included 338 infrainguinal bypasses performed in 293 patients with a mean age of 64 years, 67% of whom were male. The patient cohort had risk factors similar to those in most patients with peripheral vascular disease and included hypertension (70%), diabetes (53%), coronary artery disease (51%), hyperlipidemia (48%), and current tobacco use (30%). Indications for bypass included claudication in 26%, rest pain in 27%, tissue loss in 31%, and popliteal aneurysm in 4%. Bypass procedures included femoral to popliteal in 53%, and femoral to tibial or peroneal vessels in 43%. Autologous greater saphenous vein (61%) was the most commonly used conduit. Thirty-nine percent of patients underwent a postoperative duplex graft surveillance study one or more times.

Cumulative graft patency was 73% with mean follow-up of 17.5 +/− 14 months. The mean preoperative ABI was 0.42 and the mean postoperative ABI was 0.75. The overall rate of amputation was 13% and overall mortality during follow-up was 8%. In terms of medical therapy, 76% of patients were taking aspirin, 27% were taking clopidogrel, 30% were taking warfarin, 69% were taking a beta-blocker, and approximately 50% were taking an ACE-inhibitor and/or a statin drug. Interestingly, total cholesterol and LDL cholesterol were compared between patients receiving or not receiving a statin, and no difference was found.

Univariate analysis revealed that aspirin or warfarin, ACE inhibitors, statins, and beta-blocker use correlated with improved graft patency and decreased amputation rates. Multivariate analysis revealed a number of positive findings related to statin use. A two-to threefold improvement in graft patency was associated with postoperative graft surveillance (Odds Ratio 2.4; $p = 0.006$), male gender (OR 2.8; $p < 0.001$), and the use of statin drugs (OR 3.7; $p < 0.001$). Patients taking statin drugs had a nearly 80% decreased risk of amputation (OR 0.34; $p > 0.01$). Analysis solely for medication effect over time with Cox proportionate hazards modeling revealed that only therapy with statin drugs (Hazard Ratio 0.52; $p = 0.005$) or aspirin (HR 0.52; $p = 0.007$) was associated with significantly decreased risk for graft occlusion. Statins were not found to be significantly associated with survival in this study.

The authors concluded that among other findings, their report demonstrated the significant protective effect that statins confer on graft patency and limb salvage. This positive effect is shown by their data to be even greater than that determined by conduit type, severity of ischemia, or vascular comorbidities. As has been proposed by other authors, this report also suggests that given that the total and LDL cholesterol levels were similar between patients receiving and not receiving statins, there is a protective effect independent of their lipid-lowering activity. Both animal and human studies have shown that statins stabilize atherosclerotic plaque via matrix metalloproteinases and leukocytic matrix interactions.[17-19] Other studies have shown that statins inhibit production of inflammatory cytokines by leukocytes,[20,21] and inhibit T cell activation and antigen-presenting functions.[22,23] Statins have also been shown to lead to an increase in the expression and activity of endothelial nitric oxide synthase (eNOS).[24,25]

Abbruzzese et al. conducted a retrospective review of consecutive patients undergoing infrainguinal revascularization at Brigham and Women's Hospital from 1999–2001.[4] This report sought to determine the influence of statin therapy on graft patency after autogenous infrainguinal reconstruction. Following chart review, patients were divided into two groups: those taking a statin drug at the time of their initial procedure, and those not taking a statin drug (controls). A total of 189 grafts in 172 patients were analyzed, and were broken down into 94 grafts in the statin group and 95 grafts in the control group. While there was no difference between groups in terms of gender, diabetes, hypertension, smoking, renal failure, congestive heart failure, or COPD, there was a greater incidence of coronary artery disease and history of coronary artery bypass grafting in the statin group. As in the previous study, there was no significant difference in the cholesterol levels between the two groups.

There was no significant difference in the indication for operation between the two groups, and included claudication (8%), rest pain (24%), and tissue loss (68%). The study only included patients in whom the conduit was a single segment of saphenous vein. The sites of proximal and distal anastamosis and graft orientation were likewise similar in both groups, with the exception of grafts more commonly arising from the superficial femoral artery in the control group (47 vs. 17; $p < 0.03$).

Thirty-day mortality was 2.6% overall and not significantly different among the two groups (two deaths in the statin group, three deaths in the control group; $p = 0.51$). The overall postoperative morbidity rate was 21% and not significantly different between the two groups. Early graft thrombosis occurred in 3.7% of grafts and was not significantly different between groups. Overall, two-year patient survival was 66% with no significant difference between groups. Primary patency at two years was 72% and was not significantly different between groups. Overall, two-year primary-revised patency was 89%; 94% in the statin group and 83% in the control group ($p < 0.02$). Similar improved results were seen in the statin group for two-year secondary patency (97% in the statin group and 87% in the control group; $p<0.02$). The overall risk of graft failure was found to be 3.2-fold higher in the control group. Limb salvage at two years was 91% with no significant difference identified between the two groups.

By univariate analysis, statin use ($p = 0.03$) was the only factor found to have a significant association with secondary graft patency. No significant association was found for smoking, diabetes, hypertension, coronary disease, COPD, or renal failure. With all variables examined in a stepwise Cox proportional hazards model, the association with statins alone remained significant ($p = 0.03$). While this study did not demonstrate a significant difference in morbidity or mortality between the statin and control groups, the protective effect of statins in graft patency are quite similar to those in the report above from Michigan. Again demonstrated was no significant difference in cholesterol levels between the two groups, suggesting a protective mechanism conferred by statins that is independent of their cholesterol-lowering activity. The authors speculated that statins may reduce the overall virulence of the graft hyperplasia response, or may exert a primary antithrombotic effect.

Poldermans et al. reported on a series of patients undergoing major vascular surgery at a single center from 1991 to 2000.[6] The goal of this study was to evaluate the association between statin use and perioperative mortality in this patient population. Of 2,816 major vascular operations (abdominal aortic aneurysm repair, carotid endarterectomy, lower extremity revascularization) done during this time period, there were 160 (5.8%) perioperative deaths. Utilizing database review, two patients were selected as controls (n = 320) for each patient who died and a case control study was performed.

Case and control groups had similar rates of hypertension, diabetes, and hypercholesterolemia. There was a significantly greater incidence of renal insufficiency, congestive heart failure, history of myocardial infarction, angina pectoris, and stroke in the case group (deaths). Statin use was found to be significantly less common in cases than controls (8% vs. 25%; $p<0.001$), and the risk of perioperative mortality was reduced 4.5 times compared to those not taking statin drugs (Odds Ratio 0.22). Once again, no statistically significant difference was seen in cholesterol levels between cases and controls as well as between statin users and nonusers. Using perioperative mortality as an endpoint, this report concluded that patients on statin therapy who undergo major vascular surgery enjoy a greater than fourfold reduced risk.

LaMuraglia et al. evaluated a group of consecutive patients undergoing carotid endarterectomy at the Massachusetts General Hospital from 1989 through 1999, with the aim of evaluating determinants of anatomic durability of carotid endarterectomy.[13] This retrospective review studied 2,127 procedures performed in 1,853 patients. The primary endpoint for the study was carotid restenosis based on duplex criteria and was stratified into minimal, moderate, severe, or occlusion. Patients were further temporally divided into two groups: early (<2 years) and late (>2 years) restenosis.

Patients averaged 70.5 years of age and demonstrated many of the typical comorbidities of this patient population: hypertension (80%), diabetes (25%), coronary artery disease (55%), COPD (13%), and tobacco use (68%). Surgical characteristics included 36% symptomatic patients, shunting in 33% of patients, and patching in 50% of patients.

Univariate analysis of variables associated with early restenosis identified lipid-lowering drugs and patch use as having protective effects. Statin drugs specifically were found to confer a significantly reduced incidence of early restenosis (Odds Ratio 0.619; p = 0.0043), early failure (OR 0.466; p = 0.012), late progression (OR 0.280; $p<0.0001$), and late failure (OR 0.176; $p<0.0001$). Multivariate analysis found similarly convincing evidence of the protective effect from both early and late restenosis and failure afforded by statin drugs (Early restenosis OR 0.601; p = 0.0071, Early failure OR 0.517; p = 0.037. Late restenosis OR 0.202; p = 0.00028, and Late failure OR 0.128; p = 0.00037).

This study further bolsters the argument for statin administration in the vascular patient population as statins were found to have the greatest effect of all variables studied to protect against recurrent stenosis after carotid endarterectomy. The authors again suggested that in addition to the lipid-lowering characteristics of the statins, there are likely other beneficial mechanisms such as decreasing vessel wall inflammatory response, increasing circulating endothelial progenitor cells, and promotion of smooth muscle cell apoptosis.[29,30]

Kertai et al. reported on a series of patients who underwent open abdominal aortic aneurysm surgery from 1991 and 2001, and assessed the long-term use of statins and their association with all-cause and cardiovascular mortality in this cohort.[7] Some 519 of the 570 patients (91%) who underwent aortic aneurysm repair during this time period survived greater than 30 days and were included in the analysis. Patients were stratified into two groups based on whether on not they were taking a statin drug at the time of their operation. Among the statin users, a significantly increased percentage of patients had angina pectoris (30% vs. 15%, $p<0.001$), previous myocardial infarction (38% vs. 20%, $p<0.001$), and renal dysfunction (15% vs. 8%, $p = 0.01$).

With a median follow-up of 4.7 years, survival was significantly improved in patients using statins compared to those who did not. Patients using statins had a 2.5-fold reduction in the risk of all-cause mortality and a more than threefold reduction in the risk of cardiovascular mortality compared to patients not taking statins. This risk reduction was unchanged with multivariate analysis, and remained after adjustment for clinical risk factors and use of other drugs such as beta-blockers.

The above review of current literature strongly supports the use of statins in vascular surgery patients. There is evidence that statins improve perioperative mortality, improve long-term bypass graft patency, increase limb salvage, decrease restenosis after carotid endarterectomy, and decrease all-cause mortality and cardiovascular mortality. As nearly all of the referenced studies suggest, there are likely mechanisms separate from and in addition to the lipid-lowering activity of statins that are responsible for these beneficial effects.

STATIN USE IN A VASCULAR PRACTICE

Recognizing the clear benefit of statins for vascular patients after arterial intervention, the issue is, which group of physicians should prescribe these medications? The management of statins may be overly complex for many vascular surgery practices. The considerations include selecting a specific drug, initial evaluation of the patient's lipid profile, dose choice, serum chemistry testing, and follow-up lipid profiles and serum testing. These are routine responsibilities for primary care doctors and cardiologists, but may overwhelm a vascular clinic. On the other hand, some vascular offices may have the support and record-keeping capacity to prescribe and supervise these drugs. Depending on the local clinical circumstances, there may be no other physician who can reliably do so. From the standpoint of the supervising physician, the cognitive interaction is not a difficult one and dose adjustment with lipid profile changes can be easily learned. It is, however, necessary to follow blood chemistry patterns in patients once they are placed on statins. Therefore, it remains a personal choice, depending on circumstances and interest, for vascular surgeons to prescribe statins themselves or ask a primary care physician to assume this responsibility. The emphasis of this chapter is to highlight to the vascular surgery community the importance of placing patients on statins regardless of who manages their admistration.

PRINCIPLES OF LIPID MANAGEMENT

Traditional guidelines for managing serum lipids have focused on LDL (low-density lipoprotein) cholesterol. This is for good reason as LDL cholesterol levels and their subsequent reduction correlate, in a multitude of studies, with clinical outcome.[26] Therefore, practically speaking, LDL cholesterol is usually the target of therapy. Other markers such as triglycerides and HDL (high-density lipoprotein) cholesterol[27] are sometimes relevant. The National Cholesterol Education Program (NCEP) Adult Treatment Panel III guidelines are useful.[28] A standard approach is nicely outlined in

Harrison's Principles of Internal Medicine.[14] In brief, three layers of risk are outlined. The highest are patients with coronary artery disease. In the middle are those with no coronary artery disease but with two or more risk factors. Low risk is with no coronary artery disease and less than two risk factors. The goals of therapy are, respectively, 100, 130, and 160 mg per deciliter of LDL cholesterol. Recently, there is convincing evidence that "lower is better" and LDL cholesterol levels less than 70 mg per deciliter are recommended for very high-risk patients.[26] Specific goals for lipid management have not been formally articulated for patients with peripheral arterial disease at this point.[29] Many obviously have a degree of coronary artery disease and many risk factors. A reasonable target for patients with arterial disease requiring treatment would be LDL cholesterol less than 100. Patients with particularly prevalent disease might be considered for a goal of 70 mg per deciliter LDL cholesterol.

COMPLICATIONS WITH STATIN USE

A statin safety assessment conference sponsored by the National Lipid Association was held July 17 through 19, 2005, in Washington, D.C. The synopsis of this conference, presented by Guyton, emphasizes the profound advantage and high degree of safety of these medications.[30,31] Myositis is a known complication and patients are assessed with creatinine kinase evaluation if they have symptoms. The tremendously rare, resulting rhabdomyolysis was found to occur in three per hundred-thousand person-years during statin treatment. Fatality occurs in 9% of these patients, thus resulting in a rate of 0.3 per hundred-thousand patient-years. The comparable all-cause mortality reduction was the incredibly higher 360 per hundred-thousand person-years. It was noted that cerivastatin had been removed from distribution by the FDA due to its disproportionately higher risk of fatal rhabdomyolysis compared to the other statins. Peripheral nerve damage was seen at a rate of approximately 12 per hundred-thousand person-years and most patients recovered after the medication was withdrawn. Acute, potentially fatal liver failure was reported at a rate of 0.1 case per hundred-thousand person-years of treatment, which was felt to be approximately equal to the background rate of liver failure in the general population. Guidelines for statin use specify liver function studies before initiating therapy, generally after 12 weeks of therapy, and semiannually thereafter. Medication is withheld if the transaminases rise above three times the normal limits. Transaminase elevation is dose-related, and for example, with Lipitor, the incidence is 0.2%, 0.2%, 0.6%, and 2.3% for doses of 10 mg, 20 mg, 40 mg, and 80 mg, respectively.[32]

Another issue addressed by Guyton was whether all the currently marketed statins have a similar low risk of serious adverse effects, and the conclusion was that they did. The panel concluded that "for the vast majority of patients needing statin therapy, it suffices to know that these drugs are both very effective and very safe."[30]

CONCLUDING REMARKS

HMG Co-A reductase medications, known as statins, have been found to have a strong beneficial effect for patients with atherosclerosis. Reductions in myocardial infarction, cardiac origin mortality, and even all-cause mortality have been repeatedly demonstrated. Benefits have even been demonstrated for vascular surgery patients related to bypass graft patency and reduction in postoperative carotid artery restenosis.

Based on these findings, most vascular patients with arterial disease are likely candidates for statin use and will clearly benefit from these medications.

REFERENCES

1. Bhatt DL, Steg PG, Ohman EM, et al. International prevalence, recognition, and treatment of cardiovascular risk factors in outpatients with atherothrombosis. *JAMA*. 2006;295 (2): 180–189.
2. Giri J, McDermott MM, Greenland P, et al. Statin use and functional decline in patients with and without peripheral arterial disease. *J Am Col Cardiol*. 2006;47(5):998–1004.
3. Feringa HHH, Waning VHV, Bax, JJ, et al. Cardioprotective medication is associated with improved survival in patients with peripheral arterial disease. *J Am Col Cardiol*. 2006;47(6): 1182–1187.
4. Abbruzzese TA, Havens J, Belkin M , et al. Statin therapy is associated with improved patency of autogenous infrainguinal bypass grafts. *J Vasc Surg*. 2004;39(6):1178–1185.
5. Henke PK, Blackburn S, Proctor MC, Stevens J, et al. Patients undergoing infrainguinal bypass to treat atherosclerotic vascular disease are underprescribed cardioprotective medications: Effect on graft patency, limb salvage, and mortality. *J Vasc Surg*. 2004;39(2):357–365.
6. Poldermans D, Bax JJ, Kertai MD, Krenning B, et al. Statins are associated with a reduced incidence of perioperative mortality in patients undergoing major noncardiac Vascular Surgery. *Circulation*. 2003;107:1848–1851.
7. Kertai MD, Boersma E, Westerhout CM, et al. Association between long-term statin use and mortatlity after successful abdominal aortic aneursym surgery. *Am J Med*. 2004;116(2): 96–103.
8. Grines CL. The role of statins in reversing atherosclerosis: what the latest regression studies show. *J Intervent Cardiol*. 2006;19(1):3–9. Review.
9. Salonen R, Nyyssonen K, Porkkala E, et al. Kuopio Atherosclerosis Prevention Study (KAPS) A poplulation based primary preventive trial of the effect of LDL lowering on atherosclerotic progression in carotid and femoral arteries. *Circulation*. 1995;92:1758–1764.
10. Blankenhorn DH, Azen SP, Kramsch DM, et al. Cornary angiographic changes with lovastation therapy. The Monitored Atherosclerosis Regression Study (MARS). *Ann Intern Med*. 1993;119 (10):969–976.
11. Hodis HN, Mack WJ, LaBree L, Selzer RH, et al. Reduction in cartoid arterial wall thickness using lovastatin and dietary therapy. *Ann Intern Med*. 1996;124(6):548–556.
12. De Sauvage Nolting PRW, De Groot E, Zwinderman AH, et al. Regression of carotid and femoral artery intima-media thickness in familial hypercholesterolemia. *Arch Intern Med*. 2003;163:1837–1841.
13. LaMuraglia GM, Stoner MC, Brewster DC, et al. Determinants of carotid endarterectomy anatomic durability: Effects of serum lipids and lipid-lowering drugs. *J Vasc Surg*. 2005;41(5):762–758.
14. Fauci AS, Braunwald E, Isselbacher KJ, et al. Hypolipidemic agents . In: Fauci AS, (ed.) *Harrison's, Principles of Internal Medicine, 14th Ed*, Vol. 2. New York: McGraw Hill; 1998: 2146–2148.
15. Hardman JG, Limbird LE, Goodman Gilman AJ; Mahley RW, and Bersot TP. Drug therapy for hypercholesterolemia and dyslipidemia. In: Hardman JG, Limbird AE, (eds.) *Goodman & Gilman's, The Pharmacological Basis of Therapeutics, 10th Ed*. New York: McGraw-Hill; 2001:971–989.
16. Balk EM, Karas RH , Jordan HS, et al. Effects of statins on vascular structure and function: A systematic review. *Am J Med*. 2004;117:775–787.
17. Maron DJ, Fazio S, Liton MF. Current perspectives on statins. *Circulation*. 2000;101:207–213.
18. Bea F, Blessing E, Bennett B, et al. Simvastatin promotes atherosclerotic plaque stability in apoE-deficient mice independently of lipid-lowering. *Arterioscler Thromb Vasc Biol*. 2002;22:1832–1837.

19. Crisby M, Nordin-Fredrikson G, Shah PK, et al. Pravastatin treatment increases collagen content and decreases lipid content, inflammation, metalloproteinases, and cell death in human carotid plaques. *Circulation*. 2001;103:926–933.
20. Rosenson RS, Tangney CC, Casey LC. Inhibition of proinflammatory cytokine production by pravastatin. *Lancet*. 1999;353:983–984.
21. Ikeda U, Shimada K. Statins and monocytes (letter). *Lancet*. 1999;353:2070.
22. Kwak B, Mulhaupt F, Myit S, Mach F. Statins as a newly recognized type of immunomodulator. *Nat Med*. 2000;6:1399–1402.
23. Weitz-Schmidt G, Welzenbach K. Brinkmann V, et al. Statins selectively inhibit leukocyte function antigen-1 by binding to a novel regulatory integrin site. *Nat Med*. 2001;7:687–92.
24. Laufs U, La Fata V, Plutzky J, Liao JK. Upregulation of endothelial nitric oxide synthase by HMG CoA reductase inhibitors. *Circulation*. 1998;97:1129–1135.
25. Laufs U, Liao JK. Post-transcriptional regulation of endothelial nitric oxide synthase mRNA stability by Rho GTPase. *J Biol Chem*. 1998;273:24,266–271.
26. Jones PH. Lipids. New guidelines, intensive treatment, and future directions. *Tex Heart Inst J*. 2006;33(2):180–183.
27. Rosenson RS. Low high-density lipoprotein cholersterol and cardiovascular disease: Risk reduction with statin therapy. *Am Heart J*. 2006;151(3):556–563.
28. Grundy SM, Cleeman JI, Merz CNB, et al. Implications of recent clinical trials for the National Cholesterol Education Program Adult Treatment Panel III guidelines. *Circulation*. 2004;110:227–239.
29. Daskaloupoulou SS, Daskalopoulos ME, Liapis CD, Mikhailidis DP. Peripheral arterial disease: A missed opportunity to administer statins so as to reduce cardiac morbidity and mortality. *Curr Med Chem*. 2005;12(4): 443–52. Review.
30. Guyton JR. Benefit versus risk in statin treatment. *Am J Cardiol*. 2006;97(8A):95C–97C.
31. Gotto AM Jr. Statins, cardiovascular disease, and drug safety. *Am J Cardiol*. 2006;97(8A): 3C–5C.
32. Murry L. (ed.) *2006 Physicians' Desk Reference, 60th Edition*. Thomson Pdr: Stamford CT; 2006:2995.

6

Antiplatelet Medication in Patients with Vascular Disease and Following Interventions

Andres Schanzer, M.D., Karen J. Ho, M.D., and Michael Belkin, M.D.

In response to tissue injury, platelets have been demonstrated to play a fundamental role in the coagulation cascade and subsequent hemostasis. At the same time, arterial thrombosis is the consequence of a well-orchestrated sequence of platelet adhesion, activation, and aggregation. In the setting of advanced atherosclerosis, the sequence of plaque rupture, adhesion of platelets, activation of the extrinsic clotting cascade, platelet aggregation, and stabilization of the thrombus leads to a spectrum of acute ischemic syndromes ranging from myocardial infarction and stroke to peripheral arterial or bypass graft occlusion.[1] While countless studies had previously been conducted to address whether inhibition of platelets prevents the development and progression of atherosclerosis and acute ischemic syndromes, the first systematic evaluation to effectively address this important question was performed by the Antiplatelet Trialists' Collaboration in 1994.[2-4] This landmark meta-analysis of prospective randomized blinded trials was published in three parts. The first reported a significant reduction in overall risk of nonfatal myocardial infarction, nonfatal stroke, and vascular death in 70,000 patients with multiple cardiovascular comorbidities who were given antiplatelet therapy. Part II of the study also demonstrated that antiplatelet therapy significantly improved vascular graft and hemodialysis access patency. This chapter will concentrate on the patient with peripheral vascular disease, and will review the role of antiplatelet therapy in providing protection from major cardiovascular morbidity (myocardial infarction, stroke, or death), improved bypass graft patency, and decreased rates of restenosis and occlusion following peripheral percutaneous intervention.

ROLE OF PLATELETS IN ATHEROSCLEROSIS, ARTERIAL THROMBOSIS, BYPASS GRAFT OCCLUSION, AND RESTENOSIS AFTER PERCUTANEOUS INTERVENTION

Platelets have a role in the pathogenesis of both early and late atherosclerotic disease. Early in the disease, endothelial injury exposes underlying thrombogenic components of the matrix including collagen, laminin, and von Willebrand's factor (vWf), all of which bind to platelets through surface membrane receptors.[5] Collagen is the most thrombogenic and binds to the platelet's GPIa/IIb receptor via vWF. Once the platelet is adherent, an internal signaling network is triggered that ultimately leads to a change in the platelet's morphology. This calcium-mediated activation process leads to several amplifying feedback loops: degranulation of vesicles of adenosine dihosphate (ADP) and serotonin, synthesis of thromboxane A2 (a platelet activator and vasoconstrictor), and increased expression of GPIIb/IIIa surface receptor.

Intimately involved in the platelet's role in recognizing vessel injury is the coagulation cascade. Changes in the distribution of negatively charged phospholipids on the platelet surface during activation provide a surface for the prothrombinase complex that leads to generation of thrombin.[6] Furthermore, platelet activation promotes factor IX activation and generation of cofactors Va and VIIIa.[7]

Platelet aggregation is mediated by GPIIb/IIIa receptors, which are upregulated during platelet activation. As the cell surface density of these receptors increases, more fibrinogen can be bound and converted into fibrin by thrombin. In addition, GPIIb/IIIa receptors recruit adhesion proteins fibronectin, vitronectin, and vWf, which, in turn, attract more platelets, leading to growth of a stable thrombus and platelet aggregate (Figure 6–1).

Platelets also have a critical role in the final stages of atherosclerotic pathology. Not only is platelet deposition increased in areas of vessel stenosis, culminating in an increasingly platelet-rich thrombus that can eventually occlude the vessel, but also plaque rupture leads to rapid formation of a platelet-rich thrombus that can have acute clinical manifestations including acute coronary syndromes, stroke, and critical limb ischemia.

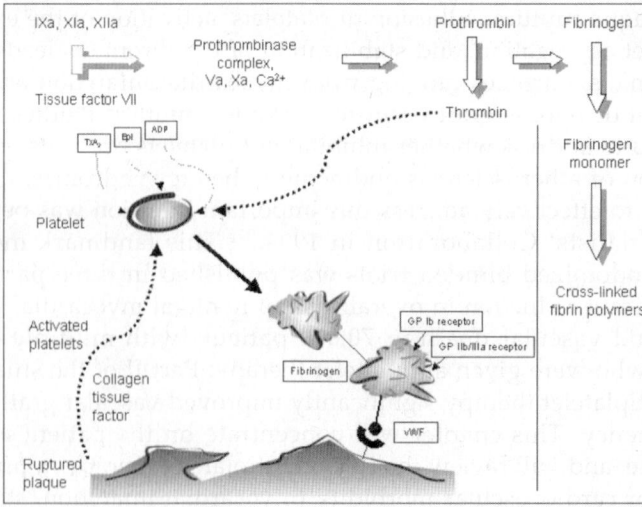

Figure 6-1. Schematic representation of the steps leading to platelet activation, aggregation, and subsequent fibrinogen binding.

ANTIPLATELET AGENTS

Antiplatelet agents, along with their mechanisms and structures, are shown in Table 6–1.

Aspirin

Aspirin is the most prescribed and widely studied antiplatelet agent in current use. It was first established as a platelet-inhibiting drug in 1967.[8] It acetylates and thereby permanently inactivates cyclooxygenase (COX)-1 and COX-2 enzymes, which are secreted by activated platelets.[9] This inactivation prevents the first step in the conversion of arachidonic acid to thromboxane A_2 and prostaglandin I_2 (inhibitor of platelet aggregation and vasodilator).[10]

Once a day dosing of aspirin irreversibly inhibits COX-1 and thereby completely blocks production of its end product, thromboxane A_2. On the other hand, prostaglandin I_2 is produced via both the COX-1 and COX-2 pathway. Its production is relatively preserved in the setting of low-dose aspirin administration, due to COX-2 partial aspirin resistance.[10] Thus, low-dose aspirin inhibits primarily thromboxane A_2 production, whereas high-dose aspirin inhibits both end products. This phenomenon, along with the side effect profile,[11] explains why low-dose aspirin (50–100 mg/d) has been shown to be as beneficial,[12] if not more so,[13] than high-dose aspirin (100–1500 mg/d).

The safety of chronic aspirin use is limited by risks of upper gastrointestinal bleeding and chronic renal failure. A history of upper gastrointestinal bleeding is the most important risk factor for subsequent bleeding, and it has been shown that 15% of patients with a history of bleeding from ulcers have recurrent bleeding within one year while on aspirin.[14] Combination therapy with proton pump inhibitors, while not completely eliminating the risk of aspirin-induced bleeding, has been shown to severely limit it.[15]

TABLE 6-1. ANTIPLATELET AGENTS, MECHANISMS, AND STRUCTURES.

Agent	Mechanism	Structure
Aspirin	Inhibits cyclooxygenase, thereby decreasing thromboxane A2 production	
Dipyridamole	Increases cyclic AMP	
Thienopyridines: Ticlopidine, Clopidogrel	Irreversibly alters the ADP receptor	
Glycoprotein IIb/IIIa Blockers: Abciximab Tifofiban Eptifibatide	Antagonizes the platelet surface receptor	

While chronic aspirin use has been shown to increase the risk of renal failure in patients with baseline kidney dysfunction,[16] no negative effects have been seen in patients with normal kidney function.[10]

Dipyridamole

Dipyridamole inhibits cyclic nucleotide phosphodiesterase and increases cyclic AMP levels, leading to both vasodilator and antiplatelet properties. Although this compound has been studied at length, the exact antiplatelet mechanism remains controversial. In the Antithrombotic Trialists' Collaboration 2002 update, 25 trials comparing dipyridamole plus aspirin with aspirin alone were reviewed. The conclusion from this analysis was that dipyridamole did not significantly reduce the number of vascular events,[12] which has thereby rendered dipyridamole primarily of historical interest.

Thienopyridines

Ticlopidine (Ticlid) and clopidogrel (Plavix) are structurally related thienopyridines that after hepatic transformation to active metabolites, function by selectively inhibiting ADP-induced platelet aggregation.[10] The ADP receptor is irreversibly modified; inhibition of aggregation, therefore, persists for the entire lifespan of the affected platelet. Although both ticlopidine and clopidogrel have been used in clinical practice and trials, clopidogrel has emerged as the thienopyridine of choice based on several factors. First, a 2002 meta-analysis demonstrated greater efficacy and superior side effect profile of clopidogrel. Bhatt and colleagues compared studies using ticlopidine to those using clopidogrel, and found clopidogrel to have a significantly lower rate of side effects leading to noncompliance (nausea, vomiting, rash, thrombotic thrombocytopenic purpura, neutropenia), major adverse cardiac events, and death.[17] Second, safety concerns about the loading dose of ticlopidine have made its use in the acute setting more challenging.[10] Finally, ticlopidine is approximately 20% more expensive than clopidogrel.

GPIIb/IIIa Receptor Antagonists

Abciximab (ReoPro), tirofiban (Aggrastat), and eptifibatide (Integrilin) target the final step of platelet activation: aggregation via surface expression of the glycoprotein (GP) IIb/IIIa and subsequent crosslinking of receptors by circulating fibrinogen molecules.[18] In addition to their antiplatelet effects, these agents have also been found to diminish thrombin generation.[10] To date, all three drugs are used primarily for patients undergoing percutaneous coronary intervention and have not been widely applied to patients with peripheral vascular disease.

PROTECTION FROM MAJOR CARDIOVASCULAR MORBIDITY (MYOCARDIAL INFARCTION, STROKE, OR DEATH)

It has been clearly established that peripheral arterial disease (PAD) is a marker for disseminated atherosclerosis. Patients with intermittent claudication, despite the relatively benign prognosis for the affected limb, experience threefold greater cardiovascular mortality than age-matched controls.[19-20] Newman and colleagues demonstrated that an inverse relationship exists between ankle-brachial index (ABI) and cardiovascular outcomes; even patients with asymptomatic reductions in ABI (0.8–1.0) are at an increased risk of experiencing cardiovascular events and premature death.[21] These data indicate that the presesence of PAD should be considered an ominous harbinger of systemic atherosclerosis akin to a previous myocardial infarction or stroke. Therefore, patients with PAD should be treated with full medical management directed toward cardiovascular event risk reduction.

The protective effect of daily aspirin treatment against stroke, MI, and death in patients with PAD was established by the Antiplatelet Trialists' Collaboration.[2] This meta-analysis included 142 randomized trials, comprised of nearly 73,000 patients at risk for cardiovascular events. They demonstrated that in patients with cardiovascular risk, aspirin reduced the risk of stroke and MI by about one-third and the risk of death by about one-sixth. When patients were stratified by risk factor, those with PAD were found to have a risk reduction similar to the other high-risk groups. As a result, the TransaAtlantic Intersociety Consensus (TASC) panel has recommended that all PAD patients be treated with an antiplatelet agent.[22]

Since the publication of this original work showing the protective benefit of aspirin, more potent antiplatelet inhibitors (thienopyridines, GPIIb/IIIa inhibitors) have come into more widespread use, primarily in patients with coronary disease. The CAPRIE trial is the only large randomized trial to compare the relative efficacy of clopidogrel with aspirin in reducing the risk of the composite endpoint of ischemic stroke, MI, or vascular death. In this trial, 19,185 patients with either a recent MI, ischemic stroke, or symptomatic PAD were randomized to receive daily aspirin or clopidogrel. The analysis revealed a significantly lower annual incidence of the composite endpoint in patients treated with clopidogrel (5.32%) than in those treated with aspirin (5.83%, $p<0.05$).[23] Of note, on subgroup analysis, the patients found to receive the greatest benefit from clopidogrel were clearly those in the PAD subgroup (Figure 6–2).

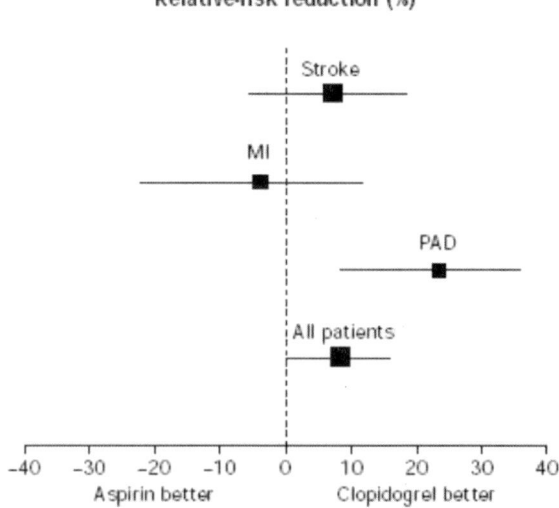

Figure 6-2. Relative-risk reduction of composite endpoint and 95% confidence interval by disease subgroup. (Adapted with permission from: A randomised, blinded, trial of clopidogrel versus aspirin in patients at risk of ischaemic events (CAPRIE). CAPRIE Steering Committee. *Lancet.* 1996;348:1329–1339.)

The CHARISMA investigators attempted to answer the question of whether dual antiplatelet therapy with aspirin and clopidogrel was superior to aspirin alone in preventing stroke, MI, and death in a broad population of patients at risk for cardiovascular events. In their randomized study of 15,602 patients, there was no significant difference in the composite outcome of MI, stroke, and death between the two groups.[24] In the group receiving dual antiplatelet therapy, there was a significantly greater rate of moderate bleeding (transfusion required) with a relative risk of 1.62 (2.1% compared to 1.3%). There was no difference in the rate of severe bleeding (hemodynamic compromise), and no difference in rates of drug discontinuation.

All patients with PAD should receive antiplatelet therapy; this should include at least daily low-dose aspirin. Additional studies that include patients with PAD need to be conducted in order to better define the role of clopidogrel in this population of patients at high risk for cardiovascular events.

ANTIPLATELET EFFECT ON BYPASS GRAFT PATENCY

Despite technical advances, improved conduit selection and handling, and careful postoperative surveillance, bypass grafts continue to fail, often with severe consequences for the affected patient. Primary, primary assisted, and secondary patency rates from a recent large multicenter trial of patients undergoing infrainguinal bypass were 61%, 77%, and 80%, respectively, at one year.[25] Although autologous and prosthetic bypass grafts demonstrate different patterns of failure, the common final pathway is thrombosis and obliteration of flow. Antiplatelet agents have been studied to determine whether they might prevent any of the steps leading ultimately to thrombosis.

A meta-analysis of approximately 3,000 patients after peripheral artery procedures who were treated with either aspirin or placebo demonstrated a reduction in the rate of vascular occlusions in the aspirin group (16%) when compared to the control group (25%, $p<0.01$).[3] Administration of aspirin conferred an odds reduction of 43% with a reduction of 90 occlusive events per 1,000 patients at 19 months. These finding were confirmed five years later in another meta-analysis of trials comparing aspirin to placebo in patients after infrainguinal bypass surgery. Although the findings were not as dramatic, the effect of aspirin remained significant: an absolute risk reduction of occlusion of 8.2% and a relative risk reduction of 22%.[26]

Only one study has investigated whether thienopyridines may play a role in improving the patency of vascular grafts. This study randomized 243 patients with lower extremity saphenous vein bypass grafts to receive two years of ticlopidine or placebo, and showed a significant difference in two-year cumulative graft patency (82% vs. 63%, $p<.01$).[27] Unfortunately, the control population did not receive aspirin, so it is impossible, based on this trial, to make any conclusions on the relative benefit of thienopyridines over aspirin. To our knowledge, although clopidogrel showed no benefit in preventing thrombosis when compared to aspirin in the setting of hemodialysis grafts,[28] no studies have been conducted using clopidogrel for lower extremity bypass grafts.

Aspirin reduces the risk of bypass graft occlusion. While thienopyridines also appear to have a protective effect, it is not known how this benefit compares with that of aspirin alone.

ANTIPLATELET EFFECT FOLLOWING PERIPHERAL PERCUTANEOUS INTERVENTION

As both coronary and peripheral percutaneous revascularization have become more common procedures, restenosis at these intervention sites has become a significant problem. Due to the lack of systematic reporting, it is difficult to establish with certainty the patency rates after percutaneous transluminal angioplasty (PTA), but the reported ranges (five-year patency rates) span 35% to 70% for the lower extremity and 54% to 78% for the aortoiliac segment.[29] Restenosis following balloon dilation occurs in four phases: elastic recoil, thrombus formation and organization, neointimal hyperplasia, and recurrent atherosclerosis. While stents can prevent elastic recoil, medical management and risk factor modification are necessary to prevent the remaining factors leading to restenosis. To date, no large trial has focused on the role of antiplatelet therapy in patients undergoing percutaneous treatment for PAD; instead, all treatment guidelines are extrapolated from the coronary literature. These data are reviewed here.

In the late 1990s, the addition of a thienopyridine to aspirin was established as protective for thrombotic complications following percutaneous coronary intervention (PCI).[30-32] The next area of investigation focused primarily on the role of preprocedure treatment with clopidogrel. The PCI-CURE trial, published in 2001, established that patients who received clopidogrel in addition to aspirin prior to PCI experienced a lower rate of the composite endpoint of cardiovascular death, reinfarction, or stroke (4.5% vs. 6.5%, 30% risk reduction) than patients receiving aspirin alone.[33] One year later, the CREDO trial was published: patients undergoing PCI were randomized to receive either clopidogrel prior to the intervention and for one year afterward, or to receive clopidogrel immediately after the intervention for a duration of only 28 days. Their results showed that pretreatment with clopidogrel given at least six hours prior was beneficial. In addition, one year of treatment with clopidogrel provided a protective effect over 28 days of treatment.[34] The PCI-CLARITY trial, published in 2005, provided further support for clopidogrel pretreatment in patients with ST-elevation myocardial infarctions undergoing PCI. These investigators observed a 46% reduction in the risk of a composite endpoint at 30 days among the pretreated group (3.6% vs. 6.2%).[35] In these three trials, none demonstrated a significantly higher rate of major bleeding in patients receiving clopidogrel .

Intravenous GPIIb/IIIa receptor blockers have also been established as a prominent therapy capable of improving outcomes with PCI. Primarily, this form of pharmacologic therapy has been shown to reduce the incidence of early events (reinfarction) while long-term therapy appears not to be beneficial and may even increase mortality.[36] Unfortunately, no randomized trials have been conducted to explore the role of GPIIb/IIIa inhibitors in the therapy of PAD.

CONCLUSIONS

The PREVENT III study is the largest and most recent trial investigating peripheral bypass surgery for critical limb ischemia.[25] In this multi-institutional study with just over 1,400 patients, at entry into the study, 67% of patients were on an antiplatelet agent. At discharge from the study—that is, after the patients underwent peripheral bypass surgery—80% of patients were on an antiplatelet medication (Figure 6–3). Not only was this clearly a patient population with PAD, but also this was the sickest subgroup

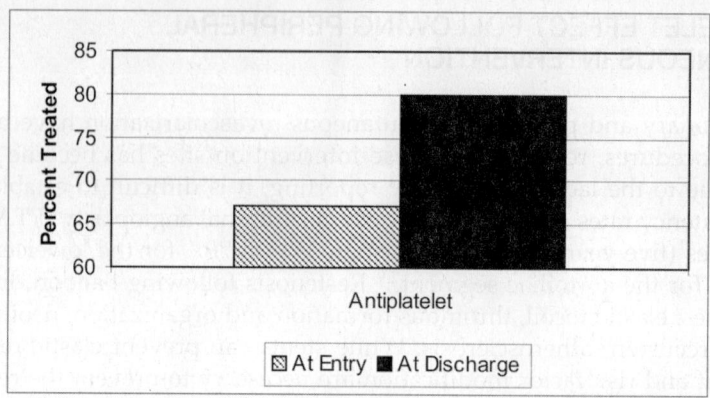

Figure 6-3. Antiplatelet usage among 1,404 patients who underwent lower extremity vein bypass for critical limb ischemia. (Adapted with permission from: Conte MS, Bandyk DF, Clowes AW, Moneta GL, Seely L, Lorenz TJ, Namini H, Hamdan AD, Roddy SP, Belkin M, Berceli SA, DeMasi RJ, Samson RH, Berman SS. Results of PRE-VENT III: a multicenter, randomized trial of edifoligide for the prevention of vein graft failure in lower extremity bypass surgery. *J Vasc Surg*. 2006;43:742–751; discussion 751.)

of PAD patients as manifested by rest pain or tissue loss. All of these patients were treated by vascular surgeons, yet 20% did not even receive aspirin. Unfortunately, this number has remained relatively constant over the last 15 years.[37]

There is abundant evidence indicating that the presence of PAD not only places the affected patient's limb at risk, but also serves as a surrogate marker for systemic atherosclerotic burden. As a result, when evaluating a patient for cardiovascular risk, the presence of PAD should be considered to be a "cardiovascular event" in much the way that a myocardial infarction is considered. A growing body of evidence, summarized in a well-conducted meta-analysis reviewed in this chapter,[2] indicates that antiplatelet therapy has a significant protective effect on the risk of development of myocardial infarction, stroke, or death in patients with PAD. However, it is not yet clear which antiplatelet agent will emerge as the drug of choice for preventing these cardiovascular events. At this time, aspirin and clopidogrel are the only therapies that have been supported by randomized controlled data. Future randomized studies that directly compare the antiplatelet agents reviewed in this chapter are necessary to answer this important question.

All patients undergoing bypass surgery, either with autologous or prosthetic grafts, should be treated with antiplatelet agents in order to improve overall patency. It remains to be investigated whether thienopyridines or even short-term therapy with GPIIb/IIIa blockers may provide added benefit, either in concert with or instead of aspirin, and whether these therapies will confer bleeding risk.

Currently, the greatest area of uncertainty centers around the role of antiplatelet agents when intervening on peripheral arteries percutaneously. Practice patterns around the country vary widely, but thienopyridine therapy before and after percutaneous intervention appears to be becoming the norm. The impetus lies with the vascular surgery community to study the utility of different antiplatelet agents directly in our patient population so that it is no longer necessary to extrapolate from the coronary literature. In particular, the arterial patency rates, bleeding risks, cost-effectiveness, and optimal timing of initiation of therapy that are associated with each antiplatelet agent need to be studied in patients with PAD.

REFERENCES

1. Platelet activation and arterial thrombosis. Report of a meeting of Physicians and Scientists, University of Texas Health Science Center at Houston and Texas Heart Institute, Houston. *Lancet*. 1994;344:991–995.
2. Collaborative overview of randomised trials of antiplatelet therapy—I: Prevention of death, myocardial infarction, and stroke by prolonged antiplatelet therapy in various categories of patients. Antiplatelet Trialists' Collaboration. *BMJ*. 1994;308:81–106.
3. Collaborative overview of randomised trials of antiplatelet therapy—II: Maintenance of vascular graft or arterial patency by antiplatelet therapy. Antiplatelet Trialists' Collaboration. *BMJ*. 1994;308:159–168.
4. Collaborative overview of randomised trials of antiplatelet therapy—III: Reduction in venous thrombosis and pulmonary embolism by antiplatelet prophylaxis among surgical and medical patients. Antiplatelet Trialists' Collaboration. *BMJ*. 1994;308:235–246.
5. Samara WM, Gurbel PA. The role of platelet receptors and adhesion molecules in coronary artery disease. *Coron Artery Dis*. 2003;14:65–79.
6. Zwaal RF, Comfurius P, Bevers EM. Lipid-protein interactions in blood coagulation. *Biochim Biophys Acta*. 1998;1376:433–453.
7. Gailani D, Ho D, Sun MF, Cheng Q, Walsh PN. Model for a factor IX activation complex on blood platelets: dimeric conformation of factor XIa is essential. *Blood*. 2001;97:3117–3122.
8. Weiss HJ, Aledort LM. Impaired platelet-connective-tissue reaction in man after aspirin ingestion. *Lancet*. 1967;2:495–497.
9. Roth GJ, Stanford N, Majerus PW. Acetylation of prostaglandin synthase by aspirin. *Proc Natl Acad Sci. U S A*. 1975;72:3073–3076.
10. Patrono C, Coller B, FitzGerald GA, et al. Platelet-active drugs: the relationships among dose, effectiveness, and side effects: the Seventh ACCP Conference on Antithrombotic and Thrombolytic Therapy. *Chest*. 2004;126:234S–264S.
11. A comparison of two doses of aspirin (30 mg vs. 283 mg a day) in patients after a transient ischemic attack or minor ischemic stroke. The Dutch TIA Trial Study Group. *N Engl J Med*. 1991;325:1261–1266.
12. Collaborative meta-analysis of randomised trials of antiplatelet therapy for prevention of death, myocardial infarction, and stroke in high risk patients. *BMJ*. 2002;324:71–86.
13. Taylor DW, Barnett HJ, Haynes RB, et al. Low-dose and high-dose acetylsalicylic acid for patients undergoing carotid endarterectomy: a randomised controlled trial. ASA and Carotid Endarterectomy (ACE) Trial Collaborators. *Lancet*. 1999;353:2179–2184.
14. Lai KC, Lam SK, Chu KM, et al. Lansoprazole for the prevention of recurrences of ulcer complications from long-term low-dose aspirin use. *N Engl J Med*. 2002;346:2033–2038.
15. Laine L. Approaches to nonsteroidal anti-inflammatory drug use in the high-risk patient. *Gastroenterology*. 2001;120:594–606.
16. Fored CM, Ejerblad E, Lindblad P, et al. Acetaminophen, aspirin, and chronic renal failure. *N Engl J Med*. 2001;345:1801–1808.
17. Bhatt DL, Bertrand ME, Berger PB, et al. Meta-analysis of randomized and registry comparisons of ticlopidine with clopidogrel after stenting. *J Am Coll Cardiol*. 2002;39:9–14.
18. Verstraete M, Zoldhelyi P. Novel antithrombotic drugs in development. *Drugs*. 1995;49:856–884.
19. Reunanen A, Takkunen H, Aromaa A. Prevalence of intermittent claudication and its effect on mortality. *Acta Med Scand*. 1982;211:249–256.
20. Howell MA, Colgan MP, Seeger RW, et al. Relationship of severity of lower limb peripheral vascular disease to mortality and morbidity: a six-year follow-up study. *J Vasc Surg*. 1989;9:691–696; discussion 696–697.
21. Newman AB, Siscovick DS, Manolio TA, Polak J, Fried LP, Borhani NO, Wolfson SK. Ankle-arm index as a marker of atherosclerosis in the Cardiovascular Health Study. Cardiovascular Heart Study (CHS) Collaborative Research Group. *Circulation*. 1993;88:837–845.

22. Dormandy JA, Rutherford RB. Management of peripheral arterial disease (PAD). TASC Working Group. TransAtlantic Inter-Society Concensus (TASC). *J Vasc Surg*. 2000;31: S1–S296.
23. A randomised, blinded, trial of clopidogrel versus aspirin in patients at risk of ischaemic events (CAPRIE). CAPRIE Steering Committee. *Lancet*. 1996;348:1329–1339.
24. Bhatt DL, Fox KA, Hacke W, et al. Clopidogrel and Aspirin versus Aspirin Alone for the Prevention of Atherothrombotic Events. *N Engl J Med*. 2006.
25. Conte MS, Bandyk DF, Clowes AW, et al. Results of PREVENT III: a multicenter, randomized trial of edifoligide for the prevention of vein graft failure in lower extremity bypass surgery. *J Vasc Surg*. 2006;43:742–751; discussion 751.
26. Tangelder MJ, Lawson JA, Algra A, Eikelboom BC. Systematic review of randomized controlled trials of aspirin and oral anticoagulants in the prevention of graft occlusion and ischemic events after infrainguinal bypass surgery. *J Vasc Surg*. 1999;30:701–709.
27. Becquemin JP. Effect of ticlopidine on the long-term patency of saphenous-vein bypass grafts in the legs. Etude de la Ticlopidine apres Pontage Femoro-Poplite and the Association Universitaire de Recherche en Chirurgie. *N Engl J Med*. 1997;337:1726–1731.
28. Kaufman JS, O'Connor TZ, Zhang JH, et al. Randomized controlled trial of clopidogrel plus aspirin to prevent hemodialysis access graft thrombosis. *J Am Soc Nephrol*. 2003;14: 2313–2321.
29. Schainfeld RM. Potential emerging therapeutic strategies to prevent restenosis in the peripheral vasculature. *Catheter Cardiovasc Interv*. 2002;56:421–431.
30. Bertrand ME, Legrand V, Boland J, et al. Randomized multicenter comparison of conventional anticoagulation versus antiplatelet therapy in unplanned and elective coronary stenting. The full anticoagulation versus aspirin and ticlopidine (fantastic) study. *Circulation*. 1998;98:1597–1603.
31. Leon MB, Baim DS, Popma JJ, et al. A clinical trial comparing three antithrombotic-drug regimens after coronary-artery stenting. Stent Anticoagulation Restenosis Study Investigators. *N Engl J Med*. 1998;339:1665–1671.
32. Schomig A, Neumann FJ, Kastrati A, et al. A randomized comparison of antiplatelet and anticoagulant therapy after the placement of coronary-artery stents. *N Engl J Med*. 1996;334:1084–1089.
33. Mehta SR, Yusuf S, Peters RJ, et al. Effects of pretreatment with clopidogrel and aspirin followed by long-term therapy in patients undergoing percutaneous coronary intervention: the PCI-CURE study. *Lancet*. 2001;358:527–533.
34. Steinhubl SR, Berger PB, Mann JT, 3rd, et al. Early and sustained dual oral antiplatelet therapy following percutaneous coronary intervention: a randomized controlled trial. *JAMA*. 2002;288:2411–2420.
35. Sabatine MS, Cannon CP, Gibson CM, et al. Effect of clopidogrel pretreatment before percutaneous coronary intervention in patients with ST-elevation myocardial infarction treated with fibrinolytics: the PCI-CLARITY study. *JAMA*. 2005;294:1224–1232.
36. Chew DP, Bhatt DL, Sapp S, Topol EJ. Increased mortality with oral platelet glycoprotein IIb/IIIa antagonists: a meta-analysis of phase III multicenter randomized trials. *Circulation*. 2001;103:201–206.
37. Efficacy of oral anticoagulants compared with aspirin after infrainguinal bypass surgery (The Dutch Bypass Oral Anticoagulants or Aspirin Study): a randomised trial. *Lancet*. 2000;355:346–351.

7

The Use of Antithrombins as Alternatives to Conventional Anticoagulation

Kenneth Ouriel, M.D.

The widespread use of peripheral arterial revascularization awaited the availability of safe anticoagulants to prevent thrombosis during the procedure. In 1916, heparin was discovered by a second year medical student at Johns Hopkins, Jay Maclean.[1] Clinical use, however, awaited adequate purification processes. In 1928, Charles H. Best at the University of Toronto purified insulin from beef lung and intestine. Best worked with Connaught Laboratories, the developer of insulin, to produce crystalline heparin that could be administered in a salt solution.[2] Human trials began in 1935. By 1937, heparin was available as a safe and effective anticoagulant agent.

Today, unfractionated heparin derived from porcine intestinal mucosa is the most commonly used anticoagulant in peripheral vascular surgery. Despite its discovery almost a century ago, heparin remains a heterogenous group of heterogenous molecules; straight-chain anionic mucopolysaccharides that only indirectly inactive thrombin thorough catalyzation of antithrombin III. The use of heparin is fraught with problems.[3] First, as a result of binding to plasma proteins, the activity and half-life of heparin is quite variable. Second, it is associated with the development of thrombocytopenia in a significant proportion of patients, especially after prolonged administration. Third, the size and other chemical properties of the molecules render them unable to efficiently penetrate into a fibrin thrombus, a property that has been associated with re-thrombosis during pharmacologic thrombolysis. As well, heparin is neutralized by platelet factor 4, accounting for reduced activity in the vicinity of platelet-rich, arterial thrombi. Lastly, heparin's dependence on antithrombin III renders it ineffective in patients with antithrombin deficiencies.

On this landscape, alternatives to heparin have been studied for decades.[4] Direct thrombin inhibitors, without dependency on antithrombin III, have been a primary focus (Table 7–1). This class of anticoagulants includes hirudin, bivalirudin, argatroban, and the orally-active agent ximelagatran. These agents offer significant potential advantages over heparin with a reduced risk of thrombocytopenia, better

TABLE 7-1. DIRECT ANTITHROMBIN AGENTS[27]

Agent	Origin	Inhibition	Clearance	$t_{1/2}$
Recombinant Hirudin	Recombinant leech proteins	Almost irreversible	Renal	
Lepirudin				1.3 hr
Desirudin				2–3 hr
Bivalirudin	Recombinant COOH-terminus of hirudin linked to D-PHE-Pro-Arg-Pro	Reversible	Renal	20–30 min
Agatroban	L-arginine analogue, synthetic	Reversible	Hepatic	45 min
Melagatran	Dipeptide that mimics cleavage site on Aα chain of fibrinogen	Reversible	Renal	2.5–3.5hr

penetration into the thrombus, no requirement for antithrombin III, and no inactivation by platelet factor 4. A drawback, however, is the lack of an antidote for reversal of the effects of the direct thrombin inhibitors similar to that of protamine for heparin.

THROMBOGENESIS

The process of thrombus formation is classically described as proceeding along one of two pathways: the extrinsic pathway and the intrinsic pathway (Table 7–2). The prothrombin time is sensitive to alterations in the extrinsic pathway and the activated partial thromboplastin time is sensitive to the intrinsic pathway. The intrinsic pathway comprises high-molecular weight kininogen, factor XII, prekallikrein, factor XI, factor IX, and factor VIII. It converges with the extrinsic pathway (comprising tissue factor and factor VII) at the level of factor X; where factor X is activated as the "prothrombinase complex" along with activated factor V assembled on a phospholipid surface. The prothrombinase complex converts prothrombin to thrombin, which in tern cleaves fibrinogen to the insoluble fibrin. Fibrin is polymerized with the aid of factor XIII to form the insoluble fibrin thrombus. Polymerized fibrin is responsible for the desirable and often lifesaving hemostatic plug, but is also the source of frequently undesirable acute vascular occlusions.

This classic mode of thrombogenesis provides an accurate representation of the processes that occur in the coagulation laboratory. A more useful model to describe in vivo coagulation is represented by a "cell-based model." This model has been described as occurring in three phases: initiation, priming, and propagation.[5] The process is initiated by a break in the endothelium and exposure of thrombogenic substances; most important in this regard is tissue factor. In the priming phase, the small amount of thrombin that has been generated binds to platelets at the site of endothelial dysintegrity. Thrombin-induced platelet activation results in degranulation, release of procoagulants, and binding of activated factor V, VIII, and XI. Lastly, in the propagation phase, a complex of activated factors X and V residing on the platelet membrane generates large amounts of thrombin. The formation of a stable fibrin plug ensues; the end result of cell-dependent thrombogenesis.

Hirudin

The prototypic thrombin inhibitor is the naturally occurring agent hirudin.[6] Originally isolated from the leech *Hirudo medicinalis*, hirudin is still the most specific thrombin inhibitor

TABLE 7-2. SIMPLIFIED PROCESS OF THROMBOGENESIS

Classical Cascade Model	
Extrinsic Path	**Intrinsic Path**
	HK, XII, and PK catalyze XI to XIa
	Catalysis of IX to IXa
Tissue factor and factor VIIa catalyze X to Xa	IXa, VIIIa, and phospholipid form the "Xase complex" and catalyze X to Xa
Xa, Va on the phospholipid surface form the "prothrombinase complex" and catalyze thrombin formation from prothrombin	

Cell-based Model	
Initiation:	
1	Factor VIIa bound to TF activates factors IX and X
2	A small amount of thrombin is generated
Priming:	
1	Thrombin activates platelets, causing degranulation
2	Cofactors bind to the platelet surface
Propagation:	
1	Factor IXa activates factor X
2	Factor Xa forms a complex with Va, resulting in a burst of thrombin generation
	Fibrinogen is cleaved to Fibrin
	Polymerized fibrin is stabilized to form a hemostatic thrombus

HK- high molecular weight kininogen
PK- prekallikrein
TF- tissue factor

known. Hirudin has a tightly folded central core that is closely approximated to a globular amino-terminal domain. The amino-terminal domain binds and inhibits the catalytic side of thrombin. As well, its carboxy-terminal domain binds to the fibrin/fibrinogen binding site of thrombin. Recombinant hirudin (lepirudin) was first produced in the mid-1980s as a 65 or 66 amino-acid polypeptide with an amino-acid sequence identical to natural hirudin. Hirudin inactivated thrombin in an almost irreversible fashion, binding in a 1:1 stoichiometric ratio. The half-life of hirudin is approximately 60 minutes, eliminated by the kidneys.[3]

Recombinant hirudin is available in two forms: lepirudin and desirudin. Recombinant hirudin was studied in the setting of acute coronary syndrome, comparing the agent to intravenous heparin in over 12,000 patients.[7] The risk of death within 24 hours was significantly lower in the hirudin group, 1.3% versus 2.1% ($P = 0.001$). Death or myocardial infarction within 30 days occurred slightly but not less often when patients received hirudin, 8.9% versus 9.8%, a difference that did not attain statistical significance ($P = 0.06$). Importantly, there were no differences in the risk of major bleeding, but hirudin was associated with a higher incidence of moderate bleeding, 8.8% versus 7.7% ($P = 0.03$). The authors concluded that recombinant hirudin provided a small, early benefit in patients with acute coronary syndrome without a concomitant increase in the risk of major bleeding complications. To date, recombinant hirudin has not been evaluated clinically for peripheral arterial revascularization.

Argatroban

Argatroban is a synthetic derivative of L-arginine. Argatroban binds to an apolar binding site adjacent to the active catalytic site of thrombin, blocking thrombin's activity. Unlike hirudin, argatroban binds to thrombin in a reversible fashion and is cleared through hepatic means with a half-life of just under one hour.[3] The molecule is small (527 Da) and has specific activity directed against thrombin and not other serine proteases. The anticoagulant activity of argatroban can be measured with an activated clotting time or aPTT. The clinical trials of argatroban have been disappointing. While the agent is an adequate alternative to heparin in patients with, for instance, heparin-induced thrombocytopenia, argatroban has not been found have any advantages over heparin in patients with acute coronary syndromes.[8-9] Argatroban has no apparent advantage over heparin with regard to major bleeding complications.[10]

Bivalirudin

Bivalirudin is a direct thrombin inhibitor that is approved in the United States as an alternative to heparin in patients undergoing percutaneous coronary revascularization. It is a recombinant agent composed of a 20 amino-acid analogue of the carboxy-terminus of hirudin. The amino-terminal D-Phe-Pro-Arg-Pro sequence binds to the active site of thrombin and is connected by four Gly residues to a carboxy-terminal dodecapeptide that interacts with exosite 1 on thrombin. Like hirudin, bivalirudin interacts with thrombin in a 1:1 stoichiometric relationship. The binding affinity of bivalirudin to thrombin, however, is of much lower affinity than hirudin. The agent is slowly degraded by thrombin as the Pro-Arg bond within the amino terminal is cleaved.[11-12] Bivalirudin is cleared by the kidney with a half-life of 20–30 minutes. Thus, dosing adjustments should be made in patients with renal insufficiency. The aPTT correlates well with the plasma concentration of bivalirudin. By contrast, the activated clotting time is only loosely correlated and should be used only to judge whether or not the agent has been successfully administered.

There have been a variety of large coronary trials of bivalirudin and several small evaluations of the agent during coronary artery bypass procedures. In a phase III study comparing bivalirudin to heparin in over 4,000 patients undergoing coronary angioplasty for acute coronary syndrome, no significant difference in the composite endpoint (in-hospital death, myocardial infarction, vessel thrombosis, or cardiac deterioration) was detected.[13] However, the risk of major bleeding was reduced with bivalirudin (3.8% versus 9/8%, $P < 0.001$). Importantly, in a prospectively-defined high-risk subset of these study group, bivalirudin was associated with a reduction in the primary endpoint (9.1% versus 14.2%, $P = 0.04$). Of note, the results of this trial were reanalyzed and published six years after the initial communication.[14] When an intent-to-treat design was implemented along with a more contemporary definition of myocardial infarction, the more commonly employed endpoint of death, myocardial infarction, or repeat revascularization at one week was significantly reduced in the bivalirudin treatment arm (3.5% versus 9.3%, $P < 0.001$).

The REPLACE-2 trial entered just over 6,000 subjects undergoing percutaneous coronary intervention into a randomized comparison of bivalirudin plus a provisional GPIIb/IIIa antagonist versus heparin and a GPIIb/IIIa antagonist. The primary endpoint was death, myocardial infarction, urgent revascularization, or major bleeding at 30 days, and no difference was detected between the two treatment arms. The rate of major bleeding was decreased in the bivalirudin group, 2.4% versus 4.1% ($P < 0.001$).

But one should note that while, by design, all patients in the heparin arm received a GPIIb/IIIa antagonist, only 7% of the patients in the bivalirudin group required such an adjunct. These findings can be interpreted two ways. First, bivalirudin was associated with similar clinical outcome to heparin, without the need for GPIIb/IIIa antagonism in the vast majority of patients. Second, the rate of bleeding may be lower with bivalirudin regimen, but possibly not as a result of bivalirudin alone; rather, satisfactory efficacy of the agent without the need for GPIIb/IIIa inhibitor may be the explanation.

Bivalirudin has been studied as an adjunct to thrombolysis in patients with acute coronary syndrome. Over 17,000 patients were randomized to IV streptokinase with bivalirudin or heparin.[15] There were no differences in 30-day mortality rate or major bleeding. The rate of reinfarction was significantly lower in the bivalirudin group, however, with an odds-ratio of 0.70 ($P = 0.001$).

Bivalirudin has been used during carotid artery stenting procedures with good results. An abstract presented at the 2003 TCT conference compared 185 patients treated with bivalirudin to 383 patients treated with heparin and found significantly lower rates of any transfusion (0.6% versus 6.4%, $P = 0.002$) and major vascular complications (2.3% versus 13.3%, $P = 0.0008$) in the bivalirudin group.

There has been a modicum of work with bivalirudin for anticoagulation during coronary artery bypass procedures. Feasibility of use was demonstrated by Koster in a series of 20 patients who underwent coronary artery bypass using bivalirudin as the sole anticoagulant.[16] Merry compared the agent to standard unfractionated heparin in 100 patients undergoing off-pump coronary artery bypass.[17] While there were no differences in the rate of bleeding complications, the investigators documented an increase in graft patency in the bivalirudin-treated group. Of interest, Mann reported on the use of bivalirudin during cardiac transplantation in a patient with heparin-induced thrombocytopenia, using ultrafiltration to remove the agent at the conclusion of the procedure.[18]

Shammas studied bivalirudin in 48 consecutive patients undergoing peripheral arterial percutaneous interventions. The authors observed an in-hospital complication rate of 4.2%, which they felt compared favorably with their historical complication rate of over 9% with unfractionated heparin.[19] Allie and colleages described their results with bivalirudin in 180 renal interventions and 75 iliac interventions.[20] The results were compared with historical unfractionated heparin-treated controls. Early technical success was uniform with bivalirudin, without thrombotic events, vascular complications, or intracranial bleeding. The authors noted benefit with respect to sheath removal time, time to ambulation, and length of stay when the bivalirudin-treated group was compared with heparin-treated patients. Subsequently, Allie published the results from a 26-site registry of bivalirudin anticoagulation during percutaneous renal, iliac, or femoral interventions.[21] Procedural success was achieved din 95% of the 505 patients enrolled. The rate of major hemorrhagic complications as defined by the protocol and by TIMI criteria were 2.2% and 0.4%, respectively.

Melagatran

Melagatran is a low-molecular weight direct thrombin inhibitor. It mimics the NH2-terminal sequence of the thrombin cleavage site on the Aα chain of fibrinogen. While melagatran is poorly absorbed when administered orally, its inactive prodrug, ximelagatran, is readily absorbed and is subsequently converted to the active form melagatran. After oral administration, melagatran reaches maximum intravascular concentration within two hours and has a half-life of approximately three hours' with predominantly renal clearance.[22] For this reason, dose adjustment is unnecessary in patients with hepatic dysfunction, but patients with renal insufficiency require a decrease in the dose or increase in the dosing interval.

Melagatran has been primarily studied for the treatment of venous thromboembolism. Several Phase II studies have been performed in postoperative orthopedic patients.[23] The THIRVE 1 study demonstrated similar outcome in patients with acute deep venous thrombosis who received four different doses of ximelagatran versus those who received dalteparin and warfarin.[24] The SPORTIF III and V trials confirmed similarity between a fixed oral dose of ximelagatran and coagulation-adjusted warfarin for nonvalvular atrial fibrillation, with almost identical rates of stroke.[25-26] The risk of major hemorrhage, however, appeared lower in the ximelagatran-treated patients.

SUMMARY

The direct thrombin inhibitors offer significant theoretic advantages over standard procedural anticoagulation with heparin compounds. These benefits have been proven for percutaneous coronary interventions. Further, registry studies suggest that the direct antithrombins may offer advantages in peripheral interventions as well. While there are no data on the use of antithrombins for open peripheral vascular surgery at present, such studies are being planned. Hopefully, the direct thrombin inhibitors will offer a class of anticoagulants superior to heparin, with the potential to limit periprocedural thrombotic and bleeding complications.

REFERENCES

1. Maclean J. The thromboplastic action of cephalin. *Am J Physiol.* 1916;41:250–257.
2. Connaught Laboratories Limited. Miracle Blood Lubricant: Connaught and the Story of Heparin, 1928–1937. Internet 2005 April 23. Available from: URL: http://www.health her-itageresearch.com/Heparin-Conntact9608.html
3. Weitz JI, Bates ER. Direct thrombin inhibitors in cardiac disease. *Cardiovasc Toxicol.* 2003;3(1):13–25.
4. Donayre CE, Ouriel K, Rhee RY, Shortell CK. Future alternatives to heparin: low-molecular-weight heparin and hirudin. *J Vasc Surg.* 1992;15(4):675–682.
5. Monroe DM, Hoffman M, Roberts HR. Platelets and thrombin generation. *Arterioscler Thromb Vasc Biol.* 2002;22(9):1381–1389.
6. Lettino M, Toschi V. Direct antithrombins: new perspectives in cardiovascular medicine. *Curr Med Chem Cardiovasc Hematol Agents.* 2004;2(3):267–275.
7. Topol EJ, For the GUSTO Investigators. A comparison of recombinant hirudin with heparin for the treatment of acute coronary syndromes. The Global Use of Strategies to Open Occluded Coronary Arteries (GUSTO) IIb investigators. *N Engl J Med.* 1996;335(11):775–782.
8. Jang IK, Brown DF, Giugliano RP, et al. A multicenter, randomized study of argatroban versus heparin as adjunct to tissue plasminogen activator (TPA) in acute myocardial infarction: myocardial infarction with novastan and TPA (MINT) study. *J Am Coll Cardiol.* 1999;33(7): 1879–1885.
9. Vermeer F, Vahanian A, Fels PW, et al. Argatroban and alteplase in patients with acute myocardial infarction: the ARGAMI Study. *J Thromb Thrombolysis.* 2000;10(3):233–240.

10. Nutescu EA, Wittkowsky AK. Direct thrombin inhibitors for anticoagulation. *Ann Pharmacother*. 2004;38(1):99–109.
11. Witting JI, Bourdon P, Maraganore JM, Fenton JW. Hirulog-1 and -B2 thrombin specificity. *Biochem J*. 1992;287(Pt 2):663–664.
12. Witting JI, Bourdon P, Brezniak DV, et al. Thrombin-specific inhibition by and slow cleavage of hirulog-1. *Biochem J*. 1992;283 (Pt 3):737–743.
13. Bittl JA, Strony J, Brinker JA, et al. Treatment with bivalirudin (Hirulog) as compared with heparin during coronary angioplasty for unstable or postinfarction angina. Hirulog Angioplasty Study Investigators. *N Engl J Med*. 1995;333(12):764–769.
14. Bittl JA, Chaitman BR, Feit F. Bivalirudin versus heparin during coronary angioplasty for unstable or postinfarction angina: Final report reanalysis of the Bivalirudin Angioplasty Study. *Am Heart J*. 2001;142(6):952–959.
15. White H. Thrombin-specific anticoagulation with bivalirudin versus heparin in patients receiving fibrinolytic therapy for acute myocardial infarction: the HERO-2 randomised trial. *Lancet*. 2001;358(9296):1855–1863.
16. Koster A, Spiess B, Chew DP, et al. Effectiveness of bivalirudin as a replacement for heparin during cardiopulmonary bypass in patients undergoing coronary artery bypass grafting. *Am J Cardiol*. 2004;93(3):356–359.
17. Merry AF, Raudkivi PJ, Middleton NG, et al. Bivalirudin versus heparin and protamine in off-pump coronary artery bypass surgery. *Ann Thorac Surg*. 2004;77(3):925–931.
18. Mann MJ, Tseng E, Ratcliffe M, et al. Use of bivalirudin, a direct thrombin inhibitor, and its reversal with modified ultrafiltration during heart transplantation in a patient with heparin-induced thrombocytopenia. *J Heart Lung Transplant*. 2005;24(2):222–225.
19. Shammas NW, Lemke JH, Dippel EJ, et al. Bivalirudin in peripheral vascular interventions: a single center experience. *J Invasive Cardiol*. 2003;15(7):401–404.
20. Allie DE, Lirtzman MD, Wyatt CH, et al. Bivalirudin as a foundation anticoagulant in peripheral vascular disease: a safe and feasible alternative for renal and iliac interventions. *J Invasive Cardiol*. 2003;15(6):334–342.
21. Allie DE, Hall P, Shammas NW, Safian R, et al. The Angiomax Peripheral Procedure Registry of Vascular Events Trial (APPROVE): in-hospital and 30-day results. *J Invasive Cardiol*. 2004;16(11):651–656.
22. Eriksson H, Eriksson UG, Frison L, et al. Pharmacokinetics and pharmacodynamics of melagatran, a novel synthetic LMW thrombin inhibitor, in patients with acute DVT. *Thromb Haemost*. 1999;81(3):358–363.
23. Evans HC, Perry CM, Faulds D. Ximelagatran/Melagatran: a review of its use in the prevention of venous thromboembolism in orthopaedic surgery. *Drug*. 2004;64(6):649–678.
24. Eriksson H, Wahlander K, Gustafsson D, et al. A randomized, controlled, dose-guiding study of the oral direct thrombin inhibitor ximelagatran compared with standard therapy for the treatment of acute deep vein thrombosis: THRIVE I. *J Thromb Haemost*. 2003; 1(1):41–47.
25. Lip GY. Preventing stroke in atrial fibrillation: the SPORTIF programme. *Pathophysiol Haemost Thromb*. 2005;34 Suppl 1:25–30.
26. Olsson SB. Stroke prevention with the oral direct thrombin inhibitor ximelagatran compared with warfarin in patients with non-valvular atrial fibrillation (SPORTIF III): randomised controlled trial. *Lancet*. 2003;362(9397):1691–1698.
27. Kaplan KL, Francis CW. Direct thrombin inhibitors. *Semin Hematol*. 2002;39(3):187–196.

8

Is Revascularization/Limb Salvage Always the Best Treatment for Patients with Critical Limb Ischemia?

Lloyd M. Taylor, Jr., M.D., Gregory L. Moneta, M.D., and Gregory J. Landry, M.D.

Vascular surgeons have spent a good part of the past 50 years developing techniques of arterial revascularization that allow restoration of improved arterial flow to ischemic lower extremities in nearly all clinical cases. This has not been a rapid process, nor an easy one. But it is reasonable to state that at present, bypass grafting usually to tibial arteries, with autogenous vein grafts, often accompanied by proximal revascularization by endovascular or surgical means, is possible in most patients, even those with severe disease, calcified arteries, and difficult vein availability problems.

The short answer to the question posed by the title of this chapter is "yes, revascularization is the best treatment currently available, but it is not a very good treatment, there are alternatives which may be more appropriate for a significant number of patients, and, most importantly, our knowledge of the true benefits or lack thereof of the various treatments is minimal, and sadly deficient.

In the remainder of this chapter, we will briefly discuss the reasoning behind this statement, including the problems that currently exist with the definition of critical limb ischemia and our lack of prospectively obtained data regarding the prognosis for patients with critical limb ischemia. We will then discuss the state of knowledge regarding current surgical treatment of critical limb ischemia, and the results of that surgical treatment in terms of patient outcomes.

DEFINITION OF CRITICAL LIMB ISCHEMIA (CLI)

CLI is a term used to indicate a disease state in which the underlying limb is at high risk for amputation due to necrosis and/or infection, the resolution of which is prevented by underlying ischemia of the limb due to arterial obstruction. By convention, the category of CLI includes patients with ischemic rest pain, ischemic ulcers, and ischemic gangrene with objective evidence of ischemia, the most commonly used indicator of which is an ankle/brachial systolic pressure index of less than or equal to 0.40. As with all categorizations, there are some problems with this definition.

First, CLI is not a category with a uniform prognosis. Although it is widely believed that CLI is inexorably progressive, not all individuals who fit this description require amputation, if the ischemia cannot be relieved. Various placebo controlled trials of treatment for CLI have clearly established that as many as one-third of individuals with CLI never demonstrate disease progression, at least for the duration of the trial.[1] Some patients experience relatively mild symptoms of ischemic rest pain intermittently, and remain stable for prolonged periods. Others may experience more severe symptoms of CLI, including episodes of ischemic ulceration followed by ulcer healing and symptomatic improvement to the point that CLI is no longer present. So from this viewpoint, our definition of CLI is too inclusive.

The second problem is that relatively moderate ischemia combined with exacerbating factors that interfere with wound healing (the most frequent of which are diabetes and chronic renal failure) may result in a limb equally at risk for amputation as one which is arguably more ischemic in another patient whose only disease is extensive atherosclerosis. So from this viewpoint, our standard definition of CLI is too exclusive.

PROGNOSIS OF CLI

These inadequacies of the standard definition of CLI point out that our current knowledge base does not allow us to accurately predict prognosis for individuals presenting with CLI. Collectively, we recognize a poor prognosis, both systemically, and with regard to the index limb. Fifteen to 25% of patients are dead within six months of their initial presentation with CLI, nearly all from advanced coronary and cerebral atherosclerosis. Fully 50% are dead within five years. For those who survive, limb loss occurs (in the absence of revascularization) in about half within a year of diagnosis, and further episodes of CLI involving the contralateral limb are common. The morbid systemic prognosis associated with CLI is emphasized by the fact that in all studies to date (all studies in which some treatment for the ischemia was rendered) *mortality exceeds limb loss*.[2] To date, there have been no prospective studies or clinical trials that have confirmed criteria that allow us to differentiate patients with CLI at high risk for early mortality, for whom the benefits of revascularization might be irrelevant from other patients who will probably survive for a number of years, for whom revascularization to achieve prolonged limb salvage might be more appropriate. Clearly, such trials are needed.

LESION-BASED TREATMENT VERSUS PATIENT-BASED TREATMENT

The current status of surgical treatment of CLI can be thought of as a good news/bad news scenario. The good news is that through several decades of development, vascular surgeons have evolved techniques that reliably result in revascularization in nearly all patients with CLI. By convention, the results of infrainguinal bypass grafting (the most commonly required form of treatment) for CLI have been evaluated in terms of operative morbidity and mortality, graft patency, and limb salvage. The results of several large contemporary series of such operations indicate that revascularization can be accomplished with operative mortality under 5%, graft patency at five years of 60–70%, and salvage of the index ischemic limb of greater than 80% at five years.[3-5] Achievement of these results requires multiple factors including detailed arteriography of distal vessels, use of autogenous vein grafts for maximum patency, and frequent postoperative graft duplex scanning to detect stenotic lesions threatening graft patency to allow them to be repaired prior to graft occlusion. Safe performance of major surgery in elderly seriously systemically ill patients requires expert anesthesia and perioperative intensive care. Once revascularization has been accomplished, ischemic foot and leg lesions require prolonged and extensive wound care to achieve healing. Need for multiple foot surgeries is common. Wound complications in the surgical incisions occur in at least 20% of patients in most series. So it appears that we can, at the price of major surgery with significant side effects and complications, achieve our goal of improving the ischemic state which results from the atherosclerotic lesions.

The bad news regarding surgical treatment of CLI is that presently, there is little evidence that successful treatment of the lesions producing CLI and relief of the ischemia is of demonstrable benefit to patients. This statement may seem heretical to vascular surgeons who observe the immediate relief of ischemic rest pain often experienced by patients with critical ischemia following successful bypass grafting, but it is based on what little information is currently available regarding changes in functional status and quality of life after revascularization in critical limb ischemia patients.

FUNCTIONAL STATUS OF PATIENTS WITH CLI

Although patients with CLI are the most severely affected of all those with lower extremity ischemia, less information is available about the degree of functional impairment associated with CLI than with any other group of patients with lower extremity ischemia. Partly this is because so few patients are so severely affected, the group with CLI representing less than 5% the entire group. The most important reason is probably that functional status and quality of life assessment is so complex in this group. Most patients with CLI are elderly and/or severely affected by other major illnesses. Many are within months of the end of life. For most, functional status has been declining rapidly, and this trend continues during the period in which they are affected by CLI. Many are nonambulatory and a significant percentage cannot stand without assistance. Nearly all of the sparse information that is available regarding functional status comes from series of patients treated by surgical revascularization, arguably the patient group with the best status, since they had to have been regarded as fit for surgery and able to benefit from the revascularization.

The largest prospective study of patients with lower extremity ischemia is being conducted by McDermott and colleagues, the Walking and Leg Circulation Study in which more than 500 individuals with abnormal ABI undergo standardized testing of functional capacity. Although only a small number of the subjects had very low ABI values (less than 0.40), it is very clear that these are the most severely affected functionally. A significant percentage of these patients were unable to walk unaided for six minutes, and all functional tests showed a clear-cut direct relationship to ABI. That is, the worse the ABI (and the ischemia) the worse the functional status.[6]

The Effect of Surgery on Functional Status and Quality of Life

The largest study of the effect of revascularization on functional status evaluated the outcome of 513 patients who underwent revascularization for CLI six months after the surgery.[7] Parameters evaluated included independence (did patients live on their own, or were they in a nursing home, etc?) and walking ability. Preoperatively, a significant number were dependent and/or nonambulatory. Postoperatively, while it appeared that very few patients experienced a decline in functional status, perhaps surprisingly, successful revascularization did not result in a return to independence or ambulation for those patients who had lost these abilities preoperatively.

Several prospective studies of revascularization in CLI patients have used standardized questionnaires such as the SF-36 and others to evaluate quality of life following surgery. Most studies have been small (50–150 patients). Follow-up intervals have ranged from six to 18 months. The mixed results of these surveys have been summarized by Nehler et al[8] and can best be described as mixed. Although some health related quality of life aspects show some improvement (pain, perception of health), there has been little documented improvement in overall quality of life following revascularization.

These results should not be surprising to vascular surgeons. If patients are already elderly, with severely impaired and rapidly declining functional status, and multiple serious disease states such as diabetes, chronic renal failure, and significant heart disease, is relief of leg ischemia really a major change in overall health status?

This specific issue was evaluated by Nicoloff and colleagues in a study designed to specifically look at the results of revascularization for CLI from the standpoint of effects on the patient.[9] These authors studied 112 patients who had undergone bypass for CLI a mean of 42 months (minimum of 24 months) prior to the study. As expected, the results of the surgery with respect to the lesions treated (patency 77%, limb salvage 87% after five years) were good.

But looked at from the point of view of the patient (and their families and referring physicians), the results could be seen in a different light. For the purposes of the study, the authors defined an "ideal result" of surgery as one in which there were no operative complications, prompt healing of operative and ischemic wounds occurred, functional status was maintained or improved, and repeat surgery was not required. Shockingly, this ideal result was achieved by only 16 (14.3%) patients. The reasons for this finding were many, and are summarized in Figure 8–1. Failure to achieve an ideal result was caused by operative death in seven patients (7%), by perioperative complications in 25 patients (26%), by failure to regain or maintain preoperative functional status in 28 patients (29%), by wound complications in 27 patients (28%), and by the need for repeat surgery in 61 patients (64%). Twenty-two patients (20%) had not achieved complete wound healing by the time of final follow-up or death.

This paper starkly defined the outcome of bypass surgery for CLI in terms familiar to most vascular surgeons and certainly to patients. Most patients with CLI required ongoing treatment for their CLI from the time of its occurrence until their death (or at least until the end of the study). Prolonged wound healing, repeat operations, and, perhaps most importantly, long-term follow-up appointments and need for continuing vascular surgery care were the rule.

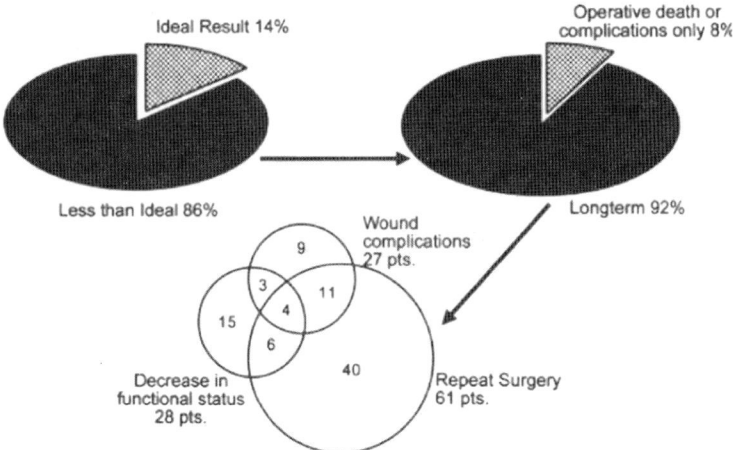

Figure 8-1. Only 16 of 112 patients (14%) achieved an ideal result. Of the 96 patients (86%) who failed to achieve an ideal result, eight (8%) failed because of perioperative death or complications only and 88 (92%) failed because of long-term factors. Sixty-one of the 96 patients (64%) required repeat surgery, 28 (29%) had a decrease in functional status (ambulatory or living status), and 27 (28%) had wound complications. (Reprinted from Nicoloff et al. Patient recovery after infrainguinal bypass for limb salvage. With permission: *J Vasc Surg.* 1998;27:256–266.)

These results are not unique. Similar studies from Great Britain have confirmed an appreciable need for ongoing care, consumption of health resources, and need for repeat surgery and the like in the CLI patient group.[10-11]

ALTERNATIVES TO REVASCULARIZATION FOR CLI

For those patients not treated by revascularization, nonoperative therapy and amputation are the remaining options. A single study from Brazil followed 31 patients with CLI treated without operation. After one year, 19 remained, the others having died, had revascularization and/or amputation. For the 19 who remained in the nonoperative group, pain and anxiety scores improved slightly.[12]

Amputation for CLI results in improvement in pain and anxiety, but numerous studies have documented that ambulation after amputation for CLI is rare. A review by Houghton et al studied the outcome of 440 major amputations performed in eight London hospitals over two years. Prior to hospital discharge, 75 patients died (17%). One hundred thirteen were not felt to have any hope of ambulation, 252 were referred to prosthetics and for rehabilitation with a goal of ambulation. Of these, after two years, 52 could walk briefly outside the home, 21 could walk within the home, and the remainder had either died or remained nonambulatory.[13]

Recent developments in mobility assistance such as motorized wheelchairs and the many infrastructure changes prescribed in the United States by the Americans with Disabilities Act have meant that in the USA, at least, nonambulatory status is not always synonymous with dependency. Nehler and colleagues have documented this relatively new phenomenon in a prospectively evaluated group of amputees.

Obviously, organized prospective study of the outcome and natural history of CLI is in its infancy. The currently available information indicates rather clearly that while nearly always possible, revascularization is not always (or even mostly) synonymous with a good outcome (as defined by an improvement in ambulatory/functional status) and that amputation is not always synonymous with a bad outcome. Noninterventional therapy is possible in a significant number of patients. The problem is that currently, we have no criteria to allow us to prospectively determine which individuals are best treated by which therapy. Prospective detailed studies of functional outcome related to treatment are clearly needed.

POSSIBLE APPROACHES TO CURRENT TREATMENT OF CLI

While we all wait for the outcome of those prospective studies, how should we approach treatment of patients with CLI? Treatment decisions at the extremes are relatively straightforward. Terminally ill patients, in the last month or two of life, may be best treated by operative palliative measures. Permanently dependent neurologically impaired nonambulatory patients should be treated by primary amputation. Fit patients, with good ambulatory status, should have aggressive attempts at revascularization and limb salvage. Between these extremes, the decision-making is less clear, and here is where one finds the majority of the patients. Nehler and colleagues[15] have suggested an approach that evaluates three separate issues: 1) the technical difficulty of the required revascularization, 2) the severity of any ischemic ulcerations/gangrenous lesions that may be present, and 3) patient comorbidities and functional status. By this approach, " . . . alternate vein conduit for a tibial bypass graft made from multiple pieces of arm vein might be reasonable for a patient with manageable toe gangrene and modest comorbidities, but would not be reasonable for a patient on home oxygen or with a large gangrenous heel ulcer."

What this suggested approach points out is that the current state of our knowledge requires that we carefully individualize surgical treatment of CLI based on the factors present in each patient. What should be clear is that universal revascularization and aggressive attempts at limb salvage are not required. Ideal outcomes are unusual with this approach, and consideration of other therapies is necessary and appropriate.

The available data allow vascular surgeons to deliver three messages very clearly to patients, families, and referring physicians. First, while it is almost always possible to achieve revascularization of a critically ischemic leg, this step in treatment should be regarded only as the beginning of a process. This treatment will include repeat visits for ongoing care, probably for the duration of the patient's life. Need for repeat operations, both on the index and contralateral legs, is common. Second, improvement in functional status following revascularization for CLI is rare. If patients are currently nonambulatory, and/or dependent, this will probably not change postoperatively. Planning for postoperative care/living status needs to take this into account. Third, and finally, other options for treatment are available. Some patients may be best served by nonoperative management and careful observation. Others are definitely best treated by amputation, despite the psychological difficulties involved.

It is important for vascular surgeons to take the time and make the effort to point out these facts to patients, their families, and to referring physicians. It may be that multiple visits and multiple talks will be required in order for patients' families and referring physicians to understand that the important aspects of a particular patient's problem are the global systemic ones rather than the lesion/limb related local ones. Revascularization for CLI should not be undertaken until patients, families, and referring physicians have heard and understood this message.

REFERENCES

1. Weitz JI, Byrne J, Claggett GP, et al. Diagnosis and Treatment of Chronic Arterial Insufficiency of the Lower Extremities: A Critical Review. *Circulation*. 1996;94:3026–3049.
2. The vascular surgical society of Great Britain and Ireland. Critical limb ischemia management and outcome. Report of a national survey. *Eur J Vas Endovasc·Surg*. 1995;10:108–113.
3. Pomposelli FB Jr, Marcaccio EJ, Gibbons GW, et al. Dorsalis pedis arterial bypass: durable limb salvage for foot ischemia in patients with diabetes mellitus. *J Vasc Surg*. 1995;21: 375–384.
4. Taylor LM Jr, Hamre D, Dalman RL, Porter JM. Limb salvage vs amputation for critical ischemia. The role of vascular surgery. *Arch Surg*. 1991;126:1251–1257.
5. Shah DM, Darling RC III, Chang BB, et al. Long-term results of in situ saphenous vein bypass. Analysis of 2058 cases. *Ann Surg*. 1995;222:438–446.
6. McDermott MM, Greenland P, Liu K, et al. Leg symptoms in peripheral arterial disease: associated clinical characteristics and functional impairment. *JAMA*. 2001;286:599–1606.
7. Abou-Zamzam AM, Lee RW, Moneta GL et al. Functional Outcome Following Infrainguinal Bypass for Limb Salvage. *J Vasc Surg*. 1997;25:287–297.
8. Nehler MR, McDermott MM, Treat-Jacobson D, et al. Functional outcomes and quality of life in peripheral arterial disease: Current Status.
9. Nicoloff AD, Taylor LM, Jr., McLafferty RB, et al. Patient Recovery After Infrainguinal Bypass for Limb Salvage. *J Vasc Surg*. 1998;27:256–266.
10. Holdsworth RJ, McCollum PT. Results and resource implications of treating end-stage limb ischaemia. *Eur J Endovasc Surg*. 1997;13:164–73.
11. Johnson BF, Singh S, Evans L, et al. A prospective study of the effect of limb-threatening ischemia and its surgical treatment on the quality of life. *Eur J Vasc Endovasc Surg*. 1997;13: 306–14.
12. Albers M, Fratezi AC, DeLuccia N. Assessment of quality of life of patients with severe ischemia as a result of infrainguinal arterial occlusive disease. *J Vasc Surg*. 1992;16:54–59.
13. Houghton AD, Taylor PR, Thurlow S, et al. Success rates for rehabilitation of vascular amputees: implications for preoperative assessment and amputation level. *Br J Surg*. 1992; 79:753–755.
14. Nehler MR, Coll JR, Hiatt WR, et al. Functional outcome in a contemporary series of major lower extremity amputations. *J Vasc Surg*. 2003;
15. Nehler MR, Hiatt WR, Taylor LM Jr. Is revascularization/limb salvage always the best treatment for critical limb ischemia? *J Vasc Surg*. 2003;37:704–708.

9

Burning Bridges: Is the Application of Emerging Technologies Deleterious to the Care of the Vascular Patient and the Nation's Financial Resources?

Michael C. Stoner, M.D. C. Steven Powell, M.D.

DEFINITION OF BURNING BRIDGES, ANATOMIC AND FINANCIAL FAILURE

The concept of burning bridges with modern vascular interventions raises two major areas of concern; one anatomic and one financial. From the anatomic standpoint, one must consider the location in the vascular system where a given intervention is to occur. This includes considering failure of an endovascular procedure and what it means in a given anatomic location for subsequent treatment options. Failure leading to a different or more difficult open procedure than one that could have been performed if there had been no endovascular procedure performed represents a burned anatomic bridge.

The second concern is the burning of financial bridges. In any given patient, this involves choosing between nonprocedural medical management of the patient's disease, and when indicated, the performance of the most durable and cost-effective interventional procedure from the outset. One burns the financial bridge when the initial procedure has a high rate of acute or chronic failure that leads to any kind of re-operative procedure. Most all endovascular failures burn a financial bridge while only some burn the anatomic bridge.

A classic example of burning both bridges is a poorly executed superficial femoral artery angioplasty with stent deployment converting what was an above-the-knee femoropopliteal bypass to a below-the-knee procedure. Burning these anatomic and financial bridges leads to a more difficult, more expensive procedure that carries a lower initial success and patency rate, and even more difficult secondary strategies in the case of failure. Burning these bridges is not unique to peripheral vascular procedures, and is readily seen in coronary artery disease where there are inferior bypass outcomes after failed percutaneous procedures.

Other examples of burning anatomic and financial bridges are encountered throughout the vascular system. These include the increased expense and higher complication rate of carotid artery stenting. Here, outside of the increased morbidity, the financial burden is also concerning. There is a high recurrence rate for subclavian angioplasty and stenting, and it eliminates the subsequent best surgical option that is the carotid-to-subclavian transposition operation. The overuse of poorly indicated renal angioplasty burns both the financial bridge and increases the subsequent risk and difficulty of open surgical revascularization, should it ever be indicated. The same is true for mesenteric angioplasty and stenting where recurrence can lead to a more difficult surgical procedure.

THE SURGICAL SAFETY NET ARGUMENT

The current use of endovascular technologies is driven by a variety of factors; these include patient demand, physician and health system reimbursement, industry influence, nonsurgeon interventionists, and a desire to seem "cutting edge". The concept of surgical fallback both in the acute setting and in a follow-up capacity assumes provision of a "safety net", and is often used to justify increasing endovascular aggressiveness and resource utilization. This is based on the premise that, with the primary use of endovascular procedures, one is extending the total time of successful revascularization. Essentially, the patient can undergo surgical revascularization once the minimally invasive options have been exhausted. There is logic to this argument as long as two criteria are met: the summation of total successful revascularization time is better in patients undergoing this serial revascularization strategy compared to those undergoing a primary open procedure, and the anatomic setup for the surgical fallback procedure must not be burned by the endovascular intervention.

We believe there is a subset of patients in whom endovascular treatment followed by open treatment is inferior to initial open treatment alone. These cases burn bridges and represent a flaw in the concept of surgical fallback since there is an increase in the cost and anatomic difficulty associated with some endovascular failures. What follows is a review of accumulated recommendations for lower extremity revascularization procedures, and our experience with failed primary lower extremity endovascular techniques that led to subsequent open procedures and their outcomes.

FEMOROPOPLITEAL: PRIMARY BYPASS VERSUS ENDOVASCULAR-FIRST

Recommendations for the treatment of femoropopliteal occlusive disease are well described in the current inter-society consensus document (TASC).[1] In brief, medical optimization is a necessity for all patients. The systemic problems of atherosclerosis are to be addressed and include smoking cessation, antiplatelet regimens, cholesterol lowering via statin-class drugs, glycemic control, and hypertension management via angiotensin blockade and beta adrenergic antagonists. One should remember that aggressive medical management of risk factors leads to better procedural outcomes, and importantly, medical management does not burn an anatomic or financial bridge! Once optimized, the performance of an intervention to treat severely symptomatic patients who have failed conservative measures may be justified.

By TASC guidelines, endoluminal treatment is justified in simple cases with short-segment stenosis or occlusions. Longer, more complex lesions can be treated if the patient does not have the physiology to support surgical revascularization. Except for this constitutional indication, the TASC document recommends surgical treatment for cases of advanced femoropopliteal disease.

Despite this well-documented consensus paper, endovascular therapy has become the de facto standard for femoropopliteal revascularization in many centers, even to the point of ignoring the TASC anatomical mandates. This is a result of the shorter hospital stay, lower morbidity and mortality, and a perceived equivalent efficacy and need for reintervention. The concept of surgical fallback has been used liberally to help justify this stance, even though the result of cases requiring surgical fallback has not been well characterized.

The bulk of the literature comparing endovascular treatment to surgical bypass has only compared the initial outcome of each procedure, and has not taken into consideration the subgroup that failed endovascular treatment and required a subsequent bypass (secondary bypass). There are several studies that demonstrate the non-inferiority of an endovascular-first plan.[2-4] These studies uniformly illustrate and seemingly ignore the inferior durability of endovascular procedures since they advocate endovascular reintervention, which is a costly endeavor that also burns the financial bridge by negating any real or perceived cost advantage of primary endovascular therapy.[5]

In a small retrospective study, Bockler et al. was one of the first to demonstrate inferior patency of surgical bypass following superficial femoral artery stenting.[6] In this paper, secondary bypass patients had significantly worse patency, limb salvage, and perioperative adverse event rates compared to those undergoing primary bypass. Other authors have demonstrated that with endovascular failure, subsequent open therapy was more likely to involve a more distal target than if the patient had undergone surgical bypass in the first place.[7]

EAST CAROLINA EXPERIENCE WITH SECONDARY BYPASS

Based on the conflicting reports noted above, and the authors' bias that there is a trend to over application of endovascular technology for lower extremity revascularization, we set out to review our experience with secondary femoropopliteal bypass grafting. We currently maintain a femoropopliteal revascularization database, which includes both open and endovascular cases. A total of 206 bypass grafts were identified in this dataset: 164 primary and 42 secondary (Table 9–1). These groups were compared using univariate statistical methods, and there was no difference with respect to operative indication (Rutherford category) or risk factors. The secondary bypass group had a higher proportion of females, and was more likely to be on perioperative antiplatelet therapy.

Primary assisted patency of the primary and secondary bypass groups was determined using the standard vascular societal guidelines. At 12 and 24 months, there was a clear superiority in the primary bypass group (Figure 9–1). In order to test the

TABLE 9-1. PATIENT AND ANATOMICAL CHARACTERISTICS OF 206 FEMOROPOPLITEAL BYPASS GRAFTS (164 PRIMARY, 42 SECONDARY).

	Primary Bypass		Secondary Bypass		
	n	%	n	%	p-value
Demographics					
Patients	164		42		
Age (years)	64 + 1		62 + 2		
Age range (years)	40−95		36−94		
Female gender	58	35	21	50	0.0287
Rutherford class					
3	74	45	15	36	
4	41	25	9	21	
5	48	29	18	43	
Anatomical					
TASC-A			2	8	
TASC-B			15	58	
TASC-C			7	27	
TASC-D			2	8	
Runoff (= 1 vessel)	83	50	21	50	
Clinical					
Diabetes mellitus	81	49	23	55	
Hypertension	148	89	36	86	
Hyperlipidemia	99	60	24	57	
Tobacco (any history)	90	56	21	50	
Coronary Artery Disease	94	56	22	52	
Serum Creatinine (>1.5)	26	16	4	10	
Dialysis	17	10	8	19	
CHF	43	26	10	24	
Medical Management					
Aspirin	120	72	36	86	0.0321
Clopidogrel	82	49	27	66	0.0236
Warfarin	19	11	4	10	
Lipid Therapy	85	51	21	50	
Follow-up					
Mean (days)	678		767		
Range (days)	1−1312		14−1541		

hypothesis that an endovascular procedure performed first results in a better overall revascularization time, we re-examined the patency data. In this analysis, the patency of the initial endovascular procedure was added to that of the secondary bypass, and again analyzed with life table technique. Again, there was a significantly worse patency in the secondary group compared to the primary (Figure 9–2). Finally, when limb salvage rates were examined, the patency differential translated into an inferior limb salvage rate in the secondary group (Figure 9–3).

There is an obvious critique to our observational study: the patients who underwent secondary bypass already represent a high-risk subgroup who have self-selected for failure based on a more aggressive atherosclerosis or intimal hyperplasia pattern.

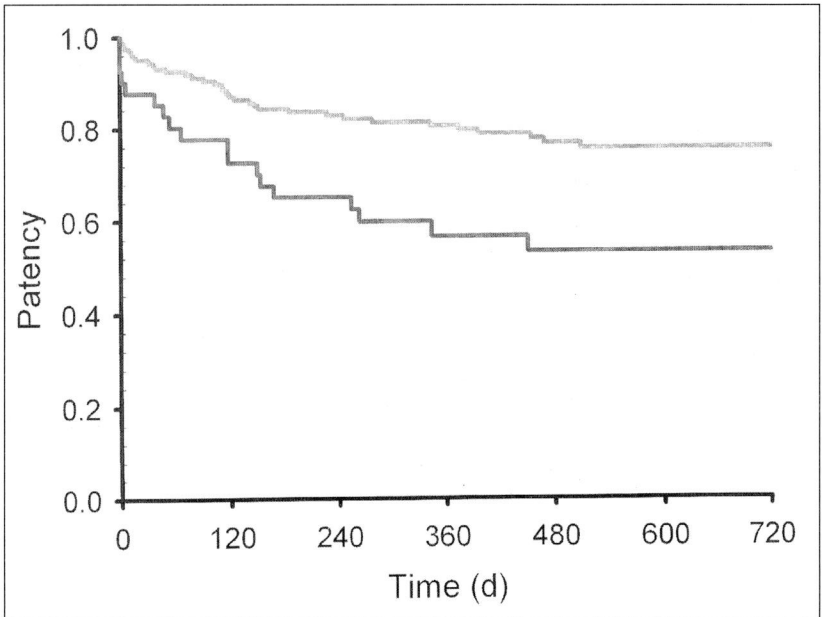

Figure 9-1. Kaplan-Meier curve demonstrating primary assisted patency of primary (grey) and secondary (black) femoropopliteal bypass grafts. Seconday bypass patency calculated from date of open procedure. (P<0.01)

Without a randomized trial designed to examine the outcomes of secondary bypass, this is impossible to answer. Our data do support the contentions that bypass grafts performed after failed endovascular procedures demonstrate inferior outcomes. At a minimum, these data can be used to counsel patients who have borderline anatomy for endovascular therapy.

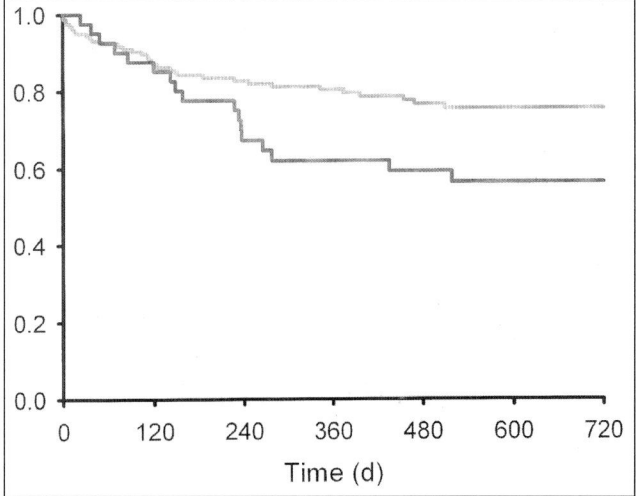

Figure 9-2. Kaplan-Meier curve demonstrating primary assisted patency of primary (grey) and secondary (black) femoropopliteal bypass grafts. Seconday bypass patency is additive, and calculated from date of initial endovascular procedure. (P<0.01)

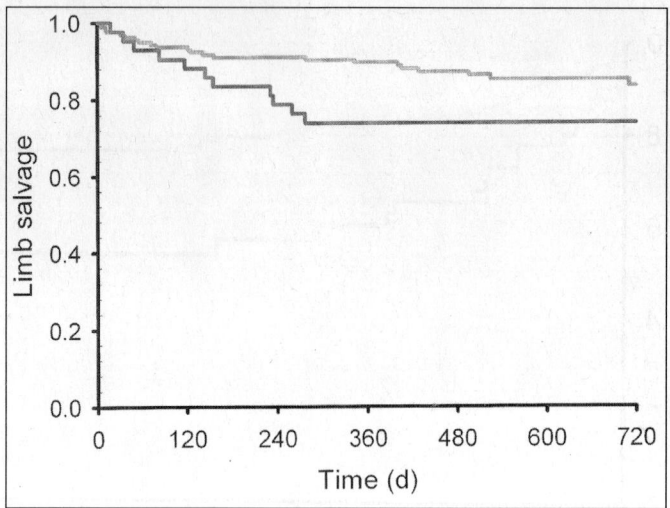

Figure 9-3. Kaplan-Meier curve demonstrating limb salvage of primary (grey) and secondary (black) femoropopliteal bypass grafts. (P<0.01)

Since realizing these data, we have taken a less aggressive posture toward endoluminal therapy in patients with suboptimal anatomy who have the constitution to undergo primary surgical bypass. It is not our contention that endovascular therapy should be abandoned, but we caution the application of endovascular tools in unproven situations where a bypass graft is a viable option. The finding that female gender was associated with secondary bypass is interesting, and follows a trend in the vascular literature citing inferior outcomes in women. This may be due to systemic and hormonal issues, or small vessel size. However, the small sample size of our review weakens this conclusion.

CONCLUSIONS

Endovascular procedures have greatly changed the specialty of vascular surgery and have permanently altered the way vascular care is delivered. These procedures reduce morbidity, and with appropriate indications, can provide outcomes comparable to traditional surgical reconstruction. However, these procedures can incur both a long-term clinical outcome and economic burden when there is inappropriate or overuse of endovascular treatment. There exists a subgroup of patients in whom an endovascular-first plan is harmful on both of these fronts. Careful case selection, and consideration of future options for revascularization both from an anatomic and financial viewpoint, is mandatory when considering endovascular therapy for all patients with vascular lesions, but most importantly, those of female gender or those who have suboptimal TASC anatomy and poor atherosclerotic risk factor control.

REFERENCES

1. Norgren L, Hiatt WR, Dormandy JA, Nehler MR, Harris KA, Fowkes FG. Inter-Society Consensus for the Management of Peripheral Arterial Disease (TASC II). *J Vasc Surg.* 2007;45 Suppl S:S5–67.

2. Adam DJ, Beard JD, Cleveland T, Bell J, Bradbury AW, et al. Bypass versus angioplasty in severe ischaemia of the leg (BASIL): multicentre, randomised controlled trial. *Lancet.* 2005;366:1925–1934.
3. Galaria II, Surowiec SM, Rhodes JM, Shortell CK, Illig KA, Davies MG. Implications of early failure of superficial femoral artery endoluminal interventions. *Ann Vasc Surg.* 2005;19: 787–792.
4. Ryer EJ, Trocciola SM, DeRubertis B, Lam R, Hynecek RL, Karwowski J, et al. Analysis of outcomes following failed endovascular treatment of chronic limb ischemia. *Ann Vasc Surg.* 2006;20:440–446.
5. Stoner MC, deFritus DJ, Manwaring ML, Carter JJ, Parker FM, Powell CS. Cost per day of patency: Understanding the impact of patency and reintervention in a sustainable model of healthcare. *J Vasc Surg.* 2008; in press.
6. Bockler D, Blaurock P, Mansmann U, Schwarzbach M, Seelos R, et al. Early surgical outcome after failed primary stenting for lower limb occlusive disease. *J Endovasc Ther.* 2005;12:13–21.
7. Joels CS, York JW, Kalbaugh CA, Cull DL, Langan EM, Taylor SM. Surgical implications of early failed endovascular intervention of the superficial femoral artery. *J Vasc Surg.* 2008;47:562–565.

Percutaneous Intervention for Limb Ischemia

Section II

Percutaneous Intervention for Limb Ischemia

10

Endovascular Therapy is the Preferred Initial Treatment for all Lower Extremity Revascularization

Glenn M. Lamuraglia, M.D.

The utilization of infrainguinal bypass surgery has been the "gold standard" for lower extremity revascularization since the 1970s. Multiple clinical series have reported excellent limb salvage and graft patency rates using vein graft conduit, with positive results in 80% or more of the patients treated. In fact, it had become the standard of care for the treatment of patients with lower extremity occlusive disease requiring therapy to improve the lower extremity perfusion.[1-3] However, since the mid-1970s when noncompliant balloons were first introduced for the use of angioplasty of occlusive arteriosclerotic disease, catheter-directed vascular intervention has significantly evolved and improved. Besides balloon angioplasty, other applications including mechanical or directional atherectomy, laser treatment, brachial therapy, and intravascular stent deployment have been or are presently in the process of evaluation as possible technical advancements in an effort to improve long-term results in selected clinical situations. Although historical series have demonstrated clearly inferior results with percutaneous interventions to bypass surgery,[4] with recent results that have demonstrated significant improvement in procedural success and long term patency, the time has come to reevaluate the paradigm for treating patients who need infrainguinal revascularization, and identify which patients should be treated initially with a percutaneous endovascular technique before considering an open bypass operative intervention as a first step.[5] Consideration of a new paradigm is not meant to discount any of the benefits and durability that surgical bypass can provide for the patient being evaluated for treatment; it just does not consider it as a first and only option.

THE BASIC QUESTION

When considering the patient for a treatment modality, the risks and benefits of a particular treatment need to be compared to the natural history of the disease process, as well as any other therapeutic options available to treat the presenting problem. For simplicity, only infrainguinal reconstructions, either open surgical or endovascular, will be considered. Therefore, in patients with peripheral vascular disease needing lower extremity revascularization, the following considerations need to be addressed to help decide the proper patient recommendation.

1. What is the natural history of the disease process as it relates to limb loss and mortality?
2. How does the natural history compare with treated patients?
3. What is the perioperative morbidity and mortality?
4. What is the functional outcome of these patients?
5. What is the patency of these revascularizations and their maintenance cost (reintervention)?
6. What is the consequence of failure?
7. Is there Level 1 evidence to support one or the other therapy?

NATURAL HISTORY

Although many initial large population studies have primarily addressed the risk factors of cardiac disease and cerebrovascular disease, more data have become available to better understand peripheral vascular disease and place this specific disease entity in proper perspective. Multiple studies have now better defined the natural history of obstructive atherosclerotic disease of the lower extremities. The general medical treatment for patients with atherosclerosis has significantly improved over the last several decades with the advent of beta blockers and other antihypertensive medicines, the Hydroxy-methyl-glutaryl CoA reductase inhibitors (statins) and other cholesterol lowering medications, and the lower prevalence of cigarette smokers. Although patients have been living longer with improvements in their medical management, it has also become evident that many of these patients with peripheral vascular disease have severe limitations to their longevity based on age-related events (such as higher incidence of cancer, organ deterioration such as dementia, or cardiac failure) or their severe cardiovascular disease.[5] Concurrent with medical advances and their positive impact on the longevity of patients with coronary and cerebrovascular disease, it has also become clearer that patients with advanced lower extremity ischemia can have very poor prognoses, likely worse than what was generally accepted. The American College of Cardiology/American Heart Association Guidelines for the Management for Peripheral Arterial Disease,[6] in delineating the natural history of patients with peripheral vascular disease (especially those with critical limb ischemia), have compiled outcomes from studies that would rival those in patient series with some cancers.

Patients with milder forms of lower extremity disease, mainly claudication, have a 15–30% five-year all-cause mortality of which 75% is related to cardiovascular causes (Table 10–1). Over the same time frame, their lower extremity symptoms remain stable except for approximately 10–20% of patients where it progresses. Only about 1–2% of patients progress to critical limb ischemia (Table 10–2), which is the subset of patients with the worst prognoses. Outcomes for patients with critical limb ischemia are evaluated based on a one-year follow-up since there is active tissue ischemia present, likely reflecting a generalized plaque activation, a high morbidity, and a CV mortality of 25% (Table 10–3).[6]

TABLE 10-1. INFRAINGUINAL OCCLUSIVE DISEASE PATIENT OUTCOMES WITH CLAUDICATION.[6]

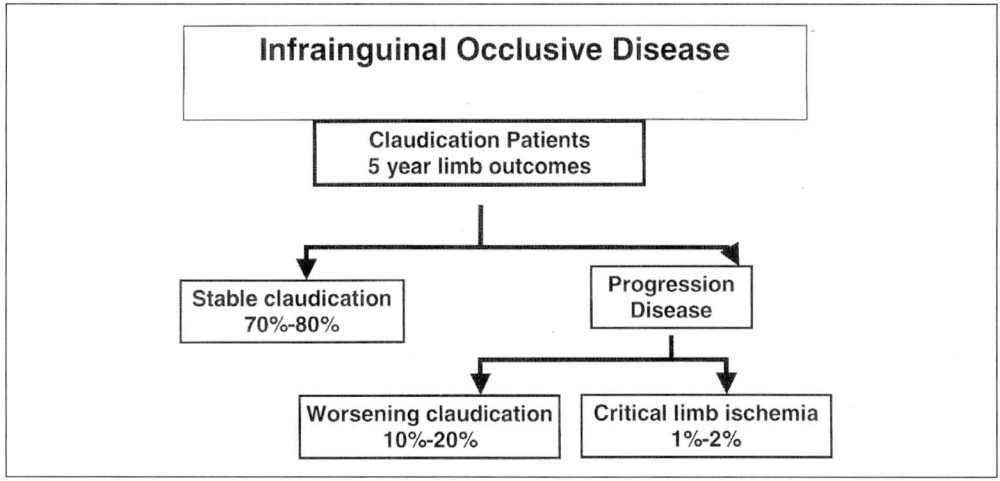

TABLE 10-2. INFRAINGUINAL OCCLUSIVE DISEASE LIMB OUTCOMES WITH CLAUDICATION.[6]

PATIENT LONGEVITY WITH LOWER EXTREMITY REVASCULARIZATION

In the era when there was significant controversy as to whether a vein bypass was better in situ or reversed, there was extensive reporting in the literature of results, including mortality of patients undergoing lower extremity bypass[1-3,7] (Table 10–4). These series, primarily reflecting patients with limb-threatening ischemia, also identified the "malignancy" of these patients with lower extremity peripheral vascular disease, identifying that close to 50% of these patients have died by five years. These results, albeit dated, are not that dissimilar to recent published results of lower extremity revascularization. A recent cohort of 189 patients undergoing vein bypass for critical limb

TABLE 10-3. INFRAINGUINAL OCCLUSIVE DISEASE PATIENT OUTCOMES WITH CRITICAL LIMB ISCHEMIA.[6]

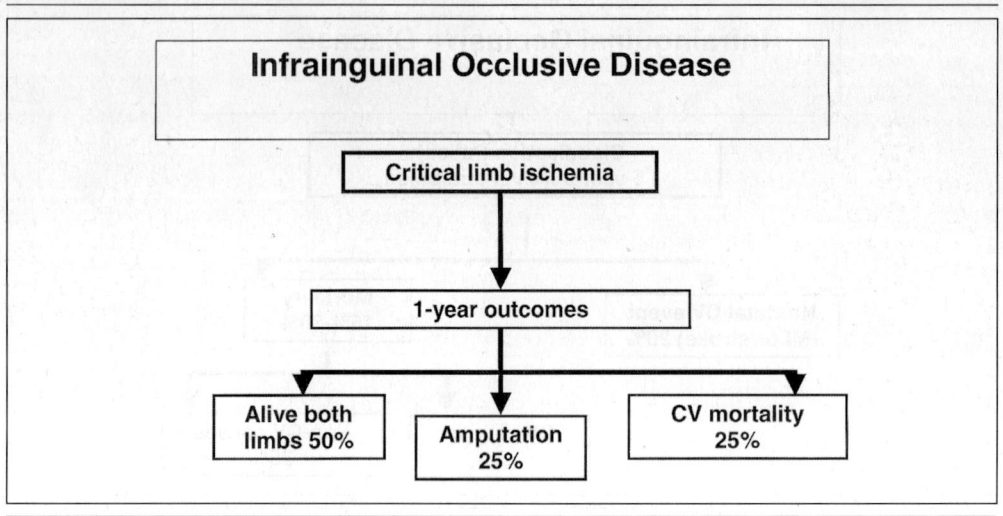

ischemia between 1999–2001 had a survival rate of 66% at two years.[8] In a similar co-hort of 208 patients who underwent a PTA of the superficial femoral or popliteal artery between 2003–2005, we reported an actuarial 78% survival in all patients; how-ever, when stratifying by claudication (94%) and critical limb ischemia (60%), the longevity was quite disparate between the groups.[5] With these findings on patient longevity, one has to strongly consider whether or not the standard "ruler" by which we determine long-term patency of an infrainguinal reconstruction should actually be five years when one-half of the patients have died and are not around to enjoy this benefit at this time frame.

PERIPROCEDURAL COMPLICATIONS

When choosing a therapy, the immediate periprocedural risks of complications and death have to be weighed against the potential benefits to the patient. These are gener-ally the most easily studied and defined. The morbidity and mortality of infrainguinal bypass surgery can be quite substantial, and reports have varied depending on

TABLE 10-4. EARLY AND LATE MORTALITY FOR PATIENTS WITH BYPASS SURGERY FOR INFRAINGUINAL ISCHEMIA.

	Early and Late Mortality for Operative Therapy for Infrainguinal Disease		
	Patients	30-day Mortality	Five-Year Survival
Taylor, 1990[7]	387	1%	28%
Bergamini, 1991[1]	322	3%	57%
Donaldson, 1991[3]	371	2%	66%
Leather, 1992[2]	2058	3%	58%
Total	3138	2%	54%

whether they were derived from governmental databases, multicenter trials, or institutions. The influences of the selected patient poplulations, operator skill, era of data acquisition, and definition of terms also can influence the results and findings. A recent study reviewed over 260,000 patients undergoing lower extremity bypass between 1994–1999 in an effort to identify differences in patient mortality between low- and high-volume hospitals.[9] The adjusted mortality was found to be 4.1–5.1% between the high- to low-volume hospitals with approximately equal numbers of patients in each group. The PREVENT III trial, though designed to evaluate an antisense gene therapy approach to prevent vein graft hyperplasia, provided important information on results of 1,404 patients from 83 centers enrolled between 2001–2003.[10] The perioperative mortality was 2.7%, with 6.2% major cardiac complications, a 1.4% stroke/TIA incidence, and a composite death, stroke, and MI event rate of 8% at 30 days. Another recent infrainguinal bypass study reported a similar mortality of 3%, major morbidity of 3%, a wound infection rate of 6.8%, and early bypass failure rate of 4% at 30 days. These results are similar to other concurrent reports.[8] These complications, especially related to the wounds, have been found in a higher rate in patients on hemodialysis and in those who were diabetic.[8-10]

It would be intuitive that a percutaneous procedure would sustain a lower morbidity and mortality rate. This has been documented in multiple studies, and most recently in our series of 238 cases in 208 patients treated for superficial femoral and popliteal angioplasty, there were no deaths and only 3% major complications including hematomas, pulmonary edema, and one patient each with arterial disruption and device malfunction requiring lower extremity bypass.[5]

Although this would cover the conventional 30-day perioperative complication rates, others have questioned if, in fact, we are not underreporting the actual problems associated with lower extremity bypass surgery since the problems likely extend out beyond the 30-day limit. This was examined in a paper that reviewed 318 patients (49% diabetic) who underwent distal bypass (84%) for critical limb ischemia (72%), and had a very high reoperative and readmission rate.[11] Reoperation at less than three months was undertaken in 49% of patients who included 16% of the claudicants, 27% of the rest pain patients, and 56% of those with tissue loss. Thirteen percent of the operations were not related to the bypass operations and included debridement and amputations. In patients readmitted within six months, 47% were admitted for problems related to the bypass, with 65% of the critical limb ischemia patients and 45% of the claudicants undergoing readmission. Care must be taken in reviewing this manuscript since those patients with tissue loss would likely require some of the same readmissions for minor amputations and debridements whether they underwent bypass surgery or a percutaneous intervention.

FUNCTIONAL OUTCOME

Another important consideration is the functional outcome of the patient. Subjecting patients to significant procedures does not have much point if they do not reach a certain level of autonomy and independent living after their recovery. As patients are living longer, and revascularization of the lower extremity becomes more of a necessity in a much older patient population that may be much more infirm than has been in the past, returning to normal independent function within a reasonable period of time is of prime importance.

One seminal study has looked into the functional status and well-being of patients after infrainguinal revascularization for critical limb ischemia.[12] In a questionnaire mailed out six months after surgery to 276 patients (84% diabetic) during one year, there were 57% responders. Several key findings were identified: those patients who lived independently preoperatively and those with limb salvage fared better than the patients who were not living independently or who underwent a major amputation. At six months, only 45% of patients felt they were back to their baseline function or independence, while only 21% of the patients who were not ambulating preoperatively were walking at six months. This not only reflects the elderly and infirm nature of the patient population at risk, but also underscores the difficulty they have at recovering from open surgical bypass procedures to the lower extremity.

PATENCY AND REINTERVENTION

The traditional teaching has been that vein graft primary and assisted primary patency at five years is 75–85%,[1-3] while that of prosthetic grafts is much less encouraging at 30% or less.[13] Contemporary results (2004) still report a 72% primary patency and a respectable 91% limb salvage rate at two years.[8] The most interesting data are that they required a 28% reintervention rate for these bypasses to obtain those patency and limb salvage rates.

In our study of PTA of the superficial femoral and popliteal arteries, assisted patency or needing to repeat the procedures, but not including failures, significantly improved the results at three years[5] (Table 10–5). Of the 69 failures of that study, 54% underwent reangioplasty to provide assisted patency while 28% underwent open bypass to obtain those results for limb salvage. We have also reviewed our results of the tibial angioplasty, and have identified similar promising results of patency and limb preservation despite a patient population survival of 54%[14] (Table 10–6).

TABLE 10-5. THREE-YEAR RESULTS OF SUPERFICIAL FEMORAL AND POPLITEAL ARTERY ANGIOPLASTY.[5]

Three-year Results of Endovascular Therapy for Superficial Femoral and Popliteal Arteries			
	All	Claudicants	CLI
Primary Patency	54%	66%	42%
Assisted Patency	93%	94%	93%
Limb Preservation	95%	100%	90%

TABLE 10-6. FOUR-YEAR RESULTS OF TIBIAL ARTERY ANGIOPLASTY.

Four-year Results of Endovascular Therapy-Tibial Arteries	
	All
Primary Patency	62%
Assisted Patency	90%
Limb Preservation	86%
Patient Survival	54%

There have been multiple studies regarding the success rate of PTA based on the lesion type (stenosis versus occlusion), lesion length (less or greater than 5 cm), and vessel runoff.[15] The utilization of stents as an adjunct to PTA of infrainguinal lesions has also not been reported to increase hemodynamic or clinical success beyond one year. However, in the situation where a flow limiting dissection has occurred, a self-expanding stent can be utilized for procedural salvage.[16]

WHAT IS THE CONSEQUENCE OF FAILURE?

The failure of a bypass graft and its consequences have been primarily related to whether the graft is a vein graft or a prosthetic graft. Vein grafts appear to fail by either a gradual narrowing of the graft itself or at the distal anastomosis. This process does not generally result in loss of the outflow by thromboembolism as is the case with prosthetic grafts.[13] These latter graft failures not infrequently result in significant clinical worsening, occasionally presenting with limb-threatening ischemia. This has not been noted in cases after balloon angioplasty.[5,17]

Restenosis has been reported to be higher in patients with balloon angioplasty than patients who have had bypass surgery. In these patients, reports vary dramatically in the reported percent restenosis, but generally 60–70% restenosis at one year has been average.[5,18] This has not precluded the retreatment of these patients, as the use of stents has also been advocated in these circumstances. In fact, patients who have been followed over long periods of time have been identified to cross over to the surgical arm for treatment with a bypass procedure when indicated. Importantly, in these series in which surgical revascularization was undertaken after primary endovascular treatment, the patients who had either a combination of both, or had initially undergone endovascular treatment before open bypass, were found to have equal or improved patency of their reconstruction in follow-up than if they had primary surgery or angioplasty alone.[18]

LEVEL 1 EVIDENCE

There has recently been published a multicenter randomized trial comparing percutaneous angioplasty versus bypass surgery as the initial treatment modality.[19] After the initial therapy, any subsequent procedures were at the discretion of the clinicians. The primary endpoint was amputation-free survival. The results of this trial demonstrated no procedural hemodynamic improvement between balloon angioplasty and bypass surgery. In addition, infrainguinal bypass and balloon angioplasty have demonstrated broadly similar outcomes regarding amputation-free survival and health related problems, while surgery was found to be the more expensive intervention.

CONCLUSIONS

Although long-term patency is clearly better with bypass surgery than with endovascular treatment for infrainguinal occlusive disease, this cannot be held alone as the prime defining factor for which therapy to choose. Surgery clearly has a higher complication rate and a higher mortality rate. These periprocedural problems, coupled with an intermediate time follow up, in which a significant number of patients do not obtain preoperative functional status by six months, raises into question the appropriateness of using bypass surgery as a first line of treatment. With the added knowledge that many of these patients have a limited life expectancy, it would make sense that these patients would not spend a significant portion of their final years in a rehabilitation institution. Furthermore, no studies have ever demonstrated that endovascular treatment for occlusive disease ultimately results in the loss of the surgical option (as opposed to prosthetic bypass that can precipitate this complication) at a later date should that become necessary for limb salvage. And, the only Level 1 evidence does not demonstrate any superiority of angioplasty versus bypass surgery. Therefore, what is there to lose by attempting to have a percutaneous approach as a first line of therapy for infrainguinal treatment? *Nothing*, but there may be very much to gain for the patient.

REFERENCES

1. Bergamini TM, Towne JB, Bandyk DF, et al. Experience with in situ saphenous vein bypasses during 1981 to 1989: determinant factors of long-term patency. *J Vasc Surg*. 1991;13 (1):137–47.
2. Shah DM, Darling RC, Chang BB, et al. Long-term results of in situ saphenous vein bypass. Analysis of 2058 cases. *Ann Surg*. 1995;222 (4):438–46.
3. Donaldson MC, Mannick Ja, Whittemore AD. Femoral-distal bypass with in situ greater saphenous vein. Long-term results using the Mills valvulotome. *Ann Surg*. 1991;213 (5): 457–64.
4. Wolf GL, Wilson SE, Cross AP, et al. Surgery or balloon angioplasty for peripheral vascular disease: a randomized clinical trial. Principal investigators and their Associates of Veterans Administration Cooperative Study Number 199. *J Vasc Interv Radiol*. 1993;4:639–48.
5. Conrad MF, Cambria RP, Stone DH, et al. Intermediate results of percutaneous endovascular therapy of femoropopliteal occlusive disease: a contemporary series. *J Vasc Surg*. 2006; 44:762–9.
6. Hirsch AT, Haskal ZJ, Hertzer NR, et al. ACC/AHA guidelines for the management of patients with peripheral arterial disease (lower extremity, renal, mesenteric, and abdominal aortic): a collaborative report from the American Association for Vascular Surgery/Society for Vascular Surgery, Society for Cardiovascular Angiography and Interventions, Society of Interventional Radiology, Society for Vascular Medicine and Biology, and the American College of Cardiology/American Heart Association Task Force on Practice Guidelines (Writing Committee to Develop Guidelines for the Management of Patients with Peripheral Arterial Disease). American College of Cardiology Web Site. Available at: http://www.acc. org/clinical/guidelines/pad/index.pdf.
7. Taylor LM, Jr., Edwards JM, Phinney ES, et al. Reversed vein bypass to infrapopliteal arteries. Modern results are superior to or equivalent to in-situ bypass for patency and for vein utilization. *Ann Surg*. 1987;205:90–7.
8. Abbruzzese TA, Havens J, Belkin M, et al. Statin therapy is associated with improved patency of autogenous infrainguinal bypass grafts. *J Vasc Surg*. 2004;39:1178–85.
9. Birkmeyer JD, Siewers AE, Finlayson EV, et al. Hospital Volume and surgical mortality in the United States. *N Engl J Med*. 2002;346:1128–37.
10. Conte MS, Bandyk DF, Clowes AW, et al. Risk factors, medical therapies and perioperative events in limb salvage surgery: observations from the PREVENT III multicenter trial. *J Vasc Surg*. 2005;42:456–65.

11. Goshima KR, Mills JL, Hughes JD. A new look at outcomes after infrainguinal bypass surgery: traditional reporting standards systematically underestimate the expenditure of effort required to attain limb salvage. *J Vasc Surg.* 2004;39:330–35.

12. Gibbons GW, Burgess AM, Guadagnoli E, et al. Return to well-being and function after infrainguinal revascularization. *J Vasc Surg.* 1995; 21: 35–45.

13. Jackson MR, Johnson WC, Williford WO, et al. The effect of anticoagulation therapy and graft selection on the ischemic consequences of femoropopliteal bypass graft occlusion: results from a multicenter randomized clinical trial. *J Vasc Surg.* 2002;35:292–98.

14. LaMuraglia GM, Conrad MF, Kang J, et al. Infrapopliteal balloon angioplasty for the treatment of chronic occlusive disease: intermediate-term results of a contemporary series. Presented at the 61st Vascular Annual Meeting, Society for Vascular Surgery, Baltimore, MD, June 8, 2007.

15. Johnston KW. Femoral and popliteal arteries: reanalysis of results of balloon angioplasty. *Radiology.* 1992;183:767–71.

16. Schillinger M, Sabeti S, Loewe C, et al. Balloon angioplasty versus implantation of nitinol stents in the superficial femoral artery. *N Engl J Med.* 2006;354(18):1879–88.

17. Kalman PG, Johnston KW. Outcome of a failed percutaneous transluminal dilation. *Surg Gynecol Obstet.* 1985;161(1):43–6.

18. Karch LA, Mattos MA, Henretta JP, et al. Clinical failure after percutaneous transluminal angioplasty of the superficial femoral and popliteal arteries. *J Vasc Surg.* 2000;31:880–7.

19. Adam DJ, Beard JD, Cleveland T, et al. Bypass versus angioplasty in severe ischaemia of the leg (BASIL): multicentre, randomised controlled trial. *Lancet.* 2005;366:1925–34.

11

Techniques to Treat Chronic Total Iliac Artery Occlusions

Raghunandan Motaganahalli, M.D.
Brian G. Peterson, M.D.

Endovascular reconstruction of the iliac arteries is increasingly being utilized as an alternative to surgery in the management of chronic total occlusions (CTOs). Surgical bypass, long held as the gold standard for the treatment of aortoiliac occlusive disease, now is more commonly performed only after failed endovascular interventions.

The aging population with multiple medical problems and the modern epidemic of obesity pose a significant challenge in revascularizing these patients with conventional surgical methods. Consistent with this change in the population, there is an increasing need to treat CTOs as disease prevalence increases. In addition to these factors, patient and physician acceptance has been the driving force for the increasing trends in endovascular management. This has resulted in a dramatic increase in the number of endovascular procedures, as well as an associated decline in the number of open procedures for extremity arterial disease.[1] However, despite the relatively less invasive nature of endovascular interventions as compared to open bypass, indications for revascularization should remain lifestyle-limiting claudication and critical limb ischemia.

The techniques for the treatment of CTOs are numerous, varied, and evolving. Along with improved techniques, there is seemingly increased technical success with newer devices. Nevertheless, the decision to bypass or to utilize an endovascular approach depends on several key determinants of success such as the site of occlusion, length of occlusion, and degree of calcification present in the arterial segment being treated.[2,3] Several key considerations including technical success rates, patient morbidity, long term patency, and patient satisfaction must be taken into account when deciding whether or not endovascular techniques are the most appropriate treatment modality. Once a decision has been made to perform an endovascular intervention, it is important to conduct that intervention with a complete understanding of how an acute or late failure of the endovascular approach might impact the options for future revascularization.[4] The keys are to minimize complications by adhering to meticulous technique, treating the intended lesion and limiting the creation of new lesions, preserving outflow and as many collaterals as possible, and keeping open the option for future open revascularization if necessary.

In the United States, more patients undergo iliac artery angioplasty and stenting than conventional open aortobifemoral bypass procedures for aortoiliac occlusive disease, likely because this was one of the first vascular beds in which results following angioplasty were nearly comparable to surgery, and morbidity and mortality were significantly reduced.[5] In a study published by Upchurch et al., the rate of iliac artery angioplasty and stenting increased 850% from 0.4 to 3.4 cases per 100,000 adults. Conversely, the rate of aortofemoral bypass declined 15.5%, from 5.8 to 4.9 cases per 100,000 adults. Interestingly, older age, white race, and higher income patients were more likely to undergo angioplasty and stenting than open surgical bypass procedure.[6]

LESION CHARACTERISTICS AND PATIENT SELECTION

The Trans-Atlantic Inter-Society consensus document on the management of peripheral arterial disease (TASC-2) stratifies lesions into various categories. TASC-A lesions represent those that yield excellent results from and should be treated by endovascular means. TASC-B lesions offer sufficiently good results with endovascular methods, and this approach is preferred first unless an open revascularization is required for other associated lesions in the same anatomic area. Open revascularization to treat TASC-C lesions produces superior long-term results, and endovascular methods should be used only in patients at high risk for open repair. Finally, TASC- D lesions do not yield good enough results with endovascular methods to justify their use as a primary treatment. To summarize, endovascular therapy is the treatment of choice for type A lesions and surgery is the treatment of choice for type D lesions. Likewise, endovascular treatment is the preferred first-line treatment for type B lesions, and surgery is the preferred treatment for good-risk patients with type C lesions.

Lesions can also be graded anatomically such that TASC-A lesions are concentric, noncalcified stenoses less than 3 cm in length; B lesions are noncalcified stenoses that are 3–5 cm in length, or calcified, eccentric lesions of less than 3 cm in length; C lesions are stenosis 5–10 cm in length, or occlusions less than 5 cm in length; and D lesions are stenoses greater than 10 cm in length, or occlusions greater than 5 cm in length.[7]

When attempting to assign a TASC grade and determine whether a patient is a candidate for endovascular revascularization, computed tomography (CT) angiography is invaluable in providing information regarding location, extent, and character of iliac arterial disease. CT angiography prevents the need for brachial arterial access when extensive aortoiliac disease makes femoral access challenging and provides information regarding distal runoff as well. Patients with occluded common femoral arteries or distal aortic occlusion are not candidates for endovascular reconstruction, and these findings are readily elucidated on preprocedural CT angiograms. In addition to CT angiograms, preprocedural arterial physiologic evaluation with ankle-brachial indices should be done not only to aid in diagnosing the presence of hemodynamically significant disease, but also to provide a baseline to help determine the effectiveness of the treatment and to assist in monitoring patients in the follow-up period.

We have previously described[4,8] the lesion characteristics that predict successful endovascular recanalization of CTOs, and found the following lesions to be most amenable to endovascular techniques: lesions that are less calcified, short segment occlusions, and the absence of collateral branches at the site of occlusion. As suggested by the TASC classification system, the presence of calcification has a bearing on the technical success of endovascular interventions. Though these assessments may be useful in the femoropopliteal segment, this finding may be of less relevance in the context of the treatment of iliac arterial disease. Interestingly, uniform, circumferential calcifications as seen in diabetic patients are less concerning than the eccentric, multisegmental, calcified lesions more commonly seen in nondiabetic patients as these lesions are more difficult to recanalize. Plaque echogenicity represented by duplex ultrasound-derived Gray scale median (GSM) can also be used to predict the success of primary angioplasty. Higher failures rates of true lumen re-entry can be anticipated if the median GSM is greater than 35.[9] And finally, the lesion length is a well-accepted factor that impacts the long- and short-term results of recanalizing a CTO.[7,10] Long lesions (i.e., TASC-C and D lesions) as determined by TASC-2 are best treated with open surgical revascularization. However, despite the TASC document recommendations significant numbers of patients are initially treated with an endovascular approach due to patient, and partly physician, preference. Along these lines, a recent survey among vascular surgeons demonstrated that for all types of aortoiliac lesions, the TASC document is generally ignored and endovascular treatment is attempted initially whenever possible (Charing cross international meeting, March 2005).

DETERMINING THE SITE OF ACCESS

Having identified the lesion, the next step in attempting recanalization of iliac CTOs involves gaining appropriate access from which one can apply enough axial force to cross the occlusion. Generally, we use an up-and-over approach from the contralateral common femoral artery when treating external iliac or distal common iliac artery occlusions; an ipsilateral, retrograde common femoral artery approach is used when the occlusion involves the more proximal common iliac artery. Although less often a major determinant in treating iliac lesions when compared to treating femoropopliteal lesions, the patient's body habitus can sometimes influence the site of access. Having decided the location of remote arterial access, we routinely utilize ultrasound-guidance and micropuncture vascular access techniques. Establishing and adhering to a meticulous routine for gaining arterial access will help to reduce the number of access-related problems encountered when treating these challenging patients who often have extensive atherosclerosis.

After having initially obtained the appropriate diagnostic images through a micropuncture catheter or 5 French sheath and catheter, a 7 French braided sheath is used when utilizing the up-and-over approach to treat contralateral distal common or external iliac lesions. When treating ipsilateral lesions, the diagnostic sheath is upsized to the appropriately sized sheath, depending on the choice of treatment modality. Patients are heparinized at the time of placement of the supporting sheath with a targeted activated clotting time (ACT) of 275–300 seconds. This level of anticoagulation is ideally achieved prior to any attempt at crossing an occlusion. Depending on the length of the procedure, repeat ACTs are obtained, and this range of anticoagulation is maintained throughout the procedure. Inadequate anticoagulation carries the risk of thrombus formation in the subintimal space, perisheath thrombosis, or clotting wherever a catheter is placed through a stenotic portion of the artery, altering flow characteristics. Furthermore, inadequate anticoagulation can lead to possible embolization once the flow is reestablished.[11]

CROSSING TOTAL OCCLUSIONS

Bolia et al. initially described the subintimal technique for crossing CTOs.[12]

The initial wire of choice is an 0.035" glidewire (Terumo, Somerset, NJ) used in combination with a 4 French straight- or angled-glide catheter. Alternatively, a variety of guide sheath and catheter combinations may be used in a co-axial fashion to provide more axial force to cross a CTO. Furthermore, if even more additional support is needed, the sheath itself can be used with its dilator placed up to the fibrous cap of the occlusion to facilitate the initial penetration with the wire. The dilator with leading wire may also be used to complete the crossing of an occlusion, but may result in a higher incidence of vessel perforation.

The wire behavior should be constantly monitored on fluoroscopy so as to create a loop no larger than the vessel diameter. Advancing the lesion with a smaller loop is preferred over a spiral formation of the wire. The traversal is done best when the glidewire is looped back several centimeters with the 180° turn near the transition of the wire from the tip to the shaft.[4] These maneuvers limit the vessel perforation and provide a better chance of gaining access back into the lumen. If the lesions are fibrotic and cannot be crossed, the back end of the standard glidewire may be used to gain access back into the true lumen. This is suited in those locations where the direction of the wire exiting the catheter is in the direction of the axis of the occluded vessel. The wire is advanced only a short distance of 5–10 mm and the catheter is advanced over the wire to that point, and the soft-tipped end of the wire is used again to push into the true lumen. Small perforations of the vessel made by the wire or catheter will typically not need treatment beyond prolonged balloon inflation across the area of perforation. Covered stents should be available if one plans to embark on treating more difficult CTOs as vessel perforation is a risk.

More concerning than vessel perforation by wire or catheter manipulation is rupture at the time of balloon angioplasty. Iliac artery rupture following balloon angioplasty is suggested by the rapid onset of profound hypotension, and outcomes can be poor if not dealt with in an expedient fashion. If iliac artery rupture is encountered, control of hemorrhage with balloon insufflation allows some time to collect your thoughts concerning the best course of action, whether that is open surgical repair or more likely endovascular repair. Endovascular repair involves the placement of a covered stent across the area of rupture, and on most occasions, requires upsizing the access sheath. Although rare, the possibility of iliac artery rupture when treating CTOs mandates familiarity of covered stent-grafts as their use can be live-saving.

MANAGEMENT OF DIFFICULTIES DURING THE RECANALIZATION OF CTOs

Failure of the glidewire and glide catheter combination in crossing CTOs or in gaining access back into the true lumen occurs in up to 7% of patients.[13] When faced with these situations, several techniques may be used to assist in crossing the lesion or in gaining access back into the true lumen As mentioned previously, the most commonly used wire to cross CTOs is the glidewire. Several other wires have been shown to be valuable when attempting to cross CTOs and these include the Miracle Asahi wire (Asahi Intec, Aichi, Japan), choice PT, and PT Graphix (Boston Scientific, Natick, MA).

Another tool that has been helpful in crossing CTOs includes the Quickcross catheter (Spectranetics, Colorado Springs, CO). This catheter is low profile and is available in 0.014, 0.018, and 0.035 configurations with catheter length varying from 65–150 cm. Not only is this catheter useful in providing extra axial support to cross the lesion, but also can be used for wire exchanges and to angiographically confirm true lumen re-entry. While no significant data are available regarding the use of this catheter in treatment of CTOs, we have found it to be a staple in our practice.

The Frontrunner catheter (Cordis, Miami Lakes, FL) is a specially designed catheter for penetrating and crossing CTOs. The end of the catheter has a small microdissector that can spread its jaws with the repetitive movement of a pistol grip mechanism. The relatively delicate manipulating action of the frontrunner sometimes is not adequate to cross heavily calcified lesions. This device is mainly utilized in the coronary bed; however, it may have a place in peripheral interventions when dealing with moderately calcified CTOs.

Additional tools and techniques are required if one is able to cross the lesion but unable to gain entry back into the true lumen. Angioplasty balloons placed in the distal end of the lesion provide extra support to the wire in an effort to penetrate into the true lumen. When this technique fails, we often resort to the use of true lumen re-entry devices. The true lumen re-entry devices facilitate precise access back into the true lumen, help preserve collateral flow, and limit the extent of vessel dissection.[4,8] Additionally, they can reduce the fluoroscopic and procedural time, but most importantly, they can virtually eliminate the most common cause of technical failure: the inability to get back into the true lumen.

One such catheter is the Outback LTD catheter (Cordis, Miami Lakes, FL). This is a 5 French catheter with a retractable nitinol hypotube that has a curved needle end. A 0.014 wire is placed through the nitinol hypotube. When the device is in place in the subintimal dissection alongside the true lumen, the wire is withdrawn back into the catheter 2–3 cm so it is within the retracted needle near the distal end of the catheter. With the wire retracted, the needle can then be advanced forward, allowing the precurved nitinol shape to point the needle tip out a side port 1.5 cm from the distal end of the catheter, and penetrate the media and intima to enter the true lumen.

The rotational orientation of the needle deployment is provided by fluoroscopic guiding marks on the catheter. Before deployment, the "L" mark is oriented to point to the true lumen and in an orthogonal view, the "T" is oriented over the true lumen. If the needle penetrates the true lumen, then the wire freely passes. The wire can then be advanced, and the device can be exchanged for a catheter or stiff wire. The extent of calcification defines the success, and sometimes the needle may have to be passed more than once to gain access to the true lumen. Available results suggest the device to be useful in difficult-to-cross lesions with a technical success of 50–80%[13-14] (Figures 11–1 through 11–4).

The Pioneer catheter (Medtronic, Santa Rosa, CA) is an intravascular ultrasound (IVUS) device that also facilitates true lumen re-entry. The tip of this device is placed beyond the occlusion. The IVUS provides an image of the vessel wall and the color flow capability of the catheter can show the flow in the true lumen. The catheter is constructed over a monorail lumen for delivery of the device over a 0.014-inch wire and a

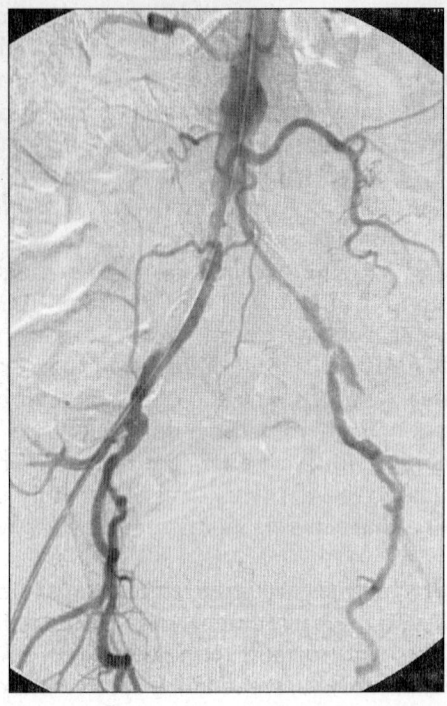

Figure 11-1. Angiogram demonstrating bilateral diffuse common iliac artery stenoses and bilateral external iliac artery occlusions.

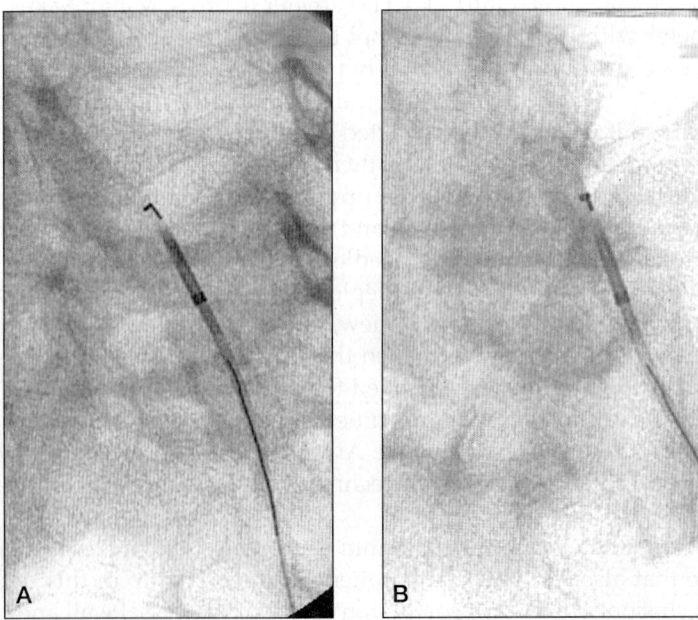

Figure 11-2. A. Outback catheter in the "L" orientation. **B.** Outback catheter in the "T" orientation in the orthogonal view.

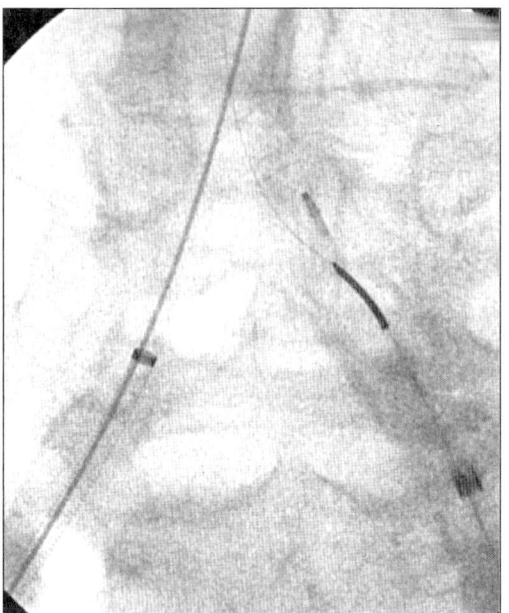

Figure 11-3. Outback catheter with nitinol needle deployed enabling true lumen re-entry.

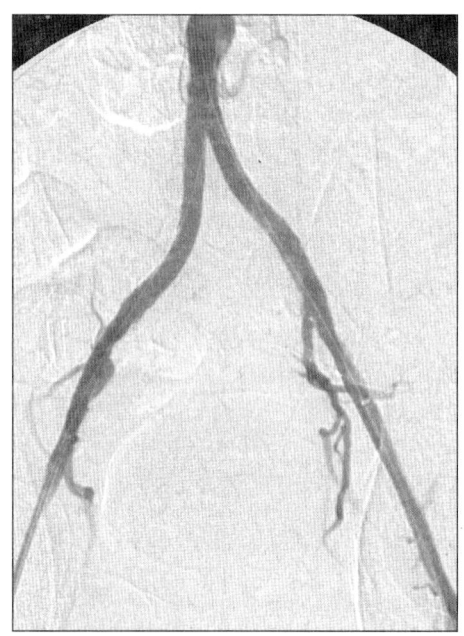

Figure 11-4. Completion angiogram following angioplasty and stenting of bilateral iliac artery disease.

second wire lumen through the end of the catheter that ends in a curved nitinol needle that is retracted in the catheter near the distal end. The needle is deployed by sliding a portion of the handle of the catheter in a calibrated fashion to cause the needle to exit a port on the side of the catheter just proximal to the IVUS transducer. The port is fixed in the 12 o'clock position and deploys the needle to penetrate from the dissection plane to the true lumen. Once the needle is deployed, the lumen of the needle is used to pass an 0.014-inch guide wire into the true lumen (Figures 11–5 through 11–8).

We have reported our initial results[8] using the pioneer catheter elsewhere. Briefly, we utilized this catheter more often in iliac occlusions than in femoral occlusions. Use of true lumen re-entry devices facilitate gaining wire passage back to true lumen and successful endovascular treatment of CTOs that would otherwise require bypass. In our own experience using this device to gain true lumen re-entry, we have had 100% technical success in both iliac and femoral arterial segments. True lumen re-entry was successful in all cases at the level of vessel reconstitution within 2 cm of the optimal angiographically defined distal target vessel. Collateral preservation is one of the main advantages associated with these re-entry devices. None of the cases in our experience required open conversion.[8] Similar results have been reported from other authors.[15]

In comparing these two re-entry devices, the outback device utilizes fluoroscopy while the pioneer catheter requires the availability of the IVUS, which adds to the cost of the procedure. In addition, the pioneer catheters are more expensive than the outback catheters; however, the IVUS guidance facilitates the accurate placement of the needle in the true lumen and limits the extent of the dissection.

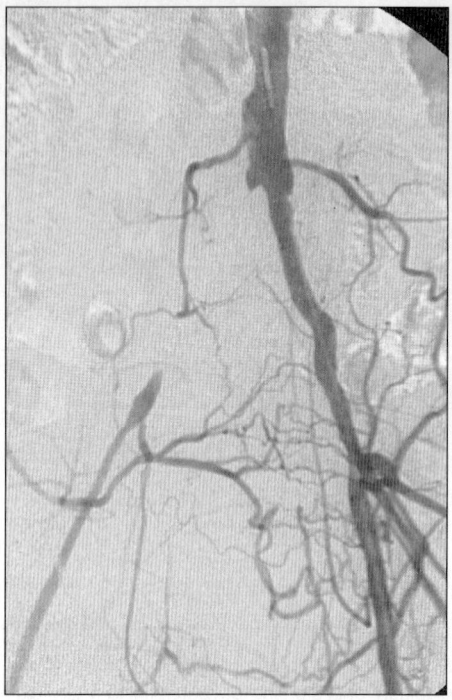

Figure 11-5. Angiogram demonstrating right common iliac artery chronic total occlusion.

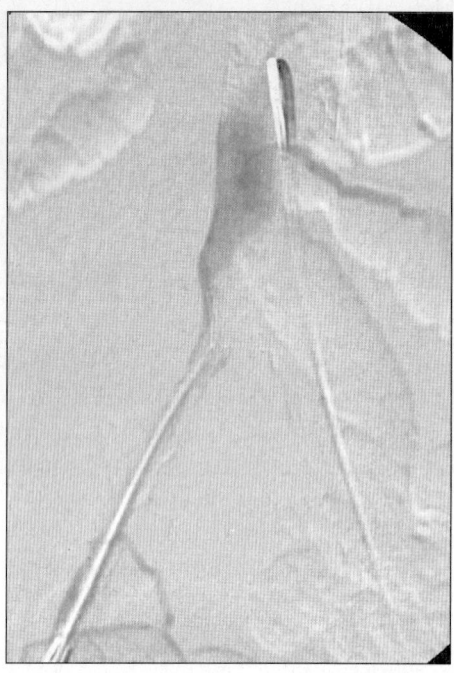

Figure 11-6. Fluoroscopic image of a multipurpose catheter in the subintimal space without true lumen re-entry.

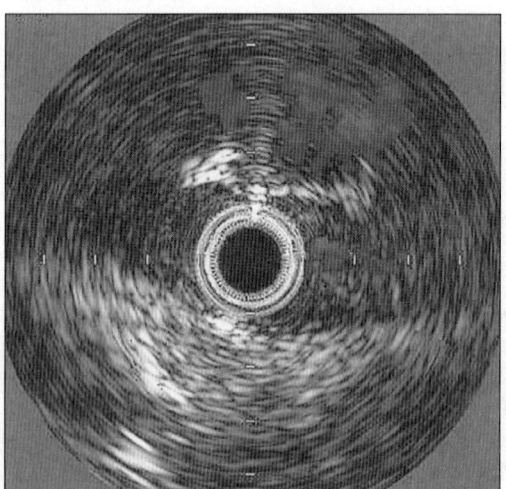

Figure 11-7. Intravascular ultrasound image obtained with Pioneer catheter demonstrating color flow in the true lumen at the 12 o'clock position, adventitia at the 6 o'clock position, and subintimal space at 3 and 9 o'clock.

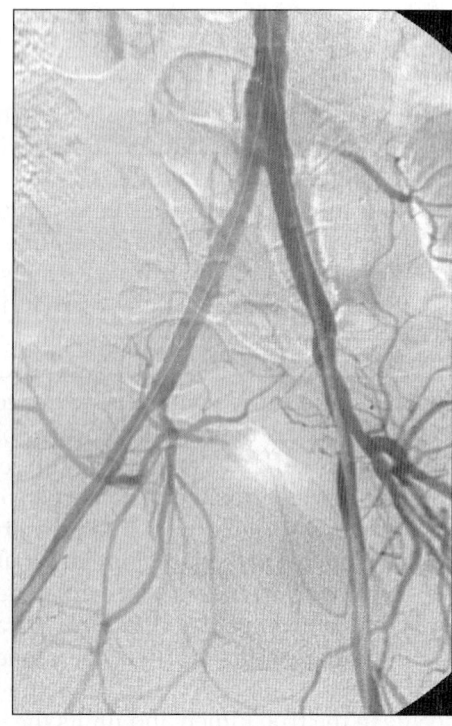

Figure 11-8. Completion angiogram following true lumen re-entry, angioplasty, and stenting of right common iliac chronic total occlusion.

RECONSTRUCTION OF ILIAC CTOs

Patients with CTOs will generally need either a bare metal stent or covered stent for reconstruction. Results with balloon angioplasty alone for occlusions demonstrate a high rate of acute occlusion. Predilatation with either balloons or with dilators may be required to advance the stents across extremely calcified lesions, and the presence of a stiff wire across these lesions will also help in delivering the stents. We generally reserve the use of covered stents to cases of iliac artery rupture. The advent of heparin-coated covered stents may ultimately show improved long-term patency compared to bare metal stents, but this has yet to be demonstrated in clinical trials.

A few caveats are important to mention when discussing actual treatment of the lesion. Balloon oversizing is generally not recommended as it can lead to significant pain and possible rupture. Patients are also not sedated heavily during the procedure as it is important to titrate the balloon inflation according to the patient's tolerance. Pain is an indicator of the adventitial stretching and may herald an arterial rupture. If severe pain is experienced, it is usually prudent to discontinue the balloon inflation or to switch to a balloon with a smaller diameter.

RESULTS OF CTO RECANALIZATION

Although aortobifemoral bypass appears to have better long-term patency than the currently available endovascular strategies for diffuse aortoiliac occlusive disease, the risk of surgery is significantly higher than the risk of an endovascular approach, not only in terms of mortality, but also in terms of major morbidity and delay in return to normal activities.[16] It is also important to understand the patient's general condition and the anatomy of the lesion before deciding which treatment modality is most appropriate, if any.

The technical and initial clinical success of percutaneous transluminal angioplasty (PTA) of iliac stenosis is about 90% in all the major reported literature. This approaches 100% for the focal iliac artery lesions. The technical success rate for recanalization of a long segment iliac occlusion is 80–85%. The recent development of devices used to cross the total occlusions will likely produce even higher technical success rates.[7] Becker et al. found a five-year patency rate of 72% in an analysis of 2,697 cases from the literature, noting even better patency (79%) in patients with claudication.[17] Further, a study by Murphy et al. found a primary patency of 74% after eight years, providing evidence for the durability of iliac artery stenting.[18] The factors that negatively affect the patency of such interventions include poor quality run-off vessels, severe ischemia, and long length of the diseased segments. Female gender has also been suggested to decrease the patency of external iliac artery stents.[19]

In a randomized trial[20] comparing open surgery to angioplasty in symptomatic iliac disease, Wolf et al. suggested that primary success favored open surgery, but limb salvage favored angioplasty, though these differences were not statistically significant. In this study of 263 patients with iliac disease and either rest pain or lifestyle-limiting claudication, participants were randomized to either surgery or angioplasty. There were three deaths in the group that underwent surgery and none in the angioplasty group. Patients in both groups had prompt and sustained improvement in their hemo-dynamics and quality of life. The study strongly favored angioplasty as outcomes between the two treatment groups were no different, but the morbidity or mortality was higher in the open surgical group. Unfortunately, one of the shortcomings of this study was that there were no women in this study.

In a study published by Ballard et al. in 1998 comparing aortoiliac stents versus surgical reconstruction, this group showed that the primary patency for bypass grafts at 30 months was 93% for bypass versus 68% for iliac stents. Further, the cost did not differ significantly between groups in this study. Multivariate analysis of this study identified that regardless of the treatment arm, female patients, patients with superficial femoral artery occlusions, patients who suffered a vascular complication, and patients with hypovolemia were more likely to suffer thrombosis.[21]

Bosch and Hunink et al. performed a meta-analysis of results comparing aortoiliac PTA versus aortoiliac stenting. The results from a database of 2,116 patients suggested the technical success was higher for stenting, whereas the complication rates and predicated mortality rates did not differ significantly. Including the technical failures, the four-year primary patency rates were 65% for PTA and 77% for stenting in patients with stenoses, and 54% for PTA and 61% for stenting in patients with occlusions, respectively. The relative risk of long-term failure was reduced by 39% after stent placement compared to PTA. Bosch et al. suggest that angioplasty with selective stent placement is a cost-effective treatment strategy compared to angioplasty alone in the treatment of intermittent claudication. Unfortunately, the results of this study cannot be applied to TASC-C and D lesions, and in our practice, patients with occlusive disease are treated with stents.[22-23]

COMPLICATIONS OF ILIAC ARTERY ANGIOPLASTY AND STENTING

Access-related problems are the most common complications seen after iliac artery interventions. There can be significant retroperitoneal bleeding without any manifestation in the groin, highlighting the importance of performing a femoral angiogram to confirm common femoral artery puncture below the level of the inguinal ligament. All patients will require close monitoring, not only during the procedure but also for several hours after the procedure.

As mentioned previously, iliac artery rupture is the most worrisome complication seen during these procedures, and several risk factors exist. Heavily calcified lesions should raise some concern for possible rupture following angioplasty. Other less common risk factors include prior mechanical trauma such as a laser recanalization, balloon angioplasty, or even balloon thrombectomy. Regardless of the etiology, recognition of arterial rupture is the most important step in managing the problem

Embolization is another complication and can occur in about 3–7% patients.[24] Primary stenting may reduce the risk of embolization; however, it does not completely eliminate the risk. Embolic material can be thrombus, cholesterol, or plaque material, and the nature of the embolic material often determines the success of the different therapeutic options. Thrombolysis is useful in treating distal embolic material that appears to be thrombus, while it works poorly if the embolic material is plaque. Percutaneous aspiration thrombectomy is a good technique for either thrombus or plaque; however, surgery may be required when percutaneous interventions are unsuccessful, and this possibility must be addressed as part of procedural informed consent.

The number of stent infections is rising with the increasing number of stents placed into the peripheral arterial system. Stent infections are generally recognized to be an underreported entity. Risk factors include multiple catheterizations through the same access site, presence of hematoma, and prolonged operative time. Patients may present with pain, elevated white cell count, bacteremia, and unexplained fever.[25] The patient may also manifest with septic emboli to the legs. This may appear as painful petechiae in the leg or in the hypogastric distribution. Although the patient is suspect of having a skin infection, the management should be very aggressive in terms of systemic antibiotics, possibility of stent excision, and bypass procedures.

CONCLUSIONS

Chronic total occlusions can be difficult lesions to treat in any vascular bed, and despite the TASC recommendations, most patients and many physicians, seem to favor the endovascular option. Technological advances have enabled the recanalization of long segment lesions that were once treated with surgical procedures. The application of these devices and wires is only going to increase due to an aging population with multiple risk factors, making conventional surgical interventions more difficult. What remains to be seen are the long-term results using this technology, and whether or not these devices can be used in a cost-effective manner.

REFERENCES

1. Solomon H, Chao AB, Weaver FA, Katz SG. Change in practice patterns of an academic division of vascular surgery. *Arch Surg.* 2007;142:733–737.
2. Spinosa DJ, Leung DA, Matsumoto AH, et al. Percutaneous intentional extra luminal recanalization in patients with chronic critical limb ischemia. *Radiology.* 2002;232:499–507.
3. Leville CD, Kashyap VS, Clair DG, et al. Endovascular management of iliac occlusions: Extending treatment to transatlantic Inter-societal classification C and D patient's. *J Vasc Surg.* 2006;43:32–39.
4. Jacobs DL, Cox DE, Motaganahalli R. Crossing chronic total occlusions of the iliac and femoral-popliteal vessels and the use of true lumen reentry devices. *Perspect Vasc Surg Endovasc Ther.* 2006;18(1):37–8
5. Murphy TP. *Introduction : Techniques in vascular and interventional radiology.* 2000;3:179
6. Upchurch GR, Dimick JB, Wainess RM, Eliason JL, Henke PK, et al. Diffusion of new technology in health care: the case of aorto-iliac occlusive disease. *Surgery.* 2004;136:812–818.
7. Norgen L, Hiatt W R, Dormandy J A, et al. Inter-Society consensus for the management of peripheral arterial disease (TASC-2). *J Vasc Surg.* 2007;45:S48–S49.
8. Jacobs DL, Motaganahalli R, Cox DE, Wittgen CM, Peterson GJ. True lumen reentry devices facilitate subintimal angioplasty and stenting of total chronic occlusions: Initial report. *J Vasc Surg.* 2006;43:1291–1296.
9. Marks NA, Ascher E, Hingorani AP, Shiferson A, Puggioni A. Gray-scale median of the atherosclerotic plaque can predict success of lumen re-entry during subintimal femoral-popliteal angioplasty. *J Vasc Surg.* 2008;47:109–116.
10. Lenti M, Cieri E, De Rango P, Pozzilli P, Coscarella C, et al. Endovascular treatment of long lesions of the superficial femoral artery: results from a multicenter registry of a spiral, covered polytetrafluoroethylene stent. *J Vasc Surg.* 2007;45:32–39.
11. Lam RC, Shah S, Faries PL, McKinsey JF, Kent KC, Morrissey NJ. Incidence and clinical significance of distal embolization during percutaneous interventions involving the superficial femoral artery. *J Vasc Surg.* 2007;46:1155–1159.

12. Bolia, Brennan J, Bell PR. Recanalisation of femoro-popliteal occlusions: improving success rate by subintimal recanalization. *Clin Radiol.* 1989;40:325.
13. Surowiec SM, Davies MG, Eberly SW, Rhodes JM, Illig KA, et al. Percutaneous angioplasty and stenting of the superficial femoral artery. *J Vasc Surg* 2005;41:269–278.
14. Desgranges P, Boufi M, Lapeyre M, Tarquini G, van Laere O, et al. Subintimal angioplasty: feasible and durable. *Eur J Vasc Endovasc Surg.* 2004;28(2):138–41.
15. Saket RR, Razavi MK, Padidar A, Kee ST, Sze DY, Dake MD. Novel intravascular ultrasound-guided method to create transintimal arterial communications: initial experience in peripheral occlusive disease and aortic dissection. *J Endovasc Ther.* 2004;11:274–280.
16. DeRubertis BG, Faries P, et al. Shifting paradigms in the treatment of lower extremity vascular disease: a report of 1000 percutaneous interventions. *Ann Surg.* 2007;246:415–422.
17. Becker GJ, Katzen BT, Dake MD. Noncoronary angioplasty. *Radiology.* 1989;170:921–940.
18. Murphy TP, Ariaratnam NS, Carney WI Jr et al. Aortoiliac insufficiency: long term experience with stent placement for treatment. *Radiology.* 2004;231:243–249.
19. Timaran CH, Stevens SL, Freeman MB ,Goldman MH, et al. External iliac and common iliac artery angioplasty and stenting in men and women. *J Vasc Surg.* 2001;34:440–446.
20. Wolf GL, Wilson SE, Cross AP, et al. Surgery or balloon angioplasty for peripheral vascular disease: a randomized clinical trial. *J Vasc Inter Rad.* 1993 Sep–Oct;4(5):639–648.
21. Ballard JL, Bergen JJ, Singh P, et al. Aortoiliac stent deployment vs surgical reconstruction: analysis of outcome and cost. *J Vasc Surg.* 1998;28:94–101.
22. Bosch JL, Hunink MG. Stent or PTA in iliac occlusive disease meta analysis of the results of PTA and stent placement in aortoiliac occlusive disease. *Radiology.* 1997;204:87–96.
23. Bosch JL. Iliac artery disease: cost effectiveness analysis of stent placement vs PTA. *Radiology.* 1998;208:641–681.
24. Dyet JF, Gaines PA, Nicholson AA , et al. Treatment of chronic iliac occlusions by means of percutaneous endovascular stent placement. *J Vasc Inter Rad.* 1997;8:349–353.
25. Hogg ME, Peterson BG, Pearce WH, Morasch MD, Kibbe MR. Bare metal stent infections: case report and review of the literature. *J Vasc Surg.* 2007;46:813–820.

12

Angioplasty-based Infrainguinal Percutaneous Interventions

Marvin D. Atkins, M.D. and David C. Brewster, M.D.

Peripheral arterial disease (PAD) of the lower extremities affects an estimated 10 million people in the United States, with an incidence of approximately 20% in patients over 75 years of age. The cornerstones of treatment for PAD are the management of systemic atherosclerosis and prevention of disease progression. Antiplatelet agents, including aspirin and clopidogrel, and reduction of serum cholesterol levels with statins are an important adjunct to reducing cardiovascular morbidity and mortality in PAD patients.[1] Smoking cessation and an exercise program have been shown in several studies to improve claudication.[2] However, the ability to implement and sustain these programs has been difficult.[3] The phosphodiesterase inhibitor cilostazol can improve walking distance in claudicants,[4] and has become an increasingly utilized medication in the medical management of patients with claudication.

The optimal treatment of patients presenting with either critical limb ischemia or failure of the above conservative medical regimen is currently a subject of intense debate. A decision between percutaneous therapy or open surgical bypass is based on various factors including the patient's overall condition, the available evidence regarding anticipated outcomes of open and endovascular therapies, and patient and surgeon preference. However, it is clear that a significant paradigm shift is occurring as percutaneous transluminal angioplasty (PTA) and associated endovascular therapies have been increasingly applied to the treatment of lower extremity occlusive disease in order to reduce the morbidity and mortality associated with open repair.

Open surgical bypass has been the gold standard of treatment for decades and has produced favorable results. Most series of autogenous reversed segment saphenous vein bypass report limb salvage rates greater than 90% at one year.[5,6] Bypass surgery is also a durable procedure with five-year limb salvage rates >80% and primary patency rates of 75%.[7,8] When alternative conduits are required, three-year limb salvage rates of 75% and primary patency rates of 55% have been achieved with prosthetic material.[9]

Open surgical bypass, however, is associated with significant morbidity, up to 25% in some series.[10-12] Recovery following infrainguinal bypass for critical limb ischemia (CLI) can be a lengthy process as well. Goshima et al. reported the time to heal lower extremity wounds exceeded three months in more than half of the patients.[10] Gibbons found the morbidity associated with open repair resulted in less than half of patients returning to normal functional status by six months.[5] One-year mortality in patients undergoing lower extremity bypass approaches 20%, secondary to significant underlying cardiovascular disease and diabetes.[13]

A variety of techniques and devices have been employed for percutaneous lower extremity interventions. In addition, differing strategies and pharmacologic agents have been utilized to hopefully overcome the problems of restenosis and recurrence of disease. Unfortunately, single-center reports with limited case numbers, short-term follow-up, no direct comparisons to currently accepted practices, variations in lesion location and length, and type of intervention performed make meaningful analysis of results impossible. The enthusiasm for several of these endovascular therapies in the lower extremity has exceeded the available data to support many of the purported conclusions. This review will present the current results of catheter-based infrainguinal percutaneous interventions, for both the femoropopliteal and infrapopliteal arterial segments, including our recent series and others. In addition, the available data for some of the novel therapies currently employed in the infrainguinal region will be considered. We conclude with a discussion of the clinical scenarios where we find open surgical therapy to still be the preferred treatment modality.

CLINICAL SERIES

Conrad et al. recently reviewed our results of PTA within the femoropopliteal and tibial arterial segments in 238 patients presenting with chronic lower extremity ischemia treated over a 30-month period at the Massachusetts General Hospital.[14] Excluded from the study were patients presenting with acute limb ischemia, a functionally unsalvageable limb, a threatened bypass graft, or patients requiring thrombectomy or thrombolysis. Fifty-four percent of patients presented with claudication and 46% presented with critical limb ischemia. Patients were categorized according to the Rutherford clinical classification[15] and by TASC lesion anatomy[16] (Table 12–1). TASC classification of the lesions found 11% TASC A, 43% TASC B, 41% TASC C, and 5% TASC D lesions. PTA was technically successful in 230/238 (97%) limbs. Stents were required in 22% of cases secondary to residual stenosis or flow limiting dissection. No deaths were attributable to the PTA procedures. There were six significant complications associated with PTA. These included two groin hematomas requiring transfusion, one thromboembolus requiring thrombolysis, one patient required intubation from pulmonary edema, and finally one SFA rupture and one device malfunction, both of which required conversion to open femoropopliteal bypass.

During follow-up, failures of primary patency occurred in 29% of patients (35% CLI, 23% claudicants). The three-year estimated Kaplan-Meier primary patency rate associated with PTA was 54% (Figure 12–1). The assisted primary patency rate was 92% at three years (Figure 12–2), and limb salvage was achieved in 89% of patients with critical limb ischemia (Figure 12–3). Of the 39 patients with critical limb ischemia and failure of primary patency, 22 patients underwent repeat PTA, 14 patients eventually

TABLE 12-1. MORPHOLOGICAL STRATIFICATION OF FEMOROPOPLITEAL LESIONS ACCORDING TO THE TASC (TRANSATLANTIC INTERSOCIETY CONSENSUS WORKING GROUP) CLASSIFICATION.

TASC type A femoropopliteal lesions

1. Single stenosis less than 3 cm of the superficial femoral artery or popliteal artery.

TASC type B femoropopliteal lesions

1. Single stenosis 3 to 10 cm in length, not involving the distal popliteal artery
2. Heavily calcified stenosis up to 3 cm in length
3. Multiple lesions, each less than 3 cm (stenosis or occlusions)
4. Single or multiple lesions in the absence of continuous tibial runoff to improve inflow for distal surgical bypass

TASC type C femoropopliteal lesions

1. Single stenosis or occlusion longer than 5cm
2. Multiple stenosis or occlusions, each 3 to 5cm in length, with or without heavy calcification

TASC type D femoropopliteal lesions

1. Complete common femoral artery or superficial femoral artery occlusions or complete popliteal and proximal trifurcation occlusions

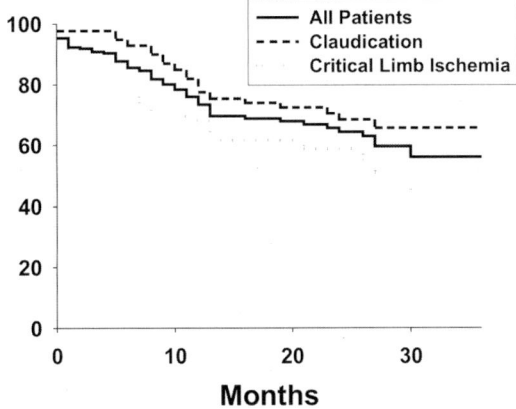

Figure 12-1. Kaplan-Meier curves for primary patency of patients undergoing PTA stratified by presentation.

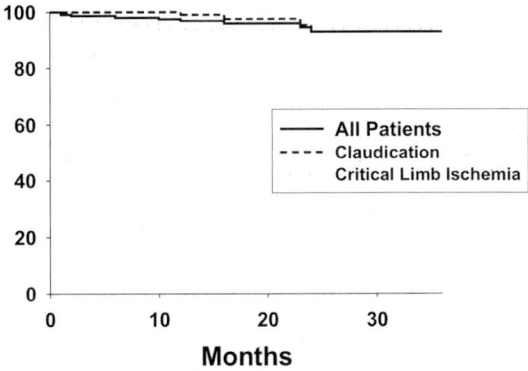

Figure 12-2. Kaplan-Meier curves for assisted patency of patients undergoing PTA stratified by presentation.

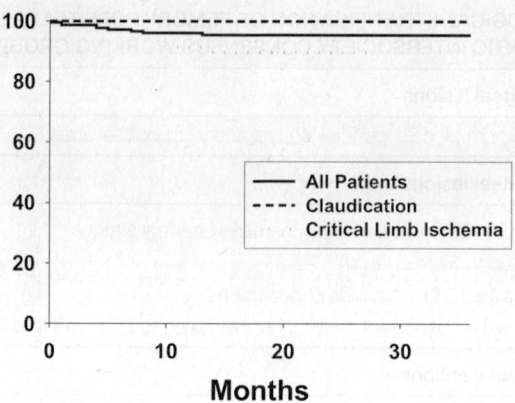

Figure 12-3. Kaplan-Meier curves for limb salvage of patients undergoing PTA stratified by presentation.

required bypass, three patients were observed, and five patients required amputation. As expected, those with claudication alone fared much better. Thirty patients had claudication and failure of primary patency. Fifteen patients required repeat PTA, 10 were observed, and five proceeded to bypass surgery. No claudicants with failure of primary patency experienced limb loss.

Predictors of primary patency failure by univariate and multivariate analysis included congestive heart failure (OR 2.0) and TASC C/D lesions (OR 2.0). Predictors of assisted patency failure included age < 65 (OR 8.3), CHF (OR 7.3), and TASC C/D lesions (OR 7.8). Predictors of limb loss included diabetes (OR 11.4) and CHF (OR 6.7).

We concluded that although primary patency rates remained low, excellent assisted patency and limb salvage rates could be achieved with careful follow-up and appropriate reintervention. Although patients with TASC C/D lesions and CHF had the worst results, the assisted patency and limb salvage rates were acceptable to justify PTA as the first line therapy in this cohort of patients. We found, as well as others, that PTA and/or other interventions did not preclude a subsequent surgical bypass. Currently, we recommend PTA as the first line therapy for most patients requiring lower extremity revascularization.

INFRAPOPLITEAL PTA RESULTS

Most patients requiring infrapopliteal intervention have limb-threatening ischemia, multilevel disease, and/or diffuse tibial lesions. Therefore, limb salvage rather than patency has been used most often to assess results. Patients presenting with critical limb ischemia usually have significant underlying diabetes, coronary disease, and renal failure, placing them at higher risk for open surgery. An endovascular solution is preferred in order to minimize morbidity and mortality in this high-risk cohort. The feasibility and technical success of infrapopliteal interventions has increased with the advent of .018 and .014 compatible low profile catheters. For success to be achieved, proper patient selection is critical. Patients with an ischemic foot due to a single focal tibial lesion interrupting flow do much better than patients with diffuse tibial disease or occlusions.

The majority of series examining infrapopliteal PTA is confounded by simultaneous interventions in the iliac or superficial femoral arteries, making direct comparisons impossible. However, an attempt at angioplasty appears justified before primary amputation and before surgical bypass in those patients at high risk for intervention.

NITINOL SELF-EXPANDING STENTS

The femoropopliteal segment is affected by a multitude of forces, which have limited the results of PTA and stenting in this region. These include significant extrinsic compressive forces with knee flexion, changes in arterial length, torsion, and flexion.[17] When stenting is required, these forces have caused significant stent fractures, which have been correlated with the development of recurrent arterial stenosis and occlusion.[18]

Mechanical compression of balloon-expandable stents led to the preferential use of self-expanding stents in the SFA and popliteal arteries. Initial results with stainless steel self-expanding stents were not very good, but more recent results with Nitinol self-expanding stents show promise. Nitinol is an alloy composed of equal parts of nickel and titanium. The elasticity and thermal shape memory properties of nitinol are more resistant to compression, and allows it to conform to tortuous vascular anatomy. However, nitinol stents still are complicated by problems of stent fracture and intimal hyperplasia. Clearly, the ideal stent design is still lacking.

Four prospective, randomized trials of femoropopliteal stent placement revealed no improvement in long-term patency compared with PTA alone. All of these trials involved balloon-expandable stents; therefore, the results may not reflect the current generation of self-expanding nitinol stents that are used by most interventionalists.

The largest experience with nitinol stents in the SFA is with the SMART nitinol self-expanding stent (Cordis). Mewissen evaluated the SMART stent in 125 limbs with either TASC B or C lesions. The hemodynamic primary stent patency rates were 92%, 76%, 66%, and 60% at 6, 12, 18, and 24 months, respectively.[19]

Currently, there is only one published prospective randomized study examining nitinol stents versus PTA in the SFA. Schillinger et al. examined the results of 104 patients (90% claudicants) randomized to PTA or self-expanding Dynalink or Absolute (Guidant) nitinol stents.[20] The mean lesion lengths were > 12cm in both groups and secondary stenting was required in 32% of the PTA group. At 12 months, duplex ultrasound documented restenosis in 37% of the nitinol stent group and 63% in the PTA group, and the restenosis was confirmed by subsequent angiography. Stent fractures at a year were identified in only 2% of patients. Based on these results, nitinol stents do appear to have a decreased fracture rate compared to other stents. Although these early results are promising, long-term data are needed to support the conclusion that primary nitinol stenting is superior to PTA of the SFA.

In summary, the intermediate term data for nitinol stents are promising as the one- and two-year primary patency rates appear superior to those for PTA and for first generation balloon-expandable stents. The durability of those results must be compared in randomized trials such as the ongoing RESILIANT trial using the Edwards Lifestent NT. Until such results are more definitive, we use nitinol stents selectively to treat post-PTA dissection or residual stenosis to avoid imminent occlusion.

NOVEL TECHNOLOGIES AND TECHNIQUES FOR INFRAINGUINAL PERCUTANEOUS INTERVENTIONS

Subintimal Angioplasty

The subintimal angioplasty technique involves the intentional creation of and entry into a dissection plane created just proximal to the occlusion using an angled glidewire and a stiff catheter. The glidewire typically forms a loop that is passed beyond the occlusion. The true lumen is then reentered, followed by PTA. Technical success rates vary significantly among operators and reentry is usually the limiting step in the technique. Several devices have been marketed to assist with reentry into the true lumen, including the Outback catheter (Cordis) and Pioneer catheter (Medtronic). The Pioneer catheter has the addition of an intravascular ultrasound probe to assist with finding the true lumen for needle puncture. These devices may be useful in limited situations following unsuccessful conventional attempts at true lumen reentry.

The one-year primary patency rates for subintimal angioplasty in the treatment of femoropopliteal disease range from 53% to 92%, with the majority of centers reporting patency rates <70%.[21] We do not routinely (or intentionally) use the subintimal angioplasty technique in the vast majority of cases and try to remain in the true lumen whenever possible.

Directed Excisional Atherectomy Devices

Percutaneous rotational atherectomy, once popularized in the early 1990s with the Simpson Athero-Cath, has seen resurgence with the development of the Silver-Hawk plaque excision system (FoxHollow, Redwood City, California). The basic principle behind such atherectomy devices are to debulk the offending plaque rather than fracturing it or displacing it, as with PTA and stenting. Percutaneous rotational atherectomy has been advocated in certain settings where the results of PTA and stenting have been suboptimal. These include lesions in areas of flexion or compression such as the common femoral artery, the adductor hiatus, and the popliteal artery. Other potential uses for atherectomy include areas of in-stent restenosis. This has been a notoriously difficult clinical problem to treat and may benefit from debulking the intimal hyperplastic response. Long lesions within the tibial vessels respond poorly to PTA and stenting, and atherectomy may have a role here as well.

Although conceptually attractive, the data supporting the Silver-Hawk device as a durable treatment are at this time lacking. FoxHollow has created the TALON (Treating Peripherals with Silver-Hawk: Outcomes Collection) registry, which is an observational, nonrandomized, multicenter, self-reporting registry. Several have questioned the validity of data in a self-reporting registry method. The TALON investigators recently presented data for the use of the Silver-Hawk device in 69 patients with critical limb ischemia.[22] Six-month follow-up data revealed a 4% reintervention rate and a 92% limb salvage rate. All of the available series concerning the device have focused on rates of initial technical success and short-term outcomes.

Problems with the technology include the relative expense of the device (~$2,900) and the fact that multiple devices may be required. The catheter is cumbersome, requiring multiple passes, and emptying the chamber is time-consuming. There is the potential for distal embolization, seen in several studies using a distal filter wire, although the clinical significance of such embolization is unknown. The device also requires a large 6 or 7 Fr sheath.

The Silver-Hawk plaque excision device appears to have high rates of initial technical success and short-term limb salvage rates. Further recommendations on the role of atherectomy using the Silver-Hawk device remain undefined until well-designed, unbiased randomized trials present data in a peer-reviewed fashion.

Excimer Laser-assisted Angioplasty

Excimer laser-assisted angioplasty uses flexible fiber-optic catheters to deliver short pulses of ultraviolet (UV) energy to ablate plaque and thrombus with a purported decreased risk of distal atheroembolization. The laser is used to establish a channel for subsequent PTA or other intervention. Data from the recently reported Laser Angioplasty for Critical Limb Ischemia (LACI) multicenter trial[23] suggests that excimer laser-assisted angioplasty results in a high rate of limb salvage (93%) at six months in patients with critical limb ischemia who were not candidates for bypass surgery. Long-term patency results for CLI may not be as relevant because the expected mortality in this patient population of 14%, 21%, and 32% at 6, 12, and 24 months respectively.[16]

The Peripheral Excimer Laser Angioplasty (PELA) trial was a U.S. and European multicenter randomized study comparing the results of excimer laser angioplasty versus PTA for long SFA occlusions.[24] No difference was found between the two groups in crossing success, adjunctive use of stents, residual stenosis, or procedural success. A reintervention rate of 57% was similar between the two groups at one year. Ultrasound follow-up at a year found no difference in the rate of vessel reocclusion (22% vs. 16%).

Excimer laser-assisted angioplasty appears to have a limited role in the armamentarium for peripheral interventions. The small laser size results in a 2.5mm channel, which requires adjuvant balloon angioplasty to achieve an adequate lumen. The device may have a role in successfully crossing chronic total occlusions.

Covered Stent Grafts

Covered stent grafts have been placed within the superficial femoral artery in order to combat problems with intimal hyperplasia and restenosis. The Viabahn (W.L. Gore, Flagstaff, Arizona) covered stent graft is currently the only approved device for use in the SFA. The ePTFE lining of the Viabahn device inhibits ingrowth of intimal hyperplasia. Failures of the device have been seen at the ends of the graft, referred to as candy wrapper stenosis. There appears to be a decreased risk of stent fractures with the ePTFE lining. The implications of the design feature are that the length of treated lesion may be a less consistent predictor of failure than bare-metal stents. Jahnke et al.[25] reported the results of a prospective, nonrandomized trial of the Viabahn device for treatment of TASC B and C lesions in 52 patients. Primary patency was 74% at two years with an assisted primary patency rate of 80%. Several series document mid- and long-term SFA primary patency outcomes for Viabahn that appear better than the results of PTA or Nitinol stenting alone.[26,27] Problems with the device include the large sheath size (8 F sheath to deploy a 6 mm Viabahn) and the unavoidable coverage of branch vessels.

W.L. Gore is currently sponsoring the Viabahn versus Bare Nitinol Stent (VIBRANT) trial. This trial randomizes patients with TASC C and D lesions to treatment with Viabahn or nitinol stents. The trial is recruiting 150 patients with plans for three-year duplex ultrasound documented follow-up. This trial will hopefully shed further light on treatment of difficult TASC C and D lesions. At present, the large profile delivery system of the Viabahn and coverage of collateral vessels have limited our use of this device in the superficial femoral artery.

Drug-eluting Stents

Drug-eluting stents (DES) in the coronary arteries have proven to be a success in the struggle against intimal hyperplasia and in-stent restenosis. The application of DES technology to the periphery was expected to be a panacea for the problem of late in-stent restenosis. The combined SIROCCO I and II trials compared the results of 93 patients with bare nitinol stents to sirolimus-eluting nitinol stent in the superficial femoral artery. At 24 months, there was no difference in restenosis (~25%), ABI, or Rutherford classification. The ongoing Zilver PTX trial will investigate the Zilver PTX paclitaxel-eluting stent in the above knee SFA. Following the Phase I feasibility study, the Phase II trial plans to randomize between PTA and the Zilver PTX stent. PTA failures will randomize to bare Zilver or Zilver PTX stents.

At present, the results of available trials suggest that DES is not superior to standard PTA or stenting. However, issues regarding optimal dosing and platform (polymer coating, nitinol) for DES are areas of ongoing research with this technology.

Cryotherapy

The cryoplasty technique was designed to address the primary problems of PTA, namely, dissection, recoil, and restenosis, by combining PTA with the delivery of cold thermal energy to the vessel wall. The prolonged inflation with nitrous oxide combined with freezing of the vessel wall has several theoretical advantages. The incidence of dissection is thought to be limited, freezing altars the elastin fiber properties of the vessel wall limiting recoil, and induction of smooth muscle cell apoptosis inhibits intimal hyperplasia. There is a paucity of clinical trials evaluating the success of cryoplasty to support the above theoretical advantages; however, initial reports are encouraging.

Laird et al. recently reported the midterm results of the 70 patients participating in the initial investigational device exemption (IDE) study for the PolarCath device (Boston Scientific).[28] They found low rates of dissection (6.9%) and of bailout stenting associated with the device (8.8%). The clinical patency rate (freedom from target vessel revascularization) was 83% at nine months and remained at 75% after 3.4 years.

Although the results of cryoplasty are promising, the results of large, randomized trial with long-term follow-up are lacking.

Cutting Balloon Angioplasty (CBA)

Cutting balloons employ three or four fixed atherotome blades to cut into atherosclerotic plaque, creating a controlled dissection. Its theoretical advantages are that it allows for lower inflation pressures, which can limit vascular injury and distal dissection during treatment. The data regarding cutting balloon angioplasty are limited, especially for native femoropopliteal disease. CBA has found a role mostly for in-stent restenosis, hemodialysis access, and vein graft stenosis. Ansel et al. reported their results of CBA in 73 patients with popliteal and infrapopliteal disease.[29] They reported 100% technical success; however, 20% required adjunctive stenting. The one-year limb salvage rate was 89.5%, similar to several series reporting conventional PTA. As long-term data are insufficient to determine the efficacy of cutting balloon angioplasty, this technique plays a limited role in our practice. In general, we employ cutting balloons for in-stent and vein graft restenoses.

FUTURE DIRECTIONS: BIODEGRADABLE STENTS

Foreign body reaction to the stent material likely plays a significant role in the pathogenesis of the intimal hyperplastic response that has limited the mid- and long-term results of stenting in the infrainguinal region. Stenting technology is moving toward the development of temporary implants composed of biodegradable materials, which mechanically support the vessel wall to seal dissection and prevent recoil over the short term. Following vessel wall healing from the initial angioplasty injury, the stent completely biodegrades over a six-week period. Bioabsorbable magnesium stents are currently in development for use in the coronary and peripheral arteries. The slow release of magnesium over a six-week period following deployment is thought to have antithrombotic and antifibroproliferative effects. This promising technology may take advantage of the short-term benefits seen with stenting without the drawbacks of late intimal hyperplasia, recurrent stenosis, and failure. Peeters et al. recently reported their short-term feasibility study of an absorbable magnesium stent in 20 patients with infrapopliteal lesions and critical limb ischemia.[30] Procedural success was 100%, clinical patency at three months was 89.5%, and all patients avoided amputation.

WHEN IS OPEN SURGERY STILL THE BEST OPTION?

Although we have found PTA to be a viable treatment modality in lower extremity arterial occlusive disease, its clinical utility and treatment durability remains a subject of debate under certain clinical circumstances. Clinical scenarios in which we recommend surgical revascularization as the primary treatment modality include (1) common femoral disease and (2) long segment (>10cm) or heavily calcified SFA occlusions (Figure 12–4). The compressive forces of hip flexion significantly limit PTA in the inguinal area, especially when secondary stenting is required. We have found the morbidity of a common femoral endarterectomy with patch angioplasty to be minimal and, therefore, have used open surgical therapy here with good results.

In reviewing our PTA results in the femoropopliteal segment, only 5% of patients had TASC D lesions. We have treated long segment and heavily calcified SFA occlusions, preferentially with open surgical bypass, and attempt PTA only in those patients who are poor surgical candidates.

Others have included multivessel disease with tissue loss or gangrene, popliteal artery disease, and diffuse tibial vessel occlusive disease as indications for first line surgical interventions.[31] Although we acknowledge the short-term durability and inferior results of endovascular therapy associated with these difficult clinical circumstances, these patients usually present with significant cardiovascular disease and diabetes, often warranting an initial attempt at PTA. Long-term patency rates in the

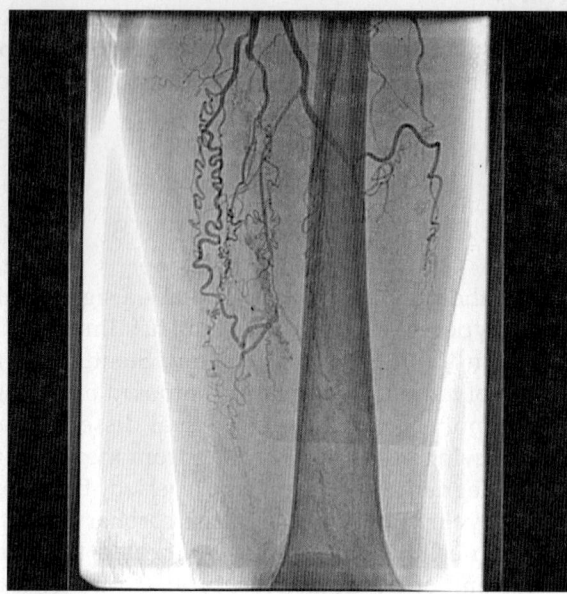

Figure 12-4. Long, calcified chronic total occlusion of the SFA in a 55-year-old man presenting with rest pain. The popliteal artery reconstitutes at the knee. This lesion is best treated by surgical bypass with reversed segment saphenous vein graft.

patient with tissue loss and CLI are less important than the clinical response to wound healing. The majority of these interventions will result in limb salvage and freedom from open surgical intervention in a patient population that is at high risk for morbidity and mortality from their underlying medical comorbidities.

CONCLUSIONS

Percutaneous infrainguinal endovascular interventions have become our first line treatment in most patients presenting with critical limb ischemia and failures of conservative treatment for claudication. The success of PTA has been correlated with a variety of anatomical factors and clinical presentations. The best results are achieved in nonocclusive short lesions in proximal, high-flow vessels. Patients with single or no runoff vessels do poorly. Patients presenting with claudication do much better than those with critical limb ischemia or tissue loss. PTA is rapidly supplanting open surgical bypass as the first line treatment for native infrainguinal disease based on its safety, technical feasibility, and the fact that a failed PTA rarely precludes subsequent surgical bypass.

We have not found atherectomy, cutting balloon angioplasty, cryoplasty, laser, or covered stent grafts to be necessary for the vast majority of cases. Until well-designed trials show a significant benefit justifying the extra expense and associated drawbacks to any of the above technologies, we will continue to employ PTA as our mainstay treatment with nitinol stenting reserved for flow limiting dissection or residual stenosis.

REFERENCES

1. Grundy SM, Balady GJ, Criqui MH, et al. Primary prevention of coronary heart disease: guidance from Framingham: a statement for healthcare professionals from the AHA Task Force on Risk Reduction. American Heart Association. *Circulation*. 1998;97(18):1876–1887.
2. Hiatt WR, Regensteiner JG, Hargarten ME, et al. Benefit of exercise conditioning for patients with peripheral arterial disease. *Circulation*. 1990;81(2):602–609.
3. Fiore MC, McCarthy DE, Jackson TC, et al. Integrating smoking cessation treatment into primary care: an effectiveness study. *Prev Med*. 2004;38(4):412–420.
4. Money SR, Herd JA, Isaacsohn JL, et al. Effect of cilostazol on walking distances in patients with intermittent claudication caused by peripheral vascular disease. *J Vasc Surg*. 1998; 27(2):267–74; discussion 74–75.
5. Gibbons GW, Burgess AM, Guadagnoli E, et al. Return to well-being and function after infrainguinal revascularization. *J Vasc Surg*. 1995;21(1):35–44; discussion.
6. Faries PL, LoGerfo FW, Hook SC, et al. The impact of diabetes on arterial reconstructions for multilevel arterial occlusive disease. *Am J Surg*. 2001;181(3):251–255.
7. Akbari CM, Pomposelli FB, Jr., Gibbons GW, et al. Lower extremity revascularization in diabetes: late observations. *Arch Surg*. 2000;135(4):452–456.
8. Kram HB GS, Veith FJ, et al. Late results of two hundred seventeen femoropopliteal bypasses to isolated popliteal artery segments. *J Vasc Surg*. 1991;14:386–390.
9. Robinson BI FJ, Tomlinson P, et al. A prospective randomized multicentre comparison of expanded polytetrafluoroethylene and gelatin-sealed knitted Dacron graft for femoropopliteal bypass. *Cardiovasc Surg*. 1999(7):214–218.
10. Goshima KR, Mills JL, Sr., Hughes JD. A new look at outcomes after infrainguinal bypass surgery: traditional reporting standards systematically underestimate the expenditure of effort required to attain limb salvage. *J Vasc Surg*. 2004;39(2):330–335.
11. Perler BA. Cost-efficacy issues in the treatment of peripheral vascular disease: primary amputation or revascularization for limb-threatening ischemia. *J Vasc Interv Radiol*. 1995;6(6 Pt 2 Su):111S–115S.
12. Treiman GS, Copland S, Yellin AE, et al. Wound infections involving infrainguinal autogenous vein grafts: a current evaluation of factors determining successful graft preservation. *J Vasc Surg*. 2001;33(5):948–954.
13. Hunink MG, Wong JB, Donaldson MC, et al. Revascularization for femoropopliteal disease. A decision and cost-effectiveness analysis. *JAMA*. 1995;274(2):165–171.
14. Conrad MF, Cambria, RP, Stone, DH, et al. Intermediate results of percutaneous endovascular therapy for femoropopliteal occlusive disease. A contemporary series. *J Vasc Surg*. 2006; In Press.
15. Rutherford RB, Baker JD, Ernst C, et al. Recommended standards for reports dealing with lower extremity ischemia: revised version. *J Vasc Surg*. 1997;26(3):517–538.
16. Dormandy JA, Rutherford RB. Management of peripheral arterial disease (PAD). TASC Working Group. TransAtlantic Inter-Society Concensus (TASC). *J Vasc Surg*. 2000;31(1 Pt 2):S1–S296.
17. Diaz JA, Villegas M, Tamashiro G, et al. Flexions of the popliteal artery: dynamic angiography. *J Invasive Cardiol*. 2004;16(12):712–715.
18. Scheinert D, Scheinert S, Sax J, et al. Prevalence and clinical impact of stent fractures after femoropopliteal stenting. *J Am Coll Cardiol*. 2005;45(2):312–315.
19. Mewissen MW. Self-expanding nitinol stents in the femoropopliteal segment: technique and mid-term results. *Tech Vasc Interv Radiol*. 2004;7(1):2–5.
20. Schillinger M, Sabeti S, Loewe C, et al. Balloon angioplasty versus implantation of nitinol stents in the superficial femoral artery. *N Engl J Med*. 2006;354(18):1879–88.
21. Treiman GS. Subintimal angioplasty for infrainguinal occlusive disease. *Surg Clin North Am*. 2004;84(5):1365–1380, viii.
22. Kandzari DE, Kiesz RS, Allie D, et al. Procedural and clinical outcomes with catheter-based plaque excision in critical limb ischemia. *J Endovasc Ther*. 2006;13(1):12–22.

23. Laird JR, Zeller T, Gray BH, et al. Limb salvage following laser-assisted angioplasty for critical limb ischemia: results of the LACI multicenter trial. *J Endovasc Ther*. 2006;13(1):1–11.

24. Laird JR. Peripheral excimer laser angioplasty (PELA) trial results. In: *Transcatheter Cardiovascular Therapeutics Annual Meeting*; 2002 September, 2002; Washington, D.C.; 2002.

25. Jahnke T, Andresen R, Muller-Hulsbeck S, et al. Hemobahn stent-grafts for treatment of femoropopliteal arterial obstructions: midterm results of a prospective trial. *J Vasc Interv Radiol*. 2003;14(1):41–51.

26. Saxon RR, Coffman JM, Gooding JM, et al. Long-term results of ePTFE stent-graft versus angioplasty in the femoropopliteal artery: single center experience from a prospective, randomized trial. *J Vasc Interv Radiol*. 2003;14(3):303–311.

27. Chopra P. 3Use of the Viabahn Stent Graft for PVD in the Femoropopliteal Arterial Segment. *Endovasc Today*. 2005(Supplement: Achieving Success in the SFA):4–8.

28. Laird JR, Biamino G, McNamara T, et al. Cryoplasty for the treatment of femoropopliteal arterial disease: extended follow-up results. *J Endovasc Ther*. 2006;13 Suppl 2:II52–59.

29. Ansel GM, Sample NS, Botti IC, Jr., et al. Cutting balloon angioplasty of the popliteal and infrapopliteal vessels for symptomatic limb ischemia. *Catheter Cardiovasc Interv* 2004;61(1):1–4.

30. Peeters P, Bosiers M, Verbist J, Deloose K, Heublein B. Preliminary results after application of absorbable metal stents in patients with critical limb ischemia. *J Endovasc Ther* 2005;12(1):1–5.

31. Kougias P. When is Surgery Still the Best Option? *Endovascular Today* 2006;5(3):78–84.

13

Remote Superficial Femoral Artery Endarterectomy

David Rosenthal, M.D., John D. Martin, M.D., Peter J. Schubart, M.D., and Eric D. Wellons, M.D.

The advent of "minimally invasive procedures" such as percutaneous transluminal angioplasty with or without stent, laser-assisted balloon angioplasty, and atherectomy, whose results have proved disappointing in the treatment of long-segment (> more than 15cm) SFA occlusive disease, stimulated a reassessment of SFA endarterectomy. With the evolution of remote superficial femoral artery endarterectomy (RSFAE), a minimally invasive technique became available that could be performed through a single incision, and allowed "debulking" of the arterial plaque, and placement of an endovascular stent.

We report results of RSFAE in an initial trial, results of RSFAE in concert with the aSpire stent that is a flexible ePTFE covered Nitinol stent with significant radial strength to withstand torsional stresses at the knee joint, and RSFAE and distal vein bypass for limb salvage.

The Portuguese surgeon Cid Dos Santos reported the first successful "desobstruction" of an atherosclerotic superficial femoral artery (SFA) in 1947 by removing the diseased inner layer of the artery wall and termed this procedure *thromboendarterectomy*.[1] Despite early promising results, the popularity of SFA endarterectomy waxed and waned, and the technique was gradually abandoned as published reports demonstrated that saphenous vein above-knee femoral popliteal (AKFP) bypass offered superior patency rates that were superior to those of SFA endarterectomy.[2, 3]

The advent, however, of "minimally invasive procedures" such as percutaneous transluminal angioplasty (PTA) with or without stent, laser-assisted balloon angioplasty, and atherectomy, the results of which have been disappointing in treatment of long-segment (> 15 cm) SFA occlusive disease, stimulated a reassessment of SFA endarterectomy.[4-8] Two reports in 1993 utilized a semiclosed endarterectomy technique with a ring stripper that achieved patency rates similar to those of AKFP bypass.[9, 10] Although this procedure required two incisions, it avoided the use of prosthetic grafts and/or harvesting of the saphenous vein, which could be used for subsequent cardiovascular or peripheral reconstructions. With the evolution of the remote superficial femoral artery endarterectomy (RSFAE) technique reported by Ho and Moll et al, a minimally invasive procedure became available that was performed through a single incision, allowed "debulking" of the arterial plaque, and placement of an endovascular stent.[11]

The aSpire stent® (Vascular Architects, San Jose, CA) (Figure 13–1) is an ePTFE covered nitinol stent, is flexible, yet has significant radial strength to withstand torsional stresses at the knee joint, seems ideal to use in concert with RSFAE. After the stent is placed across the endarterectomy end-point, it may be adjusted for diameter and length. For example, if the stent is not in satisfactory position (i.e. covering a collateral), it can be repositioned by "wrapping" it back down to a low profile and re-expanded, thereby, preserving major collaterals at the distal end-point.

The purpose of this chapter was to examine the medium-term results of RSFAE, RSFAE and distal aSpire stenting, and RSFAE and distal vein bypass for limb salvage.

RSFAE PHASE

Between March 1996 and September 2000, 60 patients underwent RSFAE as part of a retrospective multicenter study. Forty-six patients were men, and the mean patient age was 66.2 years (range, 49–81 years). The indications for operation were claudication in 52 patients and limb salvage in eight patients. Twenty-eight patients (46.7%) had a history of cigarette smoking, 29 (48.3%) had hypertension, 26 (43.3%) had diabetes mellitus, and 21 (35.0%) had coronary artery disease.

The technique for RSFAE has been previously described by Ho and Moll.[11] In summary, the SFA is exposed through a small groin incision; the common, proximal profunda femoral arteries may be exposed as well, if an open endarterectomy is necessary. After systemic heparin administration, an arteriotomy is made from the origin of the SFA distally and an endarterectomy is started between the inner and outer media. This intimal core is transversely cut at the SFA origin and threaded into the loop of a conventional ring stripper (Vollmar Dissectar, Aesalap, San Jose, CA). Under fluoroscopic surveillance, the ring stripper is advanced distally down the SFA beyond the

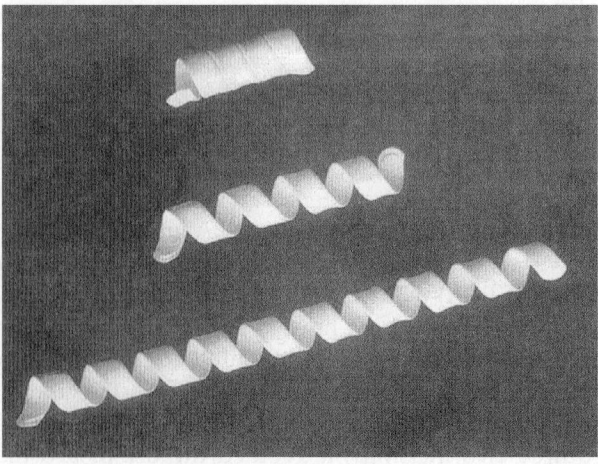

Figure 13-1. aSpire Stent.

occluded segment, the location of which has been determined by intraoperative arteriography. The ring stripper is exchanged for the MollRing Cutter device (Vascular Architects, San Jose, CA), which transects the distal atheroma core under fluoroscopic surveillance. The entire core is removed, and arteriography is performed to confirm a patent distal artery (Figure 13–2).

Under fluoroscopic guidance, a guidewire is passed across the distal SFA endarterectomy end-point and balloon/stent angioplasty is performed, "tacking" the distal plaque to prevent further dissection (Figure 13–2). Completion arteriography verifies RSFAE patency and any outflow tract obstruction. Loose debris, visualized by arteriography, may be removed with a Fogarty embolectomy or graft thrombectomy catheter (Edwards Life Sciences, Vascular Division, Irvine, CA) and the arteriotomy may be extended proximally to perform an open endarterectomy of the common femoral and/or profunda femoris ostia, as necessary.

Technical success was defined as any recanalization of an occlusive lesion on completion arteriography. All patients underwent clinical evaluation during the 30-day postoperative period with duplex color-flow ultrasound scanning. The patients were followed at three-, six-, and 12-month intervals, and at six-month intervals thereafter with color-flow duplex ultrasound scanning. Restenosis was considered significant if peak systolic velocity was higher than 300 cm/sec or the velocity ratio was greater than 3.4. RSFAE patency was confirmed with duplex scan or arteriographic evaluation. The primary end-point was any occlusion and/or radiologic or surgical intervention before occlusion. Cumulative primary and primary assisted patency rates were calculated by the actuarial life table method based on number of procedures performed. Because the study was retrospective in nature, all statistical analyses must be guarded.

RESULTS

Sixty patients underwent RSFAE and the mean length of endarterectomized SFA was 22.3 cm (range 8–37 cm). In 32 patients, a common femoral and profunda femoris ostia

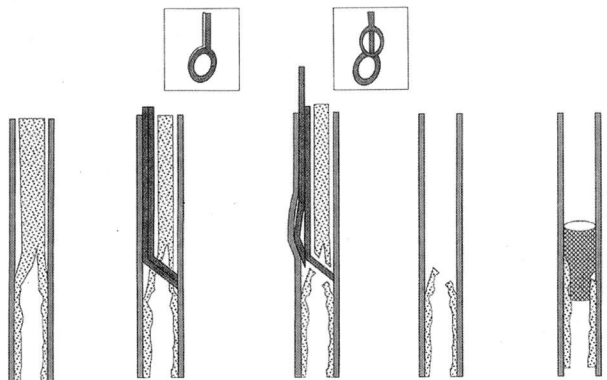

Figure 13-2. Diagram to illustrate the current technique of remote endarterectomy. **A.** Endarterectomy has been performed by ring-stripper (not shown) just distal to end of occlusion. **B.** MollRing cutter passed to same position in endarterectomy plane (inset shows ring cutter closed). **C.** Ring cutter transects atheroma at chosen level (inset shows the relative movement of rings). **D.** Atheromatous core removed proximally leaving free edge of cut atheroma. **E.** Diagrammatic representation of Palmez stent in position. (Reprinted from *Eur J Vasc.* and *Endovasc Surg.* 1998;16:254–258 with permission from WB Saunders.)

endarterectomy was performed as well. Completion arteriography demonstrated residual SFA thrombus in five cases, which was successfully removed with a Fogarty embolectomy catheter. In two other cases, arteriography demonstrated residual fractured plaque; this was removed with a Fogarty graft thrombectomy catheter. Three patients had extravasation of contrast at completion of arteriography that was self-limiting and required no intervention. Thirty-nine of the 60 arteriotomies were closed by patch angioplasty (16 with autogenous vein and 23 with prosthetic patch material).

The primary cumulative patency rate by life table analysis was 61.4% 9% (SE), (mean, 12.9 months; range, three to 36 months). Repeat radiologic intervention was necessary in 14 patients (nine PTA, five stent angioplasty), for a primary assisted patency rate of 82.6% ± 8%. The locations of the stenoses after RSFAE included six that were over the course of the SFA and four at the adductor canal in long (> 20 cm) endarterectomies, two at the SFA origin, and two at the distal stent. One below-knee amputation was performed during follow-up in a patient who was diabetic and dialysis-dependent with gangrene of the forefoot. He underwent successful RSFAE, but amputation was necessary despite a patent SFA endarterectomy. There were no deaths and one wound complication (hematoma), and the mean hospital length of stay (LOS) was 1.4 days ± 0.8 days. The ankle brachial indices rose from 0.61 (± 0.16) preoperatively to 0.97 (± 0.05) postoperatively.

RSFAE AND DISTAL ASPIRE STENTING

Between October 2000 and July 2003, 40 patients underwent RSFAE and distal aSpire stenting. All patients had documented SFA occlusions greater than 13 cm in length (TASC C) and were considered candidates for a revascularization operation. RSFAE was selected when the proximal popliteal artery was larger than 4 mm in diameter. The indications for operation were assessed using the "suggested standards for reports dealing with lower extremity ischemia" by Rutherford et al.[12] Twenty-eight patients were men, and the mean age was 64.3 (range, 43–78 years). The indications for operation were claudication in 36 patients and limb salvage in four patients. Eighteen (45.0%) had a history of cigarette smoking, 17 (42.5%) had hypertension, 16 (40.0%) had diabetes mellitus, and 13 (32.5%) had coronary artery disease.

RSFAE was performed similarly to the previous study, but the outflow track was "tacked" with the aSpire stent. All patients underwent clinical evaluation after operation, evaluation for restenosis and calculation for primary and assisted primary patency rates identical to the previous study. Prior to discharge, six patients began Plavix 75 gms and 14 patients a baby aspirin once daily.

RESULTS

The indications for operation (SVS/ISCVS-NA criteria) in the 40 patients were chronic lower extremity ischemia Category 1–3 in 36, and Category 4–5 in four patients. The mean length of endarterectomized SFAs was 26.2 cm (range, 13–41 cm), and in eight patients, a common femoral and profunda femoris endarterectomy was also performed. Completion arteriography demonstrated SFA thrombus or fractured plaque in four cases, which was successfully removed with a balloon embolectomy catheter. Twenty-six (65.0%) of the arteriotomies were closed by patch angioplasty (16 with prosthetic patch material and nine with autogenous vein). All stents were placed at the endarterectomy end-point across the residual popliteal plaque. Forty-six stents were placed in 40 patients: 29 stents were 6 mm diameter x 5 cm length, and 17 were 7 mm × 5 cm.

The primary cumulative patency rate by means of life table analysis was 68.6% ± 13.5% (SE) at 18 months (mean, 13.2 months; range, 1–31 months) (Table 13–1) (Figure 13–3). Repeat radiologic intervention was necessary in six patients (four PTA, two stent angioplasty), for a primary assisted patency rate of 88.5% ± 8.5% at 15 months (Figure 13–3). The locations of the stenoses after RSFAE included two over the course of the SFA, two at the adductor canal, and two at the distal stent. Four of the patients whose RSFAE failed underwent AKFP. There were no deaths and one wound complication occurred (skin edge slough), and the mean hospital length of stay was 2.1 ± 0.5 days. The ankle brachial indices rose from 0.58 (± 0.14) preoperative to 0.95 (± 0.04) postoperatively.

DISCUSSION

RSFAE in combination with popliteal artery balloon/stent angioplasty offers the vascular surgeon a minimally invasive endovascular alternative for the treatment of SFA occlusive disease. The reported[4-7] disappointing results for long segment (>15 cm) SFA occlusive disease, treated by PTA, with or without stent, laser assisted balloon angioplasty, and atherectomy led van der Heijden and coworkers[9] to reassess the semi-closed endarterectomy technique in the hope that "debulking" of the SFA would improve durability. They reported a 61%, five-year secondary patency rate in 259 SFA endarterectomies, which compares favorably with the results of conventional bypass operations. With this technique, a ring stripper was introduced via arteriotomies at the

TABLE 13-1. CUMULATIVE PRIMARY PATENCY RATES FOR RSFAE AND DISTAL ASPIRE STENTING

Interval	No. of grafts at risk	No. of grafts failed	Lost to follow-up	Total withdrawn	Interval patency rate (%)	Cumulative patency rate (%)	SE
0-3 mo	40	1	6	7	98.3	97.4	0
3-6 mo	33	3	5	8	90.1	88.4	2.9
6-9 mo	25	0	8	8	100.0	88.4	5.4
9-12 mo	17	0	6	6	100.0	88.4	5.4
12-15 mo	11	1	5	6	90.1	80.0	5.4
15-18 mo	8	1	0	1	87.5	68.6	9.4
18-21 mo	6	0	2	2	100.0	68.6	13.3
21-24 mo	4	0	2	2	100.0	68.6	13.3
24-27 mo	3	0	0	0	100.0	68.6	13.3
27-30 mo	2	0	1	1	100.0	68.6	13.3
30-33 mo	1	0	1	1	100.0	68.6	13.3

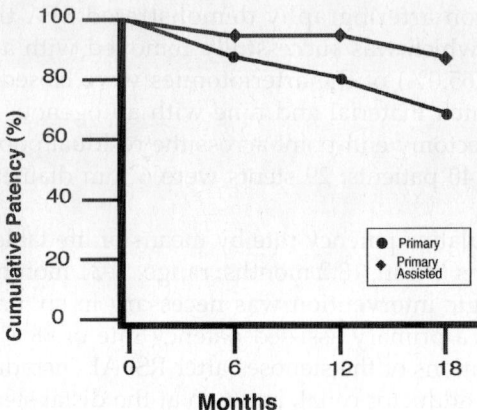

Figure 13-3. Cumulative primary and primary assisted patency after RSFAE and distal aSpire stenting.

SFA and above-knee popliteal arteries, and an endarterectomy performed; the distal popliteal artery plaque was "tacked" with sutures. The development by Ho, et al[11] of the "remote" endarterectomy technique, performed through a small inguinal incision in combination with proximal popliteal artery balloon/stent angioplasty, assisted in the complete removal of the SFA plaque and simplified treatment of the distal end-point. This technique offered several advantages: it was minimally invasive, a second distal incision was avoided, a common femoral and profunda femoris ostial endarterectomy could be easily performed, it avoided use of prosthetic material, and it could be used in the absence of saphenous vein and/or preserved the saphenous vein for use in the cardiovascular or peripheral circulation should the need arise.

In the first study, the 12-month (74.9%) and 36-month (61.4%) primary cumulative patency rates were similar to those reported by Ho and coworkers[13] and were comparable to rates expected for AKFP bypass. Part of the "learning curve" of any new procedure is patient selection and we learned that patients with heavily calcified SFAs (i.e. renal failure patients) fared poorly and were likely not candidates for RSFAE. The incidence, however, of stenosis after RSFAE was concerning in that 14 (23.3%) of 60 patients required an adjunctive procedure (nine PTA, five stent angioplasty) to maintain SFA patency. Although the incidence (23%) of early (< two years) stenosis, likely due to intimal hyperplasia, was less than that reported by Ho et al[13] (46% at one year) and by Galland and colleagues[14] (69% at 15 months), the reason is unclear but remains a concern.

In the second study, after RSFAE, the distal atheromatous plaque was "tacked" with the aSpire stent. This stent has a nitinol framework that provides excellent wall coverage and its PTFE covering eliminates metal to artery contact, one of the possible causes of neointimal hyperplasia. Yet it is flexible and has high radial strength to withstand torsional stresses proximal to the knee joint, and because of its unique design, facilitates laminar flow (Figure 13–4).[15] By adjusting the tightness of the stent spiral prior to final deployment, not only is the plaque end-point tacked, but the collateral vessels at the end point may be preserved as well (Figure 13–5). The 18-month (68.6%) primary cumulative patency rates in this study were again comparable with rates expected after AKFP bypass graft,[16] however, stenosis remained significant in that 15% (6/40) of patients required an adjunctive procedure (four PTA, two stent angioplasty) to maintain SFA patency. Although the incidence of early (< two years) stenosis in this

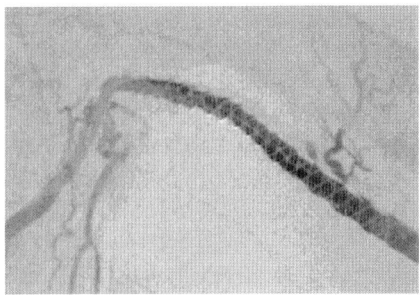

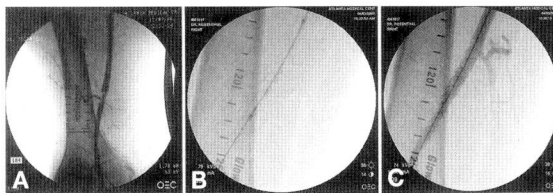

Figure 13-4. Arteriogram after RSFAE and aSpire stent angioplasty with knee flexed.

Figure 13-5. A. Arteriogram after RSFAE. Note distal "shelf" at endarterectomy endpoint. **B.** Balloon/Stent angioplasty. **C.** Completion arteriogram with collater preserved.

study (15%) was less than that reported by Rosenthal et al (23%),[17] Ho et al (46%),[18] or by Smeets et al (25%),[19] it may not be statistically different. Restenosis, due to intimal hyperplasia, remains the Achilles heel of RSFAE, but hopefully in the near future, the use of improved antiplatelet medications, drug elution therapy, endothelial cell seeding, or brachytherapy will help solve the problem of restenosis. Of interest is the observation that when RSFAE failed, the patient's symptoms were, in general, less severe than prior to operation. This was felt to be a function of collaterals being opened at the time of endarterectomy. However, this remains to be proven.

The treatment of femoropopliteal occlusive disease with RSFAE in combination with distal aSpire popliteal stent angioplasty continues to evolve. The development of new instruments, which will facilitate endarterectomy as well as guidewire passage in concert with the aSpire stent, hopefully will improve the durability of this procedure. Long segment occlusive disease of the SFA has *not* been successfully treated by radiologic minimally invasive procedures because of the SFA's long length, tortuosity, small caliber, and relatively low flow. It is incumbent on the vascular surgeon, therefore, to develop a superior minimally invasive alternative. Recanalization of the SFA by a guidewire, laser, or atherectomy in combination with PTA and/or stent angioplasty, ultimately leads to arterial recoil and remodeling, which may cause thrombosis of the artery. Debulking of the artery appears to reduce arterial recoil and remodeling[20-21] and RSFAE hopefully will offer patients a more durable procedure with comparable morbidity and patency rates, similar to those of AKFP bypass graft.

RSFAE AND DISTAL VEIN BYPASS

An interesting adjunct for RSFAE is in patients with limb threatening ischemia who require a saphenous vein bypass (SV). Saphenous vein is the conduit of choice for a femoro distal popliteal/tibial bypass,[22-24] especially in the presence of foot infection. Unfortunately, the ipsilateral greater SV has been reported to be unusable in up to 40% of cases[22] due to anatomic inadequacy (i.e. phlebitic, sclerotic), previous stripping, harvest, or intraoperative injury. Use of the contralateral SV may be an appropriate alternative; however, this vein may also be inadequate, absent, and many of these patients ultimately will require bilateral lower extremity reconstruction, therefore, tempering the enthusiasm for harvesting the contralateral SV.

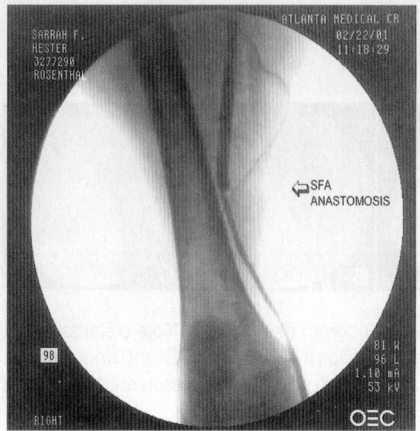
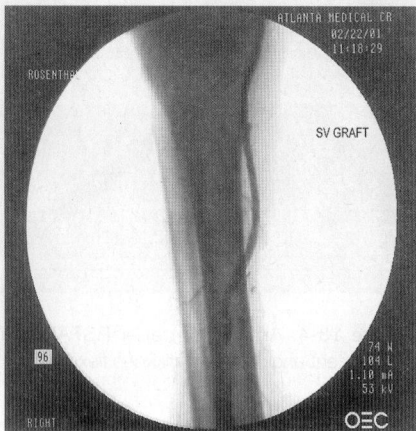

Figure 13-6. Completion arteriogram of endarterectomized SFA to saphenous vein bypass anastomosis and distal peroneal anastomosis.

RSFAE creates the ability to use the proximal popliteal artery as the "inflow" site for a distal SV bypass (Figure 13–6). If the popliteal artery beyond the endarterectomy is patent (i.e. distal "blind" popliteal segment, tibioperoneal occlusion), the distal artery may be tacked by balloon/stent angioplasty. We used RSFAE in conjunction with distal SV bypass for limb salvage in 21 patients,[25] seven SV grafts were performed in situ, eight SV segments were harvested for transposition, and six were reversed by surgeon's preference. The primary assisted patency rate was 76.5% (repeat PTA in four and stent angioplasty in two patients were necessary) and limb salvage rate 90.2% at 18 months follow-up.

When a femoro distal popliteal/tibial bypass is necessary and adequate SV is not available, RSFAE and distal bypass with residual SV bypass is a safe and moderately durable procedure, which may prove to be a useful adjunct for limb salvage, especially in the presence of foot infection where an autogenous tissue bypass is preferred.

CONCLUSION

RSFAE offers the vascular surgeon a minimally invasive alternative to catheter-based radiologic procedures that have not proven durable. RSFAE in concert with distal aSpire stenting is a safe and moderately durable procedure that allows preservation of SFA collaterals. If long-term patency rates are similar to those of AKFP bypass, RSFAE may prove to be a valuable adjunct for the treatment of SFA occlusive disease.

REFERENCES

1. Dos Santos JC. Surla desobstruction des thromboses arterieles anciennes. *Mem Acad Chir.*1947;73:409–411.
2. DeWeese JA, Barner HB, Mahoney EB, Rob CG. Autogenous venous bypass grafts and thromboendarterectomies for atherosclerotic lesions of the femoropopliteal arteries. *Ann Surg.* 1996;163:205–214.

3. Darling RC, Linton RR. Durability of femoropopliteal reconstructions: endarterectomy versus vein bypass grafts. *Am J Surg*.1972;123:472–479.

4. Matsi PJ, Manninen HI, Vanninen RL, et al. Femoropopliteal angioplasty in patients with claudication: primary and secondary patency in 140 limbs with 1-3 year follow-up. *Radiology*. 1992;191:727–733.

5. The Collaborative Rotablator Atherectomy Group (CRAG): Peripheral arthrectomy with the rotablator: a multicenter report. *J Vasc Surg*. 1994;19:509–515.

6. Diethrich EB. Laser angioplasty: A critical review based on 1849 clinical procedures. *Angiology*. 1990;41:757–767.

7. Johnston KW, Rae M, Hogg-Johnston SA, Colapinto RF, Walker PM, Baird RJ. Five-year results of a prospective study of percutaneous transluminal angioplasty. *Ann Surg*. 1987; 206:403–13.

8. Bergeron P, Pinot JJ, Poyen V, et al. Long-term results with the Palmaz stent in the superficial femoral artery. *J Endovasc Surg*. 1995;2:161–167.

9. van der Heijden FH, Eikelboom BC, van Reedt Dortland RW. Superficial femoral artery endarterectomy: a procedure worth reconsidering. *Eur J Vasc Surg*. 1993;6:651.

10. van der Heijden FH, Eikelboom BC, van Reedt Dortland RW, et al. Long-term results of semiclosed endarterectomy of the superficial femoral artery and the outcome of failed reconstruction. *J Vasc Surg*. 1993;18:271–279.

11. Ho GH, Moll FL, Joosten PP, et al. The Mollring Cutter remote endarterectomy: preliminary experience with a new endovascular technique for treatment of occlusive superficial femoral artery disease. *J Endovasc Surg*. 1995;2:278–287.

12. Rutherford RB, Flanigan DP, Gupta SK, et al. Suggested standards for reports dealing with lower extremity ischemia. *J Vasc Surg*. 1986;4:80–94.

13. Ho GH, Moll FL, Hedeman , et al. Endovascular remote endarterectomy in femoropopliteal occlusive disease: one-year clinical experience with the ring strip cutter device. *Eur J Vasc Endovasc Surg*. 1996;12:105–112.

14. Galland RB, Whiteley MS, Gibson M, et al. Remote superficial femoral artery endarterectomy: medium-term results. *Eur J Vasc Endovasc Surg*. 2000;19:278–282.

15. Wei, T. Flow model analysis comparing aSpire covered stent and the Wall stent. Dept of Mechanical Engineering 1998; Rutgers University. Personal communication 2003.

16. Abbott WM, Green RM, Matsumoto T, et al. Prosthetic above-knee femoropopliteal bypass grafting: Results of a multicenter randomized prospective trial. *J Vasc Surg*. 1997;25:19–28.

17. Rosenthal D, Schubart PJ, Kinney EV, et al. Remote superficial femoral artery endarterectomy: Multicenter medium-term results. *J Vasc Surg*. 2001;34:428–433.

18. Ho GH, Moll FL, Nolthenius RP, et al. Endovascular femoropopliteal bypass combined with remote endarterectomy in SFA occlusive disease: initial experience. *Eur J Vasc Endovasc Surg*. 2000;19:27–34.

19. Smeets L, Ho GH, Hagenaars T et al. Remote endarterectomy: first choice in surgical treatment of long segment SFA occlusive disease? *Eur J Vasc Endovasc Surg*. 2003;25:589–589.

20. Bergeron P, Chiarandini S, Nava, G, Roth O. Femoral artery endoluminal bypass grafting; indications and early results. *J Endovasc Surg*. 1997;4:404–405.

21. Morris GE, Ahn SS, Quick CRG, et al. Endovascular femoropopliteal bypass: a cadaveric study. *Eur J Vasc Endovasc Surg*. 1995;10:9–15.

22. Taylor LM, Edwards JM, Porter JM. Present status of reversed vein bypass: five-year results of a modern series. *J Vasc Surg*. 1990;11:193–205.

23. Veith FJ, Gupta SK, Ascer E, et al. Six-year prospective multi-center randomized comparison of autologous saphenous vein and expanded PTFE grafts in infrainguinal arterial reconstruction. *J Vasc Surg*. 1986;3:104–114.

24. Leather RP, Shah DM, Chang BB, Kaufman JL. Resurrection of the in situ saphenous vein bypass: 1000 cases later. *Ann Surg*. 1988;208:435–442.

25. Rosenthal D, Wellons ED, Matsuura JH et al. Remote superficial femoral artery endarterectomy and distal vein bypass for limb salvage: initial experience. *J Endovasc Therapy*. 2003; 1:121–125.

14

Subintimal Angioplasty for the Treatment of Lower Extremity Ischemia

Eric C. Scott, M.D. Jean M. Panneton, M.D.

Percutaneous methods of lower extremity revascularization have brought considerable change to the practice of vascular surgery during the last decade. Prior to the endovascular era, many elderly patients with peripheral arterial disease and multiple medical comorbidities either underwent extensive open revascularization procedures in hopes of limb salvage or were directed toward primary amputation to minimize operative risk. Today, as a result of improved guidewire and catheter technology in combination with a variety of endovascular devices and techniques, there are now numerous percutaneous strategies for lower extremity revascularization. Of these, subintimal angioplasty (SIA) has proven an essential technique in the treatment of patients with the most extensive peripheral arterial disease: those with iliac or infrainguinal arterial occlusions.

BACKGROUND

Subintimal angioplasty was first described in 1989 by Drs. Bolia, Brennan, and Bell in the United Kingdom. In the journal *Clinical Radiology*, they reported their inadvertent subintimal dissection around a 15cm popliteal artery occlusion.[1] As their wire re-entered the true lumen below the lesion, they proceeded with balloon angioplasty and successfully restored bloodflow to the distal extremity. The patient, a 58-year-old man with 100 meter claudication, remained symptom-free at the time of the report eight years later.

Subintimal angioplasty gained popularity in Europe in the 1990s following this report and others from Bolia and Bell. The technique offered durable short-term patency and achieved limb salvage in the majority of patients, yet required only an angiographic suite and conscious sedation to complete. The procedure gained popularity in the United States in the early 2000s, by which time additional reports detailed use of SIA in tibial arteries,[2-4] in patients with claudication,[5-7] and even in patients with failed bypass grafts.[8,9]

At our institution, incorporation of SIA into our endovascular surgery practice occurred in late 2002. We began use of the technique in patients with critical limb ischemia who were believed to be at prohibitive risk for open bypass and essentially referred for lower extremity amputation. As experience mounted, indications for its use were broadened to include patients with iliac or tibial artery occlusions, as well as patients who were surgical bypass candidates but preferred a less invasive approach.

TECHNIQUE

Patients with disabling claudication or critical limb ischemia are brought to an angiographic suite in anticipation of subintimal angioplasty unless a combined open and endovascular procedure is planned, for which patients are brought to an operating room. Once in an angiographic suite, moderate sedation is administered and arterial access is obtained, most commonly in a retrograde fashion in the contralateral common femoral artery. A short 4F or 5F sheath is placed and appropriate arteriography is performed in the symptomatic extremity. Following demonstration of an infrainguinal arterial occlusion, a longer 6F sheath is positioned over the aortic bifurcation and in proximity to the occlusion. Intravenous heparin is then administered.

Subintimal angioplasty begins with the creation of a dissection plane at the origin of the arterial occlusion. Using a soft, angled 0.035 inch hydrophilic guidewire and angled 4F hydrophilic catheter (Glidewire and Glidecath, Terumo Medical Corporation, Somerset, NJ), a loop is formed in the wire by advancing the wire up against the occlusion. When the stiff portion of the wire reaches the apex of the formed loop and the catheter is positioned in proximity to the beginning of the loop, the combination of wire and catheter achieves its maximal stiffness for use as a blunt dissecting tool. Using mild to moderate pressure, the looped wire is then advanced into the occlusion and a subintimal dissection plane is created. Failure to initiate the dissection plane is signaled by lengthening of the loop of wire instead of forward advancement of the loop's apex. This can be solved by repositioning the wire and catheter in a slightly new location or by using one of the numerous endovascular devices now available to assist in crossing the sometimes fibrotic or calcific cap of a chronic total occlusion (FRONTRUNNER XP, Cordis Endovascular, Warren, NJ; CROSSER Catheter, FlowCardia, Inc., Sunnyvale, CA; Excimer Laser System, Spectranetics Corp., Colorado Springs, CO).

Once the dissection plane is created, the looped wire is advanced across the length of the occlusion, stopping every 5–10cm to advance the catheter over the wire. This adds additional support to the stiff portion of the wire and may need to be done every 1–2cm for lesions that are difficult to cross. If additional support is required, a Berenstein catheter or Quick-Cross Catheter (Spectranetics Corp., Colorado Springs, CO) can be substituted. In our experience, the use of stiffer wires has increased the risk of arterial perforation, and thus are rarely used.

The distal endpoint of the occlusion must be noted prior to beginning the subintimal dissection so as to avoid extending the dissection much beyond the end of the occlusion. This can be accomplished using a radio-opaque ruler on the extremity, a roadmapping technique, or by reference to bony landmarks. Once the looped wire has crossed the endpoint of the occlusion, the wire commonly enters the true lumen of the artery spontaneously. The wire is removed from the catheter and arteriography via the catheter is used to assess its true or false lumen location. If the catheter is within the true lumen, a Benson or Rosen wire is reinserted through the catheter and balloon angioplasty is performed of the entire subintimal plane (balloon length ranging from 100 to 220 mm). If the catheter remains extraluminal, the glidewire is reinserted and the true lumen is accessed using the tip of the wire or by reforming the loop and extending the dissection plane slightly to attempt re-entry in a different location. True lumen re-entry should be achieved as close to the distal endpoint of occlusion as possible so as to avoid extending the dissection plane across the knee joint or into a tibial vessel if at all possible. If multiple attempts at true lumen re-entry fail with wire and catheter manipulation, use of a re-entry device is recommended (Outback Catheter, Cordis Endovascular, Warren, NJ; Pioneer Catheter, Medtronic Inc., Minneapolis, MN).

In our experience, selective stenting of the subintimal channel for residual stenoses greater than 30% has proven effective. Final balloon size is determined by the diameter of the adjacent patent artery and self-expanding stents are preferred. Should a primary stenting approach be taken, angioplasty of the subintimal channel must still be performed to facilitate easy passage of the stent. Completion imaging is then performed to assess antegrade flow through the subintimal channel and to ensure runoff vessels remain patent. Antiplatelet therapy is initiated with clopidogrel and continued for at least one month, followed by aspirin indefinitely.

Subintimal angioplasty of occluded iliac artery segments has also proven effective. For treatment of the iliac arteries, however, one must select between an antegrade or retrograde approach to the subintimal dissection. Proximal common iliac artery occlusions that make sheath placement over the aortic bifurcation impossible or poorly supported should be approached in a retrograde manner from a short sheath placed in the ipsilateral common femoral artery. True lumen re-entry near the aortic bifurcation can be more difficult than infrainguinal re-entry, however, due to the thicker and often more calcified plaque at this location. In addition, re-entry at the origin of the common iliac artery is optimal to avoid the creation of a distal aortic dissection flap that could impair contralateral common iliac flow and necessitate placement of kissing iliac stents. Distal common iliac or external iliac artery occlusions can successfully be approached in an antegrade fashion, similar to that used for infrainguinal occlusions.

CASE DESCRIPTIONS

Iliac Artery Occlusion

A 76-year-old male presented with rest pain in the right lower extremity, and aorto-iliac duplex imaging demonstrated a right common iliac artery occlusion. The patient desired an endovascular solution and aortography with run-off images was performed via a left common femoral artery sheath (Figure 14–1.). Following identification of the right common iliac artery total occlusion, a 6F short sheath was placed in each common femoral artery to enable a retrograde approach for SIA of the occlusion and to facilitate placement of kissing common iliac stents. A soft, angled glidewire and 4F glidecath were used to create the subintimal dissection. In this case, the loop of wire did not spontaneously enter the aortic true lumen at the bifurcation. Attempts to

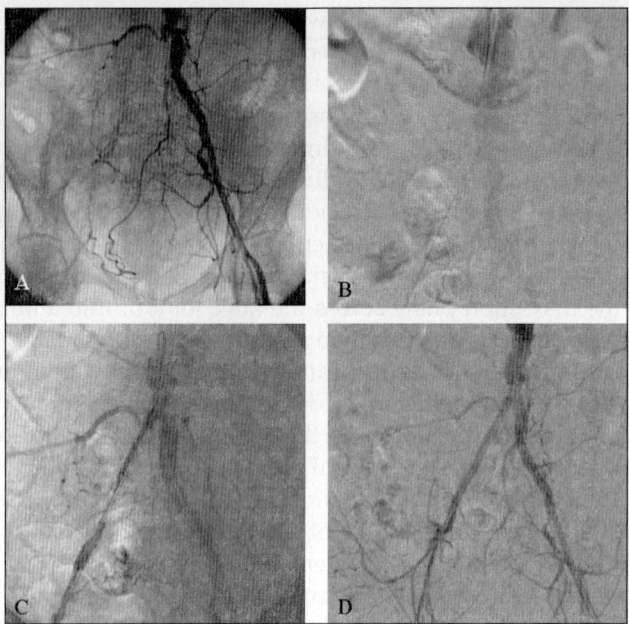

Figure 14-1. 76-year-old male with rest pain in the right foot. **(A)** Total occlusion of the right common iliac artery with faint reconstitution of external iliac and hypogastric arteries. **(B)** Right common femoral artery sheath placed and retrograde subintimal angioplasty performed. The Outback Catheter (Cordis Endovascular, Warren, NJ) was used to achieve aortic true lumen re-entry precisely at the aortic bifurcation. **(C)** Balloon angioplasty is performed on the right common iliac artery to enable placement of a stent. **(D)** Kissing balloon-expandable stents are placed in the common iliac arteries restoring flow to the right leg (right, Genesis 8mm x 79mm; left, Genesis 8mm x 29mm, Cordis Endovascular, Warren, NJ).

re-enter using the tip of the wire were unsuccessful as well. Rather than re-entering the aorta more proximally and risk creating an aortic dissection flap, the Outback Catheter was used to obtain wire re-entry precisely at the aortic bifurcation. Balloon angioplasty of the subintimal channel was then performed to enable smooth insertion of a balloon-expandable stent. Kissing stents were deployed at the aortic bifurcation and flow was restored through the right common iliac artery.

Mid-SFA Occlusion

A 63-year-old male presented with a six-month history of worsening disabling claudication in the right leg. Noninvasive studies were suggestive of superficial femoral artery (SFA) atherosclerotic disease, and arteriography was performed via a 5F short sheath placed in the left common femoral artery. A mid-SFA occlusion was demonstrated along with patent tibial vessels (Figure 14–2.). A long 6F sheath was then placed over the aortic bifurcation and advanced into the proximal right SFA. Using an angiographic roadmap, a subintimal dissection was performed and true lumen re-entry confirmed just distal to the occlusion. Balloon angioplasty was performed that resulted in a widely patent subintimal channel that was angiographically indistinguishable from the native SFA lumen. A >50% stenosis was concomitantly identified at the SFA origin and was successfully treated using the Silverhawk mechanical atherectomy device (ev3, Plymouth, MN).

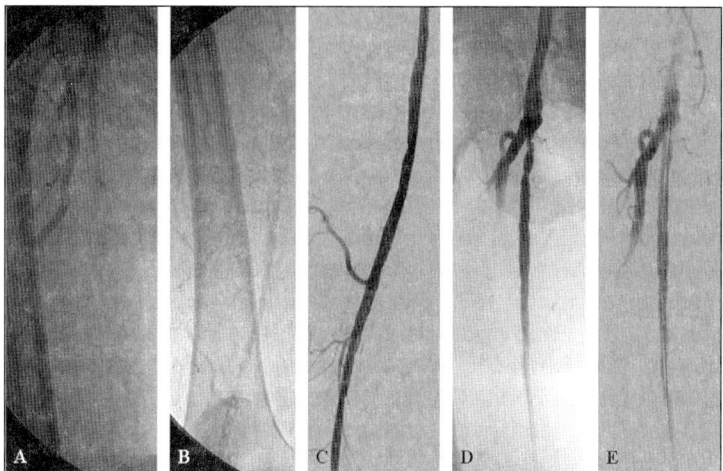

Figure 14-2. Right mid-superficial femoral artery (SFA) occlusion in a patient with disabling claudication. **(A, B)** Proximal and distal aspects of occlusion. **(C)** Widely patent distal SFA following subintimal angioplasty. **(D)** Residual stenosis at SFA origin despite balloon angioplasty. **(E)** Completion image following use of Silverhawk mechanical atherectomy catheter (ev3, Plymouth, MN) for plaque removal at femoral bifurcation.

SFA Chronic Total Occlusion

An 81-year-old diabetic female presented with ischemic ulcerations of her right toes. Arteriography demonstrated a chronic total occlusion of her right SFA with essentially no visualization of the SFA origin and reconstitution of a patent above-knee popliteal artery (Figure 14–3.). A long 6F sheath was placed over the aortic bifurcation and the tip positioned in the proximal right common femoral artery. Using a soft, angled

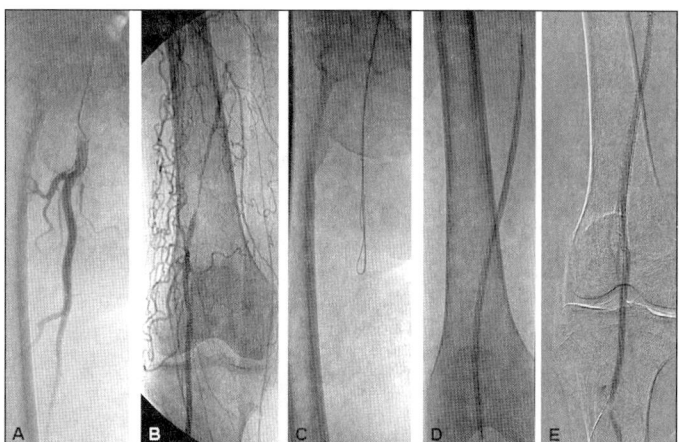

Figure 14-3. 81-year-old diabetic female with ischemic ulceration of the right toes. **(A, B)** Proximal and distal aspects of right superficial femoral artery chronic total occlusion. **(C)** Looped angled glidewire and angled glidecath are advanced through the subintimal plane. **(D)** PTA of the subintimal channel following confirmation of re-entry into the above-knee popliteal artery using Savvy 5mm x 220mm balloon (Cordis Endovascular, Warren, NJ). **(E)** Brisk flow of contrast through the distal portion of the subintimal angioplasty is seen following placement of 7mm x 150mm, 7mm x 120mm, and 6mm x 150mm PROTEGE® EndoFlex™ stents (ev3, Plymouth, MN).

glidewire and 4F angled glidecath, a subintimal dissection plane was started by positioning the catheter against the occlusion with the catheter tip angled medially toward the SFA origin. After several attempts at wire advancement, a loop of wire was formed in the SFA origin and was successfully advanced into a subintimal plane. The catheter and wire were then advanced sequentially through the occluded SFA, maintaining a distance between the apex of the looped wire and the catheter tip of 5–10cm for support. The wire spontaneously re-entered the true lumen of the above-knee popliteal artery with a characteristic release of pressure as the wire entered the patent lumen. Injection of contrast via the catheter confirmed true lumen re-entry. Balloon angioplasty was then performed of the entire subintimal channel using a Savvy 5mm × 220mm balloon (Cordis Endovascular, Warren, NJ). This failed to establish forward flow down the channel, however, and three self-expanding PROTEGE® EndoFlex™ stents were placed (ev3, Plymouth, MN). Completion imaging demonstrated brisk flow through the newly established subintimal lumen.

Tibial Artery Occlusion

A 72-year-old male presented with a nonhealing ulceration of his left foot. Following abnormal noninvasive studies, arteriography was performed (Figure 14–4.). The aortoiliac and femoropopliteal segments were widely patent. The anterior tibial artery was occluded at its origin, while the posterior tibial and peroneal arteries occluded within the proximal calf. Only the distal posterior tibial artery was seen to reconstitute at the ankle. Using this as a distal target for SIA, a long 5F sheath was brought over the aortic bifurcation from the right groin and positioned within the distal left SFA. A soft, angled glidewire and 4F glidecath were used to engage the origin of the posterior tibial artery occlusion and a subintimal dissection was started. Within the mid-calf, however, the catheter would no longer advance. At this time, a 0.018-inch V-18 guidewire

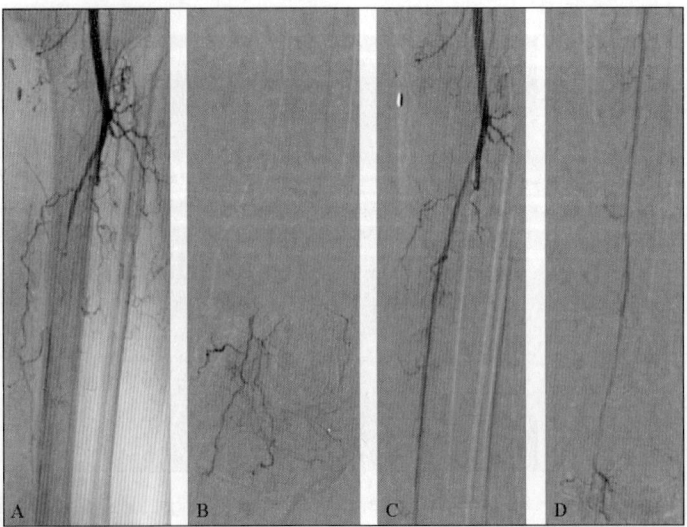

Figure 14-4. 72-year-old male with a nonhealing ulceration on the left foot. **(A)** Proximal occlusion of all three tibial vessels. **(B)** Only the posterior tibial artery reconstitutes at the ankle, perfusing the plantar branches. **(C, D)** Widely patent posterior tibial artery following subintimal angioplasty with a 0.018 inch guidewire (V-18, Boston Scientific, Natick, MA) and 0.018 inch Quick-Cross catheter (Spectranetics Corp., Colorado Springs, CO).

(Boston Scientific, Natick, MA) and 0.018 inch Quick-Cross catheter (Spectranetics Corp., Colorado Springs, CO) were exchanged and successfully used to traverse the occlusion. The V-18 wire spontaneously re-entered the true lumen of the posterior tibial artery just above the ankle. The Quick-Cross catheter was advanced to this location and arteriography confirmed the re-entry. Balloon angioplasty was then performed using 2.5mm × 120mm and 3mm × 120mm balloons. Completion imaging demonstrated brisk flow through the posterior tibial artery into the foot.

DISCUSSION

Incorporation of SIA into modern vascular and endovascular surgery practices worldwide has brought about significant changes in the way lower extremity arterial occlusions are treated. From the common iliac arteries to the most distal aspects of the tibial arteries, SIA has offered many recent patients a percutaneous revascularization instead of a major open operation. Simultaneously, it has allowed many ill patients with critical limb ischemia, who are at prohibitive surgical risk, an opportunity for limb salvage instead of amputation.

Technical Feasibility

Numerous studies now demonstrate the technical feasibility of SIA. Reports of technical success have ranged from 82–100%,[4,10] with most authors reporting successful procedures in 85–90% of patients.[5,8,11-13] The location of lower extremity arterial occlusion does not appear to significantly alter the rate of success, nor does the length of the lesion.[7,11] In our experience with SIA for SFA occlusions, 73% of immediate failure was due to our inability to re-enter the true lumen.[11] A number of devices are now available to aid in either entering the subintimal plane or to aid with true lumen re-entry that will likely improve rates of technical success in the future. Jacobs et al. recently reported on 24 cases of difficult true lumen re-entry for which either the Pioneer re-entry catheter (Medtronic Inc., Minneapolis, MN) or the Outback catheter were used.[14] In all cases, re-entry was successfully achieved.

Two factors continue to make SIA difficult or even impossible when present. The first is calcification of the arterial wall.[5] Marks et al. determined that duplex examination of the occlusion and calculation of its gray-scale median, a measure of overall plaque density, could predict failure of subintimal angioplasty.[15] In this study, the authors found a technical success rate of only 10% in patients who had lesions with a gray-scale median >35, while their overall rate of technical success was 85%. The second factor is an occlusion that begins flush at its origin. This type of lesion can make it very difficult to begin a subintimal dissection, as wires and catheters alike can easily deflect down the open adjacent vessel. We have found the use of a stiffer angled catheter pushed into the origin of the occlusion prior to wire advancement to be more effective in this circumstance.

Procedural Safety

Like other endovascular techniques, SIA can be performed under light to moderate sedation, and general anesthesia is unnecessary. This alone makes SIA an appealing alternative to open bypass in many patients, and at least partially accounts for 30-day mortality rates following the procedure that are consistently <1%.

Low rates of complication during SIA are also reported. In our recently published series of over 500 infrainguinal procedures, the cumulative complication rate was 5.5%.[11] This included a 3% incidence of arterial perforation (none of which resulted in hemorrhage), and <1% incidence of femoral pseudoaneurysm, distal embolization, arteriovenous fistula formation, groin hematoma, retroperitoneal hemorrhage, and soft tissue infection. Only one patient in this series required operative intervention to remedy a procedural complication (intimal flap raised in a common femoral artery during sheath placement).

Finally, we stress that SIA and surgical bypass procedures are not mutually exclusive. Subintimal angioplasty can be performed safely as a first-line therapy without risk to future bypass options, and we do so routinely. There are currently no published reports of prior SIA precluding surgical bypass and we know of no such occurrence in our own practice. During the procedure, it remains important to regain true lumen access proximal to or at the level of a potential distal anastomotic site so as not to extend a dissection plane across such a site. Following this tenant should safeguard all future bypass options should they be needed.

It is also possible to perform SIA following a failed surgical bypass procedure. As long as the occluded vessel remains in continuity following the bypass procedure (no end-to-end anastomoses), we and others have successfully restored distal flow using SIA. The subintimal plane is created in the portion of bypassed vessel that is suture-free and true lumen access is obtained at the appropriate level of reconstitution.

Patency

There are numerous case series and prospective studies outlining the patency of SIA. Larger series reporting primary patency data are listed in Table 14–1. One-, two-, and three-year primary patency range from 22–85%, 30–66%, and 18–58%, respectively. Primary-assisted and secondary patency rates have been substantially higher. Florenes et al. reported primary-assisted patency in 116 limbs treated for disabling claudication of 70%, 66%, and 64% at one, three, and five years, respectively.[6] In our report of 506 subintimal procedures for occlusions originating in the SFA but extending as far as the tibial vessels, secondary patency at one, two, and three years was 76%, 57%, and 50%, respectively.[11] When analyzed by extent of SIA, limbs treated for an isolated superficial femoral artery or femoropopliteal occlusion achieved secondary patency of 54% and 48% at three years, respectively. Limbs with occlusions spanning into a tibial artery achieved secondary patency of 43% at three years. Additional percutaneous procedures were required in 28% of limbs to achieve this result. In a subset of patients who were studied at three years following SIA, we calculated a percutaneous reintervention rate of only 0.21 procedures per patient per year.[8]

Numerous factors affecting patency have been examined by regression analysis. London et al. reported on 159 femoropopliteal SIA procedures and found the risk of reocclusion was 2.7 times higher in patients who continued to smoke, was 1.73 times higher for each 10cm of occlusion length, and each additional run-off vessel reduced reocclusion risk by 0.54.[7] Lazaris et al. reported on 51 consecutive infrainguinal SIA procedures and found that the length of occlusion and number of distal run-off vessels impacted primary patency.[16] In patients with more than one run-off vessel, one-year primary patency was 81% compared to 25% for patients with a single run-off vessel. The hazard ratio for reocclusion was 1.02 for each centimeter of occlusion.

In contrast, Antusevas et al. recently reported on 64 SIA procedures and identified no specific factors associated with reduced primary or primary-assisted patency.[5]

TABLE 14-1. PATENCY OF SUBINTIMAL ANGIOPLASTY AS REPORTED BY VARIOUS INVESTIGATORS

Author, Year	Limbs (n)	Artery	Indication (%)	1° Patency (%)				
				1yr	2yr	3yr	4yr	5yr
Antusevas et al., 2008	73	SFA	CLI (48) Claud (52)	69	66			
Scott et al., 2008	439	SFA Pop	CLI (63) Claud (37) Tibial	45	30	25		
Vraux et al., 2007	50	Tibial	CLI (100)	46	42			
Treiman et al., 2006	29	SFA Pop Tibial	CLI (100)	85	64	18	9	
Desgranges et al., 2004	100	SFA Pop Tibial	CLI (52) Claud (48)		61			
Florenes et al., 2004	116	SFA Pop Tibial	Claud (100)	70*		66*		64*
Yilmaz et al., 2003	67	SFA	CLI (33)	22				
Vraux et al., 2000	40	Tibial	CLI (100)	72				
Nydahl et al., 1997	28	Tibial	CLI (100)	53				
London et al., 1994	159	SFA	CLI (11) Claud (89)	71		58		

SFA, superficial femoral artery; Pop, popliteal artery; CLI, critical limb ischemia; Claud, claudication. * Primary-assisted patency.

Specifically, lesions >10cm and 0-1 run-off vessels did not significantly effect patency. Likewise, in our report, we identified femorotibial occlusions requiring SIA across the knee, as well as the presence of critical limb ischemia, to be significant factors associated with reduced primary patency.[11] We have not identified absolute occlusion length or number of run-off vessels to be associated with reduced patency.

The effect of stent placement within the subintimal channel on patency remains unclear. In early descriptions of the technique, stenting was used infrequently or not at all. Treiman et al. first reported the use of primary stenting in a series of 29 patients with critical limb ischemia and femoral or popliteal artery occlusions.[12] These patients underwent SIA followed by stent placement throughout the entire channel. Short-term primary patency was excellent at one and two years (85% and 64%, respectively) but fell precipitously in the third and fourth years (18% and 9%, respectively). We have consistently practiced selective stenting of residual stenoses >30% within the subintimal channel. Using this approach, we have placed stents in 20% of limbs and found no significant difference in either primary or secondary patency at three years.[11,17] Until a randomized trial comparing selective versus primary stenting of the subintimal channel is performed, the debate over stent use is likely to persist.

Clinical Outcomes

While nearly all published reports of SIA have been replete with patency data, fewer have assessed clinical outcomes in these patients. Nydahl et al. reported limb salvage in 85% of 28 critically ischemic limbs with infrapopliteal occlusions at one year.[2]

Lazaris et al. treated 99 patients with critical limb ischemia and achieved limb salvage of 88% at three years.[17,18] In our series, 265 limbs were treated for critical ischemia and limb salvage was achieved in 88% at one year and 75% of limbs at three years.[11] When analyzed by extent of occlusion, limbs with occlusion limited to the superficial femoral artery achieved the highest limb salvage: 88% at three years. Limbs with occlusions extending from the superficial femoral artery into a tibial artery resulted in a limb salvage of 64% at three years.

We also examined the impact of SIA on patients with disabling claudication. One hundred seventy-four patients were treated with SIA and 97% reported improvement or relief from claudication three months following the procedure. This relief proved durable as 90% and 67% of patients reported ongoing improvement at one and three years.

Finally, we have determined that only 23% of patients who undergo successful SIA require surgical bypass in the three years that follow.[11] For patients with critical limb ischemia in our series, this was substantially lower than their three-year mortality rate of 45%.

SUMMARY

Subintimal angioplasty is a versatile endovascular technique to aid in the revascularization of patients with difficult lower extremity arterial occlusions. The technique has been proven safe and effective for patients with either disabling claudication or critical limb ischemia, and results in clinical outcomes comparable to those of many surgical bypass procedures. Unlike these procedures, SIA can be performed with minimal sedation and minimal risk to patients, making the procedure particularly well suited for elderly and high surgical-risk patients.

REFERENCES

1. Bolia A, Brennan J, Bell PR. Recanalisation of femoro-popliteal occlusions: improving success rate by subintimal recanalisation. *Clinical Radiology*. 1989;40(3):325.
2. Nydahl S, Hartshorne T, Bell PR, Bolia A, London NJ. Subintimal angioplasty of infrapopliteal occlusions in critically ischaemic limbs. *Eur J Vasc Endovasc Surg*. 1997;14(3): 212–216.
3. Vraux H, Hammer F, Verhelst R, Goffette P, Vandeleene B. Subintimal angioplasty of tibial vessel occlusions in the treatment of critical limb ischaemia: mid-term results. *Eur J Vasc Endovasc Surg*. 2000;20(5):441–446.
4. Vraux H, Bertoncello N. Subintimal angioplasty of tibial vessel occlusions in critical limb ischaemia: a good opportunity? *Eur J Vasc Endovasc Surg*. 2006;32(6):663–667.
5. Antusevas A, Aleksynas N, Kaupas RS, Inciura D, Kinduris S. Comparison of results of subintimal angioplasty and percutaneous transluminal angioplasty in superficial femoral artery occlusions. *Eur J Vasc Endovasc Surg*. 2008;36(1):101–106.
6. Florenes T, Bay D, Sandbaek G, Saetre T, Jorgensen JJ,et al. Subintimal angioplasty in the treatment of patients with intermittent claudication: long term results. *Eur J Vasc Endovasc Surg*. 2004;28(6):645–650.
7. London NJ, Srinivasan R, Naylor AR, Hartshorne T, Ratliff DA, et al. Subintimal angioplasty of femoropopliteal artery occlusions: the long-term results. *Eur J Vasc Surg*. 1994;8(2): 148–155.

8. Scott EC, Biuckians A, Light RE, Scibelli CD, Milner TP, Meier GH 3rd, Panneton JM. Subintimal angioplasty for the treatment of claudication and critical limb ischemia: 3-year results. *J Vasc Surg.* 2007;46(5):959–964.

9. Walker SR, Papavassiliou VG, Bolia A, London N. Subintimal angioplasty of native vessels in the management of occluded vascular grafts. *Eur J Vasc Endovasc Surg.* 2001;22(1):41–43.

10. Hynes N, Akhtar Y, Manning B, Aremu M, Oiakhinan K, et al. Subintimal angioplasty as a primary modality in the management of critical limb ischemia: comparison to bypass grafting for aortoiliac and femoropopliteal occlusive disease. *J Endovasc Ther.* 2004;11(4):460–471.

11. Scott EC, Biuckians A, Light RE, Burgess J, Meier GH, 3rd, Panneton JM. Subintimal angioplasty: Our experience in the treatment of 506 infrainguinal arterial occlusions. *J Vasc Surg.* 2008;48:878–884.

12. Treiman GS, Treiman R, Whiting J. Results of percutaneous subintimal angioplasty using routine stenting. *J Vasc Surg.* 2006;43(3):513–519.

13. Desgranges P, Boufi M, Lapeyre M, Tarquini G, van Laere O, Losy F, Melliere D, Becquemin JP, Kobeiter H. Subintimal angioplasty: feasible and durable. *Eur J Vasc Endovasc Surg.* 2004; 28(2):138–141.

14. Jacobs DL, Motaganahalli RL, Cox DE, Wittgen CM, Peterson GJ. True lumen re-entry devices facilitate subintimal angioplasty and stenting of total chronic occlusions: Initial report. *J Vasc Surg* 2006;43(6):1291–1296.

15. Marks NA, Ascher E, Hingorani AP, Shiferson A, Puggioni A. Gray-scale median of the atherosclerotic plaque can predict success of lumen re-entry during subintimal femoral-popliteal angioplasty. *J Vasc Surg.* 2008;47(1):109–115; discussion 115–106.

16. Lazaris AM, Salas C, Tsiamis AC, Vlachou PA, Bolia A, Fishwick G, Bell PR. Factors affecting patency of subintimal infrainguinal angioplasty in patients with critical lower limb ischemia. *Eur J Vasc Endovasc Surg.* 2006;32(6):668–674.

17. Schmieder GC, Richardson AI, Scott EC, Stokes GK, Meier GH 3rd, Panneton JM. Selective stenting in subintimal angioplasty: Analysis of primary stent outcomes. *J Vasc Surg* 2008;48: 1175–1181.

18. Lazaris AM, Tsiamis AC, Fishwick G, Bolia A, Bell PR. Clinical outcome of primary infrainguinal subintimal angioplasty in diabetic patients with critical lower limb ischemia. J Endovasc Ther. 2004;11(4):447–453.

15

The Role of Atherectomy in Lower Extremity Arterial Occlusive Disease

James F. Mckinsey, M.D. Soo J. Rhee, M.D.

Endovascular treatment of lower extremity occlusive disease has greatly evolved since the first reported percutaneous intervention performed by Dotter in 1964.[1] In comparison to traditional surgical revascularization, endovascular procedures are less invasive, allowing treatment of patients who are at increased risk for adverse outcomes following lower extremity bypass, as well as allowing a more rapid return to normal activities.[2] Despite the benefits of minimally invasive techniques, maintaining patency over time has remained an uncertainty. Early results of percutaneous balloon angioplasty reported five-year patency rates ranging from 30% to 50% depending on the location of the lesion, degree of stenosis, and runoff.[3,4] Efforts to improve long-term patency have resulted in the development of alternative technologies.

Percutaneous balloon angioplasty uses a high-pressure balloon to dilate the vessel, resulting in small and occasionally large dissections and displacement of the lesion. The resultant injury to the vessel wall may lead to myointimal hyperplasia during the healing process resulting in restenosis at the lesion site. Atherectomy removes the atherosclerotic plaque from within the vessel lumen through shaving or obliterating the plaque. The debulking of the plaque results in an increase in luminal diameter without the barotrauma or injury to the outer medial and adventia that is associated with balloon angioplasty. Ikeno et al. studied the effects of atherectomy and angioplasty on luminal area using intravascular ultrasound.[5] While both modalities resulted in an increase in luminal diameter, with atherectomy this was due to a decrease in the volume of plaque within the vessel wall while with balloon angioplasty, there was an overall vessel expansion with an associated displacement of the atherosclerotic plaque. There was also a reported increase incidence of dissection associated with angioplasty.

The atherectomy devices that have been developed can be categorized into two groups based on the mechanism of removing atheroma: extirpative and ablative. Extirpative atherectomy devices shave or cut the plaque, and the resulting segments of plaque are collected and later removed. In ablative atherectomy, the atheroma is pulverized or vaporized into fragments that are small enough to be either aspirated or released to pass through the capillary system.

In 1986, Simpson et al. first reported the use of a percutaneous directional atherectomy catheter.[6] The Simpson AtheroCath (Guidant Corp, Indianapolis, IN) utilized a high-pressure balloon on one side of the catheter tip and a hollow chamber with a battery-powered rotary cutter on the other. With inflation of the balloon, the cutting blade was pushed against the arterial wall, shaving the plaque that was stored in a collection chamber. A wide range of patency rates were reported in the literature. Kim et al. reported patency at one, two, and three years of 92%, 84%, and 84%, respectively.[7] Vroegindeweij et al. reported patency with atherectomy using the Simpson catheter at one month to be 89%, but at two years, patency rates of the treated segments was 34%.[8] When compared to a second group of patients undergoing balloon angioplasty, in which the patency rates at one month and two years were 97% and 56%, respectively, results with atherectomy were not found to be as durable.

Since then, other atherectomy devices have been developed. The Transluminal Extraction Catheter (TEC device) (Interventional Technologies, San Diego, CA) used a rotating cone-shaped cutter to shave plaque that was then aspirated through a catheter into a separate collection chamber. The Trac-Wright catheter (Dow Corning Wright, Arlington, TN) and Auth Rotablator (Boston Scientific, Natick, MA) were ablative catheters that were used in the past but are no longer commonly used in the peripheral circulation clinically. Both the Trac-Wright and Rotablator catheters were found to have promising immediate success rates, but mid-term follow-up showed a significant number of restenoses.[9,10,11] An additional concern regarding the use of the Rotablator, especially in the coronary vasculature, is the not uncommon occurrence of distal no-flow after the atherectomy, presumably due to distal embolization of the atherosclerotic material and occlusion of the distal outflow capilary network. Recently introduced are two new atherectomy devices: the CSI DiamondBack 360 atherectomy device (Minneapolis, MN) and the Pathway Medical Device (Kirkland, WA). The CSI DiamondBack 360 is an orbital atherectomy device (Figure 15–1) that has a fine diamond grit embedded into a standard or solid crown that rotates on a specialized shaft at up to 200,000 rpm. The particles created are reported to be 1–2 microns in size and pass through the capillary network to be cleared by the endoreticular system. The Pathway Medical Device is a rotational atehrectomy device (Figure 15–2) that has a rotational cutting device that cuts at a smaller diameter in one direction, but when the rotation is reversed, it will engages a larger cutting disk that will create a larger lumen. The atheroma is then aspirated into the shaft of the device via an auger mechanism and negative suction. Both devices are being clinically evaluated and have promising applications.

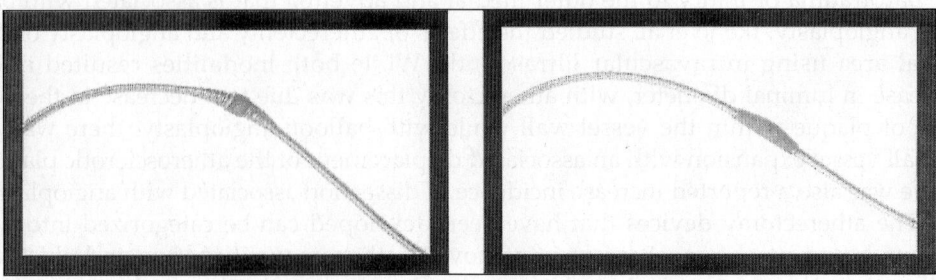

Figure 15-1. CSI DiamondBack 360 Atherectomy Devices

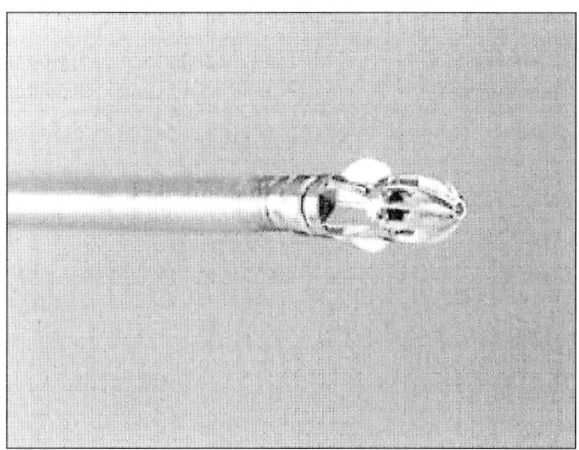

Figure 15-2. Pathway Medical Rotational Atherectomy device

The atherectomy device most commonly used currently is the SilverHawk Plaque Excision System (EV3, Minneapolis, MN). This directional extirpative atherectomy catheter was approved by the U.S. Food and Drug Administration in 2003. The catheter uses a battery-powered motor that rotates a catheter-encased drive shaft connected to a carbide circular blade at 8000 rpm. When the motor is turned on, the distal portion of the catheter deflects, allowing a portion of the rotating blade to protrude out of the catheter and shave fragments from the adjacent atherosclerotic plaque. These fragments of atheroma are directed into the enclosed nosecone of the catheter where they are stored until the catheter is removed from the artery (Figure 15–3). The opening in the blade's housing is radiopaque, allowing the operator to orient the catheter. Multiple passes are made in the lumen circumferentially, removing atheroma from the vessel wall.

The catheter is a monorail, rapid-exchange system that is used with a 0.014-inch diameter wire. The catheter comes in a variety of sizes (Table 15–1) and passes through a 6F to 8F sheath, depending on the size of the device. The catheters come with various features including flush (F) catheters that have a tip that is emptied using forceful saline flushing, as well as a specially designed cutting disk for calcium (Rockhawk). The extended tip (X) catheters have a larger nosecone, permitting an increased number of passes prior to removing the device and emptying of the nosecone. The collecting nosecone in the larger sizes of the catheters has a radiopaque packing mechanism that allows the operator to gauge the remaining capacity in the nosecone. The nosecone is emptied either by flushing with saline (flush devices) or by mechanical evacuation.

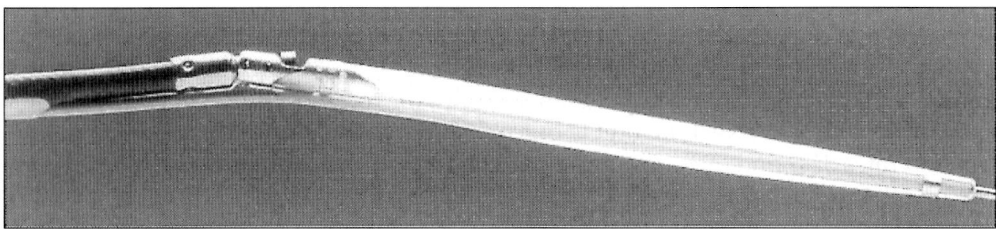

Figure 15-3. EV3 SilverHawk Directional Atherectomy Device

TABLE 15-1. TYPES AND SIZES OF SILVERHAWK DEVICES

SilverHawk Catheter Type	Target Vessel Size	Target Vessel Diameter (mm)	Crossing Profile (mm)	Tip Length (cm)
LS Large Vessel Standard Tip	Large (SFA)	4.5–7.0 mm	2.7	6.0
LS-F Large Vessel Standard Flush Tip	Large (SFA)	4.5–7.0 mm	2.7	6.0
LX Large Vessel Xtended Tip	Large (SFA)	4.5–6.5 mm	2.7	9.0
MS Medium Vessel Standard Tip	Medium (Popliteal)	3.5–5.0	2.7	6.0
MS-F Medium Vessel Standard Flush Tip	Medium (Popliteal)	3.5–5.0	2.7	6.0
SX Small Vessel Xtended Tip	Small (Tibial)	3.0–3.5	2.4	4.3
SXL Small Vessel Xtra Long Tip	Small (Tibial)	3.0–3.5	2.4	7.2
SS+ Small Vessel Standard Tip	Small (Tibial)	3.0–3.5	2.3	2.6
EXL Extra Small Vessel Xtra Long Tip	Extra small (Distal tibial)	2.0–3.0	2.0	6.0
ES+ Extra Small Vessel Standard Tip	Extra small (Distal tibial)	2.0–2.5 mm	1.9	2.2
DS Distal Vessel Standard Tip	Distal	1.5–2.0 mm	1.9	2.6

STUDIES

Early results using the Silverhawk atherectomy catheter were promising. Zeller et al. reported their mid-term results in 2004 treating 71 lesions in the femoropopliteal region.[12] These lesions were either primary stenoses (42%), native artery restenoses (38%), or in-stent restenoses (20%). At six months, the restenosis rate based on duplex ultrasound studies for primary lesions was 27%, and 20% of primary lesions required reintervention. Patients undergoing atherectomy for restenosis, both native artery and in-stent, did not have such favorable outcomes (restenosis rates 41% and 36%, reintervention rates 37% and 29%, respectively). The same group also examined their results for below-knee lesions.[13] They reported a rate of restenosis, defined as at least 70% stenosis on duplex ultrasound of 14% at three months and 22% at six months, respectively. The three- and six-month patency rates were 98% and 94%, respectively.

In 2006, the results of the TALON (Treating Peripherals with SilverHawk: Outcomes Collection) registry were reported.[14] This multicenter, prospective study looked at 601 patients with 1,258 atherosclerotic lesions in 748 limbs. The authors reported a 94.7% procedure success rate (success was defined as ≤50% residual diameter stenosis), and 41.9% of procedures required the treatment of two or more lesions. Only 26.7% of the lesions required any adjunctive therapy and 6.3% of the lesions required subsequent stent placement after atherectomy. Follow-up at six and 12 months showed 90% and 80% survival free of target lesion revascularization, respectively. Multivariate analysis found significant predictors of reintervention of atherosclerotic lesions at six months: history of MI or CABG, ≥2 lesions treated, increasing ischemia based on Rutherford classification, and length of the lesion. These results showed promising short- and mid-term results using SilverHawk atherectomy with low complication rates in population with widely varying degrees of ischemia and levels of disease.

Other single institution studies have also found that lesion characteristics and degree of ischemia effects results with atherectomy. Keeling et al. performed 70 atherectomy procedures on 66 limbs in 60 patients.[15] They reported an initial success rate of 87.1% with adjunctive procedures required in 24.3%. Postoperative surveillance was by noninvasive studies, and restenosis was based on lesion diameters seen on CTA, MRA, or angiography. Primary, primary assisted, and secondary patency were 61.7%, 64.1%, and 76.4% at one year, respectively. Limb salvage rates of patients with chronic limb ischemia (Rutherford Grade 4–6) was 86.2% at one year. Patients with TASC C or D lesions were more likely than those with TASC A or B lesions to reocclude, as were patients with higher Rutherford classification and those that required tibial atherectomy, along with treatment of more proximal disease. Though increased degrees of ischemia are associated with worse outcomes, the use of atherectomy in the treatment of critical limb ischemia has good short-term results:[16,17] avoiding amputation and allowing the treatment of patients who are high-risk for open bypass.

Recently, intermediate term results have been reported for both femoropopliteal and infrapopliteal arteries. For femoropopliteal lesions, Zeller et al. looked at eighty-four patients with 100 limbs and 131 lesions.[18] Primary patency was defined as restenosis ≤50% on duplex ultrasound. The primary patency at 12 months of patents with de novo lesions (34%), native vessel restenoses (33%), and in-stent restenoses (33%) were 84%, 54% and 54%, respectively. At 18 months, the primary patency rates were 73%, 42%, and 49% for the three groups. The rates of target lesion revascularization rate for each of the groups were 16%, 44%, and 47% at 12 months, and 22%, 56%, and 49% at 18 months. Once again, results with Silverhawk atherectomy in the treatment of de novo lesions were better than for restenosis. In terms of below-knee lesions, primary and secondary patency rates were 67% and 91% at one year and 60% and 80% at two years.[19]

We reviewed the single center prospective data at Columbia/Cornell in which 579 lesions were treated in 275 patients with claudication (36.7%) and critical limb ischemia (63.3%). Lesions were defined as primarily in the superficial femoral artery, popliteal artery, tibial vessels, or multilevel disease of femorotibial, femoropopliteal, or popliteal tibial lesions. The multilevel disease had a high instance of chronic total occlusion (CTO) between 89.5% and 100%, and the tibial lesions had a 54.6% instance of chronic total occlusion. The mean degree of stenosis in the superficial femoral artery is 88.7% + 14.1%, popliteal region of 85.6% ± 13.2%, and the tibial vessels, 92% ± 11.4%. Lesions were also divided by the TASC classification (TransAtlantic Symptomatic Stenosis Classification): TASC classification A, 120 patients; TASC B, 158 patients; TASC C, 116 patients; TASC D, 163 patients (Table 15–2).

TABLE 15-2. LESIONS CHARACTERISTICS OF THE 579 LESIONS TREATED

| | SFA | Popliteal | Tibial | Multilevel | | |
				Fem-tib	Fem-pop	Pop-tib
N	199	110	218	3	30	19
Length (mm) (SD	91.6 ± 90.8	37.7 ± 33.5	46.4 ± 51.1	395.3 ± 53.2	183.6 ± 93.7	102.3 ± 39.1
% Stenosis (SD	88.7 ± 14.1	85.6 ± 13.2	92.0 ± 11.4	100	98.8 ± 4.1	99.2 ± 2.5
# CTO (%)	73 (36.7)	33 (30)	118 (54.6)	3 (100)	27 (90)	17 (89.5)

PATENCY TABLE FOR TASC CLASSIFICATIONS:

| | Primary Patency | | Secondary Patency | | Limb Salvage | |
	12 mos	18 mos	12 mos	18 mos	12 mos	18 mos
TASC A	71.4 ± 4.7	58.6 ± 5.5	87.0 ± 3.5	79.8 ± 4.5	91.5 ± 2.9	89.9 ± 3.2
TASC B	69.7 ± 4.9	57.3 ± 5.8	85.0 ± 3.5	73.6 ± 5.3	90.8 ± 3.1	90.8 ± 3.1
TASC C	56.4 ± 5.8	50.6 ± 6.1	80.1 ± 4.4	80.1 ± 4.4	91.0 ± 3.1	91.0 ± 3.1
TASC D	53.7 ± 4.7	47.8 ± 5.1	74.1 ± 4.2	72.2 ± 4.5	86.7 ± 3.3	83.2 ± 4.0

Primary and secondary patencies as well as limb salvage is calculated for all lesions at 12 and 18 months. Primary patency for all lesions at 12 and 18 months was 62.2% ± 2.5% and 52.7% ± 2.8% respectively. Secondary patency at 12 and 18 months for all lesions was 80.3% ± 2% and 75.0% ± 2.4%, respectively. Limb salvage for all lesions was 89.7% at 12 months and 88.3% at 18 months. There was not a statistically significant difference between the primary and secondary patency of lesions based on the location and treatment: femoral, popliteal, or tibial lesions. However, there was a significant difference in those patients with extensive disease involving multilevel compared to isolated lesions. The primary and secondary patency as well as the limb salvage rates demonstrated a statistical advantage for claudicants compared to those patients with critical limb ischemia (P<0.05) (Table 15–3).

COMPLICATIONS

Immediate complications associated with Silverhawk atherectomy include perforation, dissections, occlusion and/or thrombosis, and embolism.[14] We have also observed the

TABLE 15-3. 12- AND 18-MONTH PATENCIES FOR ALL LESIONS TREATED

| | Primary Patency | | Secondary Patency | | Limb Salvage | |
	12 mos	18 mos	12 mos	18 mos	12 mos	18 mos
ALL Lesions	62.2 ± 2.5	52.7 ± 2.8	80.3 ± 2.0	75.0 ± 2.4	89.7 ± 1.6	88.3 ± 1.8
Femoral	61.4 ± 4.3	52.0 ± 4.8	85.4 ± 3.1	80.3 ± 3.9	95.4 ± 1.9	9543 ± 1.9
Popliteal	68.9 ± 5.4	59.2 ± 6.2	84.9 ± 4.1	76.7 ± 5.4	90.9 ± 3.4	88.4 ± 4.1
Tibial	62.7 ± 4.1	53.6 ± 4.8	74.2 ± 3.7	70.0 ± 4.2	83.6 ± 3.2	80.6 ± 3.7
Multilevel	50.5 ± 8.1	40.3 ± 8.3	75.7 ± 6.7	71.7 ± 7.5	89.7 ± 4.9	89.7 ± 4.9
Claudicants	67.1 ± 3.7	58.0 ± 4.3	89.4 ± 2.4	82.5 ± 3.5	98.3 ± 1.0	98.3 ± 1.0
CLI	59.1 ± 3.3	49.4 ± 3.7	74.3 ± 2.9	69.9 ± 3.2	83.9 ± 2.5	81.5 ± 2.8

formation of arteriovenous fistulas after atherectomy, most of which resolve with conservative management. Some advocate the use of distal protection device to protect the outflow from embolization. Suri et al. reported 10 cases in which a EPI Filterwire (Boston Scientific, Natick, MA) was placed distally prior to atherectomy.[20] Debris was collected in the filter in every case, with one case resulting in lack of flow distal to the filter that was restored after the protection device was removed. The size of the debris recovered ranged from 0.5 to 10 mm. Other access site complications associated with percutaneous interventions such as local hematomas, pseudoaneurysms, and retroperitoneal hematomas have also been associated with atherectomy. Rare occurrence of late pseudoaneurysm formation at the site of atherectomy has been reported.[21]

APPLICATIONS

Atherectomy is well suited for the treatment of arteries that are subject to flexion and compression such as the common femoral and popliteal arteries. Plaque debulking is favored over angioplasty and stenting since the mechanical forces in these locations could result in stent fatigue and eventual fracture. An additional advantage to using atherectomy instead of stenting at the common femoral region includes the ability to treat the lesion without covering the origin of the profunda femoris artery with a stent, which could impede flow and prevent future access to this vessel. Also, with angioplasty in this region, it is possible to push plaque into the profunda; with atherectomy, treatment can be directed instead of circumferential dilation of the region. Some prefer atherectomy over stenting in the treatment of long tibial disease since the stents in the small diameters come only in short lengths that would require the use of multiple stents. Eccentric lesions are well suited for directional atherectomy, as are cases of in-stent restenosis.

CONCLUSION

Atherectomy has been shown to be safe and effective in the treatment of lower extremity occlusive disease in a variety of clinical settings and anatomic locations. It has been used in the treatment of stenoses, occlusions, native arterial restenosis, and in-stent restenosis. There is an increased advantage in the infrapopliteal region where angioplasty and bailout stenting have limited usage. Our single center data indicate that there is acceptable 18-month primary patency, and excellent secondary patency and limb salvage for those patients treated with atherectomy. Whether atherectomy is superior to other percutaneous interventions is yet to be determined, and a prospective randomized clinical trial is needed to further define the appropriate indications for atherectomy or other endovascular therapies.

REFERENCES

1. Dotter CT, Judkins MP. Transluminal treatment of arteriosclerotic obstruction: Description of a new technique and preliminary report of its application. *Circulation*. 1964;30:654–670.

2. Feinglass J, Pearce WH, Martin GJ et al. Postoperative and amputation-free survival outcomes after femorodistal bypass grafting surgery: findings from the Department of Veterans Affairs National Surgical Quality Improvement Program. *J Vasc Surg*. 2001;34: 283–290.

3. Gallino A, Mahler F, Probst P et al. Percutaneous transluminal angioplasty of the arteries of the lower limbs: a 5 year follow-up. *Circulation*. 1984;70:619–623.

4. Johnston KW, Rae M, Hogg-Johnston SA et al. 5-year results of a prospective study of percutaneous transluminal angioplasty *Ann Surg*. 1987;206:403–413.

5. Ikeno F, Braden GA, Kaneda H, et al. Mechanism of luminal gain with plaque excision in atherosclerotic coronary and peripheral arteries: assessment by histology and intravascular ultrasound. *J Interven Cardiol*. 2007;20:107–113.

6. Simpson JB, Zimmerman JJ, Selmon RM et al. Transluminal atherectomy: initial clinical results in 27 patients. *Circulation*. 1986;74(Suppl II):203.

7. Kim D, Gianturco LE, Porter DH et al. Peripheral directional atherectomy: 4-year experience. *Radiology*. 1992;183:773–778.

8. Vroegindeweij D, Tielbeek AV, Buth J et al. Directional atherectomy versus balloon angioplasty in segmental femoropoliteal artery disease: Two-year follow-up with color-flow duplex scanning. *J Vasc Surg*. 1995;21:255–269.

9. Wholey MH, Smith JAM, Godlewski P et al. Recanalization of total arterial occlusions with the Kensey dynamic angioplasty catheter. *Radiology*. 1989;172:947–952.

10. The Collaborative Rotablator Atherectomy Group (CRAG). Peripheral atherectomy with the Rotablator: a multicenter report. *J Vasc Surg*.1994;19:509–515.

11. Jahnke T, Link J, Muller-Hulsbeck S et al. Treatment of infrapopliteal occlusive disease by high-speed rotational atherectomy: Initial and mid-term results. *J Vasc Interv Radiol*. 2001;12:221–226.

12. Zeller T, Rastan A, Schwarzwalder U et al. Percutaneous peripheral atherectomy of femoropopliteal stenoses using a new-generation device: six-month results from a single-center experience. *J Endovasc Ther*. 2004;11:676–685.

13. Zeller T, Rastan A, Schwarzwalder U et al. Midterm results after atherectomy-assisted angioplasty of below-knee arteries with use of the Silverhawk device. *J Vasc Interv Radiol*. 2004;15:1391–1397.

14. Ramaiah V, Gammon R, Kiesz S et al. Midterm outcomes from the TALON registry: Treating Peripherals With SilverHawk:Outcomes Collection. *J Endovasc Ther*. 2006;13: 592–602.

15. Keeling WB, Shames ML, Stone PA et al. Plaque excision with the Silverhawk catheter: Early results in patients with claudication or critical limb ischemia. *J Vasc Surg*. 2007;45: 25–31.

16. Kandzari DE, Kiesz S, Allie D et al. Procedural and clinical outcomes with catheter-based plaque excision in critical limb ischemia. *J Endovasc Ther*. 2006;13:12–22.

17. Yancey AE, Minion DJ, Rodriguez C et al. Peripheral atherectomy in TransAtlantic InterSociety Consensus type C femoropopliteal liesions for limb salvage. *J Vasc Surg*. 2006;44:503–509.

18. Zeller T, Rastan A, Sixt S et al. Long-term results after directional atherectomy of femoropopliteal lesions. *J Am Coll Cardiol*. 2006;48:1573–1578.

19. Zeller T, Sixt S, Schwarzalder U, et al. Two-year results after directional atherectomy of infrapopliteal arteries with the SilverHawk device. *J Endovasc Ther*. 2007;14:232–240.

20. Suri R, Wholey MH, Postoak D et al. Distal embolic protection during femoropoliteal atherectomy. *Catheter Cardiovasc Interv*. 2006;67:417–422.

21. Nikam S, Morgan JH, Zakhary EM et al. Native superficial femoral artery peripheral atherectomy site pseudoaneurysm: a case report. *J Vasc Surg*. 2007;46:565–568.

Open Surgical Revascularization in the Endovascular Era

SECTION III

Open Surgical
Revascularization in
the Endovascular Era

16

Improving Lower Extremity Bypass Patency

Peter K. Henke, M.D.

Peripheral arterial disease (PAD) is common, affecting approximately 12% of the U.S. population. Though most patients never require a bypass, the indications for such require emphasis: rest pain, tissue loss, and in *rare occasions*, lifestyle-limiting claudication.[1] The downsides of performing infrainguinal arterial bypasses for indications less than those stated (e.g. mild claudication) are significant as their durability is far from perfect. This point is particularly true when considering the relatively benign course of claudication once risk factor and medical therapy is instituted. Thus, to improve on infrainguinal bypass results, a comprehensive algorithm that encompasses all facets of care is suggested (Figure 16–1).

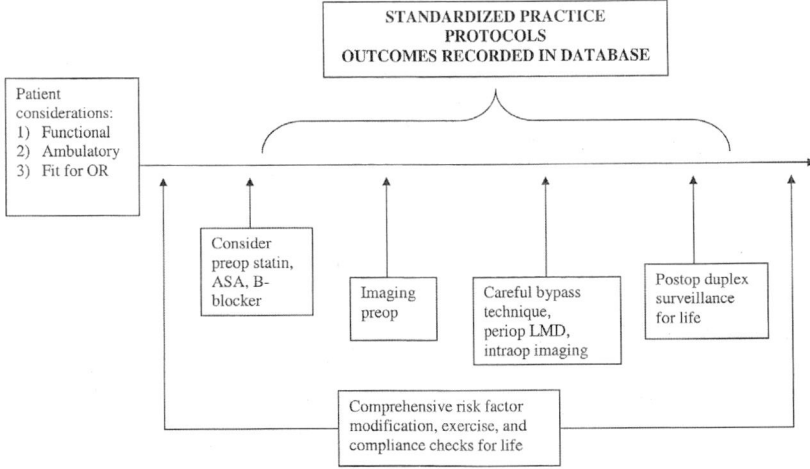

Figure 16-1. A comprehensive algorythm is suggested to include all facets of care for patients with operative PAD. LMD = low molecular weight dextran.

The problem related to lower extremity bypass grafting is primarily one of long-term patency or durability. Perioperative morbidity and mortality are acceptable, with most patients surviving beyond 30 days.[2-4] If one considers the published long-term patency rates of aortofemoral bypass, open abdominal aortic aneurysm (AAA) repair, and carotid endarterectomy (CEA), the failure rate is low, ranging from 5–15%. For example, most aortofemoral bypass surgery series report an approximate 80% patency rate at 10 years.[5] In contrast, most best series in the literature report assisted primary and secondary primary patency rates of autologous saphenous vein bypass of 80% at *five years*,[4-7] and less in prospective trials,[8-11] or those with non-saphenous venous conduit[12] (Table16–1).

Infrainguinal bypasses are compromised compared with these other vascular repairs for several reasons: 1) First, AAA and CEA is done for prophylaxis against a life-threatening condition that involve vessels that have abnormal enlargement, or encompass a short segment stenosis feeding a low resistance outflow bed, respectively; 2) Aortofemoral bypass uses a large caliber synthetic graft that tends to have high flow rates, decreasing risk of thrombosis; and 3) Infrainguinal bypasses using autologous vein, while considered the first choice of conduit, are fraught with short and long-term risk for vein intimal injury and subsequent stenoses. This is compounded by longer length bypasses, which by definition have a greater area for neointimal hyperplasia to develop.

TABLE 16-1. SELECTED INFRAINGUINAL BYPASS SERIES

Series	N	Indications	Evidence Level	Conduit	2° Patency	Limb Salvage
VEITH, ET AL[9]	845	CLAUD: 11% RP: 37% TL: 61%	I	ASV: 253 PTFE: 592	4 YR: 68% ASV 47% PTFE	75%
GREEN, ET AL[11]	240	CLAUD: 58% RP: 11% TL: 27%	I	PFTE: 120 DACRON: 120	5 Yr: 67%	95%
POMPOSELLI, ET AL[3]	1032	RP/TL: 100%	III	AV: 1030	2 YR: 63%	78%
DONALDSON, ET AL[7]	585	CLAUD: 29% RP/TL: 71%	III	AV: 447 PTFE: 138	5 YR: 72%	92%
JOHNSON, ET AL[8]	752	CLAUD: 34% RP/TL: 68%	I	PTFE: 265 AV: 226 HUV: 261	5 YR:* 73% AV 53% HUV 39% PTFE	90%
TAYLOR, ET AL[6]	553	CLAMP: 20% RP/TL: 80%	III	AV: 516 PTFE: 37	5 YR: 80% AV 68% PROTH	90%
KLINKERT, ET AL[10]	151	CLAMP: 20% RP/TL: 80%	I	AV: 75 PTFE: 76	5 YR:* 80% AV 57% PTFE	90%

AV = autologous vein; RP = rest pain; TL = tissue loss; HUV = human umbilical vein; CLAUD = claudication
*denotes significantly better outcomes with autologous vein compared with non-vein conduit

PATIENT SELECTION

It bears repeating that interventions for PAD should be nonoperative in most claudi-cants. Simply put, graft failure and the attendant sequelae do not occur in a patient who is properly selected for nonoperative management. Rest pain and tissue loss are solid indications, while claudication should only be considered in cases where good medical and risk factor reducing therapy have been tried for at least six months with no documented improvement. This includes smoking cessation and requires the pa-tient to participate in their care prior to any subsequent surgical intervention. As mod-ern vascular surgical techniques have broken down many of the technical barriers to peripheral arterial bypass, who best to select for these operations becomes paramount. For example, several authors have highlighted the typical long and involved postoper-ative course these patients endure, often requiring multiple later surgeries for wound problems (up to 17%) despite technically successful procedures and commonly a lengthy rehabilitation stay.[13-15]

In some cases, primary amputation may be best for some patients that have lim-ited functional capacity and/or otherwise have medical comorbidities.[16] For example, elderly patients with tissue loss and hemodialysis dependent renal failure represent a group with high graft failure and limited lifespan, and where bypasses are not rou-tinely recommended. In contrast, diabetic patients with even minor tissue loss should be treated aggressively to restore normal perfusion as delayed revascularization may make an infection impossible to eradicate and lead to limb loss despite a patent graft. Furthermore, graft success in diabetic patients is as good as nondiabetics.[3,17] While most series have focused on technical success and perioperative complications, the long-term functional outcome is likely worse than thought. For example, a Markov de-cision model evaluating the quality adjusted life years with peripheral arterial bypass estimated only two months, gained at a significant monetary expense.[18] Not surpris-ingly, bypasses for tissue loss and patients with multiple medical comorbidities also significantly increase costs.[19] Thus, it is incumbent on the surgeon to thoroughly eval-uate the patient (beyond merely justifying their perioperative risk) and consider their lifestyle, social support system, and mental faculty.

IMAGING CONSIDERATIONS

Operative decisions for infrainguinal lower extremity bypass surgeries are based on duplex waveforms and segmental arterial pressure screening, followed by preopera-tive contrast angiography. Some institutions have magnetic resonance angiography (MRA) scanning capabilities of sufficient sensitivity and specificity to allow operations to be based solely on this imaging modality.[20]

Duplex scanning is not only important for screening but also is a useful adjunct for determining adequacy of the recipient outflow artery. For instance, duplex scanning using a high-frequency transducer (10 MHz) can be used to assess the tibial vessels for size and flow rates, where extensive proximal disease may not allow clear arteriographic imaging.[21] Arterial bypasses are usually successful with a duplex im-aged pedal vessel larger than 1.5 mm diameter and with demonstrated diastolic flow suggesting no immediate distal occlusion (e.g. diastolic flow > 10 cm/sec). This is par-ticularly relevant for diabetic and multisegmental occlusive disease patients who often have significant infrageniculate arterial disease. Again, MRA may be helpful in this regard as it can delineate tibial vessels with greater sensitivity, but motion and phase dropout artifacts are common.

To confirm immediate technical success, an intraoperative duplex scan should be done at bypass completion to assess for native inflow artery, proximal graft, mid-graft, distal graft, and native artery outflow velocities, as well as grey scale imaging. While graft velocities vary depending on the segment interrogated, a helpful index is the mean calculated total graft flow, as higher flow rates (> 90 ml/min) have less chance of later failure than lower flow grafts (< 80 ml/min).[22] Segmental velocities within the body or distal graft of < 50 cm/sec suggest a proximal flow limiting stenosis that bears close intraoperative investigation to make sure an anatomical problem is not present. However, very slow velocities at the distal hood (e.g. 20 cm/sec) in reversed vein grafts do not seem to confer an increased risk of graft occlusion, as long as normal velocities are found in the recipient native artery. Furthermore, duplex scanning is very helpful for *in situ* bypass technique to define a residual A-V fistula or a partially lysed valve. The intraoperative duplex scanning velocities can then be used as a comparison for later follow-up studies. Many times, the absolute postoperative velocities will increase from the intraoperative values but the relationship between proximal to distal outflows usually remain similar.

Having a patient adhere to a postoperative bypass graft surveillance program is perhaps even more important than intraoperative duplex scanning. Significantly improved lower extremity bypass patencies can be achieved as hemodynamically significant stenoses can be diagnosed and interventions taken before a graft thromboses.[23-25] Most graft problems manifest within the first two years and intensive surveillance is warranted during this period (Table 16–2). Typically, a 3.5-fold increase in graft velocity compared with a proximal normal velocity suggests a critical stenosis and warrants urgent operative correction. Though no data are available to state the risk of occlusion with certainty, prolonging the repair more than four weeks once diagnosed is not suggested. Preprocedural full—dose, low-molecular weight heparin can be added to the current antiplatelet regimen if a delay is anticipated.

The use of intraoperative angioscopy is appealing as the intraluminal surface and anastomoses can be directly visualized. The stenotic areas can be directly assessed and corrected if need be. However, good visualization can be technically challenging to

TABLE 16-2. DUPLEX IMAGING

PREOPERATIVE	USED FOR VEIN MAPPING AND DESIGNATION OF ARTERIAL TARGETS
INTRAOPERATIVE	CONFIRM INFLOW, GRAFT, OUTFLOW VELOCITIES, AND EVALUATE FOR TECHNICAL DEFECTS
	*INFLOW: 60–150 CM/SEC
	GRAFT: 80–180 CM/SEC
	OUTFLOW: 60–200 CM/SEC
POSTOPERATIVE	RECOMMENDED SCHEDULE:
	Q 3 MONTHS FOR YEAR 1
	Q 6 MONTHS FOR YEAR 2
	Q YEAR THEREAFTER
	(FULL GRAFT SCAN & ABI'S)

*denotes typical flow velocities, not absolute cutoffs

achieve and the angioscope often requires a separate venotomy. Another common use for angioscopy is to directly visualize valve lysis when the *in situ* technique is used. The sensitivity and specificity of angioscopy may be better than completion angiography,[26,27] and can supplement intraoperative duplex.

CURRENT LOWER EXTREMITY BYPASS TECHNIQUES

Bypass durability is typically reported in the literature as primary and secondary patency, and is assessed by life table analysis. For practical purposes, the assisted primary or secondary patency, as well as limb salvage, are most relevant for graft success measured long term. Grafts that fail, and which were done for rest pain or tissue loss, directly decrease limb salvage.[28-30] Autologous venous bypasses are recommended without hesitation over prosthetics in *all situations*. *In situ* vein with valve lysis, reversed vein, and non-reversed translocated with valve lysis all have similar patency rates at institutions where they are done in sufficient number (e.g. > 40 bypasses per year).[31] The surgeon should be comfortable with all techniques, but perform one technique primarily, such that the volume and the subtleties that are required for a successful operation become ingrained in a systematic way. The patency rates between vein preparation techniques are comparable with advantages and disadvantages of both types. The positive association between higher volume and better outcome likely plays a role in this particular surgery, though the effect is less strong than coronary artery bypass grafting (CABG) as greater variation in technique and patient factors exist.[31]

Another common controversial situation is attempting salvage of a thrombosed bypass versus placing a new one. Currently, this means the use of thrombolysis in acute or semi-acute graft occlusions. While this is technically feasible, the long-term outcomes are variable.[28,32] Regardless of the surgeon's philosophy, the more rapid the graft is lysed, the less endothelial damage occurs, and the higher the chance of graft salvage. Others have found early graft failures (< 30 days) without an identified technical defect to be highly predictive of subsequent graft failure and placement of a new graft should be done.[33] Similarly, the author's group has also found that early graft failure confers a significant independent risk for secondary graft failure.[30]

ANATOMICAL AND TECHNICAL CONSIDERATIONS

Many factors contribute to the success of an infrainguinal arterial bypass, but simplistically, these include inflow, outflow, and conduit (Table 16–3). Adequate arterial inflow pressure is mandatory for successful infrainguinal bypass. As a practical matter, a palpable femoral pulse in the groin ipsilateral to the planned infrainguinal bypass usually indicates a sufficient arterial pressure to support a new graft. Whether one should have documented triphasic duplex waveforms confirmed for the inflow artery is speculative, and in the setting of an easily palpable pulse and a patent aortoiliac system by arteriography, is probably not necessary. Aortofemoral bypass or iliac angioplasty/stent prior to an infrainguinal procedure is reasonable if compromised inflow is present. The patency of grafts below a stented artery have not been well described in long-term follow-up studies, but as angioplasty/stent patency is dependent on adequate outflow,[34] a

TABLE 16-3. TECHNICAL CONSIDERATIONS

INFLOW ARTERY	SUPRABRACHIAL ARTERIAL PRESSURE
	TRIPHASIC DUPLEX WAVEFORM;
	NO SIGNIFICANT PROXIMAL STENOSIS BY ANGIOGRAPHY
OUTFLOW ARTERY	LARGEST PROXIMAL UNOBSTRUCTED ARTERY TO FOOT TEST WITH
	1.5–2.5 MM DILATOR AT OPERATION
CONDUIT	AK POPLITEAL: GSV > ARM VEIN > ePTFE
	BK POPLITEAL OR DISTAL:
	GSV > ARM VEIN > COMPOSITE VEIN > ePTFE WITH CUFF

AK = above knee; BK = below knee; GSV = greater saphenous vein

functioning graft should be beneficial. Conversely, in-stent intimal hyperplasia is a pervasive problem and for which predictive risk variables are not always clear.[30]

The outflow artery should be the most proximal, nonobstructed vessel that leads to the foot. The conduit should be autologous vein for any below knee bypass, including using composite vein-vein bypasses. It is the author's opinion that autologous vein should be used in almost all cases of above the knee bypasses as well. For example, if no ipsilateral or contralateral greater saphenous vein is available, adequate arm vein should be considered for above-knee popliteal bypass prior to using a prosthetic material. This tenet is *controversial* but is based on the long-term outcome data of infrainguinal bypasses (Table 16–1). While prosthetic grafts have similar two-year patency rates as compared with vein in the above the knee position, a marked divergence occurs soon after and prosthetic grafts tend to fail at a significant rate in the long term (e.g. five years).[8,9,35] This would not be so troublesome except that when prosthetic grafts fail, the patient often presents with a grade of ischemia that is significantly worse than baseline, is not favorably modified with aggressive anticoagulation, and increases limb loss risk.[35,36] If a prosthetic bypass is needed for a below knee site, it is recommended that a vein patch angioplasty of the recipient artery be performed, and the graft anastomosed to this patch. One group has reported a three-year mean assisted patency rate of nearly 70% with the concomitant use of Coumadin.[37] Another technique that may improve infrapatellar prosthetic graft patency is the creation of a distal AV fistula to accelerate blood flow velocity.[38] Larger series need to be reported before routine adaptation of these techniques, especially if adequate nonsaphenous vein is available.

The argument of "saving the vein" for a future bypass is not valid for two reasons: First, the vein in the region of where the prosthetic graft is placed may become damaged and sclerotic, rendering that vein unusable for later bypasses.[10] Second, as endovascular and medical therapy for coronary heart disease improves, many who would have previously had a CABG now never come to this intervention. Thus, the vein should be used for what is the most pressing health issue at the time.

When harvesting the vein, it is important not to deeply skeletonize the vein as this removes the arterial and venous vessels that maintain the adventitia. Harvesting a vein for a reversed vein bypass may cause more periadvential damage, as compared with the *in situ* technique, but the valvulotome causes endothelial damage and is probably why these techniques have similar long-term patencies.[6,7] In general, the shorter the bypass, the better it is. For example, it is the author's preference to base a distal bypass off an intact and minimally diseased AK popliteal as compared with the common femoral vessel, particularly in diabetics. Arterial exposure should be just enough to allow safe clamp placement but not so much as to risk damaging surrounding structures. An anastomosis length of 2–2.5 cm is usually adequate for popliteal or tibial recipient arteries. It cannot be emphasized enough not to perform blind endarterectomies on the recipient vessel as this will inevitably create an intimal-medial flap and subsequent occlusion. This creates misery for the surgeon and places the patient at risk of limb loss and operative complications.

The need for graft revision, once detected, is estimated to occur in 20–30% of grafts, regardless of the technique.[4] Graft revisions are done prophylactically for a critical stenosis to prevent a later graft failure secondary to thrombosis. Once a graft thromboses, the ability to salvage it drops significantly.[28, 29] Excellent long-term graft patencies can be achieved with operative interposition or patch angioplasty techniques, even if multiple revisions are required.[39] Less data are available to determine the safety and utility of endovascular angioplasty techniques, but short-term follow-up data are favorable.[40] Until better studies become available, the author's practice is to treat distal stenoses with primary balloon angioplasty whereas proximal stenoses are approached with an open vein angioplasty. Newer cutting balloons may provide more definitive scar release than standard angioplasty.[41] This tenet is modified by the angiographic features of the stenosis (diffuse segment lesions favor open repair), and whether the stenosis develops in the first 12 months (angioplasty) or after 24 months (open repair) as the etiologies and treatment responses differ.

MEDICAL ADJUNCTS

Several medical therapies are available which may improve bypass patency. However, these do not replace the aforementioned judgment nor the technical skill required to achieve excellent results. These medications should be considered in all patients with symptomatic PAD, as these are associated with a significant reduction in overall cardiac morbidity and mortality (Table 16–4).[42]

Antiplatelet therapy should be instituted not only to enhance bypass patency but also to afford the patient its significant cardioprotective benefits. An aspirin (ASA, 81 mg per day) regimen should be in place prior to the patient undergoing an infrainguinal bypass and should not be stopped preoperatively. Use of clopidogrel may

TABLE 16-4. MEDICAL ADJUNCTS

Agent	Action	Cardio-protective	Graft protective	Dosage	Evidence level
ASA	ANTI-PLATELET	Y	Y	81 MG EVERY DAY	I
CLOPIDOGREL	ANTIPLATELET	Y	Y	75 MG EVERY DAY	I, II
WARFARIN	ANTICOAGULANT	±	Y	TARGET INR 2-3	II
STATIN	CHOLESTEROL LOWERING	Y	Y	VARIES*	I, III
ACE I	ANTIHYPERTENSIVE	Y	N	VARIES	I, III
BETA BLOCKER	ANTIHYPERTENSIVE	Y	N	VARIES**	I
MV	METABOLISM	±	N	ONE PER DAY	I

ACE-I—angiotensin converting enzyme inhibitor; MV = multivitamin
*titrate to LDL = 70 mg/dl
**some evidence to titrate to HR > 50 < 65 bpm

provide better graft patency than ASA as extrapolated from cardiac studies[43-44] but in the author's practice, is only used for bypasses considered higher risk (e.g. redo or disadvantaged outflow). However, this medication should be ceased approximately five days prior to the patient's operation as excessive bleeding may occur. In these cases, the patient should be switched to ASA preoperatively, and then restarted on the clopidogrel postoperatively. Low-molecular weight dextran (LMD) at 20 cc/hour is instituted intraoperatively prior to protamine reversal continued for 36 hours, and the postoperative ASA begun on the first postoperative day. The LMD has a modest antiplatelet effect and is an intravascular volume expander, both which may help prevent early platelet-mediated graft thrombosis.

Intravenous heparinization is used periprocedurally, but not usually continued into the postoperative period unless the patient has a known hypercoagulable state or other medical condition where postoperative Coumadinization will be required (e.g., mitral valve). Some surgeons use the regimen of heparin followed by Coumadin for patients who undergo a redo bypass, those with disadvantaged outflows, or those with a contraindication to long-term ASA use.[45] However, a randomized controlled trial of ASA versus ASA plus Coumadin (INR 1.8–2.4) failed to show a significant patency advantage compared with ASA alone in vein grafts.[46] The bleeding risk with Coumadin is not insignificant and the need for long-term blood draws and monitoring needs to be kept in mind when choosing this therapy.

Use of an HMG CoA-reductase inhibitor (statin) is also important and can be prescribed directly by surgeons. The patient should be told of possible myalgias and is not generally prescribed to patients with liver disease. Indeed, a retrospective study suggested that perioperative statin use was associated with a three-fold increase in graft patency and three-fold decrease in limb loss.[24] Stronger evidence is extrapolated from the cardiac literature where a lower rate of need for revascularization and improved CABG patency has been shown. Statins, like beta-blockers, also seem to lower periprocedural mortality.[47] The statins seem to have beneficial effects independent from their lipid lowering effect. Experimental data suggests that statins increase circulating endothelial progenitor cells (for *in vivo* normal arterial repair), as well as have anti-inflammatory effects.[48]

Certain biomarkers are also becoming better recognized for predicting cardiovascular health.[49] These include such factors as C-reactive protein, CD40 ligand, Lipoprotein-a, and certain cell adhesions molecules, but their prognostic role in pre- and postinfrainguinal arterial bypass outcomes is unknown. One could envision in the near future a comprehensive preoperative risk analysis based on these markers to better select patients in whom a bypass has the most chance of success, as well as following postprocedure for early prognostication of graft stenosis.

E2F decoy transfection, directed antifibrotic gene therapy, and bone marrow derived endothelial progenitor cells are being actively investigated and hold promise for improving graft patency as well as perhaps delaying the need for bypasses altogether.[50] Currently, trials in related areas of lower extremity ischemic disease are ongoing.

A COMPREHENSIVE PROGRAM

As stated, the single biggest problem with infrainguinal arterial bypasses is the long-term durability. Failed grafts neither accomplish the therapeutic goal of improving limb perfusion and salvage, nor are these procedures without significant perioperative and long-term risks. Failed grafts directly increase subsequent limb loss rates, and amputees have more difficulties with activities of daily living and a higher long-term mortality.[2]

It is highly recommended that each vascular surgery practice, whether academic or private, set up a database with all patients who undergo such procedures, including those in whom only an endovascular procedure is done, to allow the surgeon to critically assess the long-term outcomes. When used for quality improvement and not published research, these databases are HIPAA compliant without need for separate patient consent. The human mind has a propensity to only remember the successes and not track failures. One team member who is invaluable to a busy vascular service is a nurse practitioner or physician assistant. They can deal with issues of pre- and postoperative patient care (in times of decreased resident coverage) as well as manage this patient database. Quarterly or bi-yearly reports allow ongoing assessment of outcomes and practice processes to change as needed.

Similarly, practice protocols to ensure the patients are taking appropriate preoperative medications such as ASA, statins, and beta-blockers should be instituted. An easy way to manage this is to have standardized preoperative and postoperative orders so the details are not forgotten. Furthermore, this can be carried into the clinic to document compliance with medications and risk factor modification.

Few things in surgery are as satisfying as having patients return ambulatory, with healed wounds, lack of rest pain, and a patent graft. If instituted systematically, the imaging, surgical, and medical adjuncts should allow for overall excellent outcomes. The goal (five-year, 90% assisted primary patency rate) should be feasible with proper patient selection, surgical techniques, medical adjuncts, and duplex imaging follow-up.

REFERENCES

1. Henke PK. Lower Extremity Ischemia. *Practic Cardiol*. 2003:493–509.
2. Feinglass J, Pearce WH, Martin GJ, et al. Postoperative and amputation-free survival outcomes after femorodistal bypass grafting surgery: findings from the Department of Veterans Affairs National Surgical Quality Improvement Program. *J Vasc Surg*. 2001;34(2): 283–290.
3. Pomposelli FB, Kansal N, Hamdan AD, et al. A decade of experience with dorsalis pedis artery bypass: analysis of outcome in more than 1000 cases. *J Vasc Surg*. 2003;37(2): 307–315.
4. Wixon CL, Mills JL, Westerband A,et al. An economic appraisal of lower extremity bypass graft maintenance. *J Vasc Surg*. 2000;32(1):1–12.
5. Brewster DC. Aortofemoral bypass for atherosclerotic aortoiliac occlusive disease. *Current Therapy in Vascular Surgery*. 2001;Fourth Edition:375–380.
6. Taylor LM, Jr., Edwards JM, Porter JM. Present status of reversed vein bypass grafting: five-year results of a modern series. *J Vasc Surg*. 1990;11(2):193–205;discussion 206.
7. Donaldson MC, Whittemore AD, Mannick JA. Further experience with an all-autogenous tissue policy for infrainguinal reconstruction. *J Vasc Surg*. 1993;18(1):41–48.
8. Johnson WC, Lee KK. A comparative evaluation of polytetrafluoroethylene, umbilical vein, and saphenous vein bypass grafts for femoral-popliteal above-knee revascularization: a prospective randomized Department of Veterans Affairs cooperative study. *J Vasc Surg*. 2000;32(2):268–277.
9. Veith FJ, Gupta SK, Ascer E, et al. Six-year prospective multicenter randomized comparison of autologous saphenous vein and expanded polytetrafluoroethylene grafts in infrainguinal arterial reconstructions. *J Vasc Surg*. 1986;3(1):104–114.

10. Klinkert P, Schepers A, Burger DH,et al. Vein versus polytetrafluoroethylene in above-knee femoropopliteal bypass grafting: five-year results of a randomized controlled trial. *J Vasc Surg.* 2003;37(1):149–155.

11. Green RM, Abbott WM, Matsumoto T, et al. Prosthetic above-knee femoropopliteal bypass grafting: five-year results of a randomized trial. *J Vasc Surg.* 2000;31(3):417–425.

12. Chew DK, Conte MS, Donaldson MC, et al. Autogenous composite vein bypass graft for infrainguinal arterial reconstruction. *J Vasc Surg.* 2001;33(2):259–264; discussion 264–265.

13. Abou-Zamzam AM, Jr., Lee RW, Moneta GL, et al. Functional outcome after infrainguinal bypass for limb salvage. *J Vasc Surg.* 1997;25(2):287–295; discussion 295–297.

14. Wengrovitz M, Atnip RG, Gifford RR, et al. Wound complications of autogenous subcutaneous infrainguinal arterial bypass surgery: predisposing factors and management. *J Vasc Surg.* 1990;11(1):156–161; discussion 61–63.

15. Goshima KR, Mills JL, Sr., Hughes JD. A new look at outcomes after infrainguinal bypass surgery: traditional reporting standards systematically underestimate the expenditure of effort required to attain limb salvage. *J Vasc Surg.* 2004;39(2):330–5.

16. Nehler MR, Hiatt WR, Taylor LM, Jr. Is revascularization and limb salvage always the best treatment for critical limb ischemia? *J Vasc Surg.* 2003;37(3):704–8.

17. Akbari CM, Pomposelli FB, Jr., Gibbons GW, et al. Lower extremity revascularization in diabetes: late observations. *Arch Surg.* 2000;135(4):452–456.

18. Hunink MG, Wong JB, Donaldson MC, et al. Revascularization for femoropopliteal disease. A decision and cost-effectiveness analysis. *JAMA.* 1995;274(2):165–171.

19. Jansen RM, de Vries SO, Cullen KA, et al. Cost-identification analysis of revascularization procedures on patients with peripheral arterial occlusive disease. *J Vasc Surg.* 1998;28(4): 617–623.

20. Hoch JR, Tullis MJ, Kennell TW, et al. Use of magnetic resonance angiography for the preoperative evaluation of patients with infrainguinal arterial occlusive disease. *J Vasc Surg.* 1996;23(5):792–800; discussion 801.

21. Hofmann WJ, Walter J, Ugurluoglu A, et al. Preoperative high-frequency duplex scanning of potential pedal target vessels. *J Vasc Surg.* 2004;39(1):169–175.

22. Ihlberg LH, Alback NA, Lassila R, Lepantalo M. Intraoperative flow predicts the development of stenosis in infrainguinal vein grafts. *J Vasc Surg.* 2001;34(2):269–276.

23. Bandyk DF. Essentials of graft surveillance. *Semin Vasc Surg.* 1993;6(2):92–102.

24. Henke PK, Blackburn S, Proctor MC, et al. Patients undergoing infrainguinal bypass to treat atherosclerotic vascular disease are underprescribed cardioprotective medications: effect on graft patency, limb salvage, and mortality. *J Vasc Surg.* 2004;39(2):357–365.

25. Mills JL, Sr. P values may lack power: the choice of conduit for above-knee femoropopliteal bypass graft. *J Vasc Surg.* 2000;32(2):402–405.

26. Woelfle KD, Kugelmann U, Bruijnen H, et al. Intraoperative imaging techniques in infrainguinal arterial bypass grafting: completion angiography versus vascular endoscopy. *Eur J Vasc Surg.* 1994;8(5):556–561.

27. Harward TR, Govostis DM, Rosenthal GJ, et al. Impact of angioscopy on infrainguinal graft patency. *Am J Surg.* 1994;168(2):107–110.

28. Whittemore AD, Donaldson MC, Polak JF, Mannick JA. Limitations of balloon angioplasty for vein graft stenosis. *J Vasc Surg.* 1991;14(3):340–345.

29. Belkin M, Donaldson MC, Whittemore AD, et al. Observations on the use of thrombolytic agents for thrombotic occlusion of infrainguinal vein grafts. *J Vasc Surg.* 1990;11(2):289–294; discussion 95–96.

30. Henke PK, Proctor MC, Zajkowski PJ, et al. Tissue loss, early primary graft occlusion, female gender, and a prohibitive failure rate of secondary infrainguinal arterial reconstruction. *J Vasc Surg.* 2002;35:902–909.

31. Birkmeyer JD, Siewers AE, Finlayson EV, et al. Hospital volume and surgical mortality in the United States. *N Engl J Med.* 2002;346(15):1128–1137.

32. Conrad MF, Shepard AD, Rubinfeld IS, et al. Long-term results of catheter-directed thrombolysis to treat infrainguinal bypass graft occlusion: the urokinase era. *J Vasc Surg.* 2003; 37(5):1009–1016.

33. Lombardi JV, Dougherty MJ, Calligaro KD, et al. Predictors of outcome when reoperating for early infrainguinal bypass occlusion. *Ann Vasc Surg*. 2000;14(4):350–355.

34. Hood DB, Hodgson KJ. Percutaneous arterial dilation for atherosclerotic aortoiliac occlusve disease. *Current Therapy in Vascular Surgery*. 2001;Fourth edition:384–390.

35. Jackson MR, Johnson WC, Williford WO, et al. The effect of anticoagulation therapy and graft selection on the ischemic consequences of femoropopliteal bypass graft occlusion: results from a multicenter randomized clinical trial. *J Vasc Surg*. 2002;35(2):292–298.

36. Jackson MR, Belott TP, Dickason T, et al. The consequences of a failed femoropopliteal bypass grafting: comparison of saphenous vein and PTFE grafts. *J Vasc Surg*. 2000; 32(3): 498–504; 505.

37. Neville RF, Tempesta B, Sidway AN. Tibial bypass for limb salvage using polytetrafluoroethylene and a distal vein patch. *J Vasc Surg*. 2001;33(2):266–271; discussion 271–272.

38. Jacobs MJ, Reul GJ, Gregoric ID, et al. Creation of a distal arteriovenous fistula improves microcirculatory hemodynamics of prosthetic graft bypass in secondary limb salvage procedures. *J Vasc Surg*. 1993;18(1):1–8; discussion 9.

39. Landry GJ, Moneta GL, Taylor LM, Jr.,et al. Patency and characteristics of lower extremity vein grafts requiring multiple revisions. *J Vasc Surg*. 2000;32(1):23–31.

40. Sanchez LA, Suggs WD, Veith FJ, et al. Is surveillance to detect failing polytetrafluoroethylene bypasses worthwhile?: Twelve-year experience with ninety-one grafts. *J Vasc Surg*. 1993;18(6):981–989; discussion 989–990.

41. Kasirajan K, Schneider PA. Early outcome of "cutting" balloon for infrainguinal vein graft stenosis. *J Vasc Surg*. 2004(39):702–708.

42. Hiatt WR. Pharmacologic therapy for peripheral arterial disease and claudication. *J Vasc Surg*. 2002;36(6):1283–1291.

43. Bhatt DL, Chew DP, Hirsch AT et al. Superiority of clopidogrel versus aspirin in patients with prior cardiac surgery. *Circulation*. 2001;103(3):363–368.

44. Becquemin JP. Effect of ticlopidine on the long-term patency of saphenous-vein bypass grafts in the legs. Etude de la Ticlopidine apres Pontage Femoro-Poplite and the Association Universitaire de Recherche en Chirurgie. *N Engl J Med*. 1997;337(24):1726–1731.

45. Sarac TP, Huber TS, Back MR, et al. Warfarin improves the outcome of infrainguinal vein bypass grafting at high risk for failure. *J Vasc Surg*. 1998;28(3):446–457.

46. Johnson·WC, Williford WO. Benefits, morbidity, and mortality associated with long-term administration of oral anticoagulant therapy to patients with peripheral arterial bypass procedures: a prospective randomized study. *J Vasc Surg*. 2002;35(3):413–421.

47. Poldermans D, Bax JJ, Kertai MD, et al. Statins are associated with a reduced incidence of perioperative mortality in patients undergoing major noncardiac vascular surgery. *Circulation*. 2003;107(14):1848–1851.

48. Wolfrum S, Jensen KS, Liao JK. Endothelium-dependent effects of statins. *Arterioscler Thromb Vasc Biol*. 2003;23(5):729–736.

49. Blake GJ, Ridker PM. Novel clinical markers of vascular wall inflammation. *Circ Res*. 2001;89(9):763–71.

50. Conte MS, Mann MJ, Simosa HF, et al. Genetic interventions for vein bypass graft disease: a review. *J Vasc Surg*. 2002;36(5):1040–1052.

17

A 20-year Experience with Infrapopliteal Prosthetic Graft

Samuel S. Ahn, M.D., Woo-Hyung Kwun, M.D., Ph.D., and Toshifumi Kudo, M.D., Ph.D.

Critical limb ischemia (CLI) is a common and often challenging entity faced by the vascular surgeon. The complexity of any lower extremity operation for ischemia increases in the setting of previous revascularization attempts and the unavailability of autogenous conduit. Specifically, the question of whether to use prosthetic conduit for revascularization to the infrapopliteal vessels when no autogenous vein is available remains unanswered and controversial. To our knowledge, no study to date has compared prosthetic distal bypass versus primary amputation of a severely ischemic limb, and looked at the outcome measures of return to ambulation, quality of life, and survival. However, clearly conducting such a prospective trial would be difficult. Concerns about the treatment of these patients undergoing distal prosthetic bypass include intraoperative technique, procedure durability, and long-term benefit. Thus, to answer these questions, establish guidelines, and elucidate factors important in the care of these patients, we reviewed our experience in the past two decades.

BYPASS CONDUIT IN LOWER EXTREMITY REVASCULARIZATION

Kunlin first described the use of autogenous saphenous vein (ASV) as a bypass conduit in the treatment of femoral arterial occlusive disease in 1949.[1] Linton introduced and popularized femoropopliteal bypass grafting in the United States starting in 1954.[2] There has been remarkable progress in the field of peripheral vascular surgery in the past few decades and the ability to salvage limbs in patients with severe atherosclerotic disease and critical ischemia has become common for the vascular surgeon. The ideal vascular graft should be biocompatible, resistant to infection, nonimmunogenic, nonthrombogenic, easy to handle, durable, and readily available.[3] In the absence of a perfect arterial substitute, autogenous vein remains the preferred substitute and acquires the characteristics of the replaced arterial segment more than any other conduit.[4] However, sometimes this conduit is unavailable due to prior use or intrinsic disease, or not of sufficient length or caliber for revascularization. The role of prosthetic conduit in lower extremity revascularization has been debated despite many studies, and controversy remains as to the indication and optimal use of prosthetic conduit in patients requiring revascularization.

PTFE grafts were first used as arterial conduits in 1976[5] and soon after, reports documented acceptable results using PTFE in the femoropopliteal position. Reports dealing with infrapopliteal prosthetic bypass were less promising. A prospective, multicenter randomized trial of ASV compared to PTFE in lower extremity revascularization was published in 1986.[6] Primary patency of ASV was 49% at four years and was significantly better than that of PTFE (12%) in the infrapopliteal location. However, limb salvage rates were similar at 3.5 years (57% versus 61%) and the group concluded that a PTFE distal bypass was preferential to a primary amputation.

Previously, Quinones-Baldrich reviewed the UCLA experience with the use of PTFE in 258 patients undergoing 322 infrainguinal revascularizations.[7] The vast majority of these patients underwent femoropopliteal bypass, but 9% of the included cases were distal infrapopliteal bypasses. Primary patency for all femoropopliteal bypasses performed with PTFE was 59% at five years and secondary patency was 74% at five years. Femoropopliteal bypasses done for limb salvage resulted in a 70% salvage rate at five years. However, femoral-infrapopliteal reconstructions using PTFE had a dismal primary patency rate of 22% at three years with a limb salvage rate of 37%. The conclusions reached after this report concluded that PTFE distal bypass plays a limited role in infrainguinal revascularization, but may be preferable to amputation in patients lacking ASV.

DATA ANALYSIS

During 1978 to 1998, 81 operations in 77 patients were identified as being lower extremity revascularization using prosthetic conduit to the infrapopliteal vessels.[8] Four patients underwent sequential bilateral leg bypass using prosthetic conduit. These 81 cases were found within a group of approximately 1,500 lower extremity revascularization operations during the same interval on the Vascular Surgery Service at the University of California–Los Angeles Center for the Health Sciences, and thus represented 5.4% of the total. Included in these 81 cases were composite grafts with a prosthetic-vein anastomosis in the mid-graft and cases where a vein patch was used at the distal anastomosis. Specifically excluded were cases where the distal anastomosis was to the popliteal artery or higher. All clinical, perioperative, and demographic data were obtained through review of original hospital, physician, and vascular laboratory records. All patients were observed at our institution with follow-up clinical examination, noninvasive testing, and occasional duplex ultrasonographic imaging (Diasonics Gateway Series, Santa Clara, CA) performed at the UCLA outpatient vascular laboratory.

All data were compiled on a spreadsheet with basic statistical analyses capability (Excel, Microsoft Corp, Redmond, WA). Patency, limb salvage, and survival curves were generated using the Kaplan-Meier method. Univariate and multivariate statistical analyses were carried out using Systat software package (SPSS Inc, Chicago, IL). A p value less than 0.05 was considered statistically significant.

Patient Population and Operative Factors

Demographic and clinical factors of patients undergoing distal lower extremity revascularization are shown in Table 17–1. Salient features include a mean age of 72 years, nearly a two-thirds male preponderance, and a smoking history in nearly three-fourths of patients. Also, 15% of patients were on dialysis or had extreme creatinine elevation and decreased renal function preoperatively. Vascular surgical history of these patients is displayed in Table 17–2. Before leg revascularization, 35% had undergone an inflow procedure, mostly aortobifemoral bypass grafting; however, some had an extraanatomic bypass. The saphenous vein had been used for coronary artery bypass graft (CABG) or prior lower extremity revascularization in a total of 86% of these patients. In the remainder, prosthetic conduit was used for the leg revascularization because of the inadequate quality of the saphenous vein (9%), or in rare instances, preferentially (5%) (early in this experience during the late 1970s).

Lower extremity revascularization originated at the femoral artery in 90% of cases with the remainder originating from the external iliac artery or limb of an aortobifemoral graft (Table 17–3). The distal anastomosis was performed to the anterior tibial artery (43%), posterior tibial artery (28%), tibioperoneal trunk (16%), or peroneal artery (12%). Other salient intraoperative factors are displayed in Table 17–3. All grafts were

TABLE 17-1. DEMOGRAPHIC AND CLINICAL FACTORS IN PATIENTS UNDERGOING DISTAL LOWER EXTREMITY REVASCULARIZATION USING PROSTHETIC CONDUIT (N = 81)

Parameter	%
Mean age	72 yr
Gender	
Male	62
Femal	38
CAD	59
Hypertension	68
Diabetes mellitus	49
Smoking	77
COPD	12
Renal failure	15

CAD, cornary artery disease; COPD, chronic obstructive pulmonary disease.

TABLE 17-2. PRIOR VASCULAR SURGICAL HISTORY IN PATIENTS UNDERGOING DISTAL LOWER EXTREMITY REVASCULARIZATION USING PROSTHETIC CONDUIT (N = 81)

Previous Surgery	N (%)
Inflow procedure	28 (35)
CABG	20 (25)
Femoro-popliteal bypass	49 (60)
Femoro-distal bypass	19 (23)
ASV utilized	70 (86)

CABG, coronary artery bypass grafting; ASV, autologous saphenous vein.

TABLE 17-3. INTRAOPERATIVE FACTORS IN PATIENTS UNDERGOING DISTAL LOWER EXTREMITY REVASCULARIZATION USING PROSTHETIC CONDUIT (N = 81)

Factor	Detail	N (%)
Type of graft	PTFE	81 (100)
	6 mm size	77 (95)
	Ring reinforced	44 (54)
	Composite graft	15 (19)
Proximal anastomosis	Femoral artery	73 (90)
	Profundaplasty	14 (17)
Distal anastomosis	Anterior tibial artery	35 (43)
	Posterior tibial artery	23 (28)
	Tibioperoneal trunk	13 (16)
	Peroneal artery	10 (12)
	Adjunctive vein patch	20 (25)
Anesthesia	General	61 (75)
	Regional	20 (25)
Mean blood loss		285 mL

PTFE, polytetrafluoroethylene.

made of polytetrafluoroethylene (PTFE) (W. L. Gore, Flagstaff, AZ), mostly of the 6 mm variety. Other prosthetic conduit choices including umbilical vein or cryopreserved vein were not used. Composite grafts with a prosthetic vein anastomosis in the mid-graft were used in 15 cases (19%). Adjunctive profundaplasty was performed in 17% of cases and a distal vein patch was done in 25%. General anesthesia was used in three-fourths of the cases.

RESULTS

Relevant postoperative details are displayed in Table 17–4. The mean length of hospital stay was 17.5 days. One-fifth of the patients developed a postoperative wound hematoma or wound infection, mostly resolving with conservative measures. A majority of these wound infections was superficial cellulitis; however, fasciitis developed in two patients early in this series, requiring operative debridement. Graft infections developed in five

TABLE 17-4. POSTOPERATIVE FEATURES IN PATIENTS UNDERGOING DISTAL LOWER EXTREMITY REVASCULARIZATION USING PROSTHETIC CONDUIT (N = 81)

Postoperative Feature	N (%)
Mean length of stay	17.5 days
Hematoma/wound cellulites	15 (19)
Graft infection	5 (6)
Acute graft thrombosis	11 (14)
Perioperative death	3 (4)
Postoperative wafarin	51 (63)

patients with three of the five undergoing operative revision. One patient was treated with antibiotics alone and the other was lost in follow-up. Operative mortality was 4%. Thirty-day postoperative graft thrombosis occurred in 11 cases or 14%. Interestingly, all graft thromboses were in patients who had undergone general anesthesia. Four of the 11 cases had successful thrombectomy and prolonged secondary patency of the initial graft. A majority of all patients (63%) were placed on warfarin postoperatively.

Graft Patency Rate and Limb Salvage Rate

Long-term follow-up has ranged from one to 144 months with a mean of 22 months. Using the Kaplan Meier method, primary patency was calculated to be 20% at 36 months. Secondary patency was 42% and limb salvage was 55% (Figure 17–1). Overall survival was 69% at 36 months with the vast majority of deaths due to cardiac disease. Univariate analyses was performed to identify possible factors that may be associated with improved patency or limb salvage (Table 17–5). Regional anesthesia was found to be significantly associated with prolonged primary patency (35% versus 15%, $p = 0.026$) (Figure 17–2). This was mostly spinal anesthesia; however, recently, epidural anesthesia has become more common. Ring-reinforced PTFE conduit was found to be significantly associated with prolonged limb salvage (65% versus 40%, $p = 0.042$) (Figure 17–3). None of the other variables including male gender, the lack of diabetes mellitus or renal failure, decade of operation, use of a vein patch at the distal anastomosis, or postoperative warfarin use were found to be significantly associated with either prolonged patency or limb salvage. Multivariate analyses also did not reveal any other significant factors associated with patency or limb salvage.

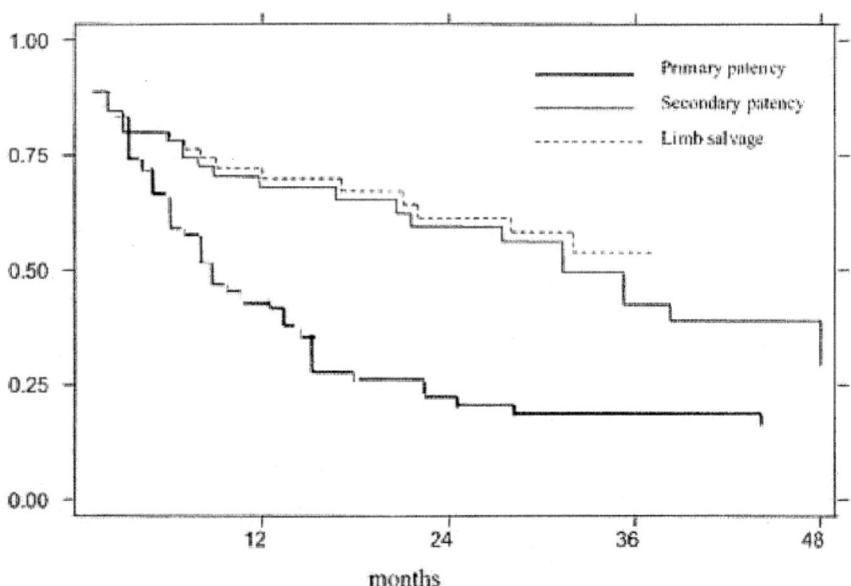

Figure 17-1. Primary, secondary, and limb salvage rates for all patients undergoing infrapopliteal bypass with prosthetic conduit (n = 81 cases). At 36 months, primary patency was 20% secondary patency 42%, and limb salvage 55% calculated by Kaplan-Meier method.

TABLE 17-5. UNIVARIATE ANALYSES OF VARIABLES ASSOCIATED WITH IMPROVED PATENCY OR LIMB SALVAGE

Variable	Associated with Primary Patency (p Value)	Associated with Secondary Patency (p Value)	Associated with Limb Salvage (p Value)
Male gender	0.94	0.74	0.48
No smoking history	0.49	0.53	0.37
No diabetes mellitus	0.47	0.46	0.85
No renal failure	0.57	0.31	0.16
Regional anesthesia	0.03*	0.07	0.18
Ring-reinforced PTFE	0.48	0.36	0.04*
Distal vein patch	0.80	0.89	0.88
Posoperative warfarin	0.60	0.47	0.55

PTFE, polytetrafluoroethylene. *$p < 0.05$.

Choice of Bypass Conduit in Infrapopliteal Revascularization

In this series, a vast majority of the patients underwent prosthetic bypass to the infrapopliteal vessels in the setting of CLI and the unavailability of autogenous vein. In recent years, given the acceptance of a poorer patency with prosthetic reconstruction in the infrapopliteal position, all available autogenous veins have been sought and harvested including the lesser saphenous and arm veins. Still, in these 81 cases in the past two decades, PTFE conduit was used as opposed to primary amputation. A majority of the patients had ASV used in previous revascularization attempts, usually in femoral to popliteal artery bypass grafting. Prosthetic conduit reconstruction to the above-knee popliteal artery remains controversial, but patency rates approximate vein bypass grafting. In some of the patients

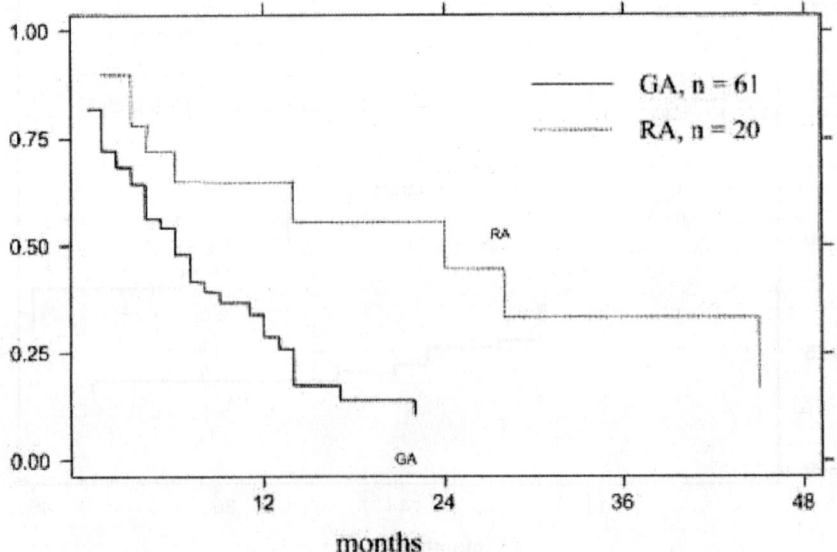

Figure 17-2. Primary patency in patients undergoing infrapopliteal prosthetic bypass under regional anesthesia is significantly higher than compared to patients undergoing operation under general anesthesia (35% versus 15%, p = 0.026).

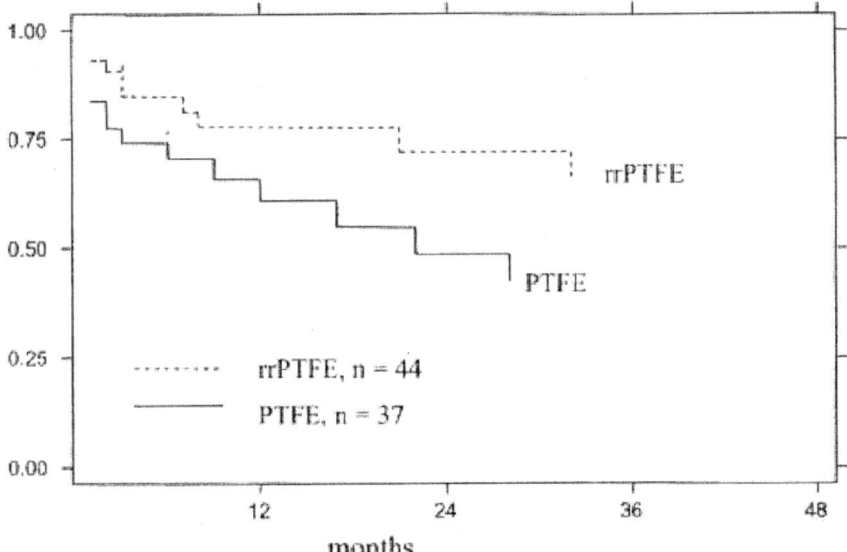

Figure 17-3. Limb salvage rates are greater in patients receiving ring-reinforced PTFE conduit versus nonringed conduit (65% versus 40%, p = 0.042).

in this series, a more favorable sequence may have been prosthetic popliteal bypass first, thus reserving ASV for distal revascularization if needed. It must be emphasized that currently at UCLA, infrapopliteal prosthetic bypass is only performed on patients with CLI where no autogenous conduit is available and amputation is the only other choice.

In this series, the use of ring-reinforced PTFE was found to be associated with prolonged limb salvage. Despite the frequent usage of ring-reinforced PTFE in long bypass grafts that cross a joint space, this finding had not been corroborated before. In this experience over two decades, ring-reinforced PTFE has been used more frequently than the nonringed variety since the early 1990s. We intuitively expected, but did not find, enhanced long-term secondary patency in these patients. Nevertheless, many authorities believe that infrapopliteal bypass with prosthetic conduit should use only the ring-reinforced variety,[9-10] and this study would support that posture.

Anesthesia

The results in this series indicate that choice of anesthetic is an important consideration for infrapopliteal prosthetic revascularization. All 11 cases of postoperative graft thrombosis occurred in patients who had undergone general anesthesia (GA). Others have also suggested that regional anesthesia (RA) may favorably influence early graft patency. Tuman and colleagues[11] conducted a prospective, randomized study in 80 patients undergoing vascular surgery comparing RA versus GA. They discovered a graft failure rate of 2.5% in the RA group versus a 20% graft failure rate in the GA group. Similarly, Christopherson and colleagues[12] randomized 100 patients undergoing lower extremity revascularization and found that patients undergoing RA had a significantly lower risk of graft thrombosis. The risk of thrombectomy or graft revision in patients receiving RA was 4% versus 22% in the patients receiving GA ($p < 0.01$). However, in a retrospective review at the Cleveland Clinic[13], the choice of anesthesia did not have any impact on graft thromboses rates in lower extremity revascularization using both vein and prosthetic conduit. Theoretically, regional anesthesia may decrease peripheral vascular resistance secondary to vasodilatation and increase intragraft blood flow in the perioperative period. Thus, the use of RA should have a beneficial impact on patency because it has been shown to increase limb blood flow during surgery[14-15] and perhaps ameliorate the hypercoagulable state seen postoperatively.[11,16]

Adjuncts to Improve Patency of Infrapopliteal Prosthetic Graft

Due to the relatively poor patency of prosthetic bypass grafts to distal popliteal or tibial target vessels, a number of techniques have been developed to improve patency when autologous conduit is not available. A number of limited retrospective series suggest that there may be an advantage in interposing autologous vein (i.e., cuffs, patches, or fistula) between the prosthetic graft and the native artery at the distal anastomosis of below-knee popliteal or tibial bypasses. Parsons and colleagues[17] looked at a 10-year interval with 66 PTFE bypasses in 63 patients without autogenous conduit who faced immediate amputation. Their three-year results were primary patency 39%, secondary patency 55%, and limb salvage 71%. This was in the face of a two-year actuarial patient survival of only 67%. They compared their results with the best reported patency and limb salvage rates for infrapopliteal prosthetic bypasses with adjunctive maneuvers (distal vein cuff, arteriovenous fistula), and found them to be no different. However, Taylor and colleagues reported an impressive 54% five-year primary patency of infrapopliteal PTFE bypasses when a distal anastomotic vein patch was used in a series of 256 patients.[18] Despite the limitations of these studies, they support the conclusion that infrapopliteal bypass remains a worthwhile option in patients without usable vein. The patency results in Parsons' report may be better than the results presented here because of their routine use of warfarin. We did not identify postoperative warfarin as a beneficial adjunct in our analysis. However, this may represent a type II error given the small numbers of patients in this series.

In the largest experience reported to date, Fichelle and colleagues[19] described the outcome of 149 infrapopliteal PTFE bypasses in 145 patients collected over a decade. Similar to the previous studies above, the vast majority of patients was in CLI without any usable autogenous vein. A composite bypass was performed in 35% of cases with the graft/vein anastomosis always above the knee. Primary patency and limb salvage at three years were 41% and 68%. No advantages were found with respect to use of composite versus all prosthetic graft, the addition of a distal vein patch, or whether the case was an initial versus repeat operation. The group concluded that the patency of infrapopliteal PTFE bypasses remained low, but that the limb salvage rate supported the policy of routine aggressive infrapopliteal revascularization, even in the absence of autogenous vein.

INFRAPOPLITEAL ANGIOPLASTY FOR CRITICAL LIMB ISCHEMIA

For comparison, we reviewed our 10-year experience of infrapopliteal angioplasty at UCLA.[20]

Methods

Between 1995 and 2005, a total of 64 limbs in 57 patients (33 men and 24 women, a mean age of 71 years) underwent percutaneous transluminal angioplasty (PTA) on tibial arteries for the treatment of CLI (rest pain in 20 [31%] and ulcer/gangrene in 44 [69%]). TransAtlantic

Society Consensus (TASC) tibial lesion types[21] were seven in type B, 34 in type C, and 23 in type D. The treated lesions were located in the tibioperoneal trunk (14 limbs), the anterior tibial (30), posterior tibial (6), peroneal (35), and dorsal pedal artery (one). Angioplasty was carried out in one tibial artery on 50 limbs (78%), in two tibial arteries on 12 (19%), in three tibial arteries on 2 (3%), and in four tibial arteries in 1 (2%). On 53 limbs (83%), concomitant proximal angioplasty was performed during the same procedure. On 11 limbs (17%), only tibial arteries were treated with PTA. No stent was inserted in the tibial lesions.

The criteria for clinical improvement were defined by the Society for Vascular Surgery and the International Society for Cardiovascular Surgery (SVERSUS/ISCVERSUS) reporting standards.[22] PTA was considered as a clinical success or clinical improvement if the symptoms improved by at least one category together with an increase in ABI of more than .10.

Results

Mortality rate within 30 days after PTA was 0%, and the complication rate was 3% (two groin hematomas). Average hospital stay was 5.5 days. Technical success rate was 95.3%.

Primary tibial PTAs were followed by subsequent distal bypass surgery in three limbs (5%) during the follow-up. The primary patency, assisted primary patency, and secondary patency rates were 34%, 62%, and 67% at 12 months, and 24%, 44%, and 48% at 36 months, respectively (Figure 17–4). Continued clinical improvement rate was 63% at 12 months and 34% at 36 months (Figure 17–5). Limb salvage rate was 87% at 12 months and 75% at 36 months.

Univariate analysis revealed that TASC types D lesion had significantly decreased primary, assisted primary, secondary patency rates, and limb salvage rates compared with TASC type B/type C (Kaplan-Meier, log-rank test, $p < 0.05$).

Thus, tibial PTA appears to be a safe and effective alternative to infrapopliteal bypass, and may be preferable.

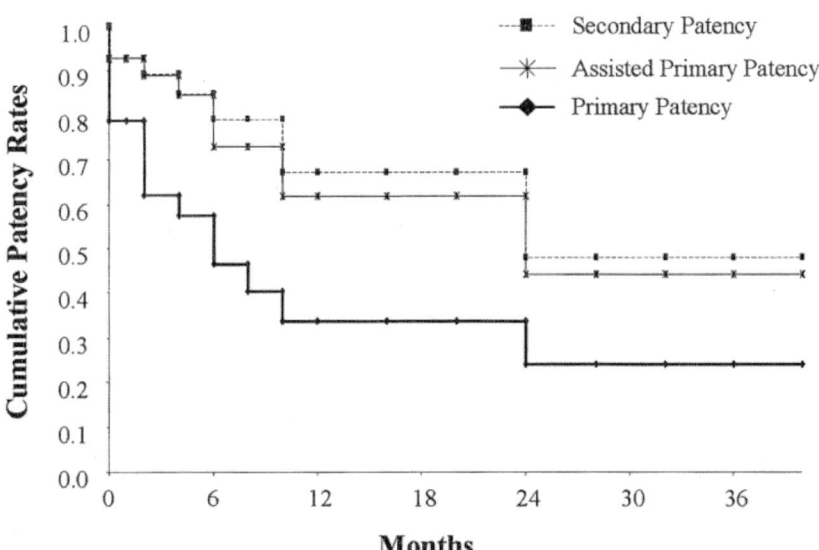

Figure 17-4. Cumulative primary, assisted primary, and secondary patency rates in 64 limbs with infrapopliteal angioplasty (Kaplan-Meier life table analysis).

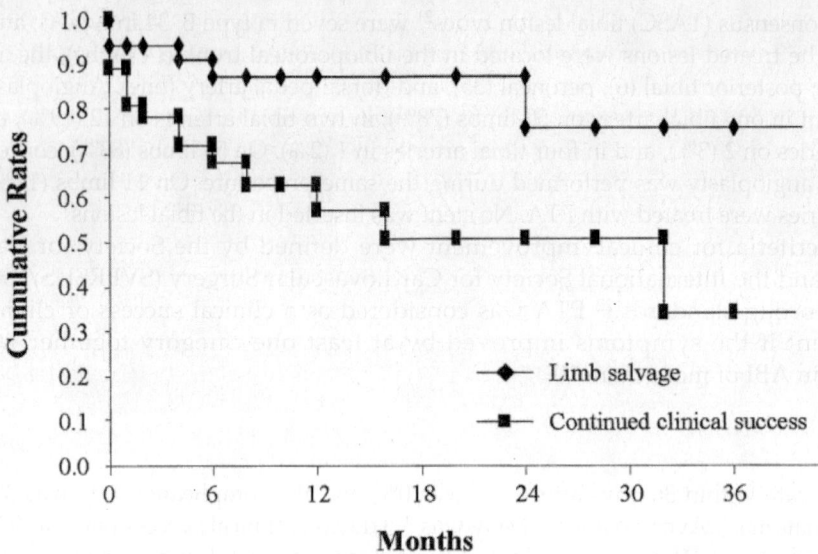

Figure 17-5. Continued clinical success and limb salvage rates in 64 limbs with infrapopliteal angioplasty (Kaplan-Meier life table analysis).

SUMMARY

In this study, we looked at our experience over the past two decades with infrapopliteal revascularization with prosthetic conduit. We found that despite poor primary patency, distal prosthetic bypass can lead to long-term limb salvage. Also, our data suggest distal anastomotic vein patches and postoperative anticoagulation may not be beneficial adjuncts. However, the use of regional anesthesia may decrease the incidence of perioperative thrombosis and the use of ring-reinforced conduit may prolong limb salvage. We believe that an aggressive posture for lower extremity revascularization remains warranted in patients facing imminent amputation and should include distal prosthetic bypass in situations where no autogenous vein is available.

PTA for the tibial arteries is a safe and effective treatment in patients with CLI. Although primary patency rates were low, the high limb salvage rates and low complication rate may support the policy of tibial PTA as the initial treatment of choice in these patients.

REFERENCES

1. Kunlin J. Le traitment de l'arterite obliterante par la greffe veneuse. *Arch Mal Coeur.* 1949;42:371–379.
2. Linton RR, Darling RC. Autogenous saphenous vein bypass grafts in femoro-popliteal obliterative disease. *Surgery.* 1962;52:62–73.
3. Brewster DC. Prosthetic grafts. In: Rutherford RB, ed. Vascular Surgery. Philadelphia: WB Saunders; 1995:492–521.
4. Szilagyi DE, Elliott JP, Hagerman JH et al. Biologic fate of autogenous vein implants as arterial substitutes. *Ann Surg.* 1973;178:232.

5. Campbell CD, Brooks DH, Webster MW et al. The use of expanded microporous polytetrafluoroethylene for limb salvage. A preliminary report. *Surgery.* 1976;9:485–491.

6. Veith FJ, Gupta SK, Ascer E et al. Six-year prospective multicenter randomized comparison of autologous saphenous vein and expanded polytetrafluoroethylene grafts in infrainguinal arterial reconstructions. *J Vasc Surg.* 1986;3:104–114.

7. Quinones-Baldrich WJ, Prego AA, Ucelay-Gomez R et al. Long-term results of infrainguinal revascularization with polytetrafluoroethylene: A ten-year experience. *J Vasc Surg.* 1992; 16:209–217.

8. Kashyap VERSUS, Ahn SS, Dorey F, Quinones-Baldrich WJ, et al. Infrapopliteal Lower Extremity Revascularization with Prosthetic Conduit: A 20-Year Experience. *Vasc Endovascular Surg.* 2002;36:255–262.

9. Suggs WD, Veith FJ. Expanded polytetrafluoroethylene graft for atherosclerotic lower extremity occlusive disease. In: Ernst CB and Stanley JC, eds. Current Therapy in Vascular Surgery. St. Louis: Mosby; 1995:480–484.

10. Schweiger H, Klein P, Lang W. Tibial bypass grafting for limb salvage with ringed polytetrafluoroethylene prostheses: Results of primary and secondary procedures. *J Vasc Surg.* 1993;18:867–874.

11. Tuman KJ, McCarthy RJ, March R et al. Effects of epidural anesthesia and analgesia on coagulation and outcome after major vascular surgery. *Anesth Analg.* 1991:73:696–704.

12. Christopherson R, Beattie C, Frank SM et al. Perioperative morbidity in patients randomized to epidural or general anesthesia for lower extremity vascular surgery. *Anesthesiology.* 1993;79:422–434.

13. Schunn CD, Hertzer NR, O'Hara PJ et al. Epidural versus general anesthesia: Does anesthetic management influence early infrainguinal graft thrombosis. *Ann Vasc Surg.* 1998;12: 65–69.

14. Cousins MJ, Wright CJ. Graft, muscle, skin blood flow after epidural block in vascular surgical procedures. *Surg Gynecol Obstet.* 1971;133:55–64.

15. Haljamae H, Holm FJ, Akerstrom G. Epidural versus general anesthesia and leg blood flow in patients with occlusive atherosclerotic disease. *Eur J Vasc Surg.* 1988;2:395–400.

16. Rosenfeld BA, Beattie C, Christopherson R. et al. The effects of different anesthetic regimens on fibrinolysis and the development of postoperative arterial thrombosis. *Anesthesiology.* 1993;79:435–443.

17. Parsons RE, Suggs WD, Veith FJ et al. Polytetrafluoroethylene bypasses to infrapopliteal arteries without cuffs or patches: A better option than amputation in patients without autologous vein. *J Vasc Surg.* 1996;23:347–356.

18. Taylor RS, Loh A, McFarland RJ et al. Improved techniques for polytetrafluoroethylene bypass grafting: Long-term results using anastomotic vein patches. *Br J Surg.* 1992;79:348–354.

19. Fichelle J, Marzelle J, Colacchio G et al. Infrapopliteal polytetrafluoroethylene and composite bypass: Factors influencing patency. *Ann Vasc Surg.* 1995;9:187–196.

20. Chandra FA, Kudo T, Ahn SS. The Effectiveness of Balloon Angioplasty as a Limb Salvage Procedure for Patients with Tibial Arterial Occlusive Disease. The Society for Vascular Surgery, the VASCULAR Annual Meeting 2004 (Endovascular Forum). Anaheim, CA. June 4, 2004.

21. Dormandy JA. Management of peripheral arterial disease (PAD). TASC Working Group. TransAtlantic Inter-Society Concensus (TASC). *J Vasc Surg.* 2000;31(suppl):S1–296.

22. Rutherford RB, Baker JD, et al. Recommended standards for reports dealing with lower extremity ischemia: revised version. *J Vasc Surg.* 1997;26:517–538.

18

Lower Limb Revascularization in Patients with Diabetes Mellitus

Jonathan B. Towne, M.D.

DISTAL BYPASS IN PATIENTS WITH DIABETES MELLITUS

With the increasing incidence of Type II diabetes, there is a greater number of patients seen with vascular occlusive diseases of the lower extremities. An understanding of the anatomic characteristics of the distribution of occlusive disease in the diabetic patient is important to understanding and treating these patients.

DISTRIBUTION OF ARTERIAL OCCLUSIVE DISEASE

The vascular system can be divided into several distinct segments. The first of these is the aortic iliac system that deals with occlusive disease of the aorta and the common and external iliac arteries. Second is the femoral popliteal tibial vessels that are the main blood vessels to the lower extremities. The third area is the large vessels of the foot including the dorsal pedal, pedal arch, and metatarsal arteries. These are often the only bypass option of choice in patients with diabetes and so visualization techniques of arteries need to be considered. Finally, the small arteries, arterioles, and capillaries need to be considered. These are not reconstructible in the traditional sense but certainly occlusive disease in these vessels can contribute to the development of ischemic ulcerations and gangrene of the toes and foot.

Patients with diabetes mellitus have a unique distribution of arterial occlusive disease.[1] Jude and associates evaluated 136 arteriograms, 43% of whom were diabetic, and classified the distribution of occlusive disease from the aorta to the foot. Diabetic patients had an increased severity of arterial disease in the profunda femoris artery and in the below-knee tibial segments. The aortoiliac segment was often spared (see Figures 18–1 through 18–5). There also was no difference in incidence of common femoral or superficial femoral arterial disease between the diabetic and nondiabetic lower extremity vascular occlusive disease group. Work by King and associates also

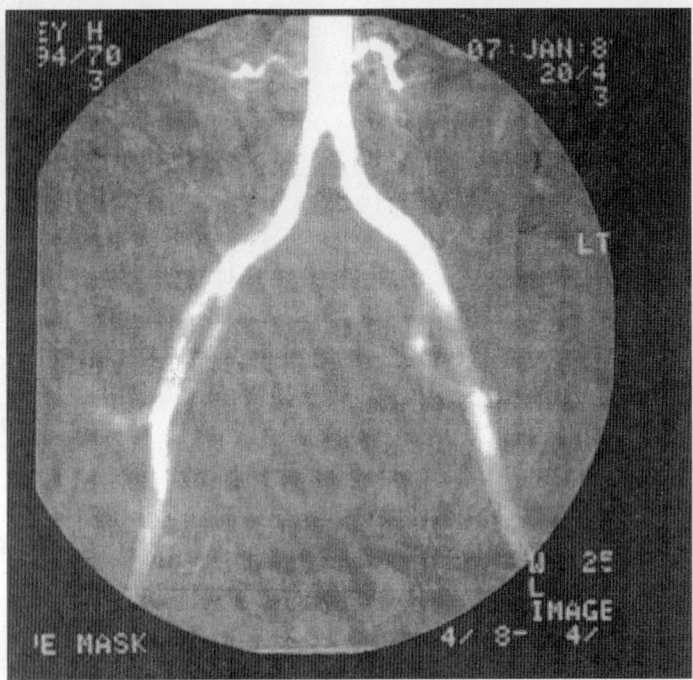

Figure 18-1. A. Classic angiogram of a patient with diabetes mellitus and limb-threatening ischemia with lack of aortoiliac involvement.

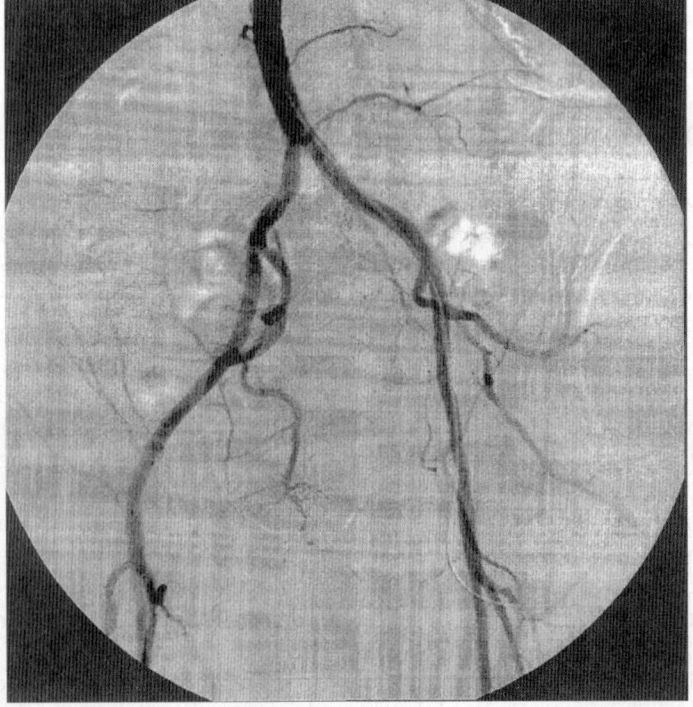

Figure 18-1. B. Classic angiogram of a patient with diabetes mellitus and limb-threatening ischemia with lack of aortoiliac involvement.

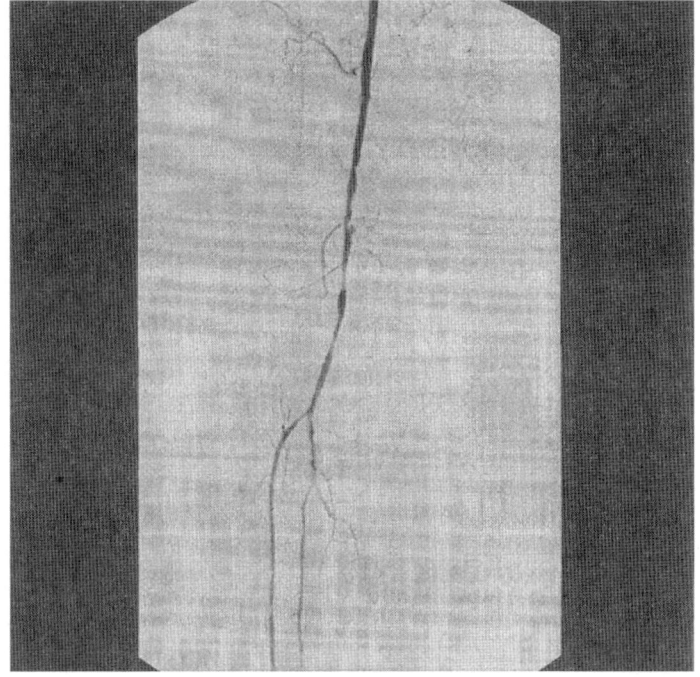

Figure 18-2. Diffuse occlusive disease of the popliteal and tibial segments.

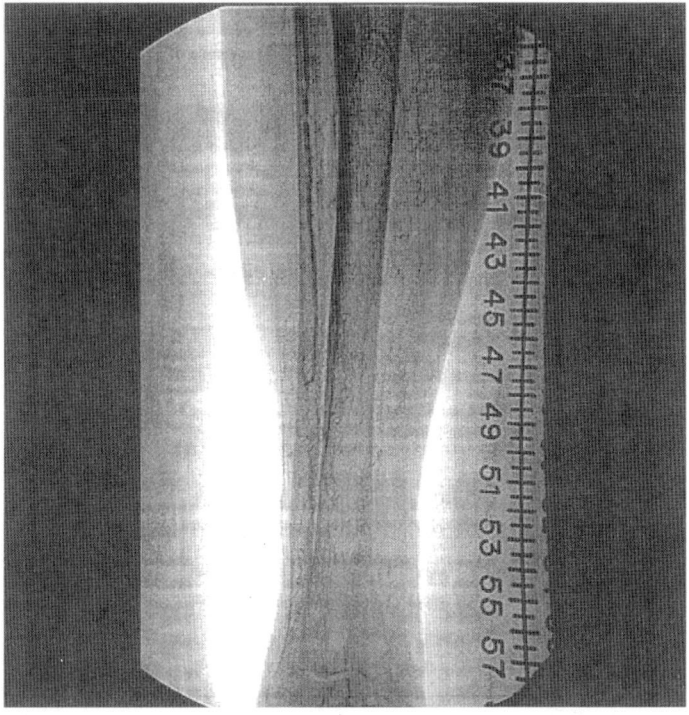

Figure 18-3. Diffuse tibial occlusive disease.

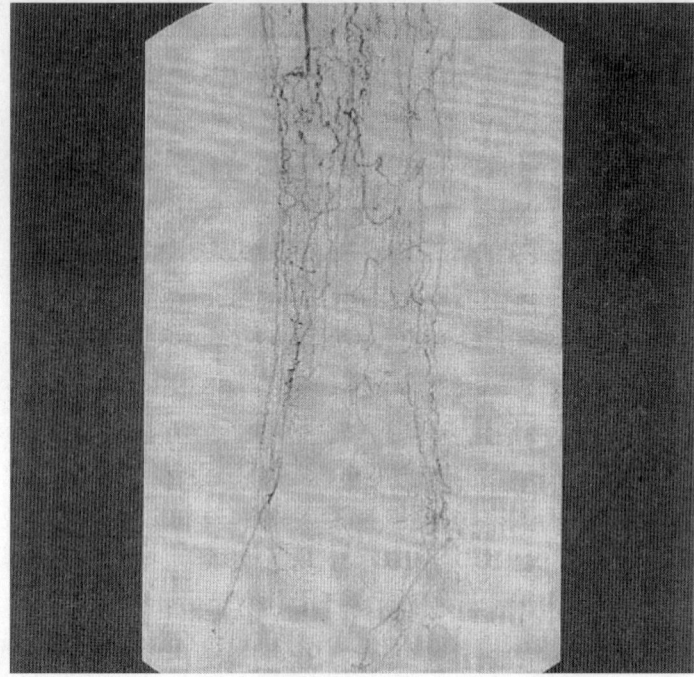

Figure 18-4. Arterial flow into foot via collateral channels.

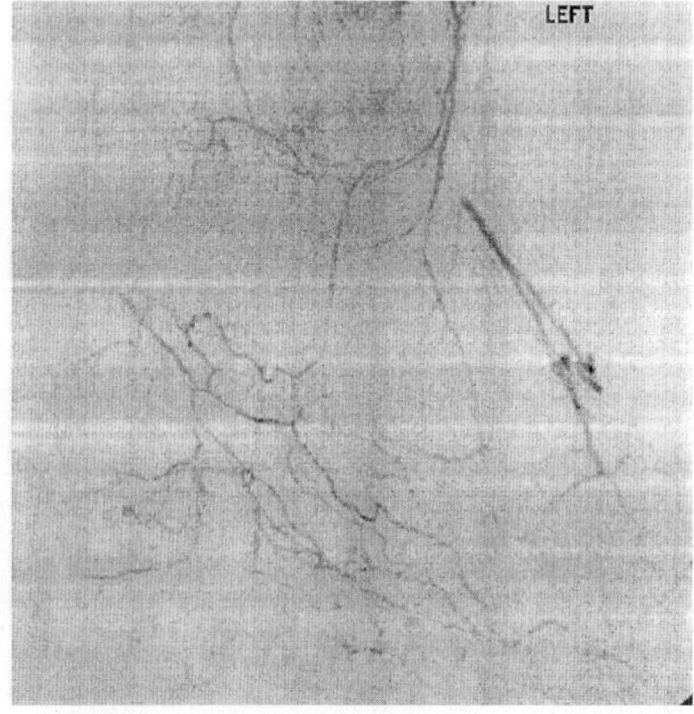

Figure 18-5. Reconstitution of doralis pedis artery on the foot.

reported an increase in incidence of occlusive disease in the profunda femoris artery in patients with diabetes mellitus. In this study, the incidence of diffuse occlusive disease throughout the profunda femoris artery was noted in diabetics as compared to nondiabetics in whom involvement at the origin of the profunda was common but disease distal in the profunda was less common.[2] These authors also found no difference in incidence of occlusive disease between diabetics and nondiabetics in superficial femoral artery and common femoral artery[2]. Haimovici and colleagues reported an incidence of atherosclerotic involvement in the profunda femoris artery in 9.5% of patients without diabetes compared to 30.5% in diabetic patients.[3]

ARTERIAL IMAGING

Since arterial reconstruction in diabetic patients often involves distal tibial and/or pedal vessels, arterial imaging is important. Over the last decade, there has been an evolution of radiographic techniques including magnetic resonance angiography and advanced digital subtraction techniques. Hoch and his group compared the operative management plans comparing magnetic resonance angiography and digital subtraction angiography in 40 patients.[4] The MRA was felt to be accurate in terms of performance of the surgical procedure in 92% of the patients. DSA was accurate in 94%. Kreitner and his group felt that MR angiography was better than DSA in revealing peripheral runoff vessels. Thirty-eight percent of the patients in his study revealed patent pedal vessels not seen on the digital subtraction angiography. In a subsequent report, they reported a perioperative patency of 93% and a 36-month patency (secondary) at 89.5% in patients with distal vessel occult to conventional angiography, but visualized by MRA.[5-6] Oser and Picus noted that DSA identified patent named vessels with a 95% sensitivity and a 92% specificity in 165 arteriograms.[7] The caveat is that MR studies are not precise in the aortic iliac segment. Also, the quality of MR and CT scans are variable, as is the expertise of the attending radiologist. The quality of the angiographic and/or MR machines is also highly variable. With vascular surgeons developing interventional skills, another option is to do duplex evaluations to map the vessels and confirm these findings with intraoperative angiograms. This is probably the most cost-effective and precise method to evaluate target vessels for bypass. The one unique characteristic of diabetic vascular occlusive disease is that the digital arteries are not calcified to the degree that the more proximal arteries are. Work of Ferrier indicates that in 60% of diabetics, the metatarsal arteries are calcified compared to 21% in nondiabetics.[8] Digital arteries are calcified in this same group of patients only 19% of the time compared to 10% in nondiabetics. Calcification of digital arteries was only seen in diabetics. Because digital arteries are often not calcified, it allows patients with diabetes who have incompressible calf vessels to have toe pressures measured as a means of quantitating the amount of ischemia. The problem with ankle/brachial indices is that they are limited by vessel wall incompressibility in diabetic patients resulting in falsely elevated pressure. Also, the ankle/brachial indices are unable to quantitate the amount of occlusive disease distal to the ankle.

The easiest way to measure toe pressures is with a digital cuff and a photoplethysmograph.[9] The cuff is placed around the base of the first or second toe. The flow pulse distal to the cuff was detected with a photoplethysmograph secured by transparent double stick tape. Three measurements are obtained: ankle/brachial index, toe ankle index, and toe/brachial index. The toe/ankle index gives a quantitative assessment of the occlusive disease between the ankle and the forefoot.[10] Normal toe pressure is 20–40 mm/Hg less than the ankle pressure. Normal toe/ankle is greater than 0.8 and toe/brachial index greater than 0.88. In a study of 85 patients, all had ulcer and/or focal gangrene at the toe or forefoot, 62 were diabetic, eight had bilateral involvement, 23 were nondiabetic patients, and all had unilateral involvement. The study evaluated whether these patients would heal an ulcer or an area of focal gangrene on the toe or forefoot. In patients who were not diabetic, the average distribution of ankle/brachial indices, patients without occlusive disease had AB indices greater than one, patient's claudication in the range of 0.65 and limb salvage less than 0.5. However, in the incompressible vessels, the determinations were of no value to determine what the actual flow was. However, if toe pressures were used, patients with claudication had an average toe/ankle index of 0.45, and those with limb salvage had a toe/ankle index of 0.2. Most important was the ability to determine healing. In general, nondiabetic patients who had a toe pressure of 40 or more went on to heal. Patients with diabetes with toe pressures of 50 or more generally went on and healed.

STRATEGIES FOR DISTAL BYPASS

The use of peroneal artery as an outflow vessel in lower extremity arterial reconstruction has historically been an area of controversy in vascular surgery.[11-15] Frequently, the peroneal artery is the only patent tibial vessel, especially in diabetic patients who have advanced tibial occlusive disease.[16-17] It is often considered the "last choice" outflow artery because it is technically the most difficult tibial bypass to construct. Earlier reports noted inferior short- and long-term patency rates with peroneal bypass grafts when compared with those for anterior and posterior tibial bypass grafts. However, with advances in vein bypass techniques, others have demonstrated equivalent patencies of peroneal, anterior tibial, and posterior tibial grafts.[16-18]

More recently, there has been a trend toward using the vessels at the ankle (anterior tibial, dorsal pedal, and posterior tibial) for the outflow artery. The superficial location of the arteries at the ankle makes these bypasses easier to construct; however, recently reported patency rates have been inferior to those of traditional tibial bypass grafts.[19] Shah et al. reported that their five-year primary patency rate for dorsalis pedis grafts was 50%. This contrasts with their own patency rate of 72% for anterior tibial and 69% for peroneal grafts. Harrington et al. reported a second patency rate at two years of 61%.[20] Pomposelli et al. reported an 18-month secondary patency rate of 82%.[21] All of these studies have patency rates that are inferior to the best series of tibial bypasses.

Through the years, we have been proponents of the use of the peroneal artery for lower limb bypass operations, and have used this conduit in approximately one-third of our cases. The purpose of our study was to evaluate our experience with peroneal artery bypass grafts. Specifically, we hoped to identify the determinants of long-term patency by evaluating such factors as the status of the pedal arch, presence of the terminal peroneal collaterals, and the quality of the autogenous vein conduit. We also compared the success of peroneal artery bypass in those patients in whom an inframalleolar bypass was an alternative. In an attempt to evaluate the peroneal artery, we evaluated 77 consecutive peroneal bypasses in 74 patients of which 80% were men and 20% women. The mean age was 71 years old.[22] Our approach to the peroneal artery is medial and was necessitated by the fact that we prefer to do in situ types of reconstruction (see Figure 18–6). We use tourniquet control for construction of distal anastomosis, and we do intraoperative spectral analysis in all cases and completion angiography in special cases.[23]

The peroneal artery bypass is a durable procedure that should be performed without reservation when the peroneal artery is the least diseased infrageniculate vessel. The primary and secondary patency rates of 61% and 92% at five years compare favorably with those reported for bypass to the tibial arteries in general, and to the peroneal artery outflow tract for distal extremity reconstruction.

Recent studies have reported acceptable results with bypasses to the paramalleolar or inframalleolar dorsalis pedis and posterior tibial arteries. We perform very few bypasses to these vessels because we prefer to bypass to a distal peroneal artery when this option exists. This is true regardless of whether the peroneal artery can be shown to directly anastomose to the pedal vessels or the pedal arch on preoperative arteriography, provided the peroneal artery itself is of adequate quality. The reasons for this policy are three-fold. First, the peroneal artery is usually richly collateralized in the leg, and its terminal collaterals potentially feed both the anterior and posterior circulation of the foot. Second, the peroneal artery bypass requires a shorter segment of vein than the equivalent pedal bypass. This increases the chances of an adequate length of good quality vein being available and decreases the length of vein at risk for iatrogenic injury, which may lead to subsequent graft failure. Finally, bypass to the peroneal artery obviates the need for incisions in the foot, which may be in proximity to contaminated wounds in a significant number of patients.

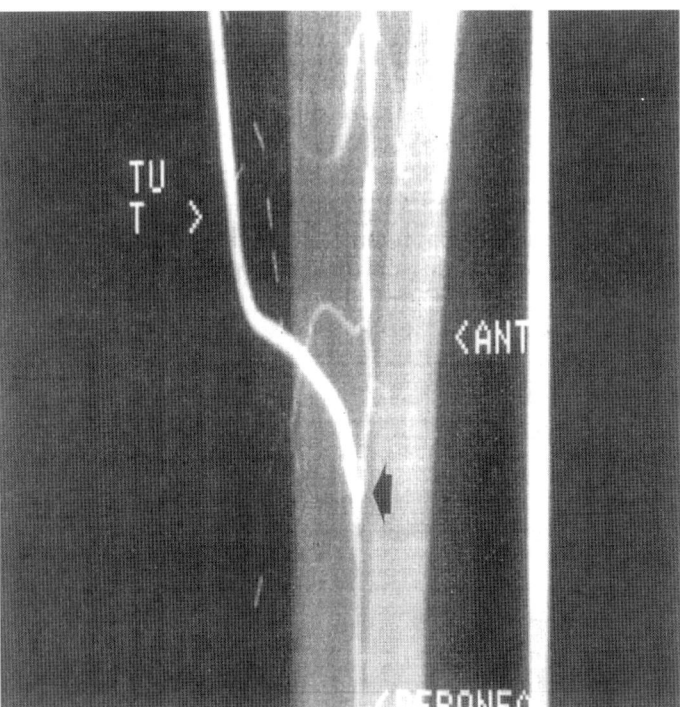

Figure 18-6. Vein bypass to peroneal Artery.

In an attempt to compare our results with those published for inframalleolar bypass, we analyzed the preoperative arteriograms for the presence of an inframalleolar vessel suitable for distal bypass. The option to bypass to an inframalleolar posterior tibial or dorsalis pedis artery existed in 59% of the patients whose arteriogram results were available for review. The secondary patency rate of 88% in these patients was not significantly different than the secondary patency of the group as a whole. Indeed, the secondary patency of those grafts in which neither the dorsalis pedis nor the posterior tibial artery was seen to reconstitute from the distal peroneal branches was slightly higher than that in the group with bypassable inframalleolar vessels. The inability to visualize direct communication between the peroneal branches and the pedal arch has led to some authors to opt for a bypass to an inframalleolar vessel over a patent distal peroneal. Klamer et al. reported that six limbs had patent peroneal arteries in their series of 68 inframalleolar bypass grafts,[24] whereas Harrington et al. opted for dorsalis pedis bypass in patients with peroneal arteries lacking direct anastomosis to the pedal vessels. The impact on patency of direct communication between the peroneal branches and the pedal arch has not been established. Our secondary patency rates for peroneal bypasses are 10%–40% higher than those recently reported for inframalleolar bypass, and this brings into question the decision to bypass distal to a patent peroneal artery.

We were unable to demonstrate any correlation between patency and a preoperative arteriogram score based on the system devised by the SVS/ISCVS Committee on Reporting Standards.[25] This system scores the peroneal branches and the pedal arch in an effort to predict relative outflow resistance. A recent report compared measured outflow resistance with the SVS/ISCVS score, and with multiple regression analysis, a modified system that statistically correlated with resistance was derived.[26] This modification is interesting in that the pedal arch score was not found to be a significant factor in their measured peroneal outflow resistance. Their findings suggest that the peroneal artery outflow is more dependent on secondary collateral channels to the foot and that direct communication with the major pedal arch may not be a good yardstick for evaluating peroneal artery outflow. In a recent review of 62 peroneal artery bypasses, Shortell et al. were unable to show any correlation between patency and the presence of a direct communication from the peroneal branches to a major pedal vessel.[27] Additionally, our study did not demonstrate a correlation between the modified angiogram score and patency. Synn et al., in a recent series that compared three angiographic scoring systems to outcome in 53 peroneal artery bypasses, came to similar conclusions.[18] This underscores the difficulty in trying to assess the quality of the outflow tract on the basis of preoperative angiography, which feeds the foot indirectly.

The factors we have found to be predictors of primary and secondary patency were the quality of the venous conduit, increased experience with the in situ bypass technique, and the postoperative ABI. History of diabetes mellitus, hypertension, coronary artery disease, and cigarette smoking did not correlate with graft survival.

The most important determinant of peroneal bypass success is the quality of the venous conduit. We initially noted this in our study of the lower extremity autogenous bypass grafts as a whole. Others have reported similar results in both in situ and reversed saphenous vein bypass grafts. This suggests that peroneal bypass grafts behave in a similar fashion to other tibial bypass grafts. The importance of a quality venous conduit is underscored by the fact that 10 (71%) of the 14 revisions involving problems with the vein graft were in patients with modified conduits. Additionally, four of the five early failures occurred in patients with modified conduits. The need to modify the venous conduit was most often due to conditions beyond the control of the surgeon (inadequate length = 9, sclerotic segment = 9). However, five of the eight conduits modified because of iatrogenic injury required subsequent revision or failed in the postoperative period. This fact emphasizes the need for meticulous handling of the venous conduit during dissection and preparation for bypass.

The secondary patency improved in the second half of the study period. Again, this is consistent with our findings for in situ bypass grafts as a whole, and is no doubt due to improvement in the technical performance of the surgeons and improvements in our clinical knowledge of the behavior of the in situ bypass graft in long-term follow-up. It is interesting to note that the primary patency for the two intervals was essentially unchanged. We believe that this is due to the implementation of our surveillance protocol during the latter half of the study period. This protocol allows us to identify grafts at risk and revise them before failure. Combined with improved technical skill, this has resulted in a 98%, five-year secondary patency rate for the second half of the study period.

The initial postoperative ABI may provide a marker for grafts at risk of failure. The mean postoperative ABI in the 22 patients whose grafts either failed or required revision in the follow-up interval was significantly lower than that in those patients whose grafts did not require revision. In addition, the ABI improved after revision and was not significantly different from the postoperative ABI of patients who did not undergo graft revision. This indicates that lesions responsible for early failure do not necessarily develop de novo in the postoperative period but are present in a subclinical form at the time of the primary procedure. Patients with postoperative ABI less than 0.90 should be observed more closely in the early follow-up period in an effort to detect correctable lesions before graft thrombosis occurs.

Bypass to the peroneal artery can be performed with excellent long-term results and should be used without reservation when it is the least diseased of the infrapopliteal vessels. The option to bypass to a dorsalis pedis or posterior tibial artery at the ankle was present in more than half our grafts. However, the patency rates reported here are superior to those reported for inframalleolar dorsalis pedis or posterior tibial artery. The factors that most affect patency are the quality of the venous conduit, and the technical and clinical skills of the surgeon. Meticulous dissection and handling of the vein and a rigorous postoperative surveillance protocol are essential for long-term success. Bypass grafts with low initial postoperative ABI require particularly close surveillance. Finally, we were unable to correlate preoperative assessment of runoff with patency. The uniqueness of the peroneal artery lies in the fact that it does not end in direct communication with the major pedal vessels. This fact has swayed many vascular surgeons to banish peroneal artery bypass to a "last choice" role in the treatment of limb-threatening ischemia. The results presented here add to a growing body of evidence that this status is unwarranted.

PROFUNDA FEMORIS ARTERY

Profunda femoris artery is of particular consequence in diabetic patients. As noted earlier, there is increased incidence of occlusive disease in the profunda femoris artery. Knowledge of this vessel, its anatomy, and the distribution of its disease is useful in evaluating and treating these patients, since it is often an overlooked vessel. However, in instances where lack of autogenous material is present for very distal bypasses, and particularly in patients who have ischemia and do not have foot necrosis, profunda femoris reconstruction is a viable option. Beals and associates in a 1971 study demonstrated that to properly evaluate the profunda femoris artery, you have to obtain oblique views.[28] The distribution of occlusive disease in profunda femoris is usually divided into three types. Type I is proximal, involving the orifice at the artery. Second is the segment from the origin to the first major penetrating artery that occurs in 74% of patients; the distal segment extends from the first perforating artery to the termination and occurs in 12%; the incidence of diffuse disease is 14%. Profundoplasty, when coupled with inflow procedures, is most effective in salvaging lower extremities. Eighty-four month patency rates exceeded 80%.[29] This is compared to approximately 30% when only profundoplasty alone was considered. At one-year, limb salvage rates are 60% with profundoplasty alone. Although these are not outstanding results, when one considers that oftentimes the alternative to a profundoplasty is a major amputation, 60% success in one year is a more favorable number. We obtained successful limb salvage in a study of 150 patients; 78% with inflow and profundoplasty verses 48% with isolated profundoplasty. We had excellent limb salvage with inflow graft (aortofemoral) thrombectomy and profundoplasty of 90%. This latter group of patients are often patients who develop fibrointimal hyperplasia at the distal end of the aortic bifemoral graft. Flow was restored by performing profundoplasty that maintains long-term graft patency.

PROCEDURES ON THE PROFUNDA

Since the profunda femoris artery can be used as a source of inflow to the lower extremity as well as an origin of distal grafts, some knowledge of its unique anatomy is necessary. The profunda artery is part of a collateral arterial network that extends from the internal iliac artery to the tibial vessels. It arises 2–4 cm below the inguinal ligament, passing posterolaterally to the superficial femoral artery. The medial and lateral circumflex femoral arteries are usually the first branches of the profunda but either can arise from the common femoral instead. The main trunk of the profunda femoris passes inferiorly just medial to the femur and gives three perforating branches. The terminal portion of the profunda anastomoses with the highest genicular branch of the popliteal artery at the adductor hiatus.

Arteriosclerotic involvement of the profunda femoris artery is most common at its origin. Since it often arises from the posterolateral aspect of the common femoral artery, stenosis at the profunda orifice may not be apparent on anterior posterior views obtained during arteriography; the profunda femoris artery may appear foreshortened, obscuring stenotic arterial lesions. Beals and associates demonstrated stenosis at the profunda femoris artery in 39% of patients. In two-thirds of patients with occlusive disease of this artery, the stenotic segment was recognized only on oblique or lateral views, demonstrating the necessity of oblique views for adequate arteriographic assessment.

There are a variety of techniques that can be used to perform a profundoplasty. Classically, if the superficial femoral artery is occluded, arteriotomy can be made from the femoral into the profunda to the end of the disease. Classically, the disease always ends at a bifurcation, although which bifurcation is variable. It can be of the medial lateral femoral circumflex or the first, second, or third perforator: all can be the point at which the disease ends. The longest profundoplasty we have done at the Medical College of Wisconsin has been 19 cm long. If one persists, generally, flow can be obtained through the profundoplasty. In terms of the type of material to use as a patch, we have used endarterectomized superficial femoral artery as a patch. We have also used saphenous vein as well as the Dacron patch.

One note is that flow can be maintained in a profundus femoral artery; therefore, the knee joint can almost always be salvaged. In patients who do require major amputation, a BK amputation has better rehabilitative potential. Likewise, in patients who already have a BK amputation who come in with an ischemic stump, this is most often due to inflow vessel occlusion. An inflow procedure with a profundoplasty can salvage the below-knee amputation.

REFERENCES

1. Jude EB, Oyibo SO, Chlamers N, Boulton AJ. Peripheral Arterial Disease in Diabetic and Nondiabetic Patients: A Comparison of Severity and Outcome. *Diabetes Care*. 2001;24(8): 1433–1437.
2. King TA, DePalma RG, Rhodes RS. Diabetes Mellitus and Atherosclerotic Involvement of the Profunda Femoris Artery. *Surg Gynecol Obstet*. 1984;159:553–556.
3. Haimovici H, Shapiro JH, Jacobson HG. Serial Femoral Arteriography in Occlusive Disease: Clinical-roentgenologic Considerations With a New Classification of Occlusive Patterns. *Am J Surg*. 1960;83:1042.
4. Hoch JR, Hollister MS, Kennell TW, et al. Comparison of Treatment Plan. *Am J Surg*. 1999; 178(2):166–172.
5. Kreitner KF, Kalden P, Neufang A, et al. Diabetes and Peripheral Arterial Occlusive Disease: Prospective Comparison of Contrast-enhanced Three-Dimensional MR Angiography With Conventional Digital Subtraction Angiography. *Am J Roentgenol*. 2000;174(1): 171–179.
6. Dorweiler B, Neufang A, Kreitner KF,et al. Magnetic Resonance Angioplasty Unmasks Reliable Target Vessels for Pedal Bypass Grafting in Patients with Diabetes Mellitus. *J Vasc Surg*. 2002;35(4) 766–772.
7. Oser RF, Picus D, Hicks ME, et al. Accuracy of DSA in the Evaluation of Patency of Infrapopliteal Vessels. *J Vasc Intervent Radiol*. 1995;6(4)589–594.
8. Ferrier TM. Comparative Study of Arterial Disease in Amputated Lower Limbs from Diabetics and Nondiabetics. *Med J*. 1967;1:5.
9. Vollrath KD, Salles-Chuna S, Vincent D, et al. Noninvasive Measurement of Toe Systolic Pressures. *Bruit*. 1980;4:27–30.
10. Vincent DG, Salles-Chuna S, Bernhard V, J. Towne. Noninvasive Assessment of Toe Systolic Pressures with Special Reference to Diabetes Mellitus. *J Cardiovasc Surg*. 1983;24(1):22–28. Jan/Feb 1983.
11. Reichel FA, Tyson RR. Femoroperoneal Bypass:Evaluation of Potential for Revascularization of the Severely Ischemic Lower Extremity. *Ann Surg*. 1975;181:182–185.
12. Dardik H, Ibrahim IM, Sprayregen S, Dardick I. Revascularization of the Peroneal Artery. *Surg Gynecol Obstet*. 1976;143:946–948.
13. Dardik H, Ibrahim IM, Dardik II. The Role of the Peroneal Artery for Limb Salvage. *Ann Surg*. 1979;189:189–198.
14. Graham JW, Hanel KC. Vein Grafts to the Peroneal Artery. *Surgery*. 1981;89:264–267.
15. Syilagyi DE, Hageman JH, Smith RF, et al. Autogenous Vein Grafting in Femoropopliteal Atherosclerosis: The Limits of its Effectiveness. *Surgery*. 1979;86:836–851.
16. Karmody AM, Leather RP, Shah DM, et al. Peroneal Artery Bypass: A Reappraisal of its Value in Limb Salvage. *J Vasc Surg*. 1984;1:809–816.
17. Leather RP, Shah DM, Chang BB, Kaufman JL. Resurrection of the in situ saphenous vein bypass: 1000 cases later. *Ann Surg*. 1988;208:435–442.

18. Synn AL, Hoballah JJ, Sharp WJ, et al. Are There Angiographic Predictors of Success for Vein Bypass for the Popliteal Artery? *Am J Surg*. 1992;164:276–280.
19. Shah DM, Darling RC, Chang BB, et al. Is Long Vein Bypass from Groin to Ankle a Durable Procedure? An Analysis of a Ten-year Experience. *J Vasc Surg*. 1992;15:402–408.
20. Harrington EB, Harrington ME, Schanzer H, et al. The Dorsalis Pedis Bypass: Moderate Success in Difficult Situations. *J Vasc Surg*. 1992;15:409–416.
21. Pomposelli FB Jr, Jepsen SJ, Gibbons GW, et al. Efficacy of the Dorsal Pedal Bypass for Limb Salvage in Diabetic Patients: Short-term Observations. *J Vasc Surg*. 1990;11:745–752.
22. Plecha E, Seabrook G, Bandyk D, Towne J. Determinants of Successful Peroneal Artery Bypass. *J Vasc Surg*. 1993;17(1):97–107.
23. Bernhardt V, Boren C, Towne J. Pneumatic Tourniquet as a Substitute for Vascular Clamps in Distal Bypass. *Surgery*. 1980;87:709–713.
24. Klamer TW, Lambert Jr GE, Richardson JD, et al. Utility of Inframalleolar Arterial Bypass Grafting. *J Vasc Surg*. 1990;11:164–170.
25. Rutherford RB, Flanigan BP, Gupta SK, et al. Suggested Standards for Reports Dealing with Lower Extremity Ischemia. *J Vasc Surg*. 1986;4:80–94.
26. Peterkin GA, Shunichiro M. LaMorte WW, Menzoian JO. Evaluation of a Proposed Standard Reporting System for Preoperative Angiograms in Infrainguinal Bypass Procedures: Angiographic Correlates of Measured Runoff Resistance. *J Vasc Surg*. 1988;7:379–385.
27. Shortell CK, Ouriel K, DeWeese JA, Green RM. Peroneal Artery Bypass: A Multifactorial Analysis. *Ann Vasc Surg*. 1992;6:15–19.
28. Beals JSM, Adcock FA, Frawley JS, et al. The Radiological Assessment of Disease of the Profunda Femoris Artery. *Br J Radiol*. 1971;44:854–859.
29. Towne J, Bernhard V, Rollins D, Baum P. Profundoplasty in Perspective: Limitations in the Long Term Management of Limb Ischemia. *Surgery*. 1981;90:1037–1345.

19

Vein Bypass Grafts to the Dorsalis Pedis Artery

Frank W. Logerfo, M.D.

The special importance of bypass grafts to the dorsalis pedis (DP) artery for preventing amputations in patients with diabetes and foot ulcers was identified over 20 years ago.[1] Since that time, there have been several reports demonstrating the international adoption of this operation. Time will tell whether DP bypass will be supplanted by newer technologies such as tibial angioplasty. However, as it stands today, all vascular surgeons providing care to patients with the lower extremity complications of diabetes mellitus should be capable of performing or providing access to this operation. The reason for this is dictated by the underlying pathophysiology of foot ulcers in diabetes and the anatomic pattern of vascular occlusion.

Virtually all diabetic patients presenting with foot ulcers have some degree of neuropathy. The motor neuropathy results in a "claw" deformity of the foot with increased pressure points under the metatarsal heads, at the tips of the toes, and the dorsum of the toes at the interphalangeal joints. The pressure is aggravated by the limited joint mobility that occurs as a consequence of disuse and glycosylation of scleral proteins. Diminished sensation at these pressure points sets the stage for ulceration with even moderate decline in arterial perfusion. The entire biology is compromised by loss of the neuroinflammatory response to injury or infection. Adding to this is the loss of sympathetic tone, with inefficient A-V shunting of blood flow around the capillary system, plus loss of apocrine and eccrine gland function. The latter results in dry, cracked skin, creating a portal of entry for bacteria.

Under these circumstances of compromised biology, the foot requires maximum perfusion to heal an ulcer or minor amputation. A good rule of thumb is to select a target artery that is in direct continuity with the arterial system in the foot. Often, this can be achieved with a standard femeropopliteal bypass, provided either the anterior or posterior tibial artery is patent all the way to the foot. The peroneal artery is a good, but not ideal, target because there is an intervening collateral system to reach the foot, especially the forefoot. It is the nature of atherosclerotic occlusive disease associated with diabetes that the occlusion involves the infrageniculate arteries, but surprisingly, spares arteries in the foot proper, most commonly the dorsalis pedis artery. Thus, for many patients with diabetes and a foot ulcer, the ideal target is the dorsalis pedis artery to achieve the goal of restoring maximum perfusion to the biologically compromised foot.

The bypass graft must be constructed with autogenous vein.[2] Inflow may be obtained from the most distal artery proximal to which there is no significant obstruction. While the common femoral artery is almost always satisfactory in terms of hemodynamics, it provides no advantage over using the superficial femoral or popliteal artery in the absence of intervening occlusive disease. In fact, just the opposite is true: the more distal inflow requires a shorter graft, allows for more effective use of limited autogenous vein, avoids incision in the groin or upper thigh where there is excessive adipose tissue, and takes less time. In our experience, we have been able to use these more distal inflow sources in about 50% of our DP bypass grafts.[3]

To achieve maximum success with these procedures, the vascular surgeon must be familiar with all aspects of autogenous vein grafting including reversed, translocated (nonreversed), and in situ techniques. Arm vein grafts are frequently appropriate, especially for shorter grafts originating from more distal inflow sites.[4] There is, perhaps, no area of vascular surgery that is more demanding of fine technical skill and creative solutions than distal vein grafting, including dorsalis pedis bypass.

With this understanding, the procedure itself is quite straightforward. There is nothing intrinsically novel to the dorsalis pedis artery that adds complexity to the procedure or results in a higher failure rate than other infrageniculate vein graft targets. The basic principles for the surgery and some technical tips are illustrated in the following example of a popliteal-to-dorsalis pedis vein graft (Figure 19–1)

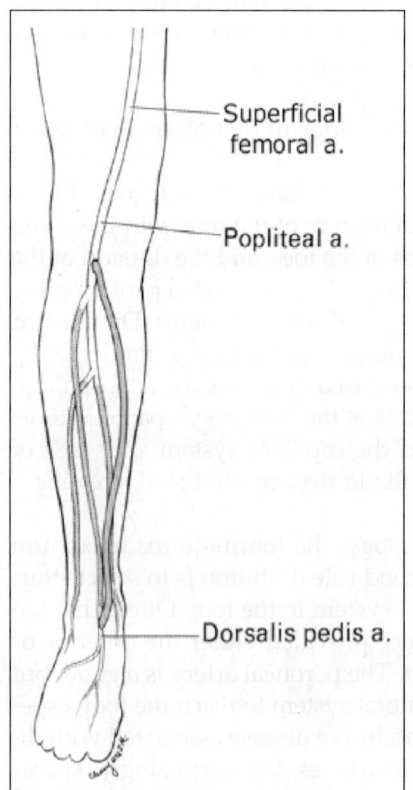

Figure 19-1. Layout of a left popliteal-to-dorsalis pedis vein graft.

The question as to whether the popliteal artery is capable of providing inflow for a pedal bypass can be accurately determined by physical examination in almost all patients. The presence of a strong, palpable popliteal pulse is sufficient evidence, even in the presence of a minor or moderate stenosis of the superficial femoral artery. Commonly, for example, a 50% stenosis of the SFA is present on arteriography. As long as a strong popliteal pulse is palpable, this is of no concern since the volume flow demand of a dorsalis pedis bypass is only about 50-60 cc/min.

On rare occasions, it may be worthwhile to measure mean pressure in the popliteal artery to ensure that it is within 10% of mean central arterial pressure. Concerns that a stenosis of the SFA will progress to late occlusion are not justified. Within the lifetime of the patient, this is an uncommon occurrence that almost never results in occlusion of an established distal bypass graft, and can easily be corrected at the time if necessary.

Assessment of the dorsalis pedis artery is, at the current time, best determined by digital subtraction arteriography, preferably with access through the opposite common femoral artery. The diagnostic catheter can then be positioned in the ipsilateral superficial femoral artery, thereby minimizing the volume of contrast agent necessary to obtain satisfactory AP and lateral views of the dorsalis pedis artery. Both views are helpful in discerning the course of the artery, sometimes distorted by degenerative neuroosteoarthropathy, and in choosing a preferred site of anastomosis. Usually, this is under the extensor retinaculum, just proximal to the origin of the lateral tarsal artery. Severe calcification of the dorsalis pedis artery does not preclude success.[5]

Ultrasound mapping of the greater saphenous vein is helpful in determining the availability of appropriate autogenous vein conduit. When ipsilateral saphenous vein is not available, it is our preference to use arm vein as a second choice because of the high likelihood of a similar problem in the opposite leg within the near future.[6]

The procedure is best carried out under general anesthesia with invasive or ultrasonic cardiac monitoring to guide fluid replacement with a goal of keeping it at a minimum. Most patients receive a total of 1200-1500 cc over the course of a two-and-a-half- to three-hour operation.

My preference is to begin the operation with an incision anterior and distal to the medial malleolus, and to cannulate the GSV with a Horsely needle. The vein is irrigated with a solution of 5000 units heparin and 120 milligrams of papaverine in 1000 cc of Normosol (or equivalent) as the incision is carried to the knee, and the tributaries are identified and ligated. The vein graft may then be excised. The distal Horsely needle is removed, the vein is irrigated from the central end, and the valves are incised with a Mills valvulotome. The Horsely needle is replaced at the distal end of the graft, a bulldog is placed on the central end, and the gently distended vein is stored in cold heparin-papaverine solution.

The popliteal artery is dissected free and secured. An incision is made along the lateral edge of the extensor hallucis longus tendon, and the dorsalis pedis artery is identified and secured (Figure 19–2)

A subfascial tunnel is constructed from the knee to lower leg (Figure 19–3). This helps to protect the vein graft in the event of superficial infection or areas of localized skin necrosis along the suture line.

A roll is placed under the foot, and a subcutaneous tunnel is constructed from the distal end of the first tunnel, anterior to the tibia, to reach the dorsalis pedis artery (Figure 19–4).

After completion of the proximal anastomosis, the graft is flushed and irrigated using the distal Horsely needle. It is then passed through the tunnels to reach the

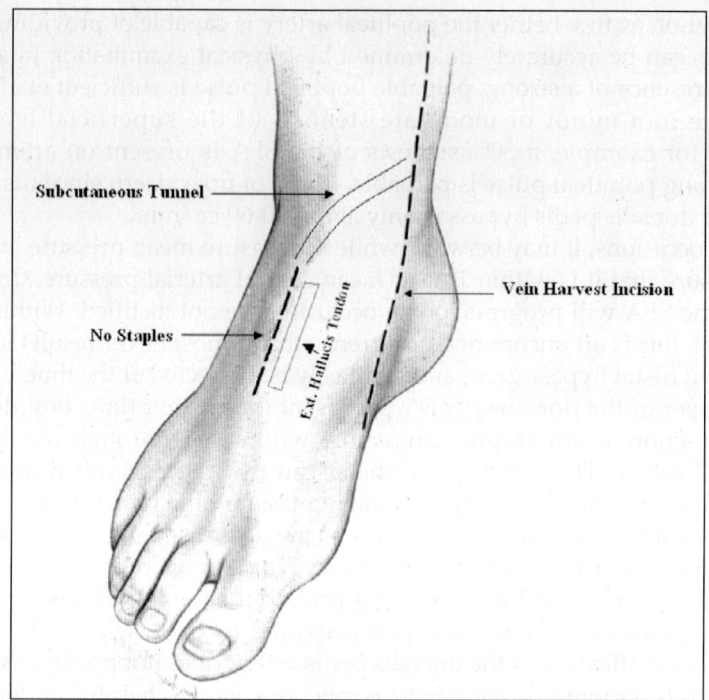

Figure 19-2. Location of incision and tunnels on the foot.

dorsalis pedis artery. It is helpful to leave the Horsely needle in the end of the vein graft to stabilize it while the anastomosis is started using 7-0 monofilament suture and the "parachute" technique (Figure 19–5).

If stay sutures are used, it is best to place them through both the vein graft and the artery. The distal excess vein graft is excised and the anastomosis is completed (Figure 19–6).

Because of the capillary leak of albumin associated with diabetes and the intense reperfusion, postoperative edema of the foot can place stress on the suture lines. For

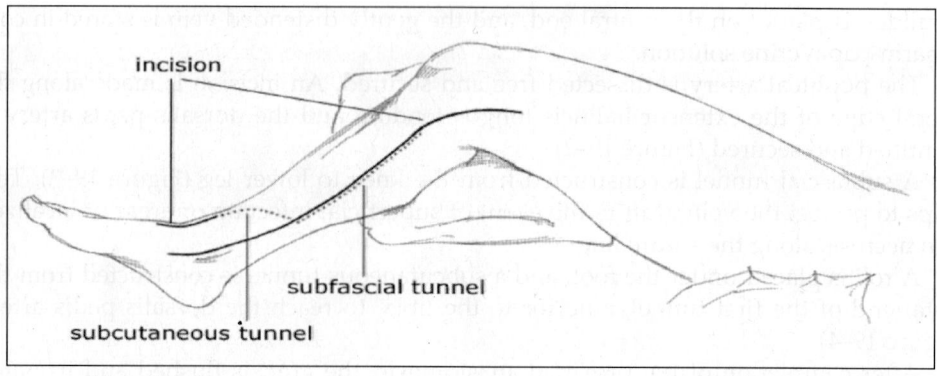

Figure 19-3. Location of the tunnels and incisions for a left popliteal-to-dorsalis pedis vein graft.

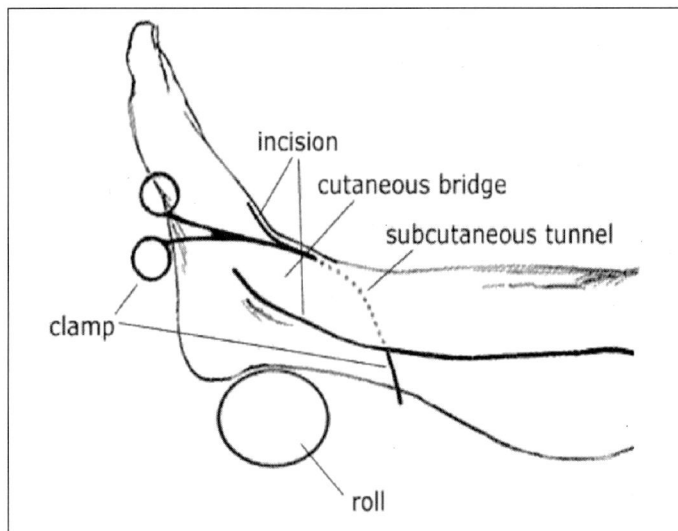

Figure 19-4. Placement of a roll underneath the heel facilitates creation of the distal subcutaneous tunnel.

this reason, the incisions on the foot are closed with subcuticular suture and/or interrupted skin sutures, taking care to minimize tension. At the completion of the procedure, while still in the operating room, the foot and leg are wrapped with an elastic bandage to help control edema. A small window is made in the bandage just over the subcutaneous segment of the graft so that the pulse in the vein graft can be palpated and monitored with Doppler ultrasound for assurance of patency (Figure 19–7). After 24 hours, the dressing is changed and an elastic bandage is applied with no further need for the window. There are no restrictions on the patient's activity as far as wound care is concerned.

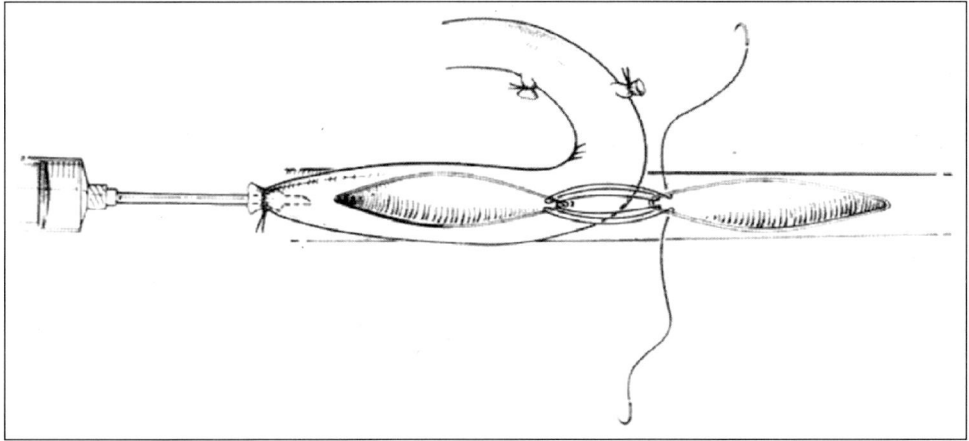

Figure 19-5. The Horsely needle is left in place to stabilize the vein graft as the "parachute" anastomosis is started.

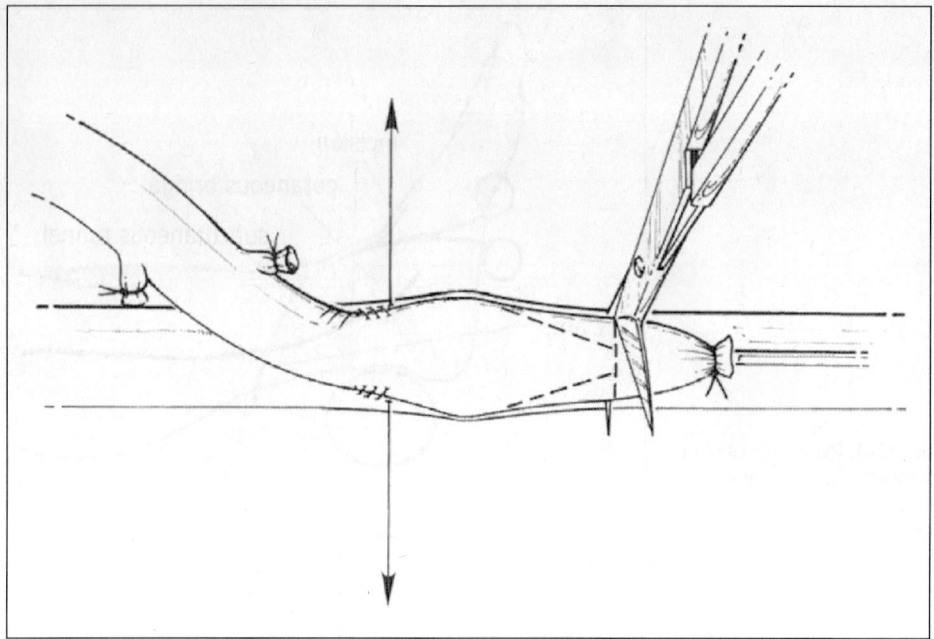

Figure 19-6. The tip of the vein graft can be precisely trimmed to fit the anastomosis.

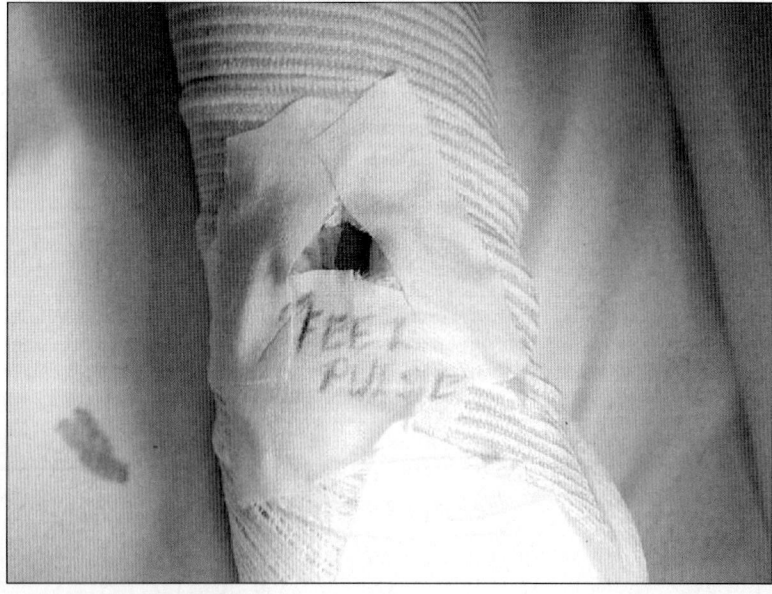

Figure 19-7. The foot and leg are wrapped with an elastic bandage with a window cut out for direct palpation and Doppler interrogation of the vein graft.

REFERENCES

1. LoGerfo FW, Coffman JD. Current concepts: Vascular and microvascular disease in the diabetic foot. Implications for foot care. *N Engl J Med*. 1984;311:1615–1619.
2. Pomposelli FB Jr, Marcaccio E, Gibbons GW, et al. Dorsalis pedis arterial bypass: Durable limb salvage for foot ischemia in patients with diabetes mellitus. *J Vasc Surg*. 1995;21: 375–384.
3. Pomposelli FB, Kansal N, Hamdan AD, et al. A decade of experience with dorsalis pedis bypass: Analysis of outcome in more than 1000 cases. *J Vasc Surg*. 2003;37:307–315.
4. Faries PL, Arora S, Pomposelli FB Jr, et al. The use of arm vein in lower extremity revascularization: Results of 520 procedures performed over eight years. *J Vasc Surg*. 2000;31:50–9.
5. Misare BD, Pomposelli FB Jr, Gibbons GW, Campbell DR, Freeman DV, LoGerfo FW. Infrapopliteal bypasses to severely calcified, unclampable outflow arteries: Two year results. *J Vasc Surg*. 1996;24:6–16.
6. Holzenbein T, Pomposelli FB Jr, Miller A, et al. Results of a policy using arm veins as the first alternative to an unavailable ipsilateral greater saphenous vein for infrainguinal bypass. *J Vasc Surg*. 1996;23:130–140.

20

Unusual Exposure for Lower Extremity Revascularization

William H. Pearce, M.D. Gale L. Tang, M.D.

Complications of either endovascular or open vascular surgery often require creative techniques to revascularize the lower extremity. In addition, heavily scarred tissue or irradiated tissue make direct surgical approach risky and unnecessary. In these situations, when the surgeon is faced with complex decisions and particularly risky interventions, it is best to avoid contaminated or scarred areas, and perform bypasses outside the area of risk (extra-anatomic). Operating in areas that are undissected reduces risks but often requires uncommon approaches. These uncommon exposures may be unfamiliar and have their own potential complications. For example, in the posterior approach to the popliteal artery, the peroneal nerve, posterior tibial nerves, and sural nerves are very superficial in the dissection and may be injured. This chapter will review unusual operative approaches including the obturator bypass, lateral approaches to the lower extremity arteries, and the posterior approach to the popliteal artery.

OBTURATOR BYPASS

The obturator bypass is used for infectious processes of the femoral triangle including mycotic aneurysm from illicit drug use and arterial infection from closure devices. The surgical principle is to bypass the scarred or contaminated area in undissected and clean surgical planes. If the groin is infected and there is associated hemorrhage, the bleeding vessels are first ligated and debrided. Unfortunately, if this tack is taken, the instruments need to be changed and the patient reprepped and draped so that the sterile obturator bypass may be performed. If the patient is not exsanguinating, the sterile procedure may be performed first with ligation of the vessels and debridement as the second procedure.

The obturator bypass was first described by Shaw and Baue[1] in 1962. While it was originally described for infectious processes, the indications have gradually broadened to include scarring, radiation, and repeated bypasses using the common femoral artery.[2] Although a variety of incisions can be made to expose the retroperitoneum in the pelvis, we prefer to use a curvilinear incision that is commonly used for kidney transplants. The key aspects of this operation are the retroperitoneal exposure of the iliac vessels, the obturator foramen, and the above-knee popliteal artery. Several key structures that are important for this operation include the lateral cutaneous nerve of the thigh, the obturator membrane, the obturator nerve, and the obturator artery. The obturator nerve and artery pass through the superior lateral aspects of the obturator foramen, and the defect in the membrane can easily be felt. Generally, the obturator artery originates from the iliac artery, but many come from the inferior epigastric. Once the retroperitoneal incision is completed, exposure of the above-knee popliteal artery is performed in a standard fashion. A medial incision is made with control of the popliteal vessels. The next step in the procedure is to create a tunnel between the knee and the pelvis. As it was originally described, the tunneling device was passed from above to the popliteal fossa. However, the angles are difficult in using this approach and DePalma[3] recommended passing the tunneling device from below. This modification provides a much easier access to the retroperitoneal structures. Often, the obturator membrane is dense and very difficult to penetrate using any tunneling device. However, because the force of the tunneling device is directed cephalad, injury to the bladder may occur. Therefore, it is essential to protect the bladder during this portion of the operation. Finally, in creating this tunnel, it is important to remain below the adductor longus, adductor brevis, and adductor magnus. These three muscles form the floor of the femoral triangle and will provide the sterile plane to separate the bypass graft from the infected field.

Operative Procedure

The operative procedure is performed by using a transverse lower abdominal incision for control of the iliac artery and proximal anastomosis. The retroperitoneum is bluntly dissected, taking care not to injure the ureter or the bladder in the process. The proximal anastomosis may be either to the common or external iliac artery. The external iliac artery may be ligated at the inguinal ligament prior to the groin exploration. With gentle retraction and blunt dissection, the obturator membrane can be palpated and visualized (Figure 20–1). Once the obturator membrane has been identified, the obturator artery and nerve that penetrate the superior medial aspect of the obturator canal should be found. Once this exposure is completed, the popliteal artery is exposed through a medial incision. With the sartorius muscle retracted, the popliteal artery is identified just as it exits the adductor canal. The tunnel from the popliteal fossa to the retroperitoneum is created by passing either the long DeBakey or the tunneling device from below (Figure 20–2). Remember that the tunnel must be below (posterior to) the adductor muscle mass. The obturator foramen is often dense and difficult to penetrate, and requires extra force. During this part of the procedure, it is essential to protect the bladder from injury, and to avoid the obturator nerve and artery. When this tunnel is created, the graft (#8 PTFE) is drawn from the abdominal incision to the popliteal fossa. Using standard techniques, the proximal and distal anastomoses are completed after the patient has been heparinized. The wounds are closed and dressing is applied. A muscle flap is frequently used to cover the infected area.

The complications associated with the obturator bypass include retroperitoneal hemorrhage, particularly if the patient is anticoagulated following the procedure.

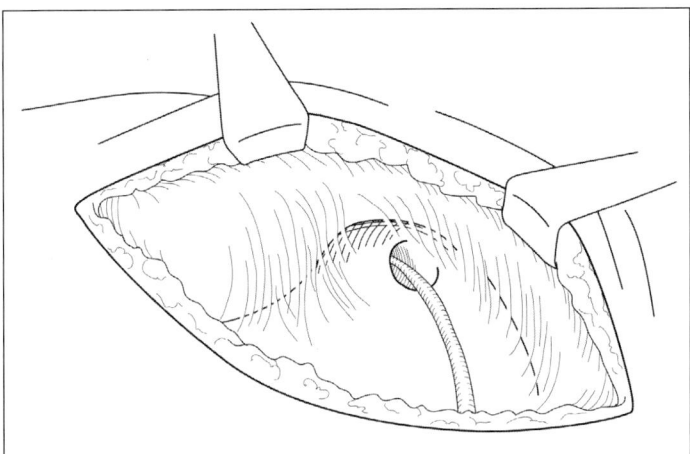

Figure 20-1. The obturator foramen, obturator nerve, and obturator artery are seen from above. It is important to note that the obturator nerve and artery penetrate the membrane in the superior lateral portion. It is often difficult to obtain this view since the obturator membrane is anterior. Often, just feeling the membrane is all that is possible in some patients with a deep pelvis.

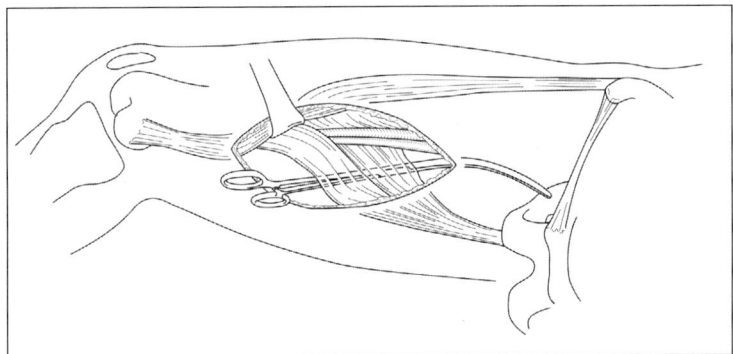

Figure 20-2. The tunneling device, either DeBakey instrument or tube tunneler, is placed from below cephalad. It is important to place the tunnel beneath the adductor muscle group, and to direct the tip away from the entrance of the obturator artery and nerve. Placing the instrument cephalad is often difficult, and the bladder should be protected.

Other complications include infection of the retroperitoneal space by direct connection. There is often little distance between the infected groin and the retroperitoneum. An incision too low in the abdominal wall may actually be contaminated by the groin incision. Finally, injury to the obturator nerve may present with an annoying groin pain, and the patient should be warned of this complication. Bladder injury has been reported rarely, but is a serious complication that can be avoided with the use of a Foley catheter and careful attention to detail during the tunneling procedure.

LATERAL APPROACHES

Lateral approaches to the arteries of the lower extremities avoid cross-contamination from medial wound infections. These approaches were described by Veith in 1987[4] and

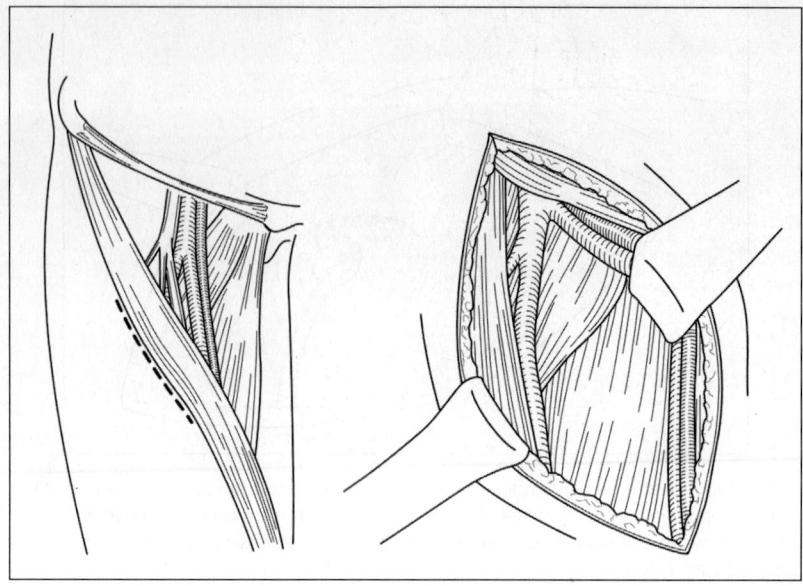

Figure 20-3. Lateral approach to the profunda femoris artery. Several incisions may be made to expose the distal profunda. In this example, an incision made just lateral to the border of the sartorius muscle is made. The sartorius muscle is reflected medially, exposing the profunda femoris artery as well as the femoral nerve. The femoral nerve is lateral in the wound.

may also be useful in repeat bypasses following graft occlusion. The lateral approach to the profunda femoris artery is also used when there is extensive dissection and scarring in the groin.[5-7]

Operative Procedures

In the proximal one-third of the thigh, an incision is made paralleling the sartorius muscle (Figure 20–3). The lateral border of the sartorius muscle is clearly identified and retracted medially to expose the profunda femoris artery. Unfortunately, in this approach, the common femoral nerve is subject to injury. In this dissection, it is important to pay careful attention to the location of the femoral nerve, which is lateral to the artery. In addition, there are numerous perforating branches of the artery, crossing veins, and lymphatics. Lymphoceles are common complications with extensive dissection of the profunda and are difficult to avoid. The proximal superficial femoral artery can be identified in this wound, and since it is often occluded, can be retracted along with the sartorius muscles. The lateral approach to the profunda is useful to avoid exposure of previously placed aortofemoral grafts. In these instances, the profunda is used as an inflow for more distal bypasses. The tunneling of the bypass originating from the profunda is often superficial or directly through the adductor muscle group. I prefer the more superficial route when using a vein, which requires careful attention to the course of the vein graft proximally as there is an abrupt change in wound depth.

The lateral approaches to the popliteal artery and peroneal arteries are generally used for open and infected medial wounds (Figure 20–4). The exception is in the exposure of the distal peroneal artery. The most distal segment of this artery is more accessible using a lateral approach. In patients with open wounds, tunneling is often

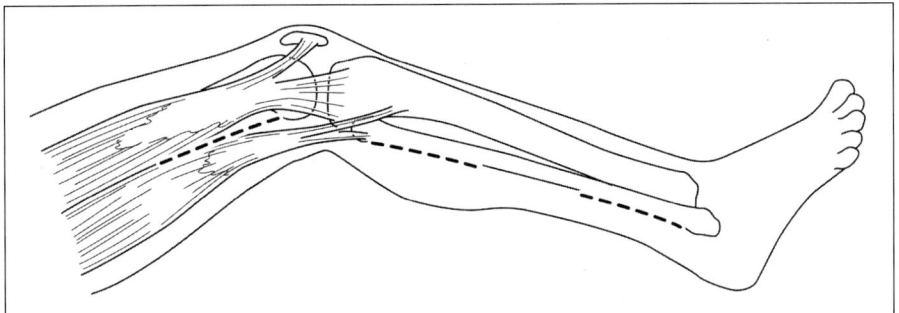

Figure 20-4. Incisions for lateral exposures of the popliteal artery and peroneal artery of the lower extremity.

subcutaneous and routed around the contaminated areas. In making these unusual tunnels, it is important to avoid boney prominences and potential impingement. Inadvertent iatrogenic entrapment may occur if the graft is accidentally placed between tendinous insertions, particularly around the knee joint.

The lateral approach to the above-knee popliteal artery begins with a lateral incision in the distal thigh just above the knee (Figure 20–5). The iliotibial tract is opened and the popliteal fossa is entered just behind the biceps femoris muscle. When entering the popliteal fossa, it is important to avoid injury to either the common peroneal nerve

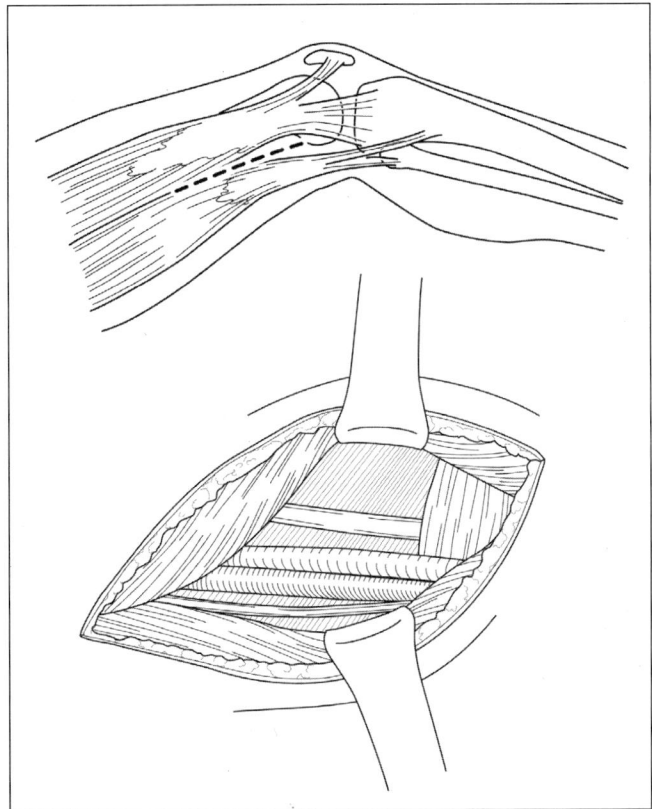

Figure 20-5. Lateral approach to the above-knee popliteal artery is made through a vertical incision through the iliotibial tract between the vastus lateralis and biceps femoris. The common peroneal nerve lies superficial in this wound, and care must be taken to avoid injuring it.

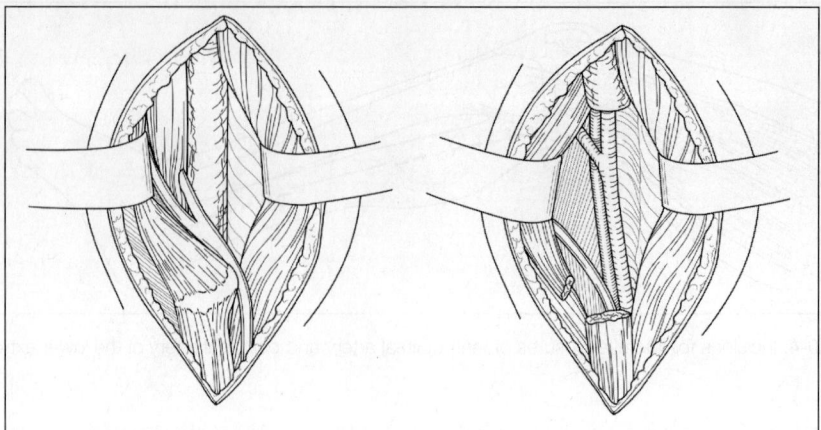

Figure 20-6. Lateral approach to the below-knee popliteal artery is made through an incision directly below the knee over the head of the fibula. The common peroneal nerve lies in close approximation to the head of fibula and beneath the biceps femoris tendon.

or the sciatic nerve. As described in the posterior approach to the popliteal artery, the sciatic nerve enters the popliteal fossa at the apex of the fossa, and then gives off the common peroneal nerve.

The lateral exposure to the below-knee popliteal artery (Figure 20–6) is via an incision that begins just above the head of the fibula and extends for 6–10 centimeters. The head of the fibula is an important landmark as well as the tendon of the bicep femoris. Since the common peroneal nerve is very superficial and prone to injury, the patient should be warned prior to the procedure. Identification of the nerve is the first step of the procedure once the skin is opened. The bicep femoris muscle tendon is resected with the peroneal nerve protected. With the peroneal nerve retracted, the head of the fibula is resected. The popliteal vessels and the tibial nerve are easily identified.

In either the lateral or posterior approach to the popliteal artery, injury to both nerves can occur. Interestingly, the popliteal artery may be more superficial in the wound than one would expect. Tunneling is variable using either a subcutaneous position or deep through the adductor muscles to the femoral triangle. If a vein graft is used and placed in the subcutaneous space, a portion of the iliotibial tract is removed to avoid compression.

The popliteal vessel and the branches can be well visualized via this approach. Tunneling is, again, generally subcutaneous, but an anatomic tunnel can be created from the below-knee incision to the above-knee space similar to a medial exposure.

Access to the distal peroneal artery is best obtained by removing the distal fibula using a lateral approach[8-9] (Figure 20–7). When entering the lateral compartment, the superficial peroneal nerve may be injured. Injury will produce anesthesia over the superolateral aspect of the foot.

POSTERIOR APPROACH

The posterior approach to the popliteal artery is useful in patients with popliteal artery entrapment, localized popliteal artery aneurysms, and popliteal trauma directly behind the knee.[10-13] In this approach, several nerves are prone to injury because of their

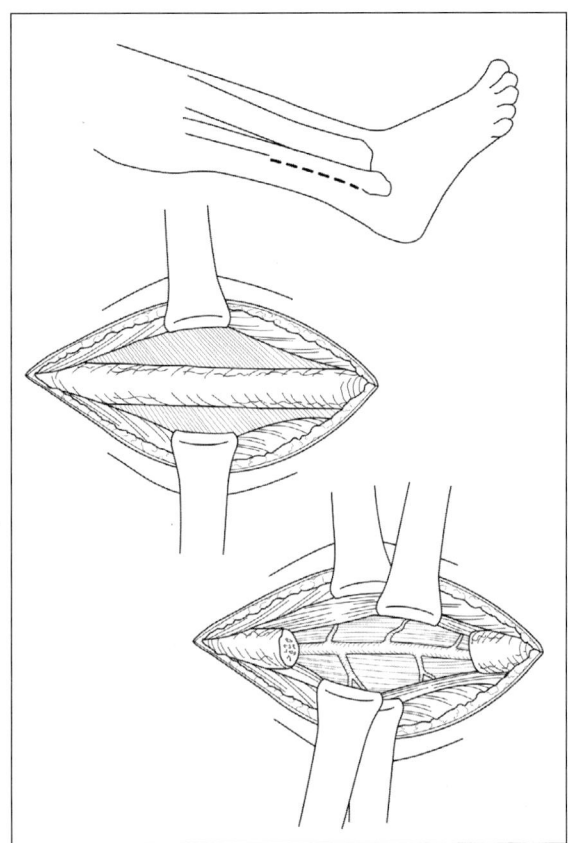

Figure 20-7. Lateral approach to the peroneal artery. The incision is made directly superior to the lateral malleolus, and approximately 7–8 cm of the fibula is removed. Just beneath the fibula is the tibial vessels and, therefore, it is important to stay close to the periosteum and to the artery when resecting this structure. The peroneal nerve superficial is located in this compartment, and care should be taken not to injure it.

superficial nature. These nerves include the sural nerve, the common peroneal nerve, and the tibial nerve. In addition, the arterial pathology must be contained within the popliteal fossa. It is difficult to dissect either more proximally or distally due to the depth of the artery, the muscle tendons, and the arboration of the tibial nerve.

Operative Procedure

With the patient in the prone position, a curvilinear incision is made from the medial aspect of the leg transversely across the knee joint, then vertically in the mid-portion of the calf (Figure 20–8). With the subcutaneous tissue divided, the deep fascia of the leg is identified. Often, the lesser saphenous vein is found in the superficial compartment, but in most instances, it is beneath the fascia. The sural nerve is identified below the fascia, often accompanying the lesser saphenous vein. Opening the deep fascia carefully is important to avoid injury to these structures. Once the deep fascia is open from the apex of the popliteal fossa to the most inferior portion, the wound is retracted gently with emphasis to not injure the common peroneal nerve. The common peroneal nerve takes origin from the tibial nerve in variable locations but passes laterally through the popliteal fossa to wrap around the fibula in the lowermost aspect of the wound. Once the sural nerve is identified, as well as the common peroneal nerve using blunt dissection, the tissue is divided down to the tibial peroneal nerve. The tibial peroneal nerve is the most superficial portion of the deep portions of the wound

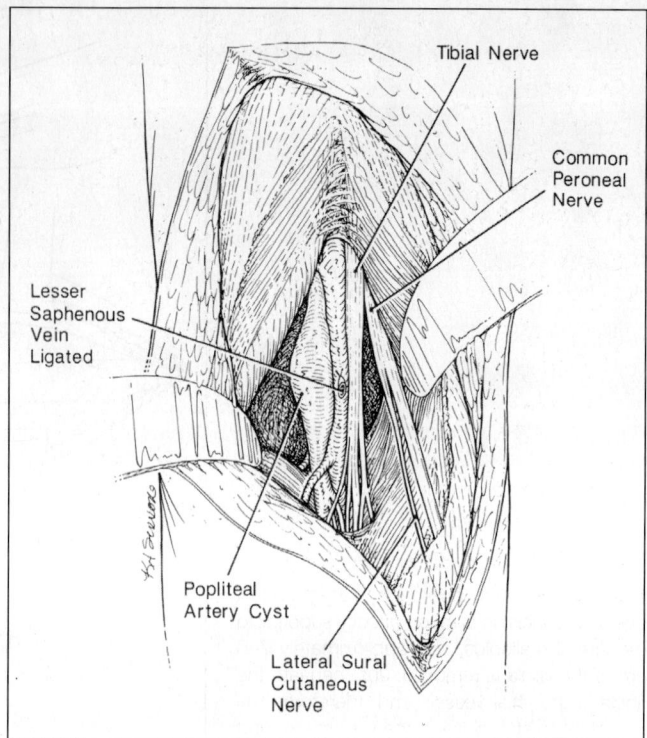

Figure 20-9. The deep fascia is carefully incised, avoiding injury to the tibial and common peroneal nerves. From: Pearce WH. Posterior approach to the popliteal artery. In: Bergan JJ, Yao JST, eds. *Techniques in Arterial Surgery*. Philadelphia: W. B. Saunders Company;1990: 180–183. Reproduced by permission.

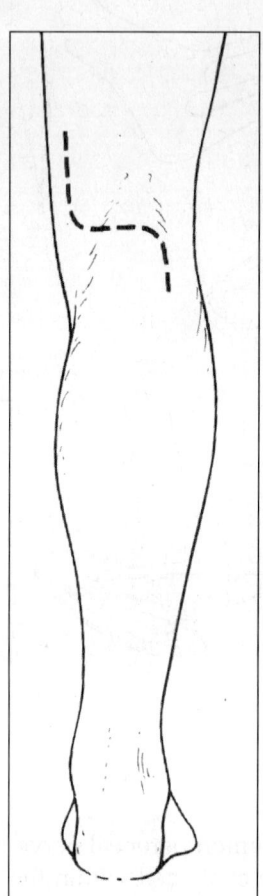

Figure 20-8. An S-shaped incision that crosses the popliteal crease is used for the posterior approach to the popliteal fossa. The inferior limb of the incision is just lateral to the midline. From: Pearce WH. Posterior approach to the popliteal artery. In: Bergan JJ, Yao JST, eds. *Techniques in Arterial Surgery*. Philadelphia: W. B. Saunders Company; 1990:180–183. Reproduced by permission.

(Figure 20–9). The tibial nerve is retracted, exposing the popliteal vein and artery. Working around both the vein and the nerve, it is possible to expose the popliteal artery from the adductor canal to the tibial peroneal trunk where it passes behind the sartorius muscle. In the inferior aspect of the wound, it is sometimes difficult to control all of the blood vessels because of the remarkable arborization of the tibial peroneal nerve. Numerous nerve branches pass to the gastrocnemius and soleus muscles. In patients who are well developed, the gastrocnemius muscles also impede the view of the more distal aspects of the popliteal artery and tibial vessels. In treating patients with popliteal artery entrapment, the medial head of the gastrocnemius muscle is traced cephalad, following its course to its insertion on the femoral condyle. As one follows the tendinous insertion, it is often possible to see the entrapment caused by the

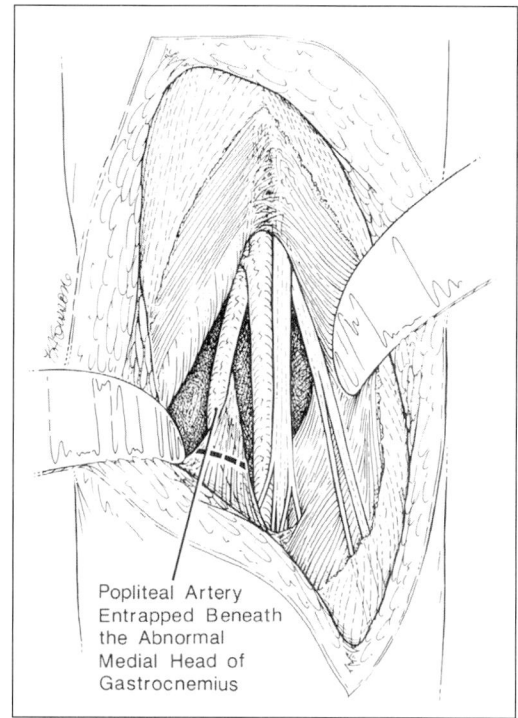

Figure 20-10. Resection of an anomalous insertion of the medial gastrocnemius muscle is made to release the entrapped popliteal artery. Note the distal branching of the tibial nerve. From: Pearce WH. Posterior approach to the popliteal artery. In: Bergan JJ, Yao JST, eds. *Techniques in Arterial Surgery.* Philadelphia: W. B. Saunders Company; 1990:180–183. Reproduced by permission.

Popliteal Artery Entrapped Beneath the Abnormal Medial Head of Gastrocnemius

lateral displacement of the medial head (Figure 20–10). The tendinous insertion is resected along with a substantial portion of the proximal muscle. In patients with damaged arteries or aneurysms, the arterial segment is replaced. A venous conduit is often harvested, either from the lesser saphenous vein or by undermining the skin medially and harvesting the greater saphenous vein at the knee. With the leg free prepped, it is possible to flex the leg and extend the leg to ensure that popliteal entrapment has been treated. The closure of the wound is often problematic. Aligning the S-shaped curve is difficult, particularly after extensive surgery when the skin may be swollen and difficult to reapproximate. Stay stitches are placed at the apex of the curvilinear incision to ensure proper alignment.

COMMENTS

Operating in undissected tissue planes to avoid contamination or perhaps lengthy operations in scarred areas is a valuable tool in the vascular surgeon's armamentarium. The lateral approaches avoid wound complications that may be associated with dense scarring or irradiated tissue. While the unusual exposures provide the ease of dissecting the artery, they also provide the opportunity for inadvertent nerve injury. It is important to describe the complications of nerve injuries to the patients prior to these procedures. Nerve complications can be problematic for both the patient and the physician, and it may take months to recover normal function. However, these unusual exposures are often used in difficult and desperate situations, and the patients are most grateful when the limb is saved.

REFERENCES

1. Shaw RS, Baue AE. Management of sepsis complicating arterial reconstructive procedures. Surgery. 1962;53:75–86.
2. Pearce WH, Ricco J-B, Yao JST, et al. Modified technique of obturator bypass in failed or infected grafts. *Ann Vasc Surg.* 1983;197:344–347.
3. DePalma RG, Hubay CA. Arterial bypass via the obturator foramen. An alternative in complicated vascular problems. *Am J Surg.* 1968;115:323–328.
4. Veith FJ, Ascer E, Gupta SK, Wengerter KR. lateral approach to the popliteal artery. *J Vasc Surg.* 1987;6:119–123.
5. Nunez AA, Veith FJ, Collier P, et al. Direct approaches to the distal portions of the deep femoral artery for limb salvage bypasses. *J Vasc Surg.* 1988;8:576–581.
6. Hershey FB, Auer AI. Extended surgical approach to the profunda femoris artery. *Surg Gynecol Obstet.* 1974;138:88–90.
7. Veith FJ, Gupta SK, Ascer E, et al. Alternative approaches to the deep femoral, the popliteal, and infrapopliteal arteries in the leg and foot. In: Bergan JJ, Yao JST, eds. *Techniques in Arterial Surgery.* Philadelphia: W.B. Saunders Company;1990:145–156.
8. McCarthy WJ, Flinn WR, Pearce, WH, Yao JST. Techniques and surgical exposures for femoral distal prosthetic graft and composite sequential bypass. In: Bergan JJ, Yao JST, eds. *Techniques in Arterial Surgery.* Philadelphia: W.B. Saunders Company; 1990:134–144.
9. Dardik H, Dardik I, Veith FJ. Exposure of the tibial-peroneal arteries by a single lateral approach. *Surgery.* 1974;75:377–382.
10. Pearce WH. Posterior approach to the popliteal artery. In: Bergan JJ, Yao JST, eds. *Techniques in Arterial Surgery.* Philadelphia: W.B. Saunders Company; 1990:180–183.
11. Rob C: Place of direct surgery in treatment of obliterative arterial disease. *Br Med J.* 1956; 2:1027–1029.
12. Arnulf G, Benichoux R. DÈcouverte large de l'artere fémoro-poplité. *Lyon Chir.* 1949;44:203.
13. Pataro EF, Acrich MW. Internal approach to the popliteal artery: Marchal's approach. *J Cardiovasc Surg.* 1971;12:402–405.

21

Surgical Management of Femoral and Popliteal Artery Aneurysms

Robert Kim, M.D., Patrick J. O'hara, M.D., F.A.C.S.

BACKGROUND AND GENERAL PRINCIPLES

Although femoral and popliteal artery aneurysms are relatively uncommon when compared to their aortic counterparts, they constitute the majority of nonaortic peripheral aneurysms (Figure 21–1). Considering the experience at The Cleveland Clinic from 1989–2001, the femoral and popliteal arteries were the most commonly involved, together compromising nearly two-thirds of all nonaortic peripheral artery aneurysms (unpublished data from the Vascular Surgery Departmental Registry).

There are two main classifications of aneurysms based on their histological appearance. True aneurysms exhibit evidence of degeneration involving all three layers in the arterial wall, are more commonly seen in men, and are often associated with aneurysms involving the aorto-iliac arteries or aneurysms present in the contralateral limb. In contrast, false aneurysms, also known as pseudoaneurysms, usually arise from trauma, anastomotic disruption, or infection (mycotic aneurysms). True femoral artery aneurysms are not as common as femoral pseudoaneurysms, but in the popliteal segment, the reverse is usually observed.

While some femoral and popliteal aneurysms are discovered by detection of an asymptomatic mass, others may present with symptoms. True aneurysms in these locations rarely rupture, but are important because of their potential to cause limb-threatening complications such as embolization or thrombosis. Large aneurysms may also cause symptoms such as swelling or dysesthesia due to their mass effect, leading to compression of adjacent venous or nerve structures. Given the paucity of peripheral aneurysms, a high index of suspicion is helpful for early diagnosis.

Treatment objectives, which are identical for both femoral and popliteal aneurysms, include elimination of complications such as rupture or emboli production, elimination of the mass effect of large aneurysms, and the maintenance of distal perfusion, all in a durable fashion. In addition, some general concepts apply to the treatment of both femoral and popliteal aneurysms. Elective repairs are usually

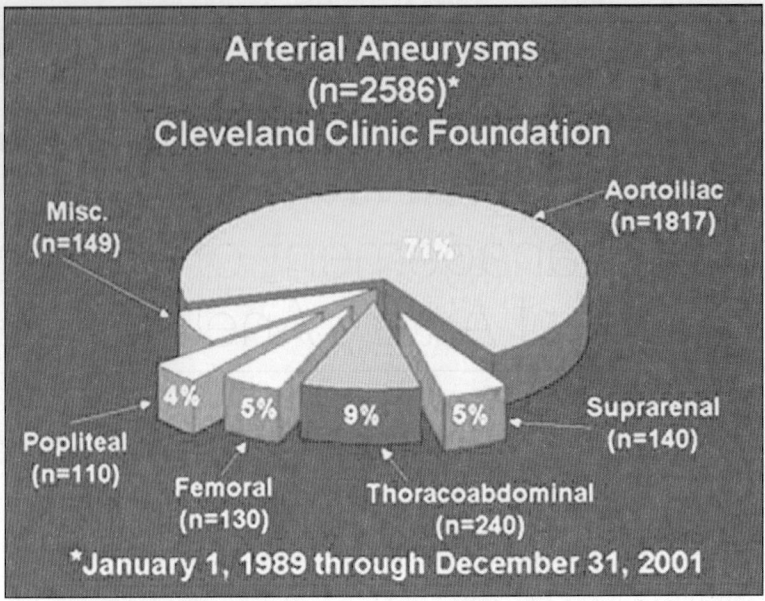

Figure 21-1. Distribution of surgical procedures performed for peripheral arterial aneurysms at The Cleveland Clinic from 1989 through 2001 (unpublished data from the computerized Vascular Surgery Departmental Registry).

associated with better outcomes than emergent aneurysm repairs, especially for limb-threatening complications. Furthermore, while there is little disagreement regarding the appropriate management of symptomatic aneurysms, controversy continues regarding the management of asymptomatic aneurysms, especially if they are small. It is also apparent that the extent of aneurysmal disease considerably influences the complexity of treatment.[1,2]

POPLITEAL ARTERY ANEURYSM

Popliteal artery aneurysms are the most commonly encountered aneurysms outside the aortoiliac system. Since 97% occur in males and the average age at diagnosis is 65 years, it is considered to be a disease of older men.[1] Popliteal aneurysms are frequently associated with aneurysms elsewhere, particularly the contralateral popliteal artery (70%) and the abdominal aorta (50%).[1,2] Conversely, 8% of people diagnosed with abdominal aortic aneurysms harbor popliteal artery aneurysms.[3]

The normal popliteal artery diameter is 0.9 ± 0.2 cm. Although some consider the vessel to be aneurysmal when the diameter exceeds 50% of the normal proximal artery, most use 2.0 cm as the clinically relevant threshold for intervention based on the observation that complications increased in frequency among patients with aneurysm sizes greater than 2.0 cm.[3,4] While the diagnosis of popliteal aneurysm may be clear if the lesion is localized, it may be difficult to define the presence of a popliteal aneurysm in the presence of generalized arteriomegaly.[1,2] Most popliteal artery aneurysms are true, degenerative aneurysms, involving all layers of the vessel wall. Popliteal entrapment syndrome, fibromuscular dysplasia, and thrombangitis obliterans have been reported as uncommon underlying etiologies.[4] Pseudoaneurysms of the popliteal artery have been described following blunt and penetrating trauma, orthopedic surgery, and osteochondromas of the femur.[5]

The importance of popliteal aneurysms is related to their predilection to cause limb-threatening ischemia if left untreated. In one series of patients with untreated popliteal aneurysms, two-thirds developed limb-threatening complications by five years.[6] Interestingly, the association of popliteal aneurysms with ischemic complications does not seem to be related to the size of the aneurysm but merely to its presence. The most common presentation of symptomatic popliteal aneurysms is the development of ischemia most commonly caused by thrombosis of the aneurysm.[7,8] The aneurysm can also be the source of emboli, which can obliterate the distal outflow to the foot leading to the blue toe syndrome or eventually, digital gangrene. If the process is gradual, claudication or chronic limb ischemia may be the end result. However, if the aneurysm suddenly occludes, the patient often presents with acute limb-threatening ischemia with rest pain, usually requiring urgent intervention for limb salvage. Less commonly, large popliteal aneurysms can compress the adjacent popliteal nerve or vein, and result in neuropathy, superficial phlebitis, or deep vein thrombosis. In contrast to many other peripheral aneurysms, rupture of a popliteal aneurysm is a distinctly uncommon event.

The diagnosis of the asymptomatic popliteal aneurysms requires a high index of suspicion. The presence of associated peripheral aneurysms or a family history of aneurysmal disease should alert the clinician to check for a prominent or widened popliteal pulse on physical examination. Occasionally, a thrombosed aneurysm may produce a firm, pulseless, popliteal mass that must be differentiated from a Baker's cyst. Unfortunately, a negative physical exam, especially in an obese patient, does not reliably eliminate the presence of a popliteal aneurysm. Popliteal duplex ultrasonography is well tolerated, inexpensive, sensitive, and readily available (Figure 21–2). These features make it arguably the best preliminary imaging method for the diagnosis of popliteal aneurysms. Contrast enhanced computerized tomographic (CT) scans (Figure 21–3) or magnetic resonance angiography (MRA) scans offer potential advantages in defining the size and extent of the aneurysm and imaging the distal runoff. Contrast angiography, while not useful to determine the size of an aneurysm, is useful

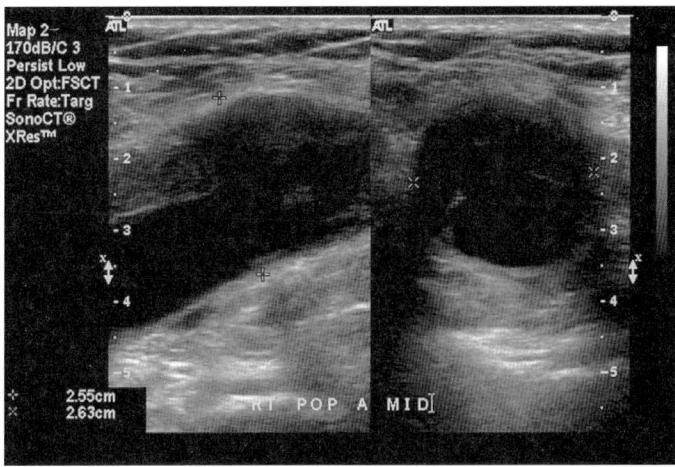

Figure 21-2. Duplex ultrasound image demonstrating longitudinal and transverse images of a popliteal artery aneurysm.

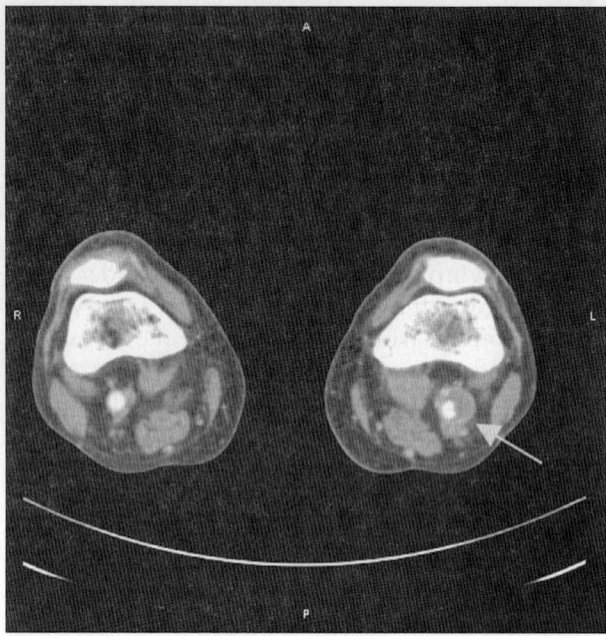

Figure 21-3. CT scan image of a left popliteal artery aneurysm with mural thrombus (arrow).

to determine the quality of the inflow and outflow vessels, as well as the extent of the popliteal aneurysm, and information necessary for preoperative planning, and it may also permit the delivery of thrombolytic agents when indicated (Figure 21–4).

While there is general agreement that all patients presenting with symptomatic or large popliteal aneurysms should undergo repair, the management of asymptomatic small popliteal aneurysms remains controversial, generally because of problems with the diagnosis of aneurysm in this setting. There seems to be consensus, however, that good risk patients with asymptomatic popliteal aneurysms should be considered for surgical repair when their aneurysms are localized and exceed 2 cm in diameter, especially if they contain thrombus. This is based on the observations that the published morbidity and mortality rates for elective surgical repair are low in general,[7-9] and the outcomes following treatment of asymptomatic popliteal aneurysms are superior to those among patients presenting with acute limb ischemia.[7,10]

Patients presenting with acute limb ischemia are particularly challenging to manage when angiography demonstrates complete occlusion of the outflow bed with poor or no suitable targets for distal bypass. Some reports have demonstrated the utility of preoperative or intraoperative thrombolytic therapy in this setting to improved patency and limb-salvage rates by opening outflow vessels or uncovering an occluded outflow vessel that may be a target for bypass.[8,10] Good clinical judgment is required, however, since thrombolysis usually requires several hours, and should only be considered when time permits such as for lesser degrees of ischemia.

Currently, the authors' preferred method for treating popliteal aneurysms involves open surgical repair unless the patient is a prohibitive surgical risk. The procedure may be accomplished through a medial or posterior approach, depending on the size of the popliteal aneurysm and its proximal and distal extent (Figure 21–5). The three commonly utilized methods of surgical reconstruction are illustrated (Figure 21–6). Proximal and distal ligation of the popliteal aneurysm eliminate it as an embolic

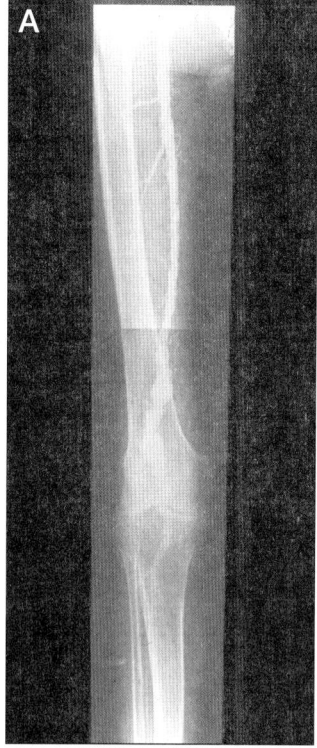 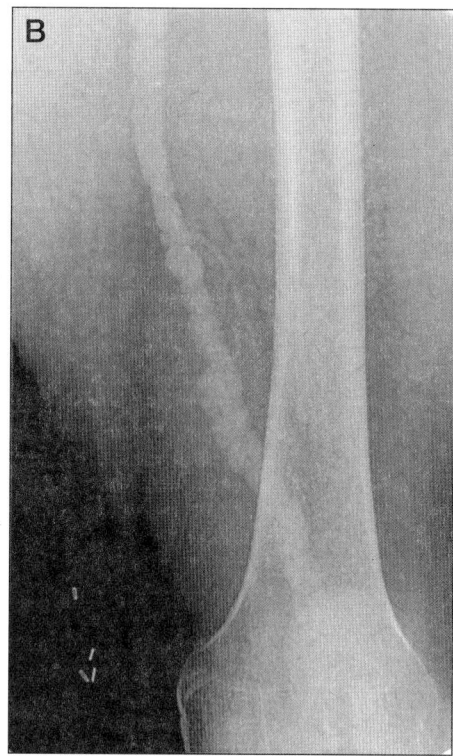

Figure 21-4. Femoral arteriograms demonstrating localized (**A**) as well as more generalized (**B**) involvement of the popliteal artery with aneurismal degeneration. The angiograms demonstrate only the opacified lumens of the involved arteries.

source while bypass around the ligated aneurysm provides distal perfusion. This procedure is usually done through a medial approach with autogenous saphenous vein as the preferred conduit, although a short synthetic graft may be required if adequate autogenous vein is unavailable. Advantages of this approach are that it offers wider exposure, which may be necessary for long aneurysms that involve the distal superficial femoral artery or encroach on the tibioperoneal trunk, and that the greater saphenous vein is easily harvested via the same incision. The proximal anastomosis may be either end to end or end to side, depending on the size disparity between the artery and the graft. Large aneurysms may require incision and decompression to eliminate the mass effect on adjacent structures. In this situation, an interposition graft may be placed within the aneurysm sac. When necessary, this maneuver may be facilitated by dividing the medial tendons, a measure that is usually well tolerated.[11] It is important to ligate all the geniculate vessels and other feeding branches to the aneurysm to prevent continued growth of the aneurysm sac despite ligation and bypass.[12] The posterior approach has been advocated by some surgeons and is most appropriate for very localized aneurysms where only limited exposure of the popliteal artery is needed.[13] In this approach, the patient is placed prone, the aneurysm sac is opened, its contents evacuated, feeding branches ligated, and an interposition graft placed within the sac. The lesser saphenous vein could be used as conduit if its size is adequate. Harvesting the greater saphenous vein, however, is more troublesome from this approach, and may require repositioning the patient as well as a separate incision. This approach is also

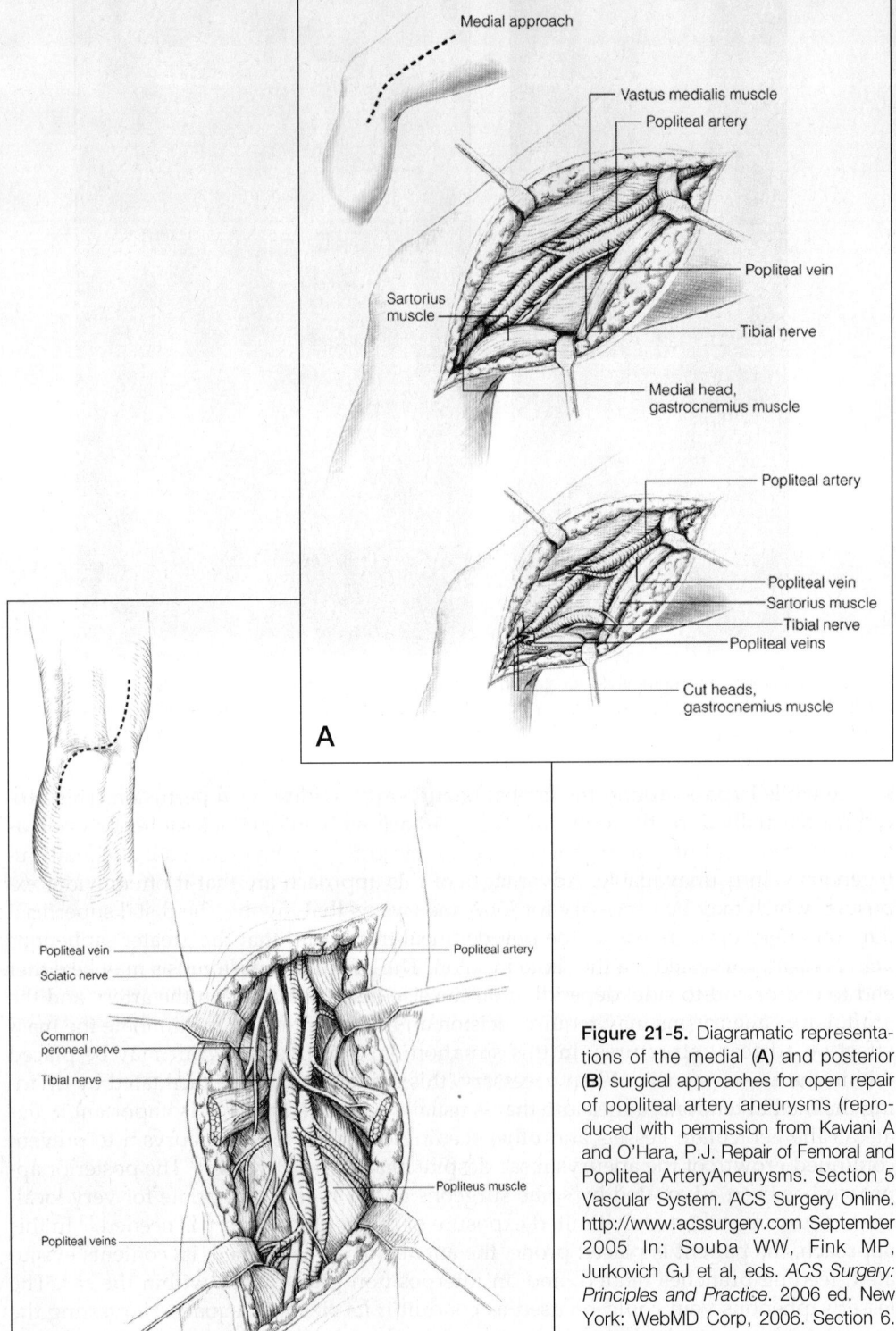

Figure 21-5. Diagramatic representations of the medial (**A**) and posterior (**B**) surgical approaches for open repair of popliteal artery aneurysms (reproduced with permission from Kaviani A and O'Hara, P.J. Repair of Femoral and Popliteal ArteryAneurysms. Section 5 Vascular System. ACS Surgery Online. http://www.acssurgery.com September 2005 In: Souba WW, Fink MP, Jurkovich GJ et al, eds. *ACS Surgery: Principles and Practice*. 2006 ed. New York: WebMD Corp, 2006. Section 6. Vascular System. Chapter 17. p. 1079–1089)[1].

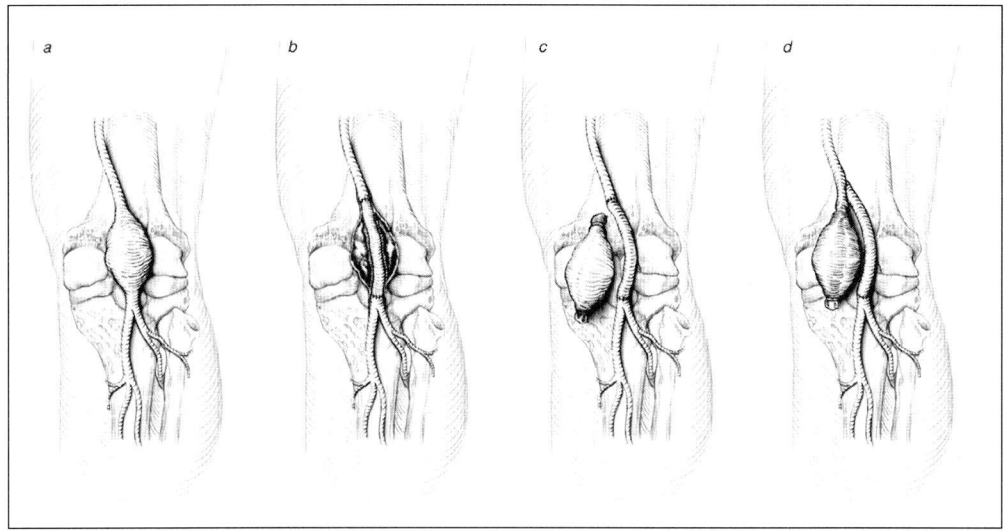

Figure 21-6. Diagramatic representations of the methods for open surgical repair of a popliteal artery aneurysm (**A**) using an interposition graft placed within the aneurysm (**B**), ligation of the aneurysm and bypass with an end-to end anastomosis (**C**), and ligation with bypass using an end-to-side anastomosis for graft/artery size disparity (**D**). Reproduced with permission from Kaviani A and O'Hara, P.J. Repair of Femoral and Popliteal Artery Aneurysms. Section 5 Vascular System. ACS Surgery Online. http://www.acssurgery.com September 2005 In: Souba WW, Fink MP, Jurkovich GJ et al, eds. *ACS Surgery: Principles and Practice.* 2006 ed. New York: WebMD Corp, 2006. Section 6. Vascular System. Chapter 17. p. 1079–1089) [1].

less useful if the aneurysm extends proximally or distally, or if the artery quality is poor. The type of presentation, the urgency of repair, the length and type of conduit, and the quality of the runoff vessels influence early and late results. As expected from experience with lower extremity bypass for occlusive disease, optimal results are associated with elective procedures done with short, autogenous bypass grafts in the presence of good runoff.[7,9]

The results of open popliteal aneurysm repair are usually good with a five-year limb-salvage rate of 95% in our own series. We also observed a five-year patency rate of 92% with good outflow and 66% in the presence of occlusive disease. With good conduit and good runoff, the 10-year patency rate was more than 80%. Early postoperative mortality (7%) resulted primarily from cardiac complications.[7]

The early results of endovascular treatment of popliteal artery aneurysms were disappointing, but over time, improvements in stent graft technology have led to wider application endografting for this purpose, especially among high-risk patients. Antonello et. al. reported a prospective randomized trial in which 30 patients with asymptomatic popliteal artery aneurysms were randomized to either open or endovascular repair.[14] It is unclear how many patients with popliteal aneurysms were excluded from randomization or unsuitable for endovascular repair. Although the sample size was too small to exclude a type II statistical error, the authors were not able to detect a significant difference in primary patency at 12 months (100% versus 87%) or secondary patency at 48 months (82% versus 100%) between the open and endovascular patients. Although further long-term follow-up is needed to assess durability, the feasibility of endovascular popliteal aneurysm repair has been demonstrated and the results are encouraging.[15] Because of the repetitive stress and angulation of the popliteal artery across the knee joint, some concerns remain regarding the propensity for migration, stent fracture, and endoleak development over the long term. The endovascular approach also does not allow for the interruption of the geniculate collaterals, and their patency may result in continued aneurysm enlargement as has been observed following open repair without aneurysm branch ligation.[12] Since anatomic considerations may preclude endovascular repair in some patients, the vascular surgeon should be familiar with open as well as endovascular techniques for the treatment of popliteal artery aneurysms.

FEMORAL ANEURYSM

True femoral artery aneurysms involving all three layers of the vessel wall are not as common as femoral pseudoaneurysms, which will be discussed separately. Femoral artery aneurysms are the second most frequently encountered peripheral aneurysm after popliteal aneurysm. True femoral aneurysms are classified according to their involvement with the profunda femoris artery as described by Cutler and Darling in 1973.[16] Type I aneurysms are confined to the common femoral artery without profunda femoris involvement, whereas type II aneurysms extend to involve the femoral bifurcation and include the profunda origin. While aneurysms isolated to the superficial femoral or the profunda femoral artery have been reported, they are extremely rare.

True femoral artery aneurysms, like those found in the popliteal artery, are usually discovered in older males in their sixth and seventh decades. Men presenting with true femoral aneurysms outnumber women by a ratio of 15 to 1. As observed among patients with popliteal aneurysms, there is an association with peripheral arterial aneurysms in other locations. In one review, 60% of patients with femoral aneurysms also had an abdominal aneurysm and 50% also had a contralateral femoral aneurysm. Interestingly, only 3% of patients in that series presenting with aortic aneurysms had associated femoral aneurysms.[17]

Femoral artery aneurysms may be discovered as an asymptomatic, pulsatile groin mass on physical examination or on imaging studies done for another purpose. Thrombosis or embolization is the most common complication and can produce signs and symptoms of lower extremity ischemia. Compression of the adjacent femoral vein or nerve by a large femoral aneurysm or one that is acutely expanding may also cause pain, leg edema, or neuropathy. Since duplex ultrasonography is reliable and usually readily available, it is usually the preferred imaging modality to confirm the diagnosis (Figure 21–7). Other imaging modalities such as CT and MR scans are also useful, and have the advantage of detection of associated aneurysms and rendering images as three-dimensional reconstructions using computer software (Figure 21–8). While catheter angiography is less useful for diagnosis, it is helpful for operative planning, and can also be used to deliver thrombolytic therapy, if indicated.

The natural history of asymptomatic femoral artery aneurysms is not well defined. In addition, there is no proven correlation between size and complication risk. Nevertheless, given the documented risk of associated thromboembolic complications leading to limb loss, there is general consensus that repair of symptomatic femoral artery aneurysms, or asymptomatic aneurysms exceeding 2.5cm in good risk patients, is indicated. This approach is supported by the low complication rates and excellent outcomes reported following elective open repair.[17,18]

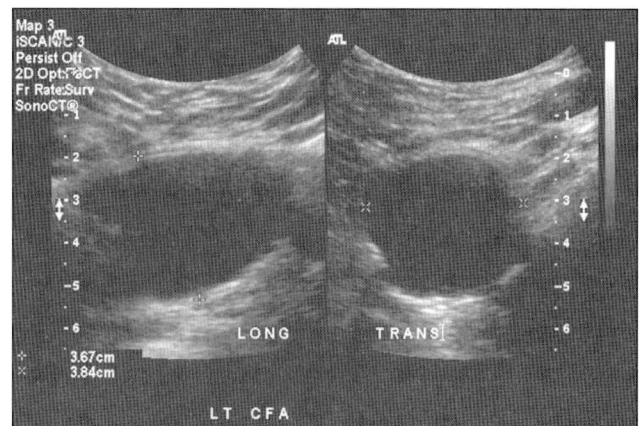

Figure 21-7. Duplex ultrasound image demonstrating longitudinal and transverse images of a femoral artery aneurysm.

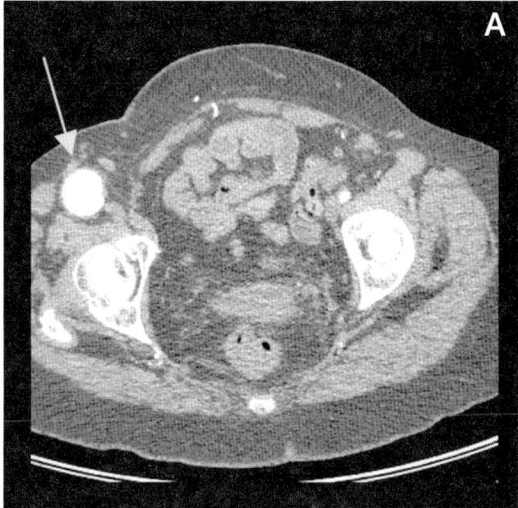

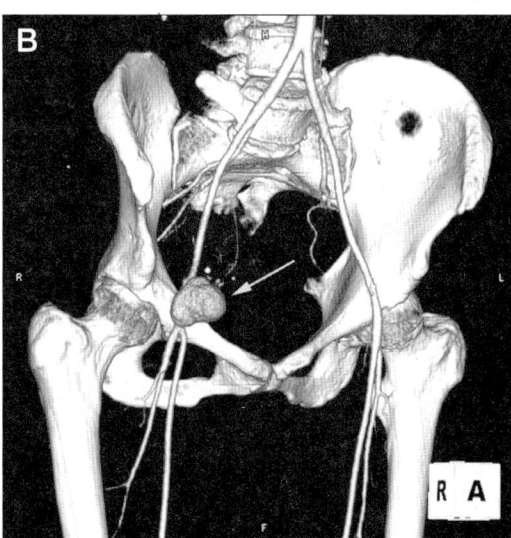

Figure 21-8. Axial CT image (**A**) of a large right femoral artery aneurysm (arrow) and a three-dimensional reconstruction (**B**) of the same aneurysm using computer software.

In addition to the usual preoperative general medical evaluation, optimum operative planning involves the careful assessment of multiple anatomic factors including the extent of the femoral aneurysm, the presence of associated aneurysms, and the presence of associated occlusive disease. Patients with extensive occlusive disease may even require distal bypass as part of the aneurysm repair. In patients with multiple aneurysms, the more threatening aneurysm should be addressed first. It is important that all anastomoses are done to healthy, uninvolved arterial wall to minimize the risk of future anastomotic pseudoaneurysm formation.

Isolated femoral aneurysms are usually approached through a longitudinal groin incision centered over the common femoral artery, an approach that offers excellent exposure for proximal and distal control, and allows cephalad extension or division of the inguinal ligament for additional proximal exposure, if needed. If necessary, an additional flank incision can be employed to access the more proximal external iliac artery in the retroperitoneum. Type I aneurysms are usually repaired with a short, synthetic common femoral interposition graft with uniformly good results. Type II femoral aneurysms, which require revascularization of both the profunda femoris and superficial femoral arteries, can be repaired by a variety of short, synthetic graft arrangements including an interposition graft from the common femoral to the profunda femoris arteries with a short jump graft to the superficial femoral artery, which is this author's preference. An alternative reconstruction involves an interposition graft placed between the common femoral and the superficial femoral arteries with a jump graft to the profunda femoris, an arrangement that is often more difficult to complete successfully since it is usually easier to work sequentially from deep to superficial tissue planes. A third option is to syndactylize the superficial femoral and profunda femoris arteries to form a common lumen, and then construct an interposition graft from the common femoral artery to the newly formed common lumen. If the superficial femoral artery is occluded, the interposition bypass can be placed directly to the profunda femoris artery (Figure 21–9).

The results of repair of true femoral artery aneurysms are uniformly good. In a recent review of 31 femoral aneurysms repaired over a 20-year period, 13 localized to the femoral artery and treated with interposition grafts had an 80% five-year patency rate. The remaining 18 femoral aneurysms were associated abdominal aneurysms and required aortobifemoral grafting with an 88% five-year patency rate.[18]

Although endovascular repair of femoral artery aneurysms with stent grafts has been reported, the experience is limited and the utility of such an approach is controversial. Early results have been disappointing because of graft thrombosis, and long-term patency may prove to be limited because of repeated hip flexion. Furthermore, since a femoral incision is usually well tolerated, even by compromised patients, the advantage conferred by the endovascular approach over open surgery in this location is small. Consequently, at the present time, endovascular repair of femoral aneurysms is not recommended except for very high-risk patients.

FEMORAL ARTERY PSEUDOANEURYSM

A pseudoaneurysm is, essentially, a hematoma arising from a defect in the arterial wall that is contained by the surrounding soft tissue. A fibrous capsule may develop, but the pseudoaneurysm does not involve the layers of the arterial wall itself.

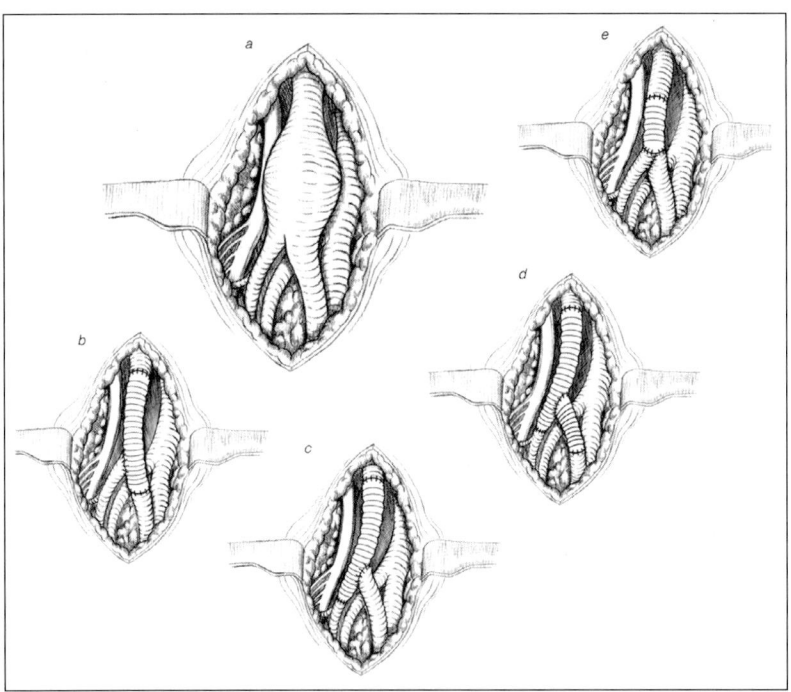

Figure 21-9. Diagramatic representation of several methods utilized for the open surgical repair of type II femoral artery aneurysms (reproduced with permission from Kaviani A and O'Hara, P.J. Repair of Femoral and Popliteal Artery Aneurysms. Section 5 Vascular System. ACS Surgery Online. http://www.acssurgery.com September 2005 In: Souba WW, Fink MP, Jurkovich GJ et al, eds. *ACS Surgery: Principles and Practice*. 2006 ed. New York: WebMD Corp, 2006. Section 6. Vascular System. Chapter 17. p. 1079–1089)[1].

Consequently, the distinctive histological feature of these aneurysms is that all three layers of the arterial wall are not involved. Pseudoaneurysms of the femoral artery usually result from trauma, anastomotic disruption, or infection. Because the fibrous capsule does not provide the strength of the native arterial wall, continuous pressurization of the sac usually leads to expansion and rupture. The therapeutic approach to a particular false aneurysm, in contrast to that for a true femoral aneurysm, is related to its etiology, and differs according to whether the pseudoaneurysm is traumatic, anastomotic, or mycotic.

The increasing utilization of catheter-based interventions has led to a concomitant increase in the occurrence of pseudoaneurysms. The reported incidence of pseudoaneurysm formation following catheterization ranges from 0.6% to 6% in retrospective series.[19] However, a prospective study, evaluating 565 consecutive patients with duplex ultrasonography following catheterization, found an incidence of pseudoaneurysm formation of 7.7%.[20] In this study, all patients who underwent catheterization were scanned, irrespective of symptoms, a feature likely leading to overestimation of the incidence of clinically significant pseudoaneurysms. Femoral pseudoaneurysms are also more common following interventional than diagnostic procedures, probably because of the use of larger sheaths and more aggressive anticoagulation measures in the interventional procedures. Other risk factors for pseudoaneurysm development include inadequate postprocedural compression, the presence of calcified arteries, obesity, and combined arterial and venous puncture. Superficial femoral or profunda femoris puncture is also thought to pose an added risk because of the lack of support surrounding these vessels when compared to that for the common femoral artery, which is easily compressed against the femoral head.

Symptomatic femoral pseudoaneurysms may present with pain and swelling from rapid expansion or rupture, eventually leading to compression of adjacent structures, skin ischemia, and necrosis. Less commonly, they can be a source of embolization or infection. Duplex ultrasonography is usually the preferred initial diagnostic test for the evaluation of femoral pseudoaneurysms because it is sensitive and specific, and also can determine useful anatomic features such as the aneurysm neck diameter, length, and the presence of multilobar anatomy. Using the color flow duplex mode, a characteristic to-and-fro flow appearance may be observed in the neck of the pseudoaneurysm. This information is useful for making therapeutic decisions such as treatment with thrombin injection, ultrasound guided compression, or direct surgical repair, as well as for later follow-up monitoring.

There are several treatment options available for noninfected, traumatic femoral pseudoaneurysms, depending on their geometry and stability. These include ultrasound guided thrombin injection or compression, endovascular repair, and primary open surgical repair. Percutaneous ultrasound guided thrombin injection is considered by some to be the treatment of choice for stable, noninfected, catheter-generated femoral pseudoaneurysms. In this technique, under ultrasound guidance, the pseudoaneurysm is localized and a needle is introduced through which thrombin is slowly injected into the sac until flow ceases within the pseudoaneurysm. Postprocedure management includes six hours of bed rest followed by a repeat duplex scan in 24 hours to confirm pseudoaneurysm thrombosis. The technical success rates reported with this procedure have ranged from 93% to 100% while complications include allergic reactions to bovine thrombin and distal embolization, which may occur in as many as 2% of patients.[19] Although intra-arterial tissue plasminogen activator to reestablish perfusion has been considered in this setting, its use may entail a risk of hemorrhage or recurrence of the pseudoaneurysm. Fortunately, most reported cases of embolization required no intervention.[19] There is consensus that pseudoaneurysms with short, wide necks, where embolization is a particular concern, are best repaired with a direct, open surgical approach.

Another treatment option for stable femoral pseudoaneurysms with suitable anatomy following catheter intervention is ultrasound guided compression. In this method, pressure is applied with the ultrasound probe over the pseudoaneurysm neck until flow in the pseudoaneurysm ceases, while still maintaining perfusion through the artery itself. If pseudoaneurysm thrombosis has not occurred after 10 minutes of compression, the procedure is repeated and several cycles of compression may be needed to achieve thrombosis. Ultrasound guided compression has a lower technical success rate, is unfavorably influenced by anticoagulation, and is less well tolerated by patients than thrombin injection. Furthermore, pseudoaneurysm rupture has been described as a complication of this technique.[19]

Although cases of endovascular repair, utilizing stent graft exclusion or coil embolization of catheter induced femoral pseudoaneurysms, have been reported, this approach has not gained wide acceptance because of a variety of disadvantages including cost and the need for synthetic material not required for open repair. Coils also may prevent pseudoaneurysm shrinkage after occlusion, a disadvantage if the pseudoaneurysm is large, and coils may serve as a nidus for infection. The disadvantages of placing stent grafts across the groin crease have been discussed in the section on true femoral aneurysms, and their use for femoral postcatheter pseudoaneurysm repair also may discourage the use of the involved groin for future catheterization access.

Open surgical repair for the treatment of postcatheterization pseudoaneurysms is indicated for failure of percutaneous treatment, for rapidly expanding pseudoaneurysms (especially those associated with hemodynamic instability), for large pseudoaneurysms with compression of adjacent neural or vascular structures, those associated with distal ischemia, those causing skin necrosis, and infected pseudoaneurysms. Open surgical repair allows prompt direct arterial repair with hematoma evacuation, and provides an opportunity for debridement and drainage when necessary. When feasible, proximal and distal arterial control is obtained before opening the pseudoaneurysm sac, allowing repair of the defect in the arterial wall with primary closure or an autogenous patch angioplasty if the defect is large. When the hematoma is large and the tissues are quite distorted, it is sometimes useful to open the pseudoaneurysm sac initially, and use digital pressure to control the bleeding site until a balloon occlusion catheter or a urethral sound can be placed in the arterial wall defect for control, then proceed with either primary or autogenous patch closure as the situation dictates.

Noninfected anastomotic femoral pseudoaneurysms are treated with reconstructions similar to those utilized for treatment of true femoral aneurysms. The repair of these lesions, however, usually involves extension of the original inflow synthetic graft using an interposition synthetic graft designed to preserve inflow to the profunda femoris artery primarily, and to the superficial femoral artery if feasible (Figure 21–10). Care must be taken to take adequate bites of solid arterial wall during these repairs to prevent another recurrence.

The treatment of infected pseudoaneurysms of either the catheter induced or anastomotic variety requires a different approach. Treatment objectives are control of the local sepsis by debridement of the infected tissue, which entails removal of all infected

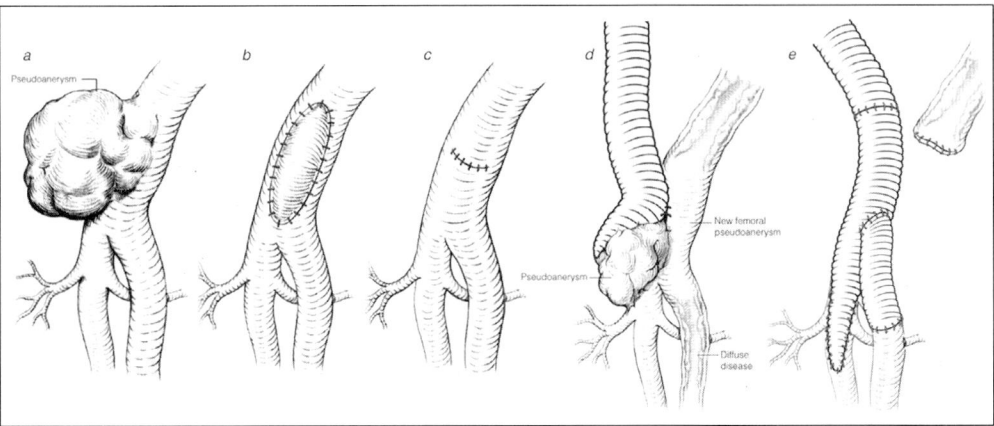

Figure 21-10. Diagramatic representation of several methods utilized for the open surgical repair of noninfested femoral artery pseudoaneurysms: (**A–C**) catheter related variety; (**D** and **E**) anastomotic (reproduced with permission from Kaviani A and O'Hara, P.J. Repair of Femoral and Popliteal Artery Aneurysms. Section 5 Vascular System. ACS Surgery Online. http://www.acssurgery.com September 2005 In: Souba WW, Fink MP, Jurkovich GJ et al, eds. *ACS Surgery: Principles and Practice.* 2006 ed. New York: WebMD Corp, 2006. Section 6. Vascular System. Chapter 17. p. 1079-1089)[1].

synthetic material and the maintenance of distal perfusion. Usually, femoral artery ligation alone will lead to severe ischemia and amputation. Depending on the extent of the infection and the pathogens involved, this approach may require either autogenous reconstruction when feasible, or extra-anatomic bypass through clean tissue beds. Adequate, specific-systemic antibiotic coverage is mandatory.

REFERENCES

1. O'Hara PJ. Treatment of Femoral and Popliteal Artery Aneurysms. In: Zelenock GB, Huber TS, Messina LM, Lumsden AL, Moneta GM (Eds). *Mastery of Vascular and Endovascular Surgery*. Philadelphia: Lippincott Williams & Wilkins Publishers; 2005.
2. Kaviani A, O'Hara PJ. ACS Surgery: Principles and Practice. Repair of Femoral and Popliteal Artery Aneurysms. Section 5 Vascular System. In: Souba WW, Fink MP, Jurkovich GJ et al, Eds. *ACS Surgery Online*. New York: WebMD Inc; 2005. http://www.acssurgery/. September 2005.
3. Szilagyi DE, Schwartz RL, Reddy DJ. Popliteal arterial aneurysms: their natural history and management. *Arch Surg*. 1981;116:724.
4. Dawson I, Sie RB, van Bockel JH. Atherosclerotic popliteal aneurysm. *Br J Surg*. 1997;84: 293–299.
5. Perez-Burkhardt JL, Gomex Castilla JC. Postruamatic popliteal pseudoaneurysm from femoral osteochondroma: case report and review of the literature. *J Vasc Surg*. 2003;37: 669–671.
6. Vermilion BD, Kimmins SA, Pace WG, et al. A review of one hundred forty-seven popliteal aneurysms with long-term follow-up. *Surgery*. 1981;90:1009.
7. Anton GE, Hertzer NR, Beven EG, et al. Surgical management of popliteal aneurysms: trends in presentation, treatment, and results from 1952 ot 1984. *J Vasc Surg*. 1986;3:125–134.
8. Varga ZA, Locke-Edumunds JC, Baird RN. A multicenter study of popliteal aneurysms. Joint Vascular Research Group. *J Vasc Surg*. 1994;20:171–177.
9. Huang Y, Gloviczki P, Noel A, et al. Early complications and long-term outcome after open surgical treatment of popliteal artery aneurysms : is exclusion with saphenous vein bypass still the gold standard ? *J Vasc Surg*. 2007;45:706–715.
10. Carpenter JP, Barker CF, Roberts B, et al. Popliteal artery aneurysms: current management and outcome. *J Vasc Surgg*. 1994;19:65–72.
11. Gryska PF, Darling RC, Linton RR. Exposure of the entire popliteal artery through a medial approach. *Surg Gynecol Obstet*. 1964;118:845–6.
12. Ebaugh JL, Morasch MD, Matsumura JS, et al. Fate of excluded popliteal artery aneurysms. *J Vasc Surg*. 2003;37:954.
13. Beseth BD, Moore WS. The posterior approach for repair of popliteal artery aneurysms. *J Vasc Surg*. 2006;43:940–945.
14. Antonello M, Frigatti P, Battocchio P, et al. Open repair versus endovascular treatment for asymptomatic popliteal artery aneurysm: results of a prospective randomized study. *J Vasc Surg*. 2005;42:185–193.
15. Tielliu IF, Verhoeven EL, Zeebgrets CJ. Endovascular treatment of popliteal artery aneurysms: results of a prospective cohort study. *J Vasc Surg*. 2005;41:561–567.
16. Cutler BS, Darling RC. Surgical management of arteriosclerotic femoral aneurysms. *Surgery*. 1973;74:764.
17. Graham LM, Zelenock GB, Whitehouse WM, et al. Clinical significance of arteriosclerotic femoral artery aneurysms. *Arch Surg*. 1980;115:502–504.
18. Sapienza P, Mingoli A, Feldhaus RJ, et al. Femoral artery aneurysms: long-term follow-up. *Cardiovasc Surg*. 1996;4:181–184.

19. Morgan R, Belli AM. Current treatment methods for postcatheterization pseudoaneurysms. *J Vasc Interv Radiol*. 2003;14:697–710.
20. Katzenshclager R, Ugurluoglu A, Ahmadi A, et al. Incidence of pseudoaneurysm after diagnostic and therapeutic angiography. *Radiology*. 1995;195:463–466.

Advances in Wound Care and Amputation

22

The Healing of Infection, Ulceration, and Minor Amputation Following Revascularization in Patients with Diabetes

Thomas S. Monahan, M.D. and Frank W. LoGerfo, M.D.

DIABETES MELLITUS AND COMPROMISED BIOLOGY

Diabetes mellitus affects roughly 12 million people in the United States and the prevalence is increasing, generating about $110 billion of health care expenditures annually.[1-2] Diabetes confers a greater risk of all forms of cardiovascular disease including peripheral arterial disease (PAD). The exact incidence of PAD in diabetics is not known; however, data from the Framingham Heart Study suggest that up to a third of diabetic patients over age fifty have PAD. This number might actually be greater due to asymptomatic disease and poor routine screening for this disease.[3]

Foot complications constitute a significant source of morbidity in diabetic patients. The lifetime incidence of foot ulcer in all diabetic patients is 15% with a three-year cumulative incidence of almost six percent. Ulceration of the foot is associated with an increase in osteomyelitis, an increase in incidence of amputation, and confers a decrease in three-year survival.[4] Patients with diabetes are more prone to foot ulcers and their attendant complications as a result of the associated neuropathy and ischemia.

The motorneuropathy associated with diabetes affects the longest, finest neurons first. This effectively denervates the intrinsic muscles of the foot including the lumbrical muscles that direct the action of the flexor digitorum longus and brevis. These deficits cause the toes to be drawn into the "claw" position, creating pressure points at the tips of the toes, the dorsum of the interphalangeal joints, and the plantar aspect of the metatarasal-phalangeal joints.

The somatic sensory neurons affected first by diabetes are also the long, fine fibers that convey the sensations of pain and temperature. With the loss of pain sensation, a patient with diabetes can sustain trauma or repetitive injury without being aware of the damage done. Typical injuries include scalding injuries, skin breakdown from improper fitting footwear, or punctures from stepping on needles or other sharp objects.

The sensory nervous system also is responsible for the neuroinflammatory response to injury. This response is mediated by the axon reflex whereby a depolarization signal in a sensory fiber travels centrally but also travels peripherally out adjacent axon branches. The sensory nerve, therefore, becomes a neuroeffector system with outbound signals. In the fine sensory fibers, this causes the release of packets of neuropeptides such as substance P which, in turn, causes the mast cells to degranulate and release histamine. Other neuropeptides are released and contribute to leukocyte chemotaxis, increased blood flow, angiogenesis, and other elements of the inflammatory response. Loss of the neuroinflammatory response occurs early in diabetic neuropathy, often prior to any detectable somatic neuropathy. Absence of neuroinflammation may explain the masked or subtle response to quite advanced infections in patients with diabetes. Autonomic neuropathy also causes dysfunction of the eccrine (sweat) and apocrine (oil) glands, resulting in fissure formation on the feet of patients with diabetes and providing a portal of entry for infection (Figure 22–1).

Patients with diabetes are at increased risk for all forms of cardiovascular disease, displaying a pattern of accelerated atherosclerosis. The pathology is histologically similar to atherosclerosis observed in patients without diabetes; however, there is a significant difference in the pattern or distribution of atherosclerotic occlusion. With diabetes, there is a specific propensity for occlusion of the tibial and peroneal arteries. One of the more recent investigations examined the amputated legs of 28 patients with and without diabetes. While arteries at 5 cm above the ankle were significantly more stenotic in diabetics, there was no difference in the arteries of the foot and ankle.[5] This relative sparing of the arteries in the foot, in spite of occluded tibial arteries, opens up the possibility of arterial reconstruction directly to arteries in the foot, especially the dorsalis

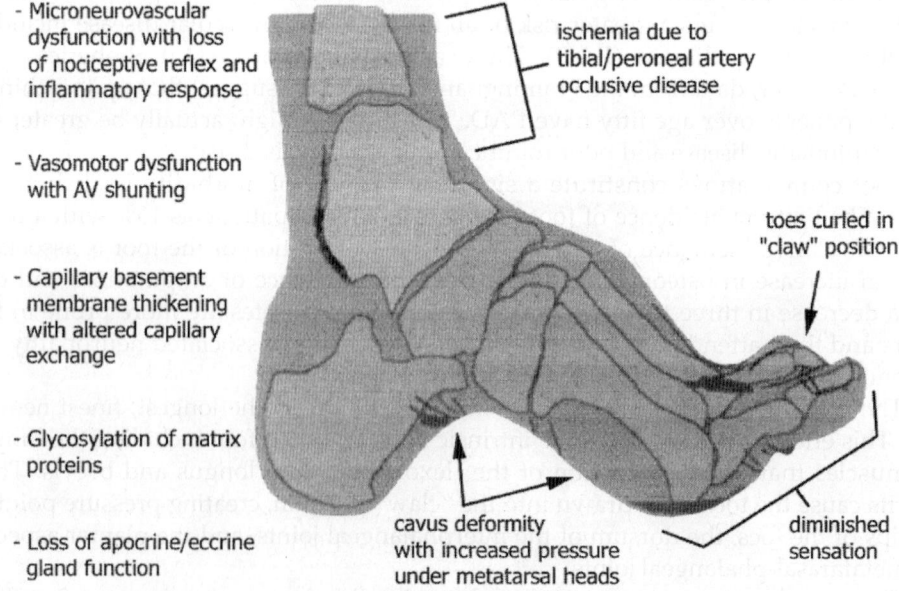

- Microneurovascular dysfunction with loss of nociceptive reflex and inflammatory response

- Vasomotor dysfunction with AV shunting

- Capillary basement membrane thickening with altered capillary exchange

- Glycosylation of matrix proteins

- Loss of apocrine/eccrine gland function

ischemia due to tibial/peroneal artery occlusive disease

toes curled in "claw" position

cavus deformity with increased pressure under metatarsal heads

diminished sensation

Figure 22-1. The compromised biology of the diabetic foot. Presented are some of the adverse effects of diabetic neuropathy on the motor, somatic, and autonomic nervous systems.

pedis. Fortunately, once perfusion of a foot artery is established, there is excellent tissue perfusion because there is no occlusion in the microcirculation, and graft patency is comparable to other distal arterial reconstructions. Because of the compromised biology associated with neuropathy, these patients are more susceptible to ulceration, even with moderate degrees of ischemia. Therefore, the presence of neuropathy argues for restoration of maximum blood flow to the foot whenever possible.

SURGICAL APPROACH TO THE PATIENT WITH DIABETES MELLITUS

As early as the 1970s, surgeons challenged the notion of small vessel disease and began attempting arterial reconstruction in diabetic patients with peripheral vascular disease using the pedal arteries. Since the first procedures, the popularity of this operation has increased and long-term outcome of large series have been reported.[6] The success of distal bypass operations has improved the outlook for diabetic patients with ulcerations of the foot.

When patients present with diabetic foot complications, it is essential to adequately drain all closed space infections and remove all necrotic, nonviable tissue. After control of local infection and debridement have been accomplished, the peripheral circulation should be assessed. If the dorsalis pedis and posterior tibial pulses are not palpable and there is sufficient evidence of ischemia as a contributing factor, arteriography should be performed. More formal, noninvasive studies are of little value in making this decision. Rather than delay to observe the wound or for further noninvasive evaluation, it is better to proceed directly to angiography, usually within 48 hours. Because of the neuropathy and compromised biology, these situations require prompt and full restoration of arterial flow to the foot to achieve maximum tissue preservation.

SEPSIS AND INFECTION

The compromised biology exhibited in diabetics and decreased perfusion from accelerated atherosclerosis renders these patients less able to clear infection than patients without diabetes. Infection in the setting of poor perfusion is a frequent presentation of a diabetic patient destined for lower extremity reconstruction. In the previously cited series of 1000 patients undergoing bypass grafts to the dorsalis pedis, almost 30% presented with active infection as evidenced by leukocytosis or fever.[6]

The compromised biology of the diabetic patients predisposes them to deceptively severe infections. Due to poor circulation, impaired leukocyte function, and minimal or absent neuroinflammation, these patients frequently mount only a mild inflammatory response to quite severe infections. This outwardly benign appearance, coupled with absence of pain from deep somatic neuropathy that frequently accompanies vascular disease in diabetics, often leads clinicians to underestimate the severity of the infection and leave deep infections incompletely drained.

Diabetic foot infections are frequently polymicrobial and deeply invasive. The first line of therapy in any patient with an infectious process of this nature is aggressive local control. These measures include initiation of parenteral broad-spectrum antibiotics, complete drainage of all deep space collections, and debridement of all necrotic, nonviable tissue. Such procedures can be frequently performed at the bedside, especially in patients with a dense neuropathy. However some patients with particularly deep seated infections will require debridement in the operating room to obtain adequate drainage. Some patients may even require partial forefoot amputation.

After aggressive local control of infection, it is essential to asses the perfusion of the limb. In a limb with threatened perfusion, the increased metabolic demand of active infection may overcome its healing capacity. Frequently, these wounds will not heal without restoration of blood flow. As has been discussed, in the diabetic patient it is often necessary to perform a bypass graft to the dorsalis pedis artery to restore circulation to the foot and thus the site of infection. It is not necessary to delay surgery until the wound is sterilized; once local control of the infection has been established, bypass surgery can be performed with acceptable results. It is often difficult to judge adequate control of infection in the diabetic patient. One of the most sensitive indicators of control is the restoration of glycemic control.

In a series of 56 patients admitted to a tertiary care referral center with an ischemic lower extremity and active infection, bypass surgery was performed as soon as local control of infection was achieved. The mean time from presentation to operation in this group was 10 days, and the procedure was performed with a 12% infection rate. Although this rate is significantly higher than in their noninfected counterparts, these patients had a 92% graft patency and 98% limb salvage rate at three-years follow-up.[7] This outcome is comparable to patients who do not have infection. The standard of care for a threatened ischemic limb with active infection involves adequate drainage of all infection, removal of necrotic tissue, and revascularization as soon as control of the infection has been achieved.

TISSUE LOSS AND ULCERATION

Tissue loss in the setting of arterial insufficiency is an indication for lower extremity vascular reconstruction. Treatment of nonhealing heel ulcers is a particularly difficult problem for the vascular surgeon. Limited availability of options for soft-tissue coverage coupled with the debilitated nature of the patients in this population makes treatment of ischemic heel ulcers a particularly difficult problem. To this end, some investigators have advocated primary amputation for selected individuals with ischemic heel ulcers.[8]

It is well established that pedal bypass operations and the ensuing restoration of pulsatile blood flow to the forefoot have been demonstrated to be beneficial in healing forefoot ischemic lesions. The role of restoration of pedal blood flow in healing heel lesions is a subject of controversy. Despite promising results of pedal bypass for forefoot lesions, some surgeons consider patients with ischemic heel ulcers better suited to amputation than to revascularization procedures.[8] At least two large studies have been conducted in recent years evaluating the role of arterial reconstruction in wound healing and limb salvage in patients with ischemic heel lesions. Treiman and colleagues evaluated the management of 91 patients with nonhealing heel wounds of at least one month duration. Patients who had a lower extremity arterial reconstruction had favorable wound healing results. A palpable pedal pulse, patent posterior tibial artery distal to the ankle, and the number of patent tibial arteries after bypass all independently predicted wound healing. Their long-term results were also quite favorable; they reported a 91% three-year primary patency. More importantly, the presence or absence of diabetes did not predict success or failure in this group.[9] This finding further dispels the myth of small vessel disease in the diabetic.

Data from our institution support the use of lower extremity reconstruction for the management of ischemic heel ulceration. During a five-year period, over four hundred pedal bypass grafts were performed for either ischemic gangrene or ulceration isolated to either the forefoot or heel. Patients in the forefoot and heel groups enjoyed similar complete healing rates, 90.5% and 86.5%, respectively. Only 10% of patients in either group ultimately required amputation during the five-year follow-up period. Given the vascular anatomy of the foot, the posterior tibial artery would seem to be a much better-suited target artery to restore perfusion to the heel (Figure 22–2). However, use of this vessel is often limited, especially in the diabetic population, by tibial atherosclerosis. The preoperative angiogram was examined and assessed for patency of the pedal arch. An intact pedal arch did not predict the success of this operation for patency rates or tissue healing.[10]

Ischemic ulceration of the hind foot should not automatically target patients for primary amputation. However, patients who have little hope of becoming ambulatory under the best of circumstances or who are so debilitated that they can not adequately protect their heel to allow healing are better served by primary amputation. In a properly selected patient population, superior healing, limb salvage, and patency rates can be achieved with a pedal bypass operation. A patent pedal arch is not necessary to achieve healing of a heel ulcer following successful dorsalis pedis bypass.

MINOR AMPUTATION

Minor foot amputations are frequently performed in patients with vascular disease. Despite this, little has been published on minor amputation performed in concert with

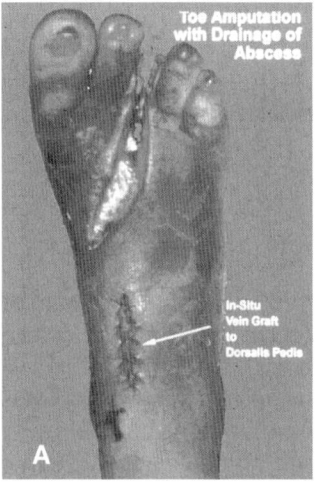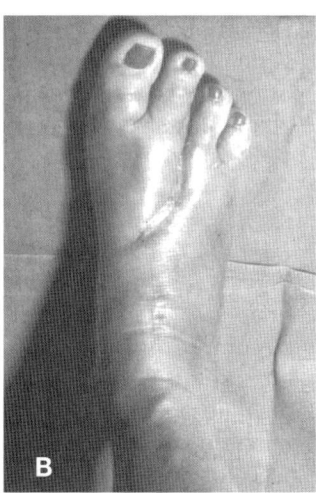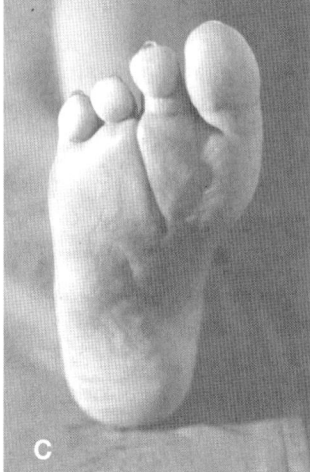

Figure 22-2. Minor amputation with revascularization. This patient presented with a deep space foot infection and a necrotic third toe. At the time of operation, she had extensive debridement of her mid and forefoot with a third toe amputation **A.** The minor amputation was performed at the same time as a bypass graft to the dorsalis pedis artery. This patient enjoyed excellent functional and cosmetic results as viewed from the dorsal **B.** and plantar **C.** surfaces.

bypass grafting. By convention, a minor amputation is considered as any amputation below the ankle including interphalangeal, ray, and transmetatarsal amputation (TMA). One of the greatest concerns facing a vascular surgeon performing a minor amputation is the viability of the often tenuous tissue flap required to close the distal amputation site. It is reasonable to postulate that increasing flow to the distal extremity will allow for a more robust flap on a minor amputation resulting in better healing rates and greater preservation of mobility. The population of patients in this situation is very heterogenous, and no prospective trial has been performed to evaluate the efficacy of revascularization and minor amputation performed in tandem. Some investigators have performed retrospective reviews to attempt to answer this question.

Campbell and colleagues investigated the effect of revascularization and amputation level or need for reamputation in their series of major amputations. In their cohort, a revascularization procedure did not have any influence on either level or need for reoperation.[11] Another investigation in a smaller group of patients examined the outcomes of patients with a TMA. In this group of 37 patients, 15 had a revascularization procedure in conjunction with TMA. Of these patients, 12 had limb preservation at three-years follow-up.[12] Although their numbers are very small, revascularization in conjunction with minor amputation might improve limb salvage rates.

Data from our institution are more equivocal than the previously cited series. In our institution, we performed 920 minor amputations on 670 patients in an 11-year period from January 1990 to December 2001. The initial amputation level was interphalangeal in 466 patients, transmetatarsal in 159 patients, and ray in 122 patients. Of all minor amputations performed, ipsilateral revascularization was performed on 65% in the month preceding the amputation, while 10% had a revascularization procedure in the 30 days following the amputation. Our 30-day mortality of just 0.7% compares favorably with other series. Limb salvage rates were 90% at one year and 80% at five years. End stage renal disease (ESRD) manifest by serum creatinine greater than 2.0 mg/dL and performance of revascularization subsequent to initial amputation were independent adverse predictors of limb salvage. ESRD and conversion to a major amputation are both poor predictors of survival in our series. There are many confounding variables making it difficult to draw conclusions from this heterogeneous population. In a well-selected patient, a distal bypass performed in conjunction with a minor amputation can provide greater limb salvage and preservation of mobility.

CONCLUSIONS

Patients with diabetes and ischemic foot complications present a unique challenge to the vascular surgeon. Because of compromised biology, deep invasive infections can often present with only subtle signs of infection. The first action is to drain all foci of infection and debride any obviously nonviable tissue. Once local control of infection is established, patients without palpable pulses should have an angiogram, generally within 48 hours. There is little need for noninvasive studies as a guide to therapy in a diabetic patient with a compromised foot and absent pedal pulses.

Revascularization, particularly a bypass to the dorsalis pedis artery, can increase limb salvage rates in patients with tissue loss to both the forefoot and hindfoot irrespective of the patency of the plantar arch. Restoring pulsatile flow to the pedal artery is a safe and often necessary procedure in patients with active infection provided there is adequate local control of infection. It is often necessary to perform a minor amputation in conjunction with revascularization in order to obtain wound closure and limb salvage. More studies are needed to identify patients, such as those with ESRD, who do not derive benefit from a combined procedure.

REFERENCES

1. Mokdad AH, Bowman BA, Ford ES, et al. The continuing epidemics of obesity and diabetes in the United States. *JAMA*. 2001;286:1195–1200.
2. Rubin RJ, Altman WM, Mendelson DN. Healthcare expenditures for people with diabetes. *J Clin Endocrinol Metab*. 1992;78:429–448.
3. Abbott, RD, Brand, FN, Kannel WB. Epidemiology of some peripheral arterial findings in diabetic men and women; experiences from the Framingham Heart Study. *Am J Med*. 1990;88:376–381.
4. Ramsey SD, Newton K, Blough D, et al. Incidence, outcomes, and cost of foot ulcers in patients with diabetes. *Diabetes Care*. 1999;22:382–387.
5. Mozes G, Keresztury G, Kadar A, et al. Atherosclerosis in amputated legs of patients with and without diabetes mellitus. *Int Angiol*. 1998:17;282–286.
6. Pomposelli FB, Kansal N, Hamdan AD, et al. A decade of experience with dorsalis pedis artery bypass: analysis of outcome in more than 1000 cases. *J Vasc Surg*. 2003;37:307–315.
7. Tannenbaum GA, Pomposelli FB, Maraccio EJ, et al. Safety of vein bypass grafting to the dorsal pedal artery in diabetic patients with foot infections. *J Vasc Surg*. 1992;15:982–990.
8. Carsten CG, Taylor SM, Langan EM, et al. Factors associated with limb loss despite a patent infrainguinal bypass graft. *Am Surg*. 1998;64:33–38.
9. Treiman GS, Oderich GS, Ashrafi A, et al. Management of ischemic heel ulceration and gangrene: an evaluation of factors associated with successful healing. *J Vasc Surg*. 2000;31:1110–1108.
10. Berceli SA, Chan A, Pomposelli FB, et al. Efficacy of dorsal pedal artery bypass in limb salvage for ischemic heel ulcers. *J Vasc Surg*. 1999;30:499–508.
11. Campbell WB, Marriott S, Eve R, et al. Factors influencing the early outcome of major lower lower limb amputation for vascular disease. *Ann Royal Coll Surg Eng*. 2001;83:309–314.
12. LaFontaine, J, Reyzelman, A, Rothberg, G, et al. The role of revascularization in transmetatarsal amputations. *J Am Podiatr Med Assoc*. 2001;91:533–535.

23

The Use of Negative Pressure Wound Therapy in Clinical Practice

Karen F. Kim Evans, M.D. Mary Ella Carter, M.D.
Christopher Attinger, M.D. Anton N. Sidawy, M.D.

The vacuum-assisted closure (V.A.C.–KCI®, San Antonio, TX) device for wound management has revolutionized wound therapy. In general, the simple application of negative pressure on a wound causes a widespread tissue response: accelerating wound contraction, increasing local blood flow, promoting wound drainage and edema resolution, encouraging granulation tissue, and stimulating cellular turnover. Since its inception approximately 18 years ago by Drs. Louis Argenta and Michael Morykwas at Wake Forest,[1,2] there have been numerous publications and presentations regarding its use, as well as comprehensive literature reviews on the subject.[3,4] This chapter is meant to provide the physiologic basis for negative pressure wound therapy, and to outline clinical applications and case studies with a focus on the vascular surgery patient population.

PHYSIOLOGIC STUDIES AND CLINICAL CORRELATION

Blood Flow

In general, the experimental studies on local tissue perfusion suggest that there is an increase in blood flow to the local environment after application of the V.A.C. In all studies, local blood perfusion was measured by laser Doppler.[5-7] There is variability within the literature on the exact timing and location of increased blood flow, as well as different animal models (swine and rabbit). Clinically, we suspect that there is an increase in local blood flow due to increased bleeding, which occurs in the wound after application of the V.A.C. Moreover, its widespread popularity and success in the diabetic population with microcirculatory pathology suggest that it is countering this physiologic derangement on some level.

Bacterial Load

The standard V.A.C. device is a closed, adherent dressing system with no true bactericidal instrumentation. To address this issue, K.C.I. has manufactured a device that allows for fluid installation so that contaminated wounds can be continuously irrigated with antibiotic fluid. There is no scientific consensus on the role of the V.A.C. in clearing bacteria from a wound.

In the initial pig studies, wounds were infected with *S. aureus* and *S. epidermidis*, and after four to five days of V.A.C. therapy, all wounds demonstrated a decrease in the number of organisms per gram of tissue.[1] In contrast, a retrospective chart review of 26 patients showed an increase in bacterial colonization with V.A.C therapy;[8] however, this study was criticized for its design flaw and lack of control.[4] A prospective randomized trial suggested that there was a decrease in *Pseudomonas* colonization after V.A.C. therapy, but an increase in *S. aureus*.[9] In general, the V.A.C. is best used after thorough surgical debridement of any contaminated wound, and if it is applied on an infected wound, the dressing must be changed every 12–24 hours.[10]

Granulation Tissue

The clinical sign of a healthy, healing wound is granulation tissue. Granulation tissue is highly vascularized and rich in fibroblasts. It forms the intermediary between injury and a re-epithelialized surface. In essence, the V.A.C. promotes and accelerates the formation of granulation tissue and allows wounds to heal by secondary intention at a faster rate. By using alginate impressions of wounds, Morykwas et. al. showed a 63% increase in granulation tissue in vacuum treated wounds compared with those left to heal by secondary intention.[1] The exact mechanism by which the subatmospheric pressure causes mechanical stimulation leading to cellular proliferation is being actively studied. This principle of mechanochemical stress to stimulate angiogenesis and mitosis has been elucidated elsewhere in other physiologic models such as the Ilizarov technique and tissue expansion.[1,11,12] Interestingly, maximal granulation tissue formation occurs at a specific negative pressure, 125 mmhg, which is the standard V.A.C. setting.[13]

Graft and Flap Survival

Due to the physiomechanical properties of the V.A.C., it is no surprise that it has been used to increase the blood supply to flaps and secure skin grafts. There have been many studies showing the effectiveness of the V.A.C. at increasing the take of a skin graft and it is now a commonly accepted practice to use the V.A.C. over split thickness or full thickness skin grafts.[14-18] Because the failure of skin grafts is usually due to infection, shear stress, or fluid collection between the graft and the recipient bed, the suction device most likely creates a stable interface between the graft and the bed, promoting adherence and eliminating fluid collection interference. This concept was studied in a pig model showing an increase in the success rate of V.A.C. applied skin grafts over bolster alone.[19]

All flaps are dependant on blood supply for survival. Local, regional, and free tissue transfer depends on both vascular inflow and outflow for viability. The V.A.C. has been studied as a means of increasing the blood supply in muscle flaps.[20] In addition, we have used the V.A.C. with random, local tissue rearrangement to increase the local blood supply.

CELLULAR STUDIES AND MICRO DEFORMATIONAL WOUND THERAPY

The therapeutic effectiveness of the V.A.C. has led many researchers to study its role on wound healing on a cellular level. Mechanical stress is known to stimulate cellular responses such as microtubular deformation and may lead to gene regulation.[21,22] The concept of microdeformational wound therapy suggests that the application of force to wounds acts on a cellular level to stimulate cellular response such as proliferation, angiogenesis, and wound healing.[23,24] In addition, the optimal sponge pore size and suction negative pressure is an important consideration that has been studied to maximize the cellular effect.

CLINICAL INDICATIONS AND CASE STUDIES

General Application Techniques

The V.A.C. is a simple wound dressing that can be applied over most wounds in nearly every clinical situation. The V.A.C. is packaged with a foam sponge (made of polyurethane ether open-pore foam, 400-600 microns), transparent closed system adhesive dressing (made of polyurethane), suction tubing, a collecting reservoir, and the suction machine. The sponge is cut to fit into the wound, the adhesive dressing is placed over the sponge, and the tubing placed into the closed system and attached to the collecting reservoir within the suction machine. To protect vital structures such as blood vessels, mediastinal structures, bowel, etc., xeroform or other nonadherent dressings can be placed under the sponge.

Recent innovations in the product include lightweight devices that are battery powered and transportable (Study Case #5). Large units are also available for large volume fluid disposal. For contaminated wounds, K.C.I. has manufactured a device that allows the instillation of fluids such as antibiotic fluids during the V.A.C. treatment. In addition, there are also silver coated sponges available that may aid in decreasing the bacterial load of infected wounds. There are also alarms on the system that warn of suction leaks, excessive fluid removal, and overfilling of the reservoir.

Diabetic Foot Wounds

Diabetic foot wounds account for major morbidity and cost; they may commonly result in amputation. Due to the microcirculatory problems and infection in the diabetic foot, the V.A.C. is an ideal wound healing adjunct. The overall success of the V.A.C. in this population has been studied extensively and has transformed the treatment of this disease.[25-30] When compared with moist saline gauze dressings, the V.A.C. has been studied extensively both retrospectively and prospectively, and has been shown to be much more effective at healing rates. In one series, the V.A.C. allowed for more rapid granulation tissue formation and healed 28% versus 9% treated with saline alone.[30] And in another series, the vac healed 59% versus 0% treated with standard saline wet to dry dressings.[29] In these series, the wounds treated with the V.A.C. healed in 22 days compared with 42 days with the standard dressings (Case 1)[30] (Figure 23–1).

While the V.A.C.'s success is unparalleled by other standard dressings, standard wound healing principles should remain. All diabetic wounds should undergo thorough debridement of necrotic tissue, and a complete vascular exam should dictate whether vascular studies should be pursued. In those selected patients, vascular

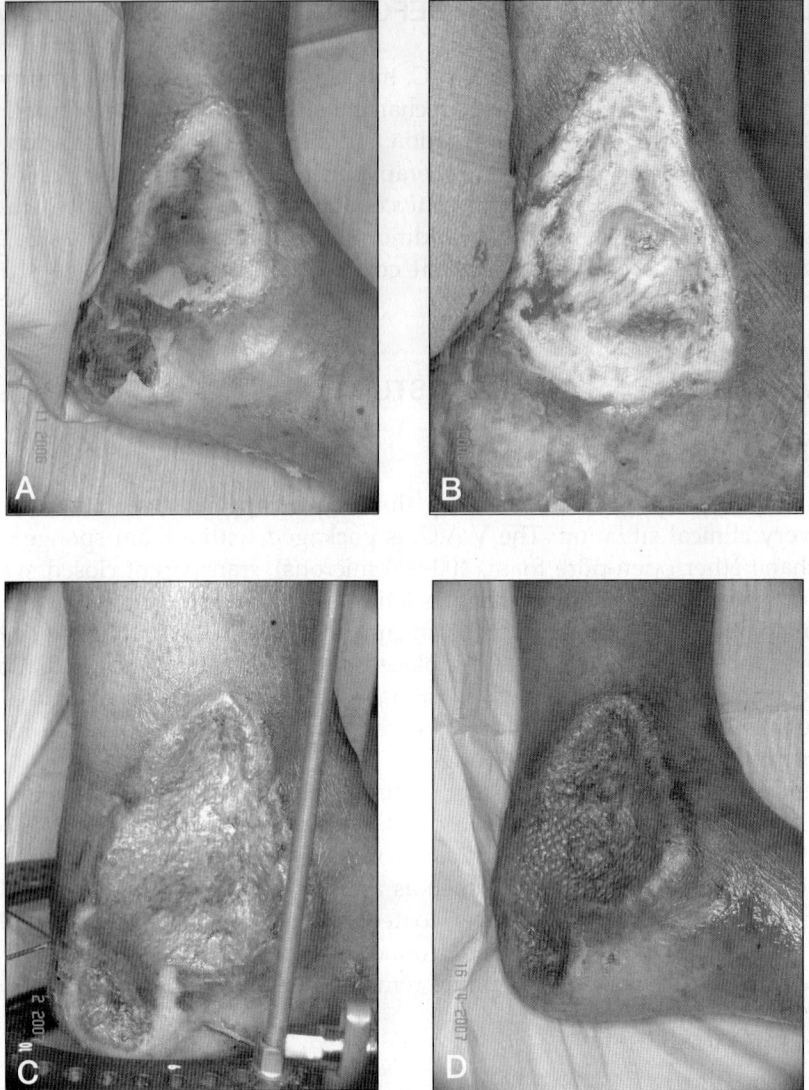

Figure 23-1. Case 1: 40-year-old who left his CAM walker on his leg for three weeks after undergoing an Achilles lengthening procedure. (**A**) Medial ankle wounds; (**B**) patient underwent multiple debridements and V.A.C. therapy; (**C**) Ilizarov external fixator in place for ankle stability and skin graft; (**D**) five months after presentation with healed wound.

bypass should precede any wound therapy. Culture directed systemic antibiotics should also be administered. The V.A.C. should be used to promote granulation tissue and fill large defects that eventually may need flaps or grafts for stable coverage (Case 2) (Figure 23–2).

Wounds with Exposed Bone, Tendon, or Hardware

The V.A.C. has become a popular modality for treatment of lower extremity wounds with exposed bone, tendon, or hardware. The V.A.C. has revolutionized how we treat these types of wounds. As stated previously, the V.A.C. has been shown to greatly

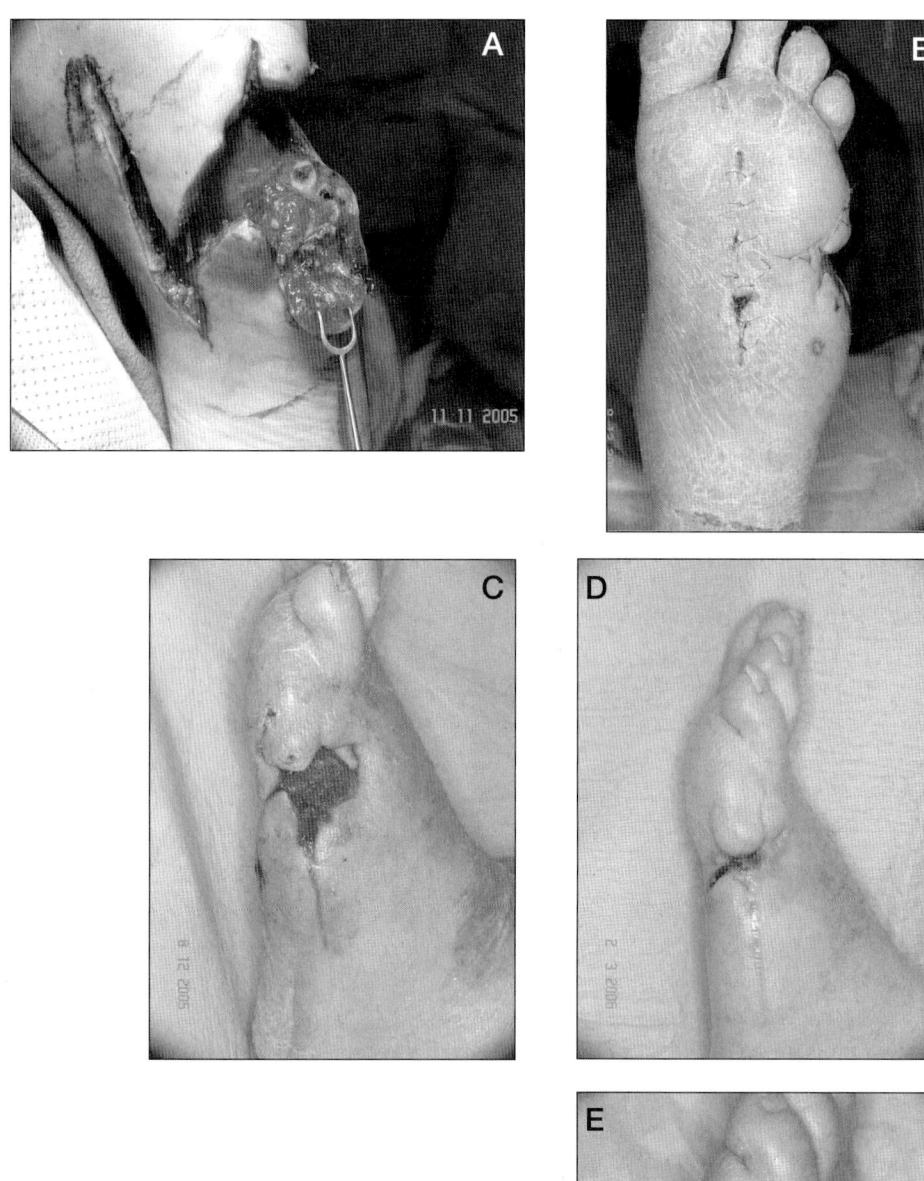

Figure 23-2. Case 2: 59-year-old with chronic renal insufficiency, diabetes mellitus, and peripheral arterial disease who presented with gangrene and osteomyelitis of the left foot. He required multiple operative debridements and culture-directed antibiotics. (**A**) Intraoperative picture; (**B,C**) approximately one month after partial closure of plantar wounds and V.A.C. therapy to lateral wound; (**D**) nearly completely healed wound with eight weeks of V.A.C. therapy; (**E**) healed foot eight months after presentation.

reduce tissue edema, thereby reducing the circumference of the extremity and thus decreasing the surface area of the wound. Before the advent of negative pressure therapy, lower extremity wounds with exposed bone, especially on the lower one-third of the leg, required microvascular free tissue transfer for coverage of the defect. It should be noted that smaller wounds have shown tremendous success with V.A.C. therapy, while the larger surface wound still require free tissue transfer (Case 3) (Figure 23–3). Some wounds with prosthetic bypasses can be healed if the bypass is rerouted away from the wound, which can be treated with V.A.C. therapy, and later skin grafted or closed primarily (Case 4) (Figure 23–4).

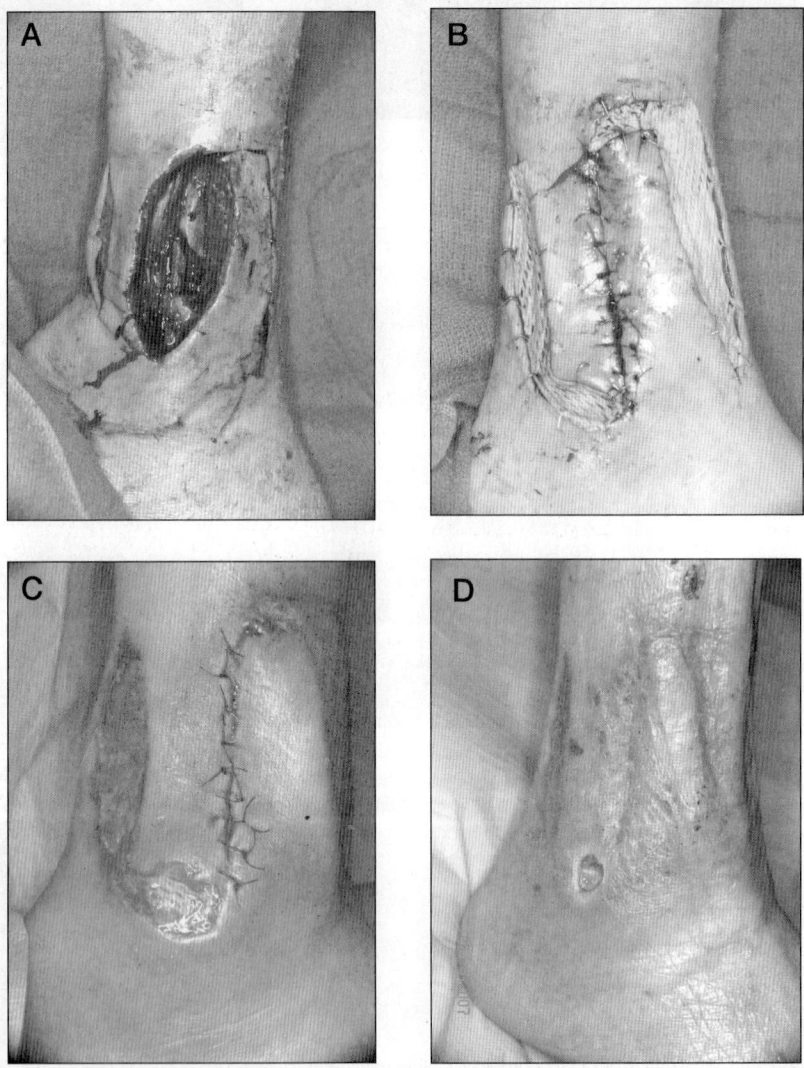

Figure 23-3. Case 3: 78-year-old diabetic with an open ankle fracture and soft tissue loss. (**A**) Intraoperative view of open fractured distal fibula and the design of local rotational flaps to cover the bone; (**B**) two flaps were used, anterior flap was based on the ascending branch of the anterior tibial artery and the posterior flap was based superiorly, the donor site soft tissue was covered with a skin graft and the V.A.C., (**C**) approximately one month after partial closure and V.A.C. therapy with nearly 100% take of the skin graft and flap survival; (**D**) two months postoperatively with a nearly healed wound.

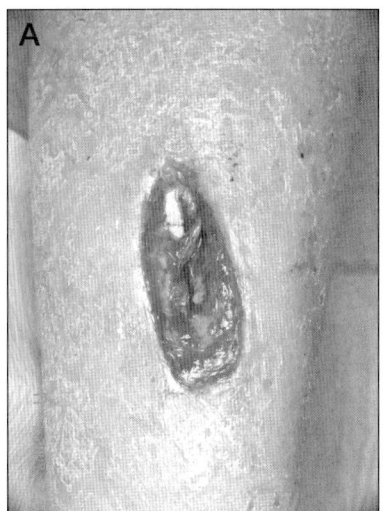

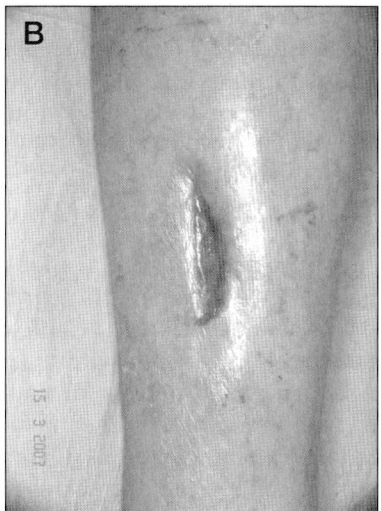

Figure 23-4. Case 4: 66-year-old smoker with chronic renal insufficiency, diabetes mellitus, and peripheral arterial disease presented with failed multiple bypasses; the last bypass was a prosthetic femoral-peroneal bypass with distal vein patch. (**A**) Patient developed wound breakdown with visible graft material, the graft was re-routed to a different arterial target and the wound was treated with V.A.C.; (**B**) wound healing approximately two months after V.A.C. placement; (**C**) completely healed wound and limb salvage.

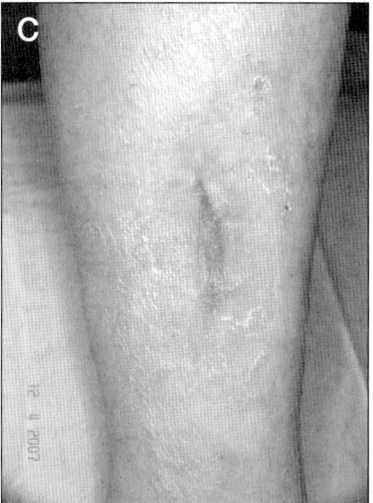

In a landmark study out of Winston Salem, North Carolina, A.J. DeFranzo et. al. treated 75 patients with open wounds of the lower extremity with exposed bone, tendon, or hardware, but without frank purulent osteomyelitis. Of these wounds, 52 were below the knee and orthopedic hardware was exposed in 12 wounds. Seventy-one out of the 75 wounds were able to be managed with V.A.C. therapy. They were able to appreciate granulation tissue by the second sponge change. Twelve wounds were treated by delayed primary closure. Fifty-eight wounds were closed with split thickness skin graft.[31] Fortunately, complications with vacuum-assisted closure are rare if wound patients are appropriately selected. Four wounds in this series that failed treatment with the V.A.C. were because of late infection.

In addition, there are published data from the Iraq war studying the use of V.A.C. on high-energy, contaminated soft tissue injuries. This retrospective review of 88 war injuries showed that all patients were discharged from the hospital with healed wounds (0% complication rate). The blast effect of high-energy missiles causes an unpredictable zone of ischemia and stasis that may or may not undergo transformation into necrosis, thrombosis, and devitalization.[32] These authors suggest that the use of negative pressure protects these wounds, which are undergoing significant physiologic changes.

The Use of V.A.C. with Other Wound Healing Adjuncts

Several biologic dressings are available to promote wound healing such as Integra bilayer matrix wound dressing (Integra Life Sciences Corporation, Plainsboro, NJ) and Apligraf (Organogenesis Inc., Canton, MA). Integra is bovine tendon collagen and glycosaminoglycan covered with a semipermeable silicone layer. It acts as the tissue ground substance and dermis, promoting cellular ingrowth and wound healing, and has been widely accepted in the management of burn injuries.[33] Integra is most useful over tendon or bone where granulation tissue is scarce; in complicated wounds it can be combined with V.A.C. to allow maximal granulation tissue formation (Case 5) (Figure 23–5). Another wound healing adjunct is Apligraf, which is a bilayered skin substitute made from bovine collagen and cultured epidermal cells approved for use on venous stasis ulcers and diabetic foot ulcers. Apligraf can also be combined with V.A.C. therapy and has been very useful for complicated, recalcitrant wounds (Case 6) (Figure 23–6).

Other Indications

As stated previously, V.A.C. has been extensively studied and shown to be useful in the management of sternal wounds,[34-44] open abdominal wounds,[45-47] and decubitus ulcers.

Expanding Indications for V.A.C. Therapy

The V.A.C. system was developed for the treatment of decubitus ulcers and wounds associated with vascular insufficiency.[2] The indications for use of this system are expanding rapidly and showing great success.

While V.A.C. therapy has shown remarkable progress with treating chronic wounds, we are now seeing evidence of success with the V.A.C. when used on infected wounds. Infections are known to complicate the treatment of wounds and impede the healing process by damaging tissue, reducing wound tensile strength, and inducing an undesirable inflammatory response. This inflammatory response negatively impacts wound healing by increasing peripheral edema. Increased bacterial burden in a wound increases the metabolic requirements of the tissues, stimulates a proinflammatory environment, and encourages the in-migration of monocytes, macrophages, and leukocytes, all of which negatively impact wound healing. Bacteria are also notorious for secreting harmful cytokines, which can lead to direct vasoconstriction and decrease blood flow to the wound.

A pilot study at Loma Linda University in California treated infected wounds with great success using a silver foam dressing along with vacuum assisted closure. The investigators found the silver foam dressing to be most useful in cases of complex, colonized, or infected wounds postdebridement, as well as for acute traumatic wounds for reduction of bacterial burden.[48]

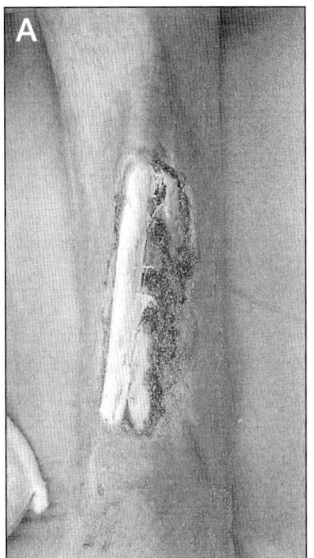
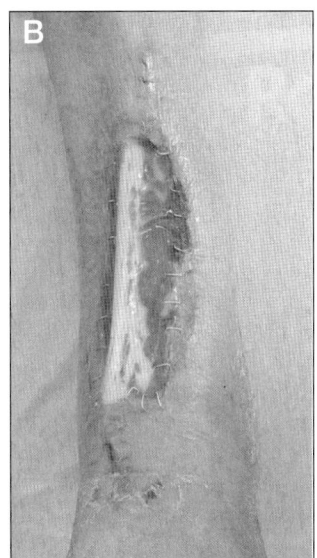
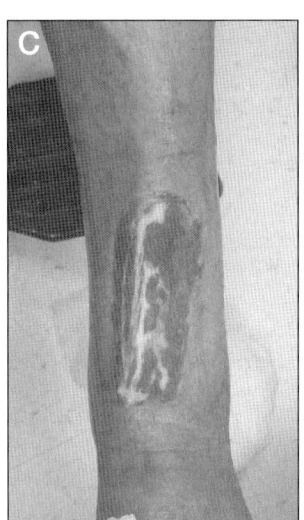
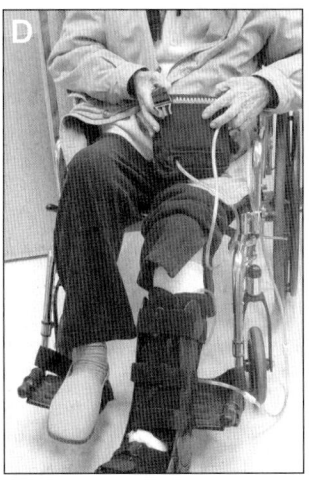
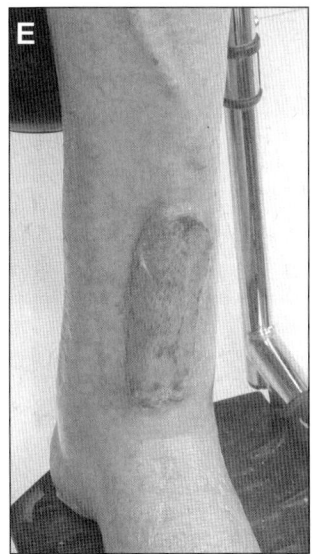

Figure 23-5. Case 5: 69-year-old with diabetes mellitus and peripheral arterial disease status post left femoral-anterior tibial bypass with reversed saphenous vein. The patient developed a wound in the distal anterior lower leg, which was treated initially with a skin graft that failed. (**A**) The lower extremity wound after failed skin grafting and exposed anterior tibialis tendon; (**B**) the tendon was covered with integra and the V.A.C.; (**C**) four weeks after integra and V.A.C. treatment with increased granulation tissue on the tendon; (**D**) the patient with his portable V.A.C. pump; (**E**) the wound was then skin grafted and the V.A.C. was used for five days after the skin graft, wound healed approximately six weeks after skin grafting over the tendon.

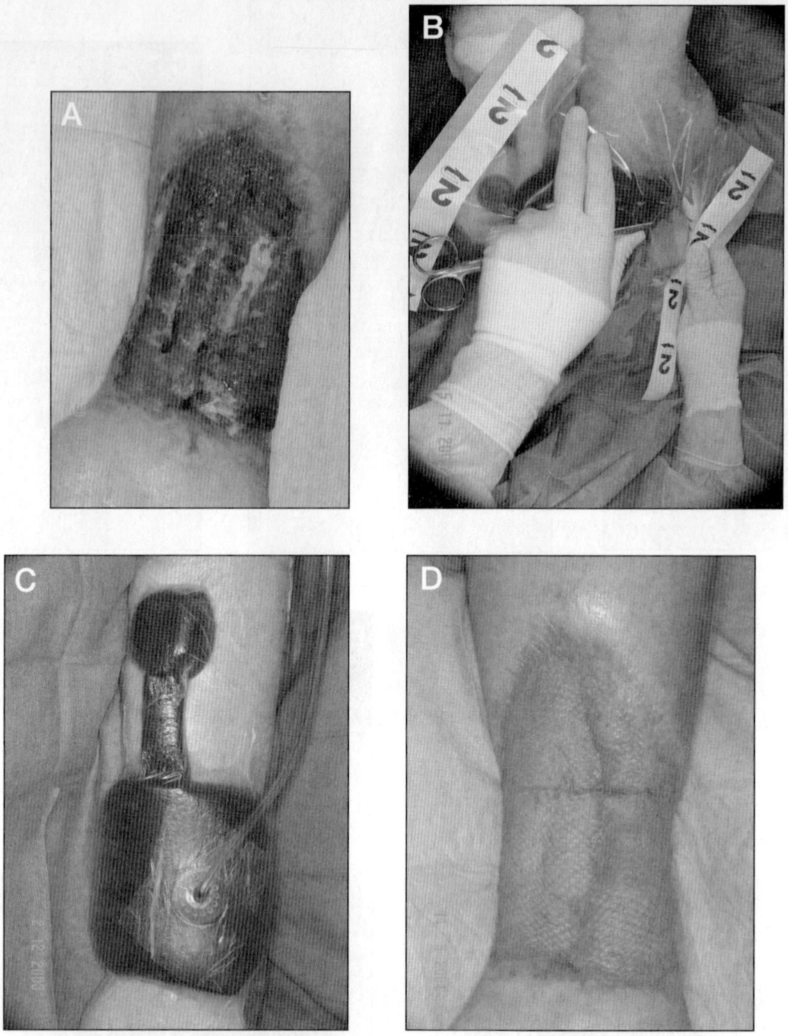

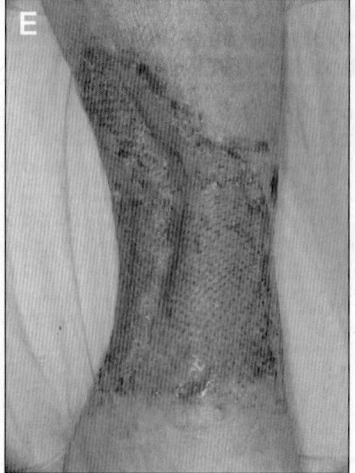

Figure 23-6. Case 6: patient with large venous stasis ulcer. (**A**) Wound on presentation; (**B**) one week s/p operative debridement, placement of Apligraf and V.A.C. therapy. (**C**) healing wound two weeks s/p operative debridement, placement of apligraf and V.A.C. therapy; (**D**) nearly completely healed wound three weeks postoperative debridement, placement of Apligraf and V.A.C. therapy; (**E**) wound healed completely in five weeks.

CONCLUSION

The V.A.C. is an example of how a simple therapeutic modality can enhance the treatment of complicated wounds. While it is not a "cure-all," this device can be applied to a variety of wounds from many etiologies with minimal complications. We have found it extremely useful in healing diabetic lower extremity wounds and complicated wounds with exposed tendon, bone, and other vital structures.

REFERENCES

1. Morykwas, MJ, Argenta, LC, Shelton-Brown EI, et al. Vacuum-assisted closure: a New method for wound control and treatment: A new method for wound control and treatment: Animal studies and basic foundation. *Ann Plast Surg.* 1997;38:553.
2. Argenta LC and Morykwas, MJ. Vacuum assisted closure a new method for wound control and treatement: clinical experience. *Ann Plast Surg.* 1997;38:563.
3. Argenta LC, Morykwas MJ, Marks MW, et al. Vacuum-assisted closure: state of clinic art. *Plast Reconstr Surg.* 2006;117(7 Suppl):127S–142S.
4. Morykwas MJ, Simpson J, Punger K, et al. Vacuum- assisted closure: state of basic research and physiologic foundation." *Plast Reconstr Surg.* 2006; 117(7 Suppl):121S–126S. Review.
5. Chen S, Li J, Li X, et al. Effects of vacuum-assisted closure on wound microciruation; An experiemental study. *Asian J Surg.* 2005:28;211.
6. Xu L, Chen SZ, Qiao C, et al. Effects of negative pressure on wound blood flow. *J Fourth Milit Med Univ.* 2000;21:967.
7. Wackensfors, A, Sjorgren J. Gustafsson R, et al. Effects of vacuum-assisted closure therapy on inguinal wound edge microvascular blood flow. *Wound Repair Regen.* 2004;12:600.
8. Weed T, Ratliff C, Dake DB. Quantifying bacterial bioburden during negative pressure wound therapy: Does the wound VAC enhance bacterial clearance? *Ann Plast Surg.* 2004;52:276.
9. Wagner S, Coerper S, Fricke J, et al. Comparison of inflammatory and systemic sources of growth factors in acute and chronic human wounds. *Wound Repair Regen.* 2003;11:253.
10. VAC therapy Clinical Guidelines, KCI
11. Ilizarov GA. The tension-stress effect on the genesis and growth of tissues. Part II. The influence of the rate and frquence of distraction. *Clin Orthop Relat Res.* 1989;238:249–81.
12. Argenta LC, Marks MW. Tissue expansion. In: Georgiade N, ed. *Essentials of plastic, maxillofacial and reconstructive surgery, 2nd ed.* Baltimore: Williams and Wilkins; 1990:103–113.
13. Morykwas MJ, Faler BJ , Pearce DJ, et al. Effects of varying levels of subatmosphereic pressure on the rate of granulation tissue formation in experimental wounds in swine. *Ann Plastic Surg.* 2001;47(5);547–551.
14. Schnieder AM, Morykwas MJ, Argenta LC. A new reliable method of securing skin grafts to the difficult recipient bed. *Plast Reconst Surg.* 1998;102:1195.
15. Backburn JH, Boemi L, Hall WW, et al. Negative-pressure dressings as a bolster for skin grafts. *Ann Plast Surg.* 1998;40:453.
16. Sherer. LA, Shiver, S, Chang M, et al the vacuum assisted closure device a method of securing skin grafts and improving graft survival. *Arch Surg,* 137; 930, 2002.
17. Moisidis E. Heath T, Boorer C, et al. A prospective, blinded randomized controlled clinical trial of topical negative pressure use in skin grafting. *Plast Reconstr Surg.* 2004;114:917.
18. Hallberg H, Holmstrom H. Vaginal construction with skin grafts and vacuum assisted closure. *Scand J Plast Reconstru Surg Hand Surg.* 2003;37:97.
19. Simman R, Forte R, Silverberg B, et al. A Comparative histological study of skin graft take with tie-over bolster dressing versus negative pressure wound therapy in a pig model: A preliminary study. *Wounds.* 2000;16:76.

20. Marks MW, Schneider AM, Capizzi M, et al. Muscle Flap survival after complete venous occlusion by application by application of a negative pressure device. Presented at the 66th Annual Meeting of the American Society for Plastic and Reconstructive Surgery. San Fransico, Calif. September 21–24, 1997.
21. Chen CS, Mrksich M, Huang, s, et al. Micropatterned surfaces for control of cell shape, position and function. *Biotechnol Prog*. 1998;14:356.
22. Huang S, Chen CS, Ingber, DE. Control of cyclin d1, p 27 and cell cycle progression in human capillary endothelial cells by cell shape and cytoskeltal tension. *Mol Biol Cell*. 1998;9:3179–93
23. Saxena V, Hwang CW, Huang S et al. Vacuum assisted closure: microdeformations of wounds and cell proliferation. *Plast Reconstr Surg*. 2004;114(5):1086–96; discussion 1097–8
24. Greene AK, Puder M, Roy R, et al. Microdeformational wound therapy effects on angiogenesis and matrix metalloproteinases in chronic wouds of 3 debilitated patients. *Ann Plas Surg*. 2006;56 (4):418–22.
25. Etoz A, Ozgenel Y, Ozcan M. The use of negative pressure wound therapy on diabetic foot ulcers; A preliminary controlled trial. *Wounds*. 2004;16:264.
26. Armstrong DG, Lavery LA, Abu-Rumman P et al. Outcomes of subatmospheric pressure dressing therapy on wounds of the diabetic foot. *Ostomy Wound Manage*. 2003;48:64.
27. Armstrong DG, Attinger CE, Boulton AJ, et al. Guidelines regarding negative wound therapy (NPWT) in the diabetic foot. *Ostomy Wound Manage*. 2004;50:3S.
28. Clare, MP, Fitzgibbons TC, McMullen ST, et al. Experience with the vacuum assisted closure negative pressure technique in the treatment of non-healing diabetic and dys-vascular wounds. *Foot Ankle Int*. 2002;23:896.
29. Expensen EH, Nixon BP, Lavery LA, et al. Use of subatmospheric (V.A.C.) therapy to improve bioengineered tissue grafting in diabetic foot wounds. *J Am Podiatr Med Assoc*. 2002;92:395.
30. McCallon SK, Knight CA, Valiulus JP, et al. Vacuum-assisted closure versus saline-moistened gauze in the healing of post operative diabetic foot wounds. *Ostomy Wound Mange*. 2000;46:28.
31. De Franzo AJ, Argenta LC, Marks MW, et al. The use of Vacuum- assisted Closure Therapy for the Treatment of Lower - Extremity Wounds with Exposed Bone. *Plast Reconstr Surg*. 2001;108:5.
32. Leininger BE, Rasmussen TE , Smith DL, et al. Experience with the wound vac and delayed primary closure of contaiminated soft tissue injuries in Iraq. *J Trauma Inj Infect Crit Care*. Vol 61 (5) Nov 2006.
33. Heimbach D, Warden G, Luterman A, et al. Multicenter post approval clinical trial of integra dermal regeneration template for burn treatment. *J Burn Care Rehab*. 2003;24:42–48.
34. Agarwal, JP, Ogilvie, M, Wu LC, et al. Vacuum-assisted closure for sternal wounds: A first line therapeutic management approach. *Plast Reconst Surg*. 2005;116:1035.
35. Tang ATM, Ohri SK, Haw MP. Novel application of vacuum-assisted closure technique to the treatment of sternotomy wound infection. *Eur J Cardiothorac Surg*. 2000;17:482–4.
36. Scholl L, Chang E, Reitz B. Sternal osteomyelitis: Use of vacuum- assisted closure device as an adjunct to definitive closure with sternectomy and muscle flap reconstruction. *J Card Surg*. 2004;19:453.
37. Oconnor J, Kells A, Henry S, et al. Vacuum assisted closure for the treatment of complexd chest wounds. *Ann Thor Surg*. 2005;79:1196.
38. Orgill DP, Austen WG, Butler CE, et al. Guidelines for treatment of complex chest wounds with negative pressure wound therapy. Presented at the Negative Pressure Wound Therapy Consesnsus Conference, Boston, MA; Sept 11, 2004.
39. Orgill DP. Avancing the treatment options of chest wounds with negative pressure wound therapy. *Ostomy Wound Manage*. 2005;51:39.
40. Immer FF, Durrer M, Muhlemann KS. Deep sternal wound infection after cardiac surgery modality of treatment and outcome. *Ann Thor Surg*. 2005;80:957.

41. Hersh RE, Jack JM, Dahman MI, et al. The vacuum-assisted closure defice as a bridge to sternal wound closure. *Ann. Plast. Surg.* 46, 250, 2001.
42. Katshka I, Frauendorfer P, Harrington W. Vacuum assisted closure therapy improves early post operative lung function in patients with large sternal wounds. *Zentrabl Chir.* 2004;129:33.
43. Fuchs U, Zittermann A, Stuettgen B, et al. Clinical outcome of patients with deep sternal wound infection managed by vacuum - assisted closure compared to conventional therapy with open packing: A retrospective analysis. *Ann Therac Surg.* 2005;79:526.
44. Song DH, Wu LC, Lohman RF, et al. Vacuum assisted closure for the treatment of sternal wounds. The bridge between debridement and definitve closure. *Plast Reconst Surg.* 2003;111:92.
45. Quah HM, Maw A,Young T, et al. Vacuum assisted closure in the management of the open abdomen: a report of a case and initial experiences. *J Tissue Viab.* 2004;14:59.
46. Stone PA, Hass SM, Flaherty SK, et al, Vacuum-assisted fascial closure for patients with abdominal trauma. *J Trauma Inj Infect Crit Care.* 2004;57:1082.
47. Miller, PR, Thompson, JT, Faler, BJ et al. Late fascial closure in lieu of ventral hernia; the next step in open abdomen management. *J Trauma.* 2002;53:843.
48. Gabriel A, Heinrich C, Shores J et. al. Reducing bacterial bioburden in infected wounds with vacuum-assisted closure and a new silver dressing-a pilot study. *Wounds.* 2006;18 (9);245–255.

24

Practical Strategies for Debridement, Off-loading, and Healing the Diabetic Foot Wound

David G. Armstrong, D.P.M., Ph.D.,
Stephanie C. Wu, D.P.M., M.S., and Ryan Crews, M.S.

An estimated 18.2 million people in the United States—8.7 percent of the population—have diabetes mellitus, a serious, lifelong condition.[1] Of those, 13 million have been diagnosed, and an alarming 5.2 million people are not even aware that they have this disease. Each year, approximately 1.3 million adults are diagnosed with diabetes. Type 2 diabetes is becoming more common among children and adolescents, particularly in American Indian, African American, and the Hispanic populations. Foot ulceration is one of the most common complications associated with diabetes and often plays a central role in the causal pathway to lower extremity amputation.[2] Well over 80,000 nontraumatic lower limb amputations are performed on people with diabetes annually within the United States alone.[1] Postamputation mortality rates for persons with diabetes are often worse than those for most malignancies, and range from 13% to 40% at one year, 35% to 65% at three years, and 39% to 80% at five years.[3] Development of a foot ulceration is one of the primary factors in the etiology of these amputations. While studying lower extremity amputation in people with diabetes, Adler et al. noted that "the odds ratio associated with first ulcer for a subsequent ipsilateral amputation was 5.7 (CI 1.6-30.2)."[4]

Current research has suggested the lifetime incidence rate of foot ulceration in people with diabetes may be as high as 25%.[5] Additionally, foot ulcers have been demonstrated to elicit substantial emotional, physical, productivity, and financial losses.[6-9] Fortunately, the etiology of the diabetic foot ulcer is fairly well understood and lends credence to treatment of ulcers by debridement and off-loading.

DIABETIC FOOT ULCER ETIOLOGY

Neuropathic diabetic foot wounds develop in response to the application of focal pressure and repetitive stress to the plantar aspect of the foot.[10] Stress to the foot is a product of the ground reaction force generated during weight-bearing activity. This force is composed of vertical, anteroposterior, and mediolateral components. The vertical force is much greater than the other two. At a fast walk, the vertical force amplitude reaches ~ 1.5 times body weight[11] and increases to ~5 times body weight when running.[12] The vertical force damages healthy tissue by compressing and deforming it. Shear is the mechanical stress collectively generated by the anteroposterior and mediolateral components of ground reaction force. It causes tissue to tear by stretching it. Shear is as equally damaging as vertical compression and is evident in peripheral undermining of poorly off-loaded diabetic foot wounds.

The gait cycle is the duration that occurs from the time the heel of one leg strikes the ground to the time at which the same leg contacts the ground again. It consists of two phases: the stance or support phase, and the swing or the recovery phase. During the support phase of gait, different portions of the foot are in contact with the ground. Ground reaction forces generally progress from the heel at touchdown to the hallux at push-off.[11] In addition to being applied at different areas, the magnitude of the ground reaction force varies throughout the support phase according to a bimodal pattern. Force initially rises at heel strike, then drops as the foot rolls forward and proceeds to rise a second time during push-off. Due to the variation in site of application and magnitude of the ground reaction force, the heel and forefoot generally experience much more pressure than the midfoot. Subsequently, these are the two sites most prone to ulceration. Spreading force out over the entire foot, and potentially even the leg, has been a strategy for clinicians treating this condition.

TREATMENT

With sufficient vascular supply, the primary modes of healing a diabetic foot ulcer are pressure dispersion and appropriate debridement. Pressure dispersion, commonly referred to as "off-loading," is most successful when force is spread over a wide area and compliance is ensured by means such as a total contact cast.[13] In order to reduce chronic inflammatory by-products in a wound, debridement may be as important as off-loading.[14-16] In a randomized control study on becaplermin, Steed and coworkers[17] found a significantly greater proportion of patients healed in centers that frequently debrided wounds. Despite a general consensus that surgical debridement is often warranted for diabetic foot ulcers, there is sparse literature detailing technique.[18-19] Thus, the following section provides instructions for surgical debridement of diabetic foot ulcers that are neither infected nor ischemic.

Debridement

With the patient seated comfortably, the wound may be approached with either a sterile scalpel and forceps (Figure 24–1), or for smaller wounds, a tissue nipper (Figure 24–2). The skin may be incised or the nipper may be introduced to the fullest extent of the undermining between the epidermis and dermis (the extent of damage caused by shear). Excision of this undermined tissue should be performed circumferentially about the wound until the periphery of the wound exhibits a firm connection between epidermis and dermis. Any nonviable tissue should be removed centrally from the wound, as required, through sharp excision or curretage. Digital pressure may be applied to the wound to achieve hemostasis.

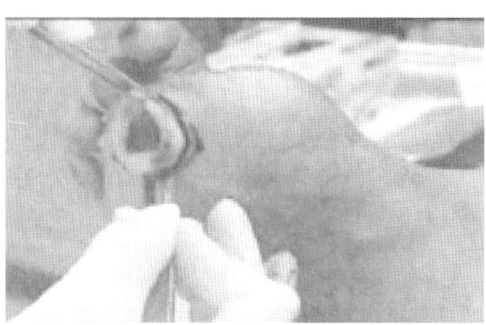
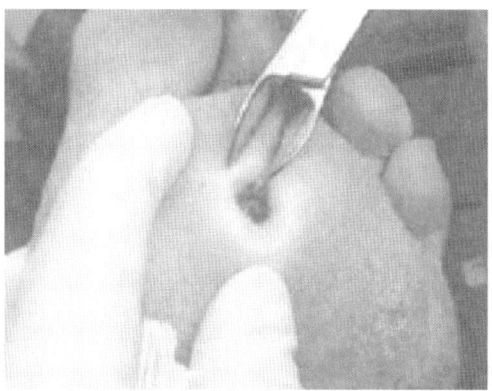

Figure 24-1. Wound debridement with scalpel.   **Figure 24-2.** Wound debridement with tissue nipper.

The wound may then be probed to assess involvement of underlying tissue and for the presence of occult infection. Following adequate debridement, one may dress and off-load the wound in an appropriate fashion. The hallmark of an appropriately off-loaded wound is the noticeable lack of undermining of the wound edges at follow up.

Off-loading

A smorgasbord of off-loading modalities is currently available to practitioners. However, a proportionately robust knowledge base of the frequency and rate of wound healing attributable to the various off-loading methods is lacking. The ensuing review describes the modalities most commonly employed by clinical practices and the evidence available to substantiate their use.

Total Contact Casts

Total contact casts (TCCs) are considered by most diabetic foot specialists to be the gold-standard off-loading modality (Figure 24–3).[19] Plaster casting to treat neuropathic foot wounds was first described for the treatment of the neuropathic wound by Milroy Paul,

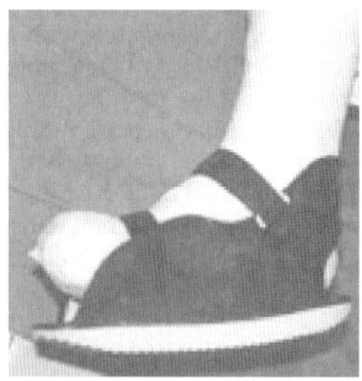

Figure 24-3. Ambulatory total contact cast.

and later popularized in the United States by Dr. Paul Brand at the Hansen's Disease Center in Carville, Louisiana.[20] The technique has come to be known as total contact casting because it employs a well-molded, minimally padded cast that maintains contact with the entire plantar aspect of the foot and the lower leg. Total contact casting is quite effective in treating the majority of noninfected, nonischemic plantar diabetic foot wounds, with healing rates ranging from 72% to 100% over a course of five to seven weeks.[21-26] Throughout the gait cycle, the averaged peak plantar pressures are highest in the forefoot, while they tend to be generally less significant in the rearfoot and medial arch. Shaw[27] and coworkers, and our own group,[28] have noted that a large proportion of the pressure reduction realized in

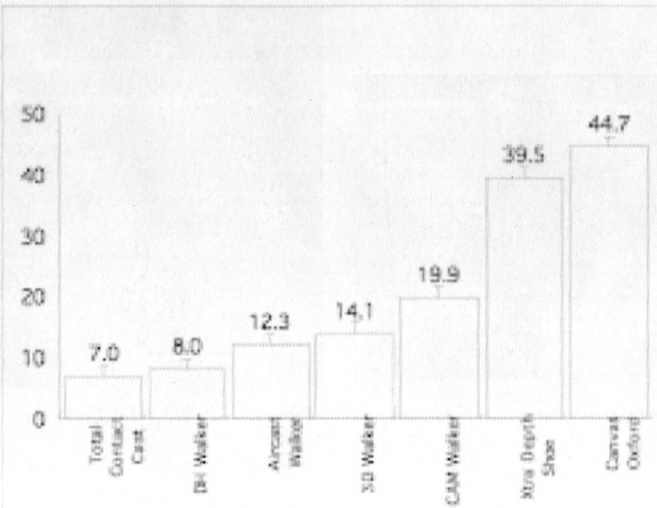

Figure 24-4. Mean peak pressure For ulcers under the metatarsal heads. Mean peak pressure (N/cm2) under the metatarsal heads among various removable cast walkers35 Values are given as N/cm2 DH Walker (Centec Orthopaedics, Camarillo, CA) is also licensed under the name Easy Step Pressure Relief Walker by Kendall Orthopaedics, Mansfield, MA, Darco International, Inc. Huntington, WV, and Aircast, Summit, NJ; and 3-D Walker, DeRoyal Orthopedic, Powell, TN.

the forefoot of the total contact cast is transmitted along the cast wall or to the rearfoot. This supports the postulate of several authors who have suggested that the total contact cast is effective because it permits walking by uniformly distributing pressures over the entire plantar surface of the foot (Figure 24–4).[20-24, 29-31]

Total contact casts are effective for a number of other reasons besides their ability to off-load. They may help reduce or control edema that can impede healing and potentially protect the foot from infection.[32] However, the most important attribute of this technique may be its ability to ensure appropriate patient compliance. In other words, the device is not easily removable. Therefore, the patient has no option other than to adhere to the regimen prescribed by the clinician.

Certainly, the above-described advantages make the total contact cast an attractive choice to off-load the diabetic foot ulcer. However, there are a number of potential negative attributes that may dissuade some clinicians from using this modality. The application of total contact casts are time-consuming and are often associated with a learning curve. Most centers do not have a physician or cast technician available with adequate training or experience to safely apply a total contact cast. Because improper cast application can cause skin irritation and in some cases even frank ulceration, this can be its single biggest negative feature. In addition, TCCs do not allow patients, family members, or health care providers to assess the foot or wound on a daily basis and are, therefore, often contraindicated in cases of soft tissue infections or osteomyelitis. Other patient complaints may include difficulty sleeping comfortably as well as bathing difficulties to avoid getting the cast wet. Certain designs of TCCs may exacerbate postural instability.[33]

Half-Shoes.   Commonly used to treat diabetic foot ulcers, the half-shoe (Figure 24–5) was developed to decrease postoperative pressure on the forefoot.[34] In a retrospective

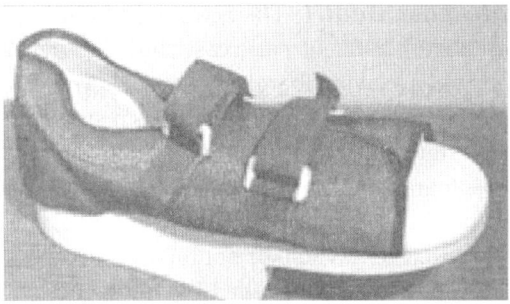

Figure 24-5. Half-shoe.

study comparing half-shoes to crutch-assisted gait in the treatment of diabetic foot ulcers, Chantelau et al. found half-shoes yielded a faster healing rate.[34] Patients treated with half-shoes also incurred fewer serious infections requiring hospitalization (4% versus 41%). In addition to their healing capabilities, half-shoes are inexpensive and easily applied. Although they have shown some promise as off-loaders, they do not work as well as other modalities. Gait lab analysis has shown half-shoes to be less effective in reducing pressure than total contact casts and certain types of removable cast walkers.[35] Additional research has shown half-shoes to heal fewer wounds than total contact casts and removable walkers.[13] Furthermore, wounds healed by half-shoes require more time to achieve healing than the other methods.[13] As can be said with the other modalities discussed in this review, additional research evaluating outcomes, patient satisfaction, costs, and complications are required.

Healing Sandals. Certainly, application of a rigid rocker to the sole of a specially designed sandal may theoretically limit dorsiflexion of the metatarsophalangeal joints, thereby limiting plantar progression of the metatarsal heads during the propulsive phase of gait. In addition, the molded nature of a "healing sandal" facilitates a greater distribution of metatarsal head pressures and may theoretically provide for a shorter pressure-time integral. This device is lightweight, stable, and reusable. It does, however, require a significant amount of time and experience to produce the rigid sole rocker design and other modifications. Most facilities do not have the time or expertise to modify these devices. Finally, these devices do not off-load as well as other modalities (such as removable cast walkers) that take less effort to produce or procure.[36] Recently, a cross between a healing sandal and a removable cast walker has been introduced. This de vice, known as the MABAL shoe, is removable, but perhaps maintains more contact with the foot than does a standard healing sandal. In a study by Hissink and coworkers, this devices howed a similar time to healing when compared to studies of total contact casting.[37] However, this device also has many of the same downfalls of the contact cast and healing sandal as it requires special expertise for its fabrication and application.

Therapeutic Footwear (Depth Inlay Shoes). Many patients are prescribed therapeutic shoes in an effort to assist in pressure reduction and wound healing. However, these devices have not proven to be effective in this role. Gait lab studies suggest that therapeutic shoes allow up to 900% more pressure in areas of the forefoot compared to total contact casts and some removable cast walkers[35] Furthermore, even the most optimistic studies using shoes as a primary offloading mechanism suggest that half of the noninfected, nonischemic, superficial wounds (UT Grade 1A[38-39]) will heal at 12 weeks.[40] We may, therefore, postulate that the true value of therapeutic shoes and insoles is in the prevention of ulceration, not during active ulceration.

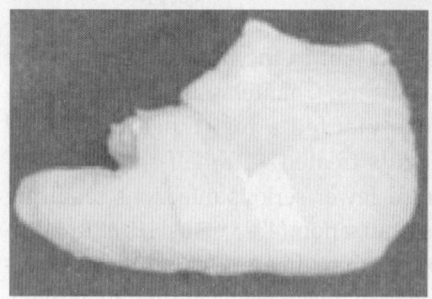

Figure 24-6. Scotchcast boot.

Scotchcast Boot. The Scotchcast boot is an alternative plaster of paris cast, and was developed when newer fiberglass materials were introduced (Figure 24–6). Scotchcast is a substitute for plaster of paris; it is much lighter and has high integral strength.[41] The Scotchcast boot is a well-padded cast cut away by the ankle, and made either removable or nonremovable by cutting away the cast over the dorsum of the foot, and making a closure of padding and tape with velcro straps. Windows are cut over the ulcers as needed, whereas a removable heel-cap of fiberglass is added for large heel ulcers. Basic functions of the cast boot are to reduce pressure on the lesion, maintain patient mobility, and to protect the remaining foot. The boot is worn with a cast sandal to increase patients' mobility while the Scotchcast protects the ulcer from any pressure and keeps the patient ambulant.

Once the ulcer has healed, the patient can gradually start increasing the time of wearing normal protective footwear while decreasing the wearing time of the Scotchcast boot. The patient usually keeps the boot and the sandal, as this can be worn if an ulcer reoccurs.

The main advantage of this type of casting is that it is removable; yet concomitantly, this is also one of its major disadvantages. A removable cast allows for regular inspections and redressing of the wound; however, it also allows for noncompliance. An alternative cast for the noncompliant patient would be a nonremovable Scotchcast boot.

Although the Scotchcast boot has been used very successfully for more than a decade in several clinics in Great Britain, predominantly treating neuropathic and sometimes neuro-ischaemic ulcers, to date there is no evidence available of comparisons of healing rates of this type of cast with the more standard casts such as the TCC. Preliminary data of healing rates ranging from 61 to 88% with a mean healing time of between 10 and 13 weeks have been reported.[41-42] A comparison study is now warranted to investigate the efficacy of this cast against other currently used methods of off-loading.

Removable Cast Walkers. This type of pressure reduction device offers several advantages over the traditional total contact cast (Figure 24–7A and B). Removable walkers are, as their name implies, easily removed for self-inspection of the wound and application of topical therapies that require frequent administration. Patients can bathe and sleep more comfortably. Because they are removable, they can be used for infected wounds as well as superficial ulcers.

The best feature of the removable cast walker is also paradoxically its potential downfall. The ability to remove the device eliminates the element of "forced compliance" that is the finest attribute of the TCC. Patients may remove the cast for dressing changes, sleeping, and showers, but they can also choose to use the walker only when they leave the house or walk excessively. While data from gait lab studies suggest that the amount of pressure reduction for certain removable cast walkers is equivalent to TCCs, data supporting their use have been disappointing. In a randomized clinical

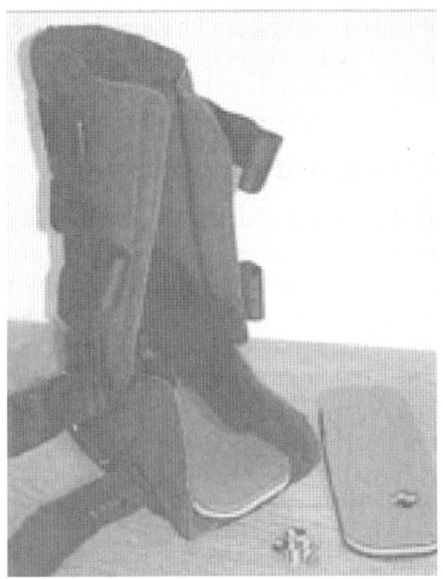

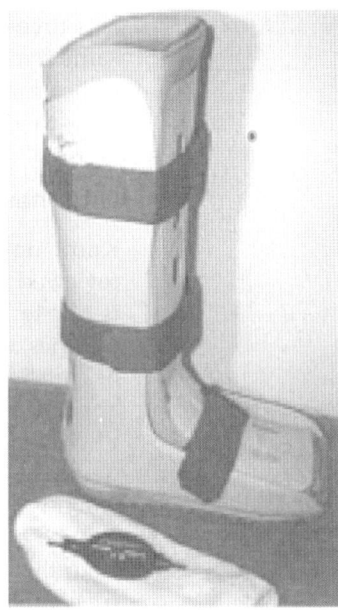

Figure 24-7. A. Removable cast walker (DH pressure relief walker).

Figure 24-7. B. Removable cast walker (Aircast).

trial comparing the RCW to the TCC and the half-shoe, we reported a significantly greater prevalence and rate of healing in the TCC.[13] Certainly, these results can, at first glance, seem puzzling. This has led us to investigate this area further and suggest a possible solution, discussed below.

Compliance with Removal Devices and the "instant" Total Contact Cast (iTCC)

We have postulated that, although the RCW and TCC may off-load (more or less) equally well, patients, because of their dense neuropathy, might not strictly adhere to a standard pressure off-loading regimen. In a recently conducted study, we evaluated the activity of patients with diabetic foot ulcers and their adherence to their off-loading regime. This study, using accelerometers worn on the patients' waist and (hidden) on the RCW, suggested that patients wore their off-loading device for less than 30% of their total daily activity.[43] This disappointing result has prompted us to search for simple solutions.

Understanding that most centers either do not have the infrastructure, expertise, or personnel to apply TCCs, in light of the previous data, we have suggested that a potential alternative might be to make the RCW less easily removable. This simple modification involves simply wrapping the RCW with either a layer of cohesive bandage or plaster/fiberglass (Figure 24–8). This solution, it might be postulated, could have the benefit of adequate off-loading (on par with the TCC) and adequate adherence to the prescribed course of pressure reduction. We have termed this modification to an RCW an "instant Total Contact Cast (iTCC)"[44] Two recent studies conducted by our group and our colleagues at University of Miami suggest that the iTCC may be as effective at healing nonin-fected, nonischemic diabetic foot wounds as the TCC, and is far more effective than the removable cast walker.[45-46] In addition, the iTCC is much

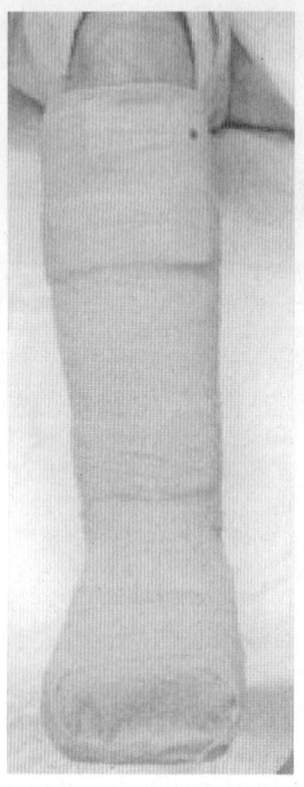

less time-consuming to apply and remove, and since the same removable cast walker can be reused, the overall cost of healing an ulcer with an iTCC is also less than it would be with a TCC.

Crutches, Walkers, and Wheelchairs

Knowing that the purpose of all the off-loading devices reviewed is a reduction in the pressure applied to ulcers, it is fair to ask, "why not remove all pressure by means of crutches, walkers, or wheelchairs?" One reason is that the use of crutches and walkers may cause additional pressure to be applied to the contralateral limb, thus putting it at risk for ulceration.[47] The answer also lies in the practicality of these devices. The majority of patients suffering diabetic foot wounds do not have the upper body strength or endurance to use these devices. They also do not have the "gift" of pain from their ulcers to promote compliance. This is especially concerning with wheelchairs. Most patients' homes are not designed for them, and this can lead to large amounts of non-compliant activity.

Figure 24-8. Removable cast walker wrapped in cohesive bandage to convert to "instant Total Contact Cast."

CONCLUSION

There is a high occurrence of foot ulcers within the population of people with diabetes. In order to diminish the detrimental consequences associated with these ulcers, a high standard of care must be provided. The direct cause of these ulcers is the ground reaction forces encountered during weight-bearing activities. Therefore, proper treatment must address these forces. The two primary means to treat nonischemic and noninfected wounds are debridement and off-loading. They form a formidable team in healing ulcers and potentially averting lower limb amputations. As our understanding of wound care advances and the development of new adjunctive treatments continues, debridement and off-loading will remain the foundation of treatment.

REFERENCES

1. Diabetes Public Health Resource, National Center for Chronic Disease Prevention and Health Promotion. April 4, 2005. Available at: http://www.cdc.gov/diabetes/statistics/lea/table1link.htm. Accessed April 7, 2005.
2. Singh N, Armstrong DG, Lipsky BA. Preventing foot ulcers in patients with diabetes. *Jama.* 2005;293(2):217–228.
3. Reiber GE. Epidemiology of foot ulcers and amputations in the diabetic foot. In: Bowker JH, Pfeifer MA, eds. *The Diabetic Foot.* St. Louis: Mosby; 2001:13–32.
4. Adler AI, Boyko EJ, Ahroni JH, Smith DG. Lower-extremity amputation in diabetes. The independent effects of peripheral vascular disease, sensory neuropathy, and foot ulcers. *Diabetes Care.* 1999;22(7):1029–1035.

5. International Consensus on the Diabetic Foot. Paper presented at: International Working Group on the Diabetic Foot, 2003; Noordwijkerhout, Netherlands.
6. Vileikyte L. Diabetic foot ulcers: a quality of life issue. *Diabetes Metab Res Rev*. 2001;17(4): 246–249.
7. Meijer JW, Trip J, Jaegers SM, et al. Quality of life in patients with diabetic foot ulcers. *Disabil Rehabil*. 20 2001;23(8):336–340.
8. Vileikyte L, Boulton AJM. Psychological/Behavioral issues in diabetic neuropathic foot ulceration. *Wounds*. 2000;12(6 Suppl B):43B–47B.
9. Boulton AJ, Kirsner RS, Vileikyte L. Clinical practice. Neuropathic diabetic foot ulcers. *N Engl J Med*. 2004;351(1):48–55.
10. Brand PW. The diabetic foot. In: Ellenberg M Rifkin H, ed. *Diabetes mellitus, theory and practice. 3rd ed*. New York: Medical Examination Publishing; 1983:803–828.
11. van Deursen R. Mechanical loading and off-loading of the plantar surface of the diabetic foot. *Clin Infect Dis*. Aug 1 2004;39 Suppl 2:S87–91.
12. Hamill J, Hardin EC. Special Topics in Biomechanics. In: Kamen G, ed. *Foundations of Exercise Science*. Baltimore: Lippincott Williams & Wilkins; 2001:177–189.
13. Armstrong DG, Nguyen HC, Lavery LA, et al. Off-loading the Diabetic Foot Wound: A Randomized Clinical Trial. *Diabetes Care*. 2001;24:1019–1022.
14. Armstrong DG, Jude EB. The Role of Matrix Metalloproteinases in Wound Healing. *J Amer Podiatr Med Assn*. 2002;92:12–18.
15. Jude EB, Rogers AA, Oyibo SO, et al. Matrix metalloproteinase and tissue inhibitor of met-alloproteinase expression in diabetic and venous ulcers. *Diabetologia*. 2001;44 (suppl 1):A3.
16. Nwomeh BC, Liang HX, Cohen IK, Yager DR. MMP-8 is the predominant collagenase in healing wounds and nonhealing ulcers. *J Surg Res*. 1999;81(2):189–195.
17. Steed DL, Donohoe D, Webster MW, Lindsley L. Effect of extensive debridement and treatment on the healing of diabetic foot ulcers. Diabetic Ulcer Study Group. *J Am Coll Surg*. 1996;183(1):61–64.
18. Armstrong DG, Lavery LA, Nixon BP, Boulton AJ. It's not what you put on, but what you take off: techniques for debriding and off-loading the diabetic foot wound. *Clin Infect Dis*. Aug 1 2004;39 Suppl 2:S92–99.
19. American Diabetes Association. Consensus Development Conference on Diabetic Foot Wound Care. *Diabetes Care*. 1999;22(8):1354.
20. Coleman W, Brand PW, Birke JA. The total contact cast, a therapy for plantar ulceration on insensitive feet. *J Am Podiatr Med Assoc*. 1984;74:548–552.
21. Armstrong DG, Lavery LA, Bushman TR. Peak foot pressures influence the healing time of diabetic foot ulcers treated with total contact casts. *J Rehabil Res Dev*. 1998;35(1):1–5.
22. Walker SC, Helm PA, Pulliam G. Chronic diabetic neuropathic foot ulcerations and total contact casting: healing effectiveness and outcome probability (abstract). *Arch Phys Med Rehabil*. 1985;66:574.
23. Walker SC, Helm PA, Pulliam G. Total contact casting and chronic diabetic neuropathic foot ulcerations: healing rates by wound location. *Arch Phys Med Rehabil*. 1987;68:217–221.
24. Sinacore DR, Mueller MJ, Diamond JE. Diabetic plantar ulcers treated by total contact casting. *Phys Ther*. 1987;67:1543–1547.
25. Myerson M, Papa J, Eaton K, Wilson K. The total contact cast for management of neuropathic plantar ulceration of the foot. *J Bone Joint Surg*. 1992;74A(2):261–269.
26. Helm PA, Walker SC, Pulliam G. Total contact casting in diabetic patients with neuropathic foot ulcerations. *Arch Phys Med Rehabil*. 1984;65:691–693.
27. Shaw JE, Hsi WL, Ulbrecht JS, et al. The mechanism of plantar unloading in total contact casts: implications for design and clinical use. *Foot Ankle Int*. 1997;18:809–817.
28. Armstrong DG, Stacpoole-Shea S. Total Contact Casts and Removable Cast Walkers: Mitigation of Plantar Heel Pressure. *J Amer Podiatr Med Assn*. 1999;89:50–53.
29. Boulton AJM, Bowker JH, Gadia M, et al. Use of plaster casts in the management of diabetic neuropathic foot ulcers. *Diabetes Care*. 1986;9(2):149–152.

30. Kominsky SJ. The ambulatory total contact cast. In: R F, ed. *The high risk foot in diabetes mellitus. 1 ed*. New York: Churchill Livingstone; 1991:449–455.

31. Lavery LA, Armstrong DG, Walker SC. Healing Rates of Diabetic Foot Ulcers Associated with Midfoot Fracture Due to Charcot's Arthropathy. *Diabetic Medicine*. 1997;14:46–49.

32. Mueller MJ, Diamond JE, Sinacore DR, et al. Total contact casting in treatment of diabetic plantar ulcers. Controlled clinical trial [see comments]. *Diabetes Care*. 1989;12(6):384–388.

33. Lavery LA, Fleishli JG, Laughlin TJ, et al. Is postural instability exacerbated by off-loading devices in high risk diabetics with foot ulcers? *Ostomy Wound Manage*. 1998;44(1):26–32, 34.

34. Chantelau E, Breuer U, Leisch AC, et al. Outpatient treatment of unilateral diabetic foot ulcers with 'half shoes'. *Diabetic Medicine*. 1993;10:267–270.

35. Lavery LA, Vela SA, Lavery DC, Quebedeaux TL. Reducing dynamic foot pressures in high-risk diabetic subjects with foot ulcerations. A comparison of treatments. *Diabetes Care*. 1996;19(8):818–821.

36. Giacalone VF, Armstrong DG, Ashry HR, et al. A Quantitative Assessment of Healing Sandals and Postoperative Shoes in Off-loading Diabetic Foot. *J Foot Ankle Surg*. 1997;36:28–30.

37. Hissink RJ, Manning HA, van Baal JG. The MABAL shoe, an alternative method in contact casting for the treatment of neuropathic diabetic foot ulcers. *Foot Ankle Int*. 2000;21(4): 320–323.

38. Armstrong DG, Lavery LA, Harkless LB. Validation of a diabetic wound classification system. The contribution of depth, infection, and ischemia to risk of amputation [see comments]. *Diabetes Care*. 1998;21(5):855–859.

39. Oyibo SO, Jude EB, Tarawneh I, et al. A comparison of two diabetic foot ulcer classification systems. *Diabetes*. 2000;49 (Suppl 1):A33.

40. Gentzkow GD, Iwasaki SD, Hershon KS. Use of Dermagraft, a Cultured Human Dermis, to Treat Diabetic Foot Ulcers. *Diabetes Care*. 1996;19:350–354.

41. Burden AC, Jones GR, Jones R, Blandford RL. Use of the "Scotchcast boot" in treating diabetic foot ulcers. *Br Med J (Clin Res Ed)*. 1983;286(6377):1555–1557.

42. Knowles A, Boulton AJM. Use of Scotchcast boot to heal diabetic foot ulcers. Paper presented at: Proceedings of 5th European Conference of Advanced Wound Care, 1996; London.

43. Armstrong DG, Lavery LA, Kimbriel HR, et al. Activity Patterns of Persons with Diabetic Foot Ulceration: Persons with Active Ulceration May Not Adhere to a Standard Pressure Off-loading Regimen. *Diabetes Care*. 2003:In Press.

44. Armstrong DG, Short B, Nixon BP, Boulton AJM. Technique for Fabrication of an "Instant" Total Contact Cast for Treatment of Neuropathic Diabetic Foot Ulcers. *J Amer Podiatr Med Assn*. 2002;92:405–408.

45. Armstrong DG, Lavery LA, Wu SC, Boulton AJM. Evaluation of removable and irremovable cast walkers in the healing of diabetic foot wounds: a Randomized Controlled Trial. *Diabetes Care*. 2005;28:551–554.

46. Katz IA, Harlan A, Miranda-Palma B, et al. A Randomized Trial of Two Irremovable Off-loading Devices in the Management of Neuropathic Diabetic Foot Ulcers. *Diabetes Care*. 2005;28:555–559.

47. Armstrong DG, Liswood PL, Todd WF. The contralateral limb during total contact casting: a dynamic pressure and thermometric analysis. *J Amer Podiatr Med Assn*. 1995;85(12): 733–737.

25

Advances in Amputation and Prosthesis

*Laura A. Miller, Ph.D., C.P., Mark L. Edwards, M.H.P.E.,
C.P., and Todd A. Kuiken, Ph.D., M.D.*

DEMOGRAPHICS AND CAUSES

Amputation remains a leading source of disability despite advances in medicine, industry, and technology. About 130,000 lower limb amputations are performed each year, and peripheral vascular disease accounts for the vast majority of lower limb amputations.[1] Vascular diseases that led to amputation accounted for 82% of limb loss discharges with incidence increasing by 27% from 1988 to 1996. The incidence of amputations is not expected to subside anytime soon, for a number of reasons, including the aging of the population and the increased incidence of diabetes in the United States. As the population ages, the number of amputations in persons older than 65 is expected to double.[2] Diabetes creates the greatest risk of amputation, surpassing the risks created by both smoking and hypertension. Diabetes is related to 67% of all amputations.[3] The age-adjusted amputation rate for persons with diabetes is as high as 18 to 28 times more than that of persons without diabetes.[4]

Older studies have shown that patients with diabetes are at greater risk for a second amputation, with rates as high as 18% at two years and 45% at four years.[5] The second operation is shown by more recent studies to be a conversion to a more proximal amputation level in 9%, with amputation of the contralateral limb in 11%–20% of the general amputee population.[6-7]

Surgical

When amputation is necessary, a well-planned surgery will improve the potential for a positive prosthetic outcome. Though anterior, medial-lateral, and skew flaps are possible, the most common transtibial surgical technique in the United States uses a posterior flap of gastrocnemius to cover the distal end, with a fibula cut slightly shorter than the tibia and the anterior tibia beveled.[8-9] In the 1960s and 1970s, Jan Ertl proposed a new transtibial amputation technique. This technique utilized a tibiofibular synostosis to join the distal tibia and fibula. The main advantage proposed was that the limb would have distal end weight-bearing. Also, additional advantages were to seal the intermedullary system, prevent bony overgrowth, and stabilize the fibula. Although this technique has not gained wide use, there has been a recent revisiting of this technique with new variations including the addition of pins by some surgeons.[10-11]

Little research has been conducted to investigate alternative amputation techniques for transfemoral amputation. The most recent work is that by Gottshalk.[12-13] He recommends preservation of the adductor magnus and myodesis of the muscle to the residual femur to achieve maintenance of the femoral shaft axis close to normal, and then myoplasty of the hamstrings and quadriceps to the adductor magnus. This provides better muscular balance to the residual limb and assurance that there will be adequate soft tissue covering the end of the femur.

Perhaps the most innovative research in amputation surgery is direct skeletal attachment of prostheses or "osseointegration." Osseointegration has been proposed as a way to load the bone directly for weight-bearing and eliminate the majority of the socket. Osseointegration is a technique designed by P.I. Branemark[14-15] in Sweden to allow the bone surrounding an implanted device to grow to the exterior of the implant for optimal stability. When applied to limb prostheses, the surgical technique implants a rigid connector into the long axis of the amputated limb. This connector is implanted and the limb is allowed to heal for a period of months to allow the bone to attach to the titanium framework. The structure is then exposed and the skin surrounding the implant is fused to the bone (Figure 25–1). This expose portion of the implant is used to attach an external prosthesis (Figure 25–2). The advantages of this system are that the weight of the body is borne through the normal anatomical structures. This eliminates the need to weight-bear through soft-tissue and minimizes the socket component, which may be especially advantageous for those with short residual limbs or tissue that has difficulty with bearing weight (burns, scars, and the like).

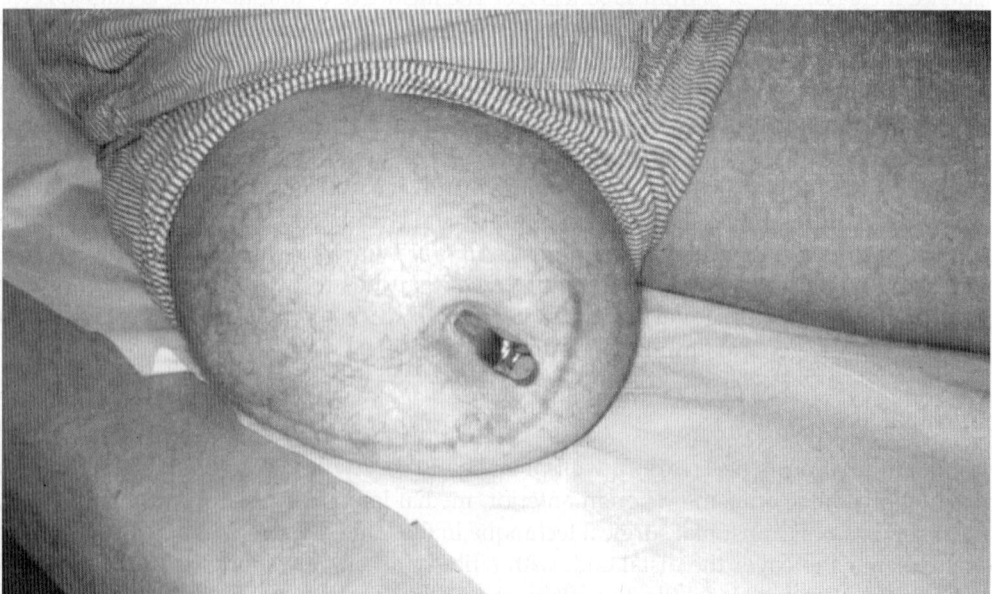

Figure 25-1. Photograph of osseointegration for a transfemoral amputation showing metal abutment exposed through skin. Photograph courtesy of R. Branemark.

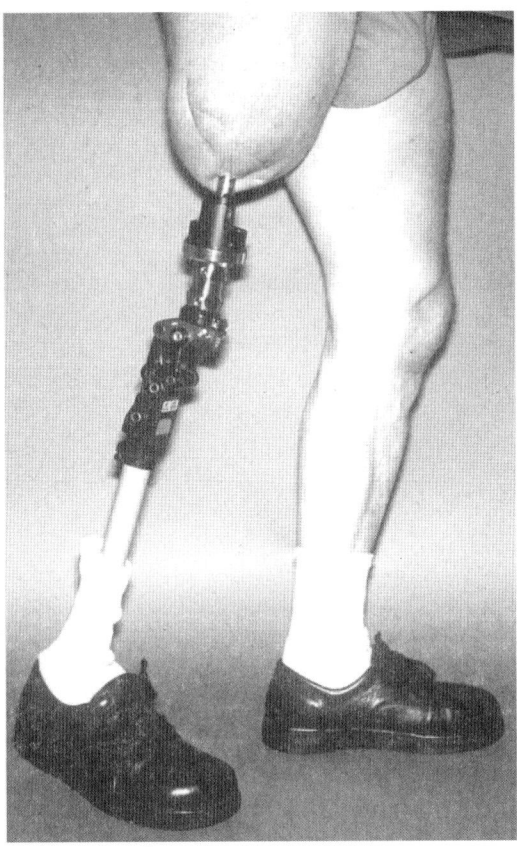

Figure 25-2. Transfemoral prosthesis connected to exposed osseointegrated metal attachment seen in Figure 25–1. Photograph courtesy of R. Branemark.

However, this technique requires additional surgeries and the chance of infection is always present. Results were presented in 1998 on 16 patients with an average follow-up of 4.7 years. Of these 16, 12 had experienced a superficial infection and six had experienced a deep infection with loosening in four. A total of seven had fixtures that loosened. Despite the concerns with infection, the authors state that "patient satisfaction was very high."[15] Vibrametry tests were also done and it was found that osseoper-ception was increased, which may help to improve function.

Postsurgical Management

Postsurgical management is extremely important to support a successful prosthetic outcome. The time felt to be necessary until initial fitting varies widely. Some surgeons and prosthetists work together to fit individuals with a postoperative prosthesis in the surgical theater. An adjustable and removable socket is fit onto the patient while anesthetized, and is mounted to a pylon and prosthetic foot (Figure 25–3). These systems may also be fit a few days or weeks following surgery. This type of treatment will require careful supervision to ensure that weight-bearing on the limb does no further damage. Properly fit, these systems have been found to reduce the healing time and complication rate.[16] More conservative treatments include removable rigid dressings (RRDs) that are fit three to five days

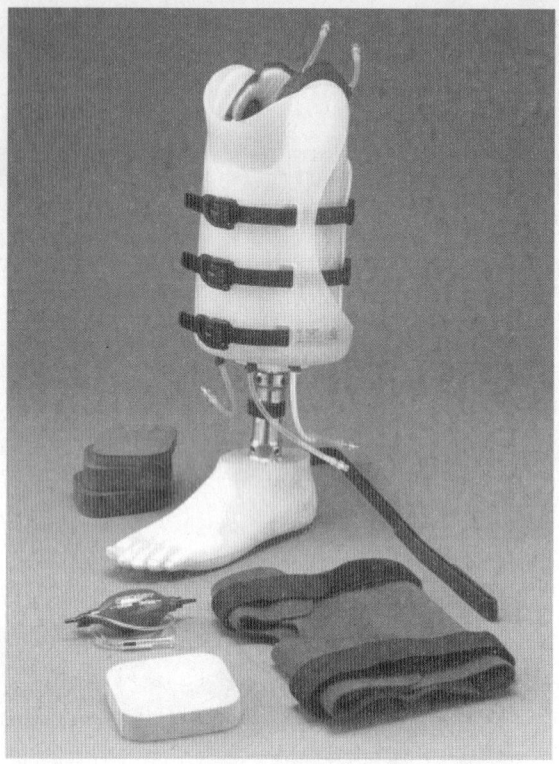

Figure 25-3. Immediate postoperative prosthesis (Air-Limb). Air bladders are used to compress the limb and distribute weight-bearing. Limited weight-bearing can begin a few days after surgery. Photograph courtesy of AirCast

after surgery when the postsurgical cast is removed.[17] This cast is removable for wound inspections, contains the limb to help reduce edema and prevent swelling, allows the addition of socks as volume is reduced to maintain compression, and is more reliable to don than traditional ace wraps. Because the RRD is rigid and can be worn at all times, it protects the limb during transfers and initial therapy. It can also be used to begin weight-bearing prior to prosthetic fitting.

Silicone liners, which are also used as an interface to a prosthetic socket, have been suggested as a postsurgical management tool.[18] The liner is rolled onto the limb and the tension in the liner helps reduce edema, similar to the RRD. Because the liners are more flexible, they may provide increased comfort. Since most of these liners are relatively thick, they may help protect the limb, but not as efficiently as the rigid dressing. The long-term efficacy of these liners as a postoperative treatment has not yet been determined.

Prosthetic Sockets and Interfaces

Traditionally, prostheses have been fabricated through a very hands-on, low-tech process. A cast of the amputee's residual limb is taken using plaster bandage. This cast is then filled with plaster, creating a positive mold of the limb. The prosthetist then modifies the positive mold by adding plaster in areas were relief is desired and removing plaster in areas where additional loading is desired. The socket is then fabricated over this positive mold.

This process of modification is learned though years of practical experience. Recent computer technology has influenced the fabrication and design of the sockets though the methods known as computer-aided design/computer-aided manufacturing (CAD/CAM), and finite element modeling (FEM). Computer control of the design and manufacturing processing has many potential advantages: files can be kept of patients to track changes over time, sockets can be easily replaced, sizes can be uniformly increased or decreased due to volume changes, and the modification process may become more standardized. As computers have become more affordable and adaptable, the use of CAD in design is becoming more common. Systems have been developed to take external scans of the residual limb. The digitized model is then modified on the computer through templates and the prosthetist.[19-20] The file can then be kept, and reused or compared to previous sockets over time. This digitized model can then be sent to a carver to create a modified positive model, which is then used to make the socket using conventional methods.

In the future, these CAD/CAM processes could take a scan of the limb (MRI or CT scan) and use known material properties of the tissue and bone to create an optimal loading pattern. This process is still only a research idea due to the challenges in modeling the nonlinear material properties of human tissue, the difficulty on obtaining scans, and the dynamic nature of weight-bearing on a socket. This process could reduce the time needed by the prosthetist and could potentially make fitting of prosthetic limbs by those with less training possible (e.g., in developing countries where a lack of trained personnel is a problem).

Changes have also taken place in the liner materials and the suspension technique. The liner is a layer of material that fits between the amputee's residual limb and the prosthetic socket. Traditional liners have been made from a foam comprised of expanded polyethelene. Newer socket liner materials are made of silicone, thermoplastic elastomers, and urethanes. All liners provide cushioning. This cushioning from the soft liner is especially beneficial for those with vascular deficiencies with associated neuropathy who may not perceive and accommodate with socks the change in socket fit due to limb volume change over the course of the day. The benefit of the newer liners is that the gel properties help reduce shear forces on the limb. These liner materials have been tested to understand how their material properties compare to human soft tissue. Depending on the characteristic tested, most of the liners have properties that compare human soft tissue.[21-23] Though many of the liners come in standards sizes, some of the new gel liners can be custom-made for individuals with atypical limbs.

Usually, the liner is rolled directly on the skin and then socks are worn over the liner to accommodate small volume changes. With this design of liner for transtibial amputees, the socket is often held on through a pin mounted into the liner at the distal end, and this pin engages a locking mechanism built into the end of the socket. Pushing a button on the side of the socket will release the mechanism. Or, instead of a pin, a sleeve can be worn over the socket and up onto the thigh section to seal the limb inside the socket. A one-way expulsion valve that lets air out, but not in, can be used to increase the suction suspension. A newer design of liner called the "ICEROSS Seal-In" liner (ÖSSUR) is now available and incorporates a hypobaric sealing membrane (HSM™) that adheres to the socket when the prosthesis is donned. This liner and membrane eliminate the need for either a pin or external sleeve. The "Seal-In" liner can be used on both transtibial and transfemoral levels of amputations (Figure 25–4).

A suction system has been further developed by Tec Industries (Otto Bock Healthcare) in the manufacture of the VASS system (Figure 25–5). The VASS (Vacuum Assisted Socket System) uses a spring-mounted shock in the support structure of the

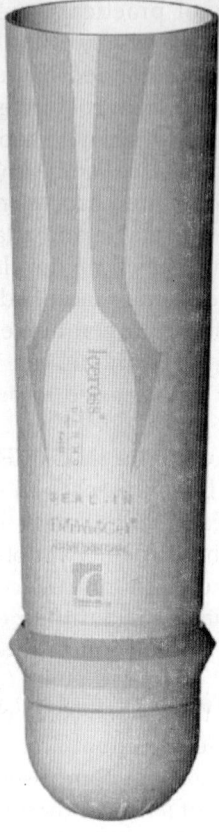

Figure 25-4. The "Seal-In" liner uses a hypobaric sealing membrane that adheres to the socket wall providing suspension without the use of a pin. Photograph courtesy of Össur North America.

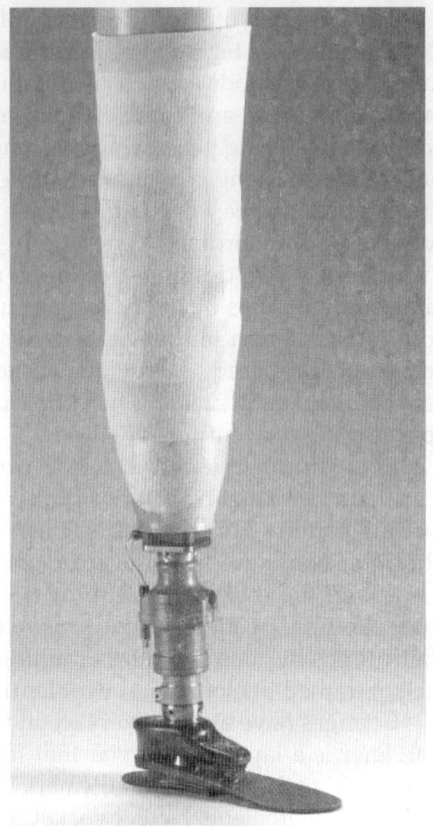

Figure 25-5. Harmony System. This system is connected to the socket to provide vacuum within the socket. The system is connected to a multiaxial dynamic response foot (Luxon Journey). Two carbon plates are connected through a layer of urethane to allow the multiaxial movement. Photograph courtesy of Otto Bock Healthcare

prosthesis to act as a pump. This pump generates a vacuum in the area around the residual limb. It is claimed that the vacuum alters the flow of fluid in the residual limb and helps reduce pistoning of the limb in the socket. The results of a study performed on 10 amputees using this system found that the residual limb gained an average of 3.7% in volume compared to an average loss of 6.5% of its volume without vacuum.[24] The authors also claim that the vacuum system helps encourage blood flow, and that by maintaining the volume, the socket fits more appropriately throughout the day, making it ideal for vascular amputees. However, the long-term effects of this system have not yet been determined.

Prosthetic Feet and Ankles

With the advent of many new materials, the number of prosthetic feet has burgeoned in the past 20 to 30 years. The Seattle Foot was the first dynamic response foot, designed to respond like a diving board, storing and releasing energy.[25] The Flexfoot, developed shortly thereafter, was based on similar ideas but was constructed out of carbon fiber technology taken from the defense and snow ski industries.[26] From these first feet, hundreds of designs are now available. The current trends in prosthetic feet are toward multiaxial capabilities simulating normal ankle motion. Some of the feet are designed to move though compression of foam or other rubber type materials (Figure 25–5), and others through joints and bumpers (Figure 25–6). Due to the increasing rates of obesity, there are also trends to design components that will be appropriate for individuals of larger mass. Most prosthetic components are rated to a mass of 100kg (220 pounds), though a limited number are warranted up to 150kg (350 pounds). Unfortunately, this may sometimes limit the componentry that can be fit to certain individuals.

Another component that has grown in popularity is the shock absorbing pylon (SAP). SAPs are designed to reduce the forces on the limb, in the same manner that shock absorbers reduce the transmitted forces in a car. Many of these shock absorbers also have rotational movement to reduce the shear forces on the limb (Figure 25–7), especially for activities such as golf where the body pivots over the limb. A recent study of these pylons has found that users who walk at faster speeds often prefer these components and a reduced transient force on the limb was measured for these users when using the SAP.[27]

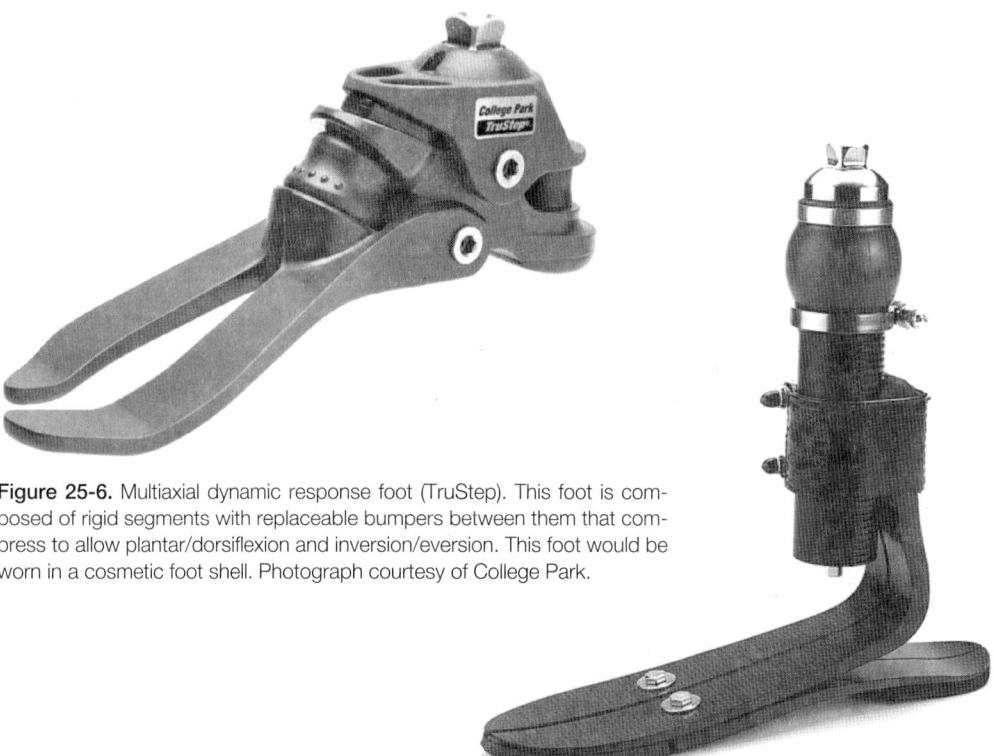

Figure 25-6. Multiaxial dynamic response foot (TruStep). This foot is composed of rigid segments with replaceable bumpers between them that compress to allow plantar/dorsiflexion and inversion/eversion. This foot would be worn in a cosmetic foot shell. Photograph courtesy of College Park.

Figure 25-7. Dynamic response foot with vertical shock pylon (Ceterus). The vertical shock pylon also allows rotation. This foot would be worn in a cosmetic foot shell. Photograph courtesy of Össur North America.

Prosthetic Knees

Prosthetic knees are designed and aligned to remain extended during the stance phase of gait when the foot is on the ground, and then bend during swing. Until recently, the most high-tech knees used hydraulic resistances to provide swing phase control, and some also proved stance phase control. High tech does not always mean new; one of the most commonly used hydraulic systems for highly active individuals, the Mauch SNS, has been available since the 1960s.[28] The hydraulic swing phase control provides a smoother gait for variable cadence ambulators because it prevents the knee from bending excessively at higher speeds. Stance phase control provides a higher amount of resistance to flexion. It is beneficial because it provides momentary stability if the user stubs the toe, and the higher friction allows the user to go down steps and curbs step-over-step.

The most recent designs have begun to utilize computer technology to assist in the control. The C-leg, produced by Otto Bock Health Care, has sensors in the knee and pylon to sense the point in time during the gait cycle (Figure 25–8). This information can be used to determine the friction levels in the knee. For example, the knee is held fixed until the sensors determine weight is on the toe of the foot and the user will be initiating swing phase. The computer can then control small motors to adjust valve settings, altering the ease of fluid flow through the system. Initial studies have found

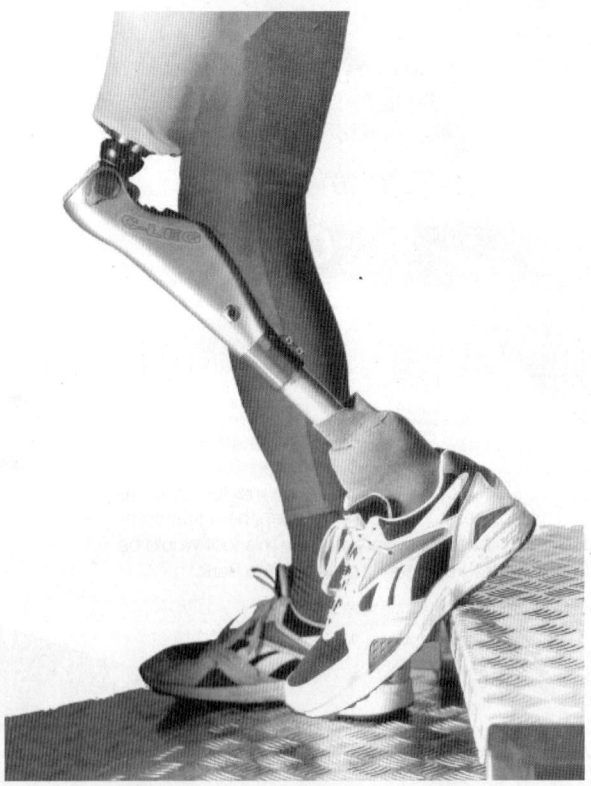

Figure 25-8. Computerized hydraulic prosthetic knee component (C-leg). The knee can be connected to a computer and adjusted for each patient. The sensors in the unit are designed to detect the phase in the step so that gait is optimized. The sensors also help detect when the user stubs the toe and requires the knee to lock, or when the user is going down stairs and requires different behavior. Photograph courtesy of Otto Bock Healthcare.

that this type of system can reduce the energy cost of ambulation.[29] Another new computerized knee component uses magnetorheological materials that change properties when exposed to a magnetic field.[30] The Rheo Knee from ÖSSUR (Figure 25–9) uses magnetic fields to vary the knee's resistance. Unlike existing hydraulic systems, magnetorheological resistance is activated only when the individual needs it most, thereby allowing more natural motion. The newest development in knee components is the Power Knee from ÖSSUR. It uses an advanced form of artificial intelligence to control the prosthesis. The electromechanical power source has the ability to replace muscle function around the knee joint. Where previously available prosthetic knee components have been limited to the imitation of excentric muscle work, the Power Knee also

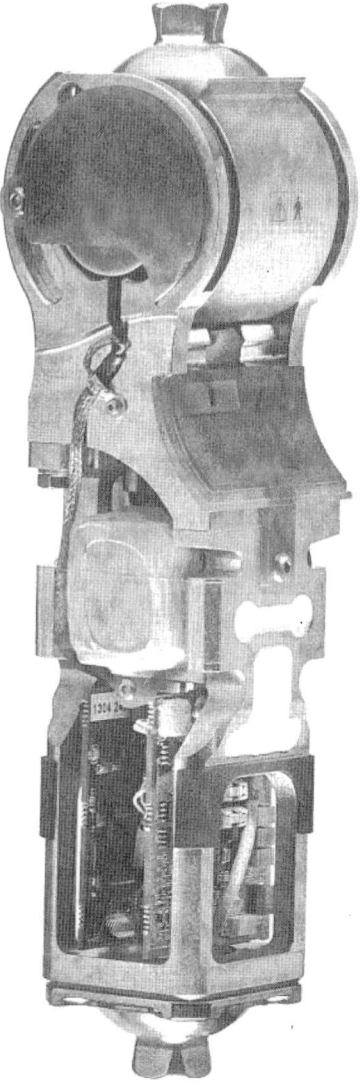

Figure 25-9. The Rheo Knee has magnetorheological materials that change properties when exposed to a magnetic field to make gait changes possible. Photograph courtesy of Össur North America.

replaces concentric muscle activity. The result is improved function such as allowing the user to ascend stairs and cover longer distances with significantly reduced effort.

Outcome Measurements and Documentation

With the pressure for outcome measurement in the health care field, there is also a desire to measure the success of various treatment modalities in prosthetics. There are multiple studies that compare various components (e.g., brands and types of knees, feet, sockets), but personal preferences often make biomechanical analyses difficult and consistent differences between components have not been found.[31]

Often, prior to amputation, there is an attempt to reconstruct or salvage the limb. Recent studies have shown that the two-year outcome results for reconstruction are similar to amputation.[32] However, limb salvage is not always the best alternative. Two editorials, by Nehler et al. and Sherman et al., discuss the considerations regarding limb salvage versus amputation. Nehler et al. examine the risks and considerations associated with revascularization for critical limb ischema, including patient morbidity and long-term function.[32] Sherman et al. describe issues related to traumatic injury that may affect the outcome of a limb reconstruction. These predictive factors include patient compliance to protocols, the type and severity of the fracture, the neurological status of the patient, and any other comorbidities.[33]

If limb reconstruction or salvage is not deemed appropriate, the potential for a successful outcome following amputation is high. With a well-healed residual limb, most amputees can expect an active lifestyle. If the need for amputation was due to long-term ulceration or a nonhealing fracture that limited function, the activity level may even increase following amputation. Pinzur et al. evaluated 95 patients with peripheral vascular insufficiency for the level of independent walking before amputation, and again at a minimum two-year follow-up using a seven-level functional grading system. Eight-four percent ambulated within one functional level of their pre-amputation status.[34] Geetzen presents a thorough 10-year review of the literature related to rehabilitation in amputation with issues related to functional outcomes, predictive factors, and phantom pain.[35]

Though many elderly vascular amputees may never run or participate in competitive sports, the accomplishments of amputee athletes highlights the successful possibilities of amputation. For example, as of April 2003, Marlon Shirley held the world record for the 100 m by a male with a transtibial amputation at 11.08s (from Disabled Sports USA at http://www.dsusa.org). That is only a few short steps behind the able-bodied time of 9.87s by Maurice Greene at the 2002 Sydney Olympics.

REFERENCES

1. Dillingham TR, Pezzin LE, MacKenzie EJ. Limb amputation and limb deficiency: Epidemiology and recent trends in the United States. *South Med J.* 2002;95(8):875–883.
2. Fletcher DD, Andrews KL, Hallett Jr JW, et al. Trends in rehabilitation after amputation for geriatric patients with vascular disease: Implications for future health resource allocation. *Arch Phys Med Rehabil.* 2002;83(10):1389–1393.
3. Resnick HE, Valsania P, Phillips CL. Diabetes mellitus and nontraumatic lower limb amputation in black and white Americans: The national health and nutrition examination survey epidemiologic follow-up study, 1971–1992. *Arch Intern Med.* 1999;159(20):2470–2475.

4. Trautner C, Haastert B, Giani G, et al. Amputations and diabetes: A case-control study. *Diabet Med.* 2002;19(1):35–40.

5. Fletcher DD, Andrews KL, Butters MA, et al. Rehabilitation of the geriatric vascular amputee patient: A population-based study. *Arch Phys Med Rehabil.* 2001;82(6):776–779.

6. Aulivola B, Hile CN, Hamdan AD, et al. Major lower limb amputation: Outcome of a modern series. *Arch Surg.* 2004;139(4):395–399; discussion 399.

7. Ebskov B, Josephsen P. Incidence of reamputation and death after gangrene of the lower limb. *Prosthet Orthot Int* 1980;4(2):77–80

8. Bowker JH, Goldberg B, Poonekar PD. Transtibial Amputation. In: Bowker JH, Michael JW, eds. *Atlas of Limb Prosthetics, 2nd edition.* Chicago: Mosby Year Book; 1992:429–452.

9. Persson B. Lower limb amputation. Part 1: Amputation methods—a 10 year literature review. *Prosthet Orthot Int.* 2001;25:7–213.

10. Drvaric DM, Kruger LM. Modified Ertl osteomyoplasty for terminal overgrowth in childhood limb deficiencies. *J Pediatr Orthop.* 2001;21:392–394.

11. Pinzur MS, Pinto MA, Schon LC, Smith DG. Controversies in amputation surgery. *Instr CourseLect.* 2003;52:445–451.

12. Gottschalk F. Transfemoral amputation. Biomechanics and surgery. *Clin Orthop.* 1999;361:15–22.

13. Gottschalk FA, Stills M. The biomechanics of trans-femoral amputation. *Prosthet Orthot Int.* 1994;18:12–17.

14. BrÂnemark R, BrÂnemark P-I, Rydevik B, Myers RR. Osseointegration in skeletal reconstruction and rehabilitation. *J Rehabil Res Dev.* 2001;38;175–182.

15. Gunterberg G, Branemark P-I, Branemark R, Bergh P, Rydevik B. Osseointegrated prosthesis in lower limb amputation: The development of a new concept. The 9th World Congress of the International Society for Prosthetics and Orthotics. Amsterdam, The Netherlands. June 1998. SY58.

16. Schon LC, Short KW, Soupiou O, Noll K, Rheinstein J. Benefits of early prosthetic management of transtibial amputees: a prospective clinical study of a prefabricated prosthesis. *Foot Ankle Int* 2002;23:509–514.

17. Wu Y, Keagy RD, Krick HJ, et al. An innovative removable rigid dressing technique for below-the-knee amputation. *J Bone Joint Surg.* 1979;61A:724–729.

18. Larsson G-U. Postoperative treatment with silicone liner in 176 ampuations. The 10th World Congress of the International Society for Prosthetics and Orthotics. Glasgow, UK. July, 2001. MO4.1.

19. Smith DG, Burgess EM. The use of CAD/CAM technology in prosthetics and orthotics—current clinical models and a view to the future. *J Rehabil Res Dev.* 2001;38:327–334.

20. Zachariah SG, Sanders JE. Interface mechanics in lower-limb external prosthetics: a review of finite element models. *IEEE Trans Rehabil Eng.* 1996;4:288–302.

21. Mak AF, Zhang M, Boone DA. State-of-the-art research in lower-limb prosthetic biomechanics-socket interface: a review. *J Rehabil Res Dev.* 2001;38:161–174.

22. Sanders JE, Greve JM, Mitchell SB, Zachariah SG. Material properties of commonly-used interface materials and their static coefficients of friction with skin and socks. *J Rehabil Res Dev.* 1998;35:161–176.

23. Covey SJ, Muonio J, Street GM. Flow constraint and loading rate effects on prosthetic liner material and human tissue mechanical response. *J Prosthet Orthot.* 2000;12:15–32.

24. Board WJ, Street GM, Caspers C. A comparison of trans-tibial amputee suction and vacuum socket conditions. *Prosthet Orthot Int.* 2001;25:202–209.

25. Hittenberger DA. The Seattle Foot. *Orthot Prosthet.* 1986;40:17–23.

26. Schuch CM. Dynamic alignment options for the flex-foot. *J Prosthet Orthot.* 1988;1:37–40.

27. Gard SA, Konz RJ. The effect of a shock-absorbing pylon on the gait of persons with unilateral transtibial amputation. *J Rehabil Res Dev* 2003;40:109–124.

28. Mauch HA. Stance control for above-knee artificial legs—design considerations in the S-N-S knee. *Bull Prosthet Res.* 1968;Fall:61–72.

29. Schmalz T, Blumentritt S, Jarasch R. Energy expenditure and biomechanical characteristics of lower limb amputee gait: the influence of prosthetic alignment and different prosthetic components. *Gait Posture*. 2002;16:255–263.

30. Herr H, Deffenbaugh B, Pratt G. A Hybrid Magnetorheological and Friction Brake for an External Knee Prosthesis. in Preparation Through the MIT Artificial Intelligence Laboratory 2001, http://www.ai.mit.edu/research/abstracts/abstracts2000/pdf/z-Herr1.pdf .

31. Bosse MJ, MacKenzie EJ, Kellam JF, et al. An analysis of outcomes of reconstruction or amputation after leg-threatening injuries. *N Engl J Med*. 2002;347:1924–1931.

32. Nehler MR, Hiatt WR, Taylor LM Jr. Is revascularization and limb salvage always the best treatment for critical limb ischemia? *J Vasc Surg*. 2003;37:704–708.

33. Sherman R. To reconstruct or not to reconstruct? *N Engl J Med*. 2002;347:1906–1907.

34. Pinzur MS, Littooy F, Daniels J, Arney C, Reddy NK, Graham G, et al. Multidisciplinary preoperative assessment and late function in dysvascular amputees. *Clin Orthop*. 1992; 281:239–243.

35. Geertzen JH, Martina JD, Rietman HS. Lower limb amputation. Part 2: Rehabilitation—a 10 year literature review. *Prosthet Orthot Int*. 2001;25:14–20.

Management of Complications after Revascularization

26

Management of Arterial Closure Device Complications

Christopher G. Carsten, III, M.D
and Eugene M. Langan, III, M.D.

The management of arterial access sites, whether for diagnostic or therapeutic procedures, can be handled in a number of clinically acceptable manners. This includes manual compression, the use of arterial closure devices, and possibly arterial cut-down for control and repair of the arterial access site. The development of arterial closure devices was designed to aid in more precise arterial hemostasis, limit postarterial access complications, and allow earlier postprocedure ambulation, as well as to facilitate earlier patient discharge.[1-2] The use of arterial closure devices can be both safe and effective at obtaining earlier arterial hemostasis.[3-4] Arterial closure devices also can be the etiology of arterial complications requiring appropriate, and at times, unique procedures for treatment.[5-11]

The rate of arterial complications after access for either peripheral or coronary angiography or intervention range from 1% to 6%.[12] Arterial complications increase in incidence with the use of larger caliber sheath sizes and/or the use of potent anticoagulation agents. Complications after arterial access with or without the use of a closure device include infection, arterial occlusion and/or dissection, pseudoaneurysms, bleeding, hematomas, and device malfunction with entrapment.

ARTERIAL INFECTIONS

Infections following the use of an arterial closure device can either be minimal, requiring observation and oral antibiotics, or major, necessitating arterial debridement and extraanatomical bypass. A postprocedural access groin infection after the use of an arterial closure device requires careful physical examination and a clinical decision to be made if it is a superficial or deep infection. A superficial cellulitis can be managed with oral antibiotics and observation, and if more severe, IV antibiotics may be possibly required.

A deeper more hostile infection can call for more aggressive treatment options including surgery (Figure 26–1). Arterial debridement with removal of the closure device remnants and patch angioplasty or bypass is often needed.[13] Depending on the

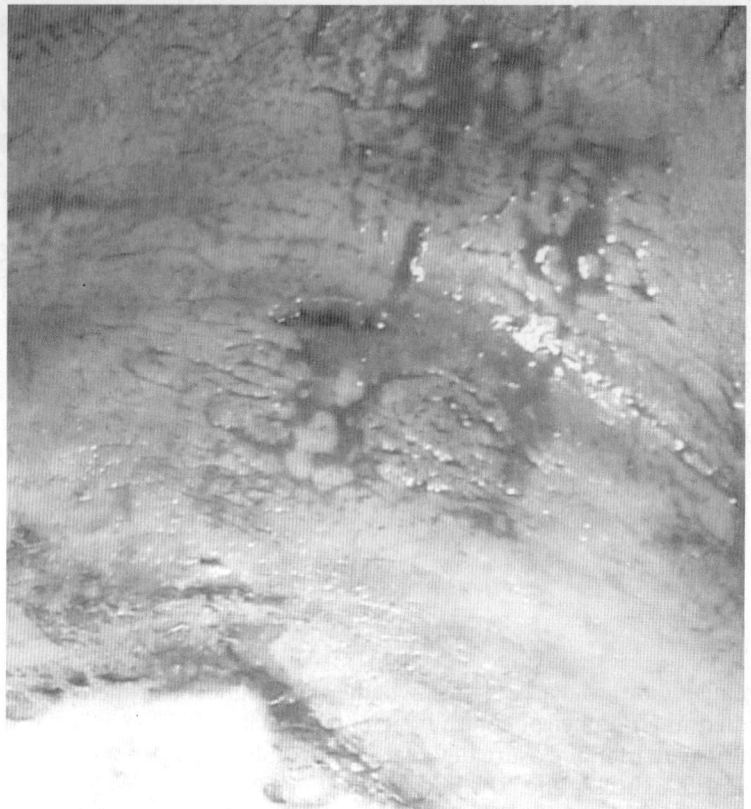

Figure 26-1. Deep hostile wound infection requiring surgical treatment.

amount of arterial destruction and hostile nature of the infection, an extraanatomic by-pass may be necessitated. An obtorator bypass is an excellent option, and allows adequate arterial and soft tissue debridement and arterial in-line flow in a noninfected tissue plane.[14] If only the anterior artery is involved with the infectious process, debridement and a vein patch repair is often adequate. In more aggressive infections involving more tissue planes, a muscle flap may be required to facilitate healing and add arterial protection. A sartorius muscle flap is an easy surgical option and can accomplish most clinical goals.

In an emergent situation, the patients' clinical status decides treatment options. At times, arterial debridement and ligation may be the only and best option, and treatment mimics that of an arterial trauma situation. Care should be taken to ensure that the profunda femoral artery remains in circulation to allow co-lateral flow to sustain the limb. Usually, the limb will remain viable and can undergo revascularization at a later date when the patient is more clinically stable and the infection is better controlled.

ARTERIAL OCCLUSION AND DISSECTION

Acute arterial occlusion and dissection after placement of an arterial closure device can be secondary to direct access site occlusion or an arterial flap and/or distal embolization[7,10]

(Figure 26–2). This complication can be treated with advanced endovascular techniques if recognized while still in the endovascular suite. This requires contralateral access and use of angioplasty/stenting and possibly thrombolysis to ensure a revascularized limb. Revascularization should not be significantly delayed to attempt endovascular salvage. In most situations, open surgical treatment is the best and safest option. It can be as simple as the release of an arterial stitch or as complicated as a bypass procedure for revascularization and limb salvage.

At the time of diagnosis, the patients' location dictates the first step in the treatment algorithm. If the patient is still in the endovascular suite and angiography can be immediately obtained, the treatment can be based on those findings. If the patient is not in the endovascular suite, a decision has to be made as to the best diagnostic tool. Physical exam may be all that is required or noninvasive imaging may add all the information to make the clinical decision. In some situations, an obligatory return to an angiography suite may be indicated to make the final diagnosis and establish a treatment plan.

Open surgical procedures to revascularize the limb depend on the findings at exploration. If a suture has caused the occlusion, it can be released, the arteriotomy primarily repaired, and circulation restored. An arterial flap may need an endarterectomy and patch angioplasty, or at times, a small interposition bypass graft. These procedures are best performed on an angiography-capable operating table to allow for completion angiography and possible angiography-directed thromboembolectomy. If the closure device has caused distal embolization, then thromboembolectomy may be all that is needed with primary arterial repair. In the rare instance that an arterial inflow or groinbased procedure cannot restore a viable limb, the clinical situation may demand a distal bypass for limb revascularization and salvage, and is based on angiographic findings.

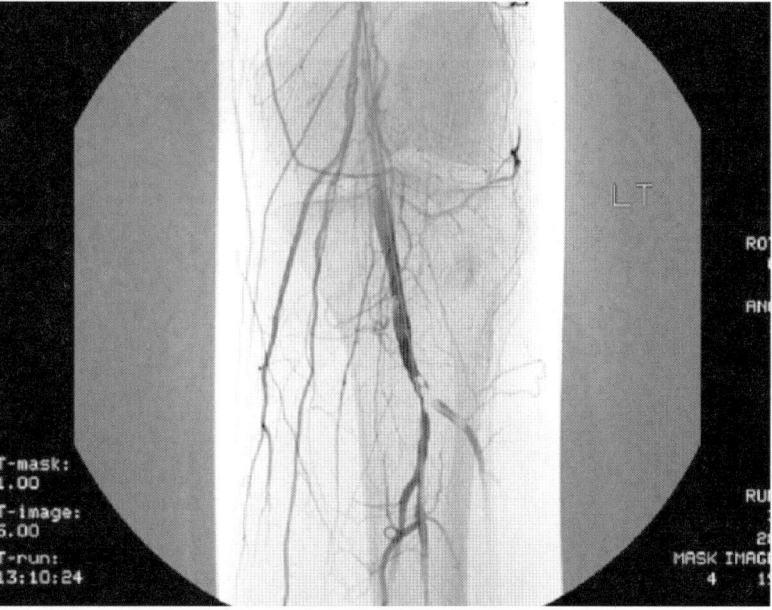

Figure 26-2. Popliteal and tibial thromboembolism after placement of arterial closure device.

PSEUDOANEURYSMS

One of the most common complications is the arterial access site pseudoaneurysm. The treatment of femoral artery pseudoaneurysms is usually nonsurgical. Some small pseudoaneurysms will thrombose without treatment, and can be managed with observation and repeat duplex scanning. Most pseudoaneurysms that require treatment can be managed with direct thrombin injection under duplex guidance[15] (Figure 26–3) or with duplex probe compression causing thrombosis.[16] In some instances, nonoperative management fails and direct surgical repair via a femoral cut-down is required with suture repair of the arteriotomy. The treatment of infected pseudoaneurysms is described above and managed as an infected artery.

BLEEDING

Arterial bleeding is more common following failed or incomplete direct arterial manual compression for arterial hemostasis than with the use of arterial closure devices. If there is acute arterial bleeding following the use of an arterial closure device, it should be considered a failure of the device. A second or different device can then be used to achieve hemostasis or manual compression can be attempted to gain hemostasis. Rarely, arterial cut-down will be needed to control postaccess arterial bleeding. The periprocedural use of anticoagulation increases the opportunity for postprocedure bleeding.

HEMATOMAS

Most hematomas can be managed nonoperatively with observation, serial hemaglobins, and possibly transfusion. Anticoagulation can be implicated as the etiology in many groin

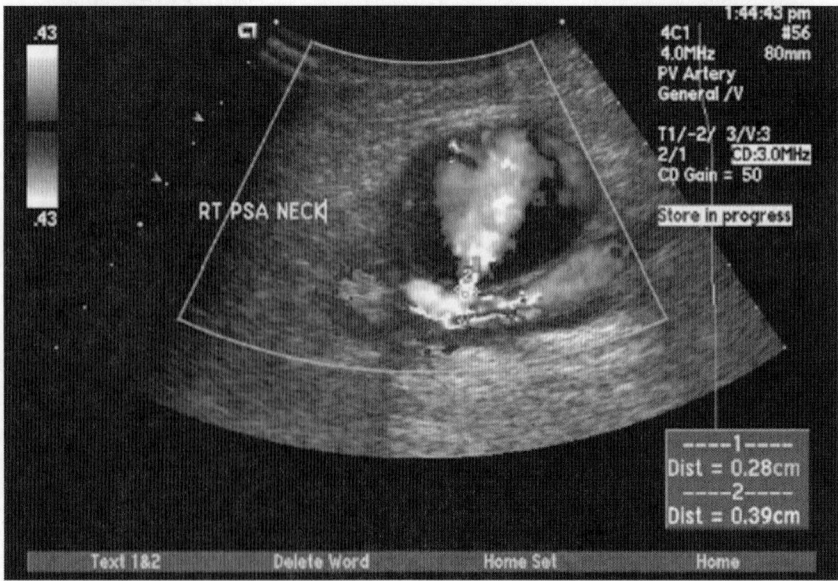

Figure 26-3. Common femoral artery pseudoaneurysm **A.** before and

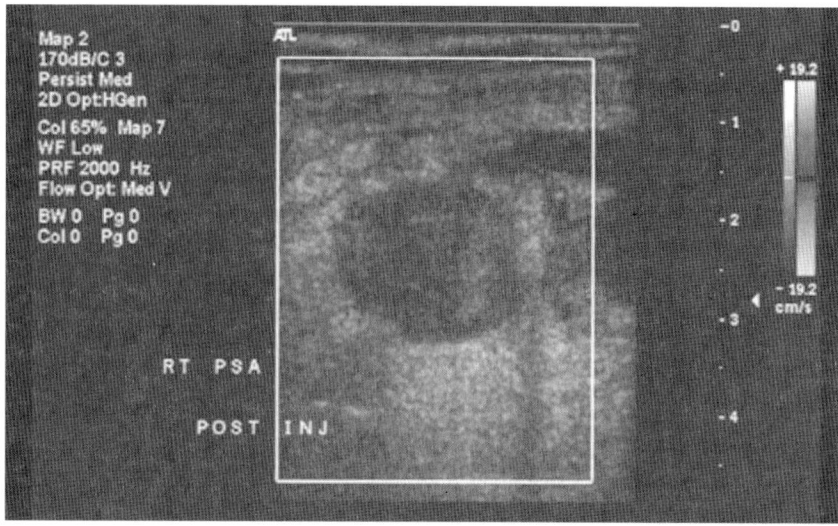

Figure 26-3. B. after thrombin injection.

and retroperitoneal hematomas, and if the patient becomes hemodynamically/clinically unstable, all anticoagulation should be discontinued immediately. Some large hematomas may require evacuation, and obviously, infected hematomas dictate open surgical care. Evacuation, debridement, and possible arterial repair may be forced as described above.

DEVICE MALFUNCTION/ENTRAPMENT

Arterial closure devices can malfunction, and at times, crack or break along the devices' shaft and become entrapped within the artery. This demands arterial cut-down, device removal, and arterial repair. There is no way to prevent this complication, and once the device is entrapped, open exposure is the only safe manner to remove it. It is our experience that this also increases the incidence of groin wound infection.

CONCLUSION

Complications of arterial access sites secondary to arterial closure devices can require innovative clinical thinking to allow the best diagnostic and treatment options to be employed. At times, nonoperative or endovascular techniques can be used, but in more complicated situations, open surgical repair is necessitated.

REFERENCES

1. Hoffer EK, Bloch RD. Percutaneous arterial closure devices. *J Vasc Interv Radiol.* 2003;14: 865–885.
2. Tron C, Koning R, Eltchaninoff H, et al. A randomized comparison of a percutaneous suture device versus manual compression for femoral artery hemostasis after PTCA. *J Interven Cardiol.* 2003;16:217–221.

3. Mackrell PJ, Kalbaugh CA, Langan EM III, et al. Can the Perclose suture-mediated closure system be used safely in patients undergoing diagnostic and therapeutic angiography to treat chronic lower extremity ischemia. *J Vasc Surg*. 2003;38:1305–1308.

4. Starnes WB, O'Donnell SD, Gillespie DL, et al. Percutaneous arterial closure in peripheral vascular disease: a retrospective randomized evaluation of the Perclose device. *J Vasc Surg*. 2003;38:263–271.

5. Chevalier B, Lancelin B, Koning R, et al. Effect of a closure device on complication rates in high-local-risk patients: results of a randomized multicenter trial. *Cathet Cardiovasc Intervent*. 2003;58:285–291.

6. Hollis HW Jr, Rehring TF. Femoral endarteritis associated with percutaneous suture closure: New technology, challenging complications. *J Vasc Surg*. 2003;38:83–57.

7. Nehler MR, Lawrence WA, Whitehill TA, Charette SD, Jones DN, Krupski WC. Iatrogenic vascular injuries from percutaneous vascular suturing devices. *J Vasc Surg*. 2001;33:943–947.

8. Toursarkissian B, Mejia A, Smilanich RP, et al. Changing pattern of access site complications with the use of percutaneous closure devices. *Vasc Surg*. 2001;35:203–206.

9. Nikolsky E, Mehran R, Halkin A, et al. Vascular complications associated with arteriotomy closure devices in patients undergoing percutaneous coronary procedures: a meta-analysis. *J Am Coll Cardiol Tech*. 2004;44:1200–1209.

10. Lewis-Carey MB, Kee ST. Complications of arterial closure devices. *Tech Vasc Interv Radiol*. 2003;6:103–106.

11. Sprouse LR II, Botta DM Jr., Hamilton IN Jr. The management of peripheral vascular complications associated with the use of percutaneous suture-mediated closure devices. *J Vasc Surg*. 2001;33:688–693.

12. Meyerson SL, Feldman T, Desai TR, et al. Angiographic access site complications in the era of arterial closure devices. *Vasc Endovasc Surg*. 2002;36:137–144.

13. Johanning JM, Franklin DP, Elmore JR, Han DC. Femoral artery infections associated with percutaneous arterial closure devices. *J Vasc Surg*. 2001;34:983–985.

14. Patel A, Taylor SM, Langan EM III, et al. Obturator bypass: a classic approach for the treatment of contemporary groin infection. *Am Surg*. 2002;68:653–659.

27

Treatment of Infected Bare Metal Stents: The Naked Truth about Problems Bugging Our Patients

Melissa E. Hogg, M.D. Melina R. Kibbe, M.D.

Percutaneous transluminal angioplasty (PTA) and endovascular stent placement in the peripheral vasculature is becoming a prevalent treatment option for atherosclerotic disease. For the past 20 years, endoluminal stenting has been frequently performed in the iliac arteries, central veins, and coronary and renal arteries. Indications for these procedures include claudication, rest pain, limb threatening ischemia, hemodialysis access stenosis, angina, and refractory hypertension and renal insufficiency secondary to renal artery stenosis (RAS). More recently, infra-inguinal, subclavian, and carotid stenting have gained popularity, and bare metal stents have been placed for treating peripheral vascular occlusive disease, subclavian steal, and carotid stenosis. According to the American Heart Association's Heart Disease and Stroke Statistics, about 1,285,000 angioplasty procedures were done according to coding data, and at least for coronary interventions, 84% of these also had stents placed at time of angioplasty.[1] The number of stents place annually, therefore, is now about one million per year: 615,000 coronary stents,[1] 400,000 peripheral arterial interventions,[2] and 40,000 interventions for RAS.[3] These procedures are performed by a range of specialties including interventional radiology, interventional cardiology, interventional neuroradiology, neurosurgeons, and vascular surgeons.

As the number of procedures increases, more complications will need to be addressed by surgical subspecialists. Problems and complications associated with these procedures include puncture site hematoma, vessel thrombosis, distal embolization, arterial dissection, arterial rupture, failure of stent expansion, stent displacement, stent malposition, neurologic injury, and pseudoaneurysm formation.[4-9] These complications reportedly occur approximately 9.9% of the time.[10] However, infection of bare metal stents in the peripheral vasculature is not well reported. The majority of reports in the literature on infectious complications following percutaneous stenting does not involve the stent site, but rather involves the common femoral artery access site. These access site complications are thought to be more common with prolonged indwelling catheters or following procedures associated with repeat ipsilateral punctures.[11] Albeit uncommon, previous case reports have demonstrated the morbidity and fatality associated with bare metal stent infections. Between 1991 and 2007, we identified nearly 40 case reports regarding infectious complications following placement of bare metal stents (Table 27–1).[2,4,7-10,12-41] If recognized early, treatment of bare metal stent infection can be initiated and have a dramatic effect on outcome, potentially preventing morbid and limb disfiguring operations.

RISK FACTORS

On review of published reports, risk factors for bare metal stent infection include breaks in sterile technique, occult glove perforation, inadequate skin preparation, less than ideal aseptic environment of angiographic suites, increased procedure time, puncture site hematoma formation, longer wires and catheters, passing wires or catheters through previously deployed stents, repeat puncture of the same arterial access site causing needle tract contamination, prolonged use or reuse of an indwelling catheter, deployment of multiple stents or multiple interventions on the same or adjacent sites, and other sources of coincident bacteremia.[7,9,24-27,29,34] Many of these are factors regarding periprocedural habits and can be avoided. Health care providers accustomed to the stringent sterile environment of an operating room should have no trouble avoiding these pitfalls. Improvements in technique regarding passing of wires and postoperative hematomas is another potential area of improvement. For patients with recurrent problems that need either repeat interventions or multiples stents, few alternatives exist to reusing indwelling catheters and reaccessing previous access sites. Both of these represent significant risk factors toward developing a stent infection. Therefore, when patients with stents develop bacteremia or sepsis from another source, it should raise a high index of suspicion for stent infection if the patient subsequently develops infectious symptoms at a later date.

PATHOPHYSIOLOGY

The natural history of stent infections involves progressive arterial destruction, stent thrombosis, septic embolization, pseudoaneurysm formation, arterial disruption, and hemorrhage.[42] The exact pathology of arteritis from angioplasty and stenting is not completely understood, but studies in animal models suggest that stents act as a nidus for colonization or a vector for iatrogenic introduction.[42-44] This occurs either through arterial trauma incurred during the procedure (i.e. denudation of the endothelial lining, which exposes the arterial media) or through the stent, which acts as a bacterial medium and sequesters bacteria beneath the struts and then spreads to the arterial wall. The resulting inflammation causes necrosis and destruction of the arterial wall, leading to pseudoaneurysm formation and subsequent rupture, which promotes platelet adherence and thrombus formation, and possibly septic emboli.[42]

Animal models suggest that poor stent incorporation predisposes the artery to infection and infection predisposes to stent thrombosis. Hearn et. al. and Thibodeaux et. al. suggested that poorly incorporated stent/artery complexes developed infections and intra-arterial stent infection affected arterial patency. They found that all thrombosed stents in their swine model were culture positive and only culture negative

TABLE 27-1. CASE REPORTS OF STENT INFECTIONS LISTED BY LOCATION

Author	Date	Vessel Location	Indication	Stent
CAROTID				
Kaviani[12]	2006	Left internal carotid artery	Amaurosis fugax	Precise[a]
SUBCLAVIAN				
Myles[2]	2000	Left subclavian artery	Coronary subclavian steal syndrome	Palmaz[a]
Malek[13]	2000	Left subclavian artery	Transient ischemic attack and vertebral-basilar insufficiency from subclavian steal	Palmaz and Multi-Link[b] SMART[a] and
Pruitt[7]	2002	Right subclavian artery and brachiocephalic artery	Tissue loss right index finger	Palmaz
Bates[14]	2005	Left subclavian artery	Coronary subclavian steal syndrome	Unknown
CORONARY				
Gunther[15]	1993	RCA	Local dissection and high grade stenosis	Palmaz-Schatz[c]
Leroy[16]	1996	LAD	Angina	Palmaz-Schatz
Bouchart[17]	1997	Left circumflex artery	Unstable angina	Palmaz-Schatz
Grewe[18]	1999	LAD	Angina	Micro stent[d]
Rensing[19]	2000	Obtuse marginal and RCA	Unstable angina	Unknown
Liu[20]	2003	LAD	Myocardial infarction	NIR[e]
Singh[21]	2005	LAD and RCA	Acute coronary syndrome	ProNOVA[f] and Prolink[f]
Alfonso[22]	2005	RCA	Angina from focal in-stent restenosis	Rapamycin-eluting
RENAL				
Rees[23]	1991	Renal artery	RAS and HTN	Palmaz
Deitch[24]	1998	Renal artery	Acute renal failure and renal artery occlusion	Unknown
Gordon[25]	1996	Left renal artery	RAS	Palmaz
DeMaioribus[26]	1998	Left renal artery	RAS and chronic renal insufficiency	Palmaz
Bukhari[27]	2000	Bilateral renal arteries	RAS and HTN	Palmaz
ILIAC				
Chalmers[28]	1993	Right CIA	Rest pain	Palmaz
Therasse[9]	1994	Left CIA, Right EIA	Tissue loss	Palmaz
Liu[4]	1995	Bilateral CIA	Claudication	Palmaz
Deiparine[29]	1996	Right CIA, Right CFA, Right EIA	Rest pain and tissue loss	Unknown
Weinberg[30]	1996	Bilateral CIA	Claudication	Palmaz
Hoffman[31]	1997	Right iliac artery	Claudication	Wallstent[e]
Bunt[32]	1997	Left EIA	Rest pain	Palmaz
Muller[33]	1998	Left CIA	Claudication	Palmaz
Schachtrupp[8]	1999	Left CIA	Claudication	Self-adjusting nitinol Angiomed[g]

(Continued on next page)

TABLE 27-1. CASE REPORTS OF STENT INFECTIONS LISTED BY LOCATION (Continued)

Author	Date	Vessel Location	Indication	Stent
Myles[2]	2000	Bilateral CIA and LAD	Claudication	Palmaz
Dosluoglu[34]	2001	Right EIA and right CIA	Claudication	Palmaz
Sternbergh[35]	2005	Right CIA	Rest pain	Unknown
Kondo[10]	2007	Left EIA	Rest pain	Palmaz
SFA				
Giannoukas[36]	1999	Left SFA, Left popliteal artery	Claudication	Strecker and Palmaz
Walton[37]	2003	Left SFA	Limb ischemia	Unknown
Hogg[38]	2007	Left SFA	Claudication	Unknown
Hogg[38]	2007	Bilateral SFA	Claudicatoon	Viabahn[h] and Protégé[i]
VEINS				
Quinn[39]	1992	Unknown vein	Venous stenosis preventing HD	Gianturco[i]
Guest[40]	1995	Right subclavian vein	Arm edema and trouble with HD	Wallstent
Naddour[41]	2000	Right inominate vein and right subclavian vein	Arm edema and pain	Wallstent
Dosluoglu[34]	2001	Left CIV	May-Thurners	Palmaz

Abbreviations: CFA = common femoral artery, CIA = common iliac artery, CIV = common iliac vein, EIA = external iliac artery, HD = hemodialysis, HTN = hypertension, LAD = left anterior descending, RAS = renal artery stenosis, RCA = right coronary artery, SFA = superficial femoral artery.

[a] Cordis Endovascular, New Brunswick, NJ, [b]Guidant/ACS, Santa Clara, CA, [c]Johnson & Johnson Interventional, Warren, NJ, [d]AVE, Santa Clara, CA, [e]Boston Scientific, Galway, Ireland, [f]Vascular Concepts, Bangalore, India, [g]C.R. Bard, Inc., Murray Hill, NJ, [h]W.L. Gore & Associates, Flagstaff, AZ, [i]ev3, Plymouth, MN, [j]Cook, Bloomington, IN.

arteries remained patent.[43,44] It appears that neointima formation may serve as a protective measure against infection and delayed bacterial challenge after arterial wall incorporation is less likely to result in infection. However, it cannot be definitively determined which occurs first; infection prohibiting incorporation or incorporation prohibiting infection.[42] In 18 of 21 infections reported by Dosluoglu et. al., the infections occurred immediately following the procedure. The other three cases of stent infection occurred after a second intervention through the stented artery several months after the original procedure.[34] A diseased human artery most likely does not form a protective neointima by three months following stent placement like a healthy swine artery. Therefore, stents may never be excluded completely.[42] Another contributing factor that prevents neointimal formation is poor apposition of the stent to the arterial wall or multiple overlapping stents covering a significant length of vessel.[10]

Animal models show that stents are more strongly associated with inflammation than angioplasty alone because they induce a greater degree of injury to the endothelium.[44] However, native arterial infections following PTA alone have been reported. One report is of a 39-year-old patient with claudication who underwent PTA of the right external iliac artery. The patient presented 14 days later with fever, malaise, sweats, hematuria, right iliac fossa pain, and a right inguinal bruit. He subsequently underwent ligation of the right external iliac artery and a femoral-femoral artery bypass secondary to an infection of the right external iliac artery.[45] Krupski et. al. reported on a 60-year-old patient with claudication who underwent PTA of the left common femoral artery that was complicated by a right common iliac artery dissection. He presented six days later with right foot pain, a swollen right knee, an erythematous rash over the entire right leg, malaise, anorexia, rigors, and a fever. He was treated with intravenous antibiotics for six weeks. On completion, his symptoms recurred, requiring arthroscopic intervention of his right knee and another course of antibiotics. He never underwent revascularization.[46] Hearn et. al. theorize that it is the arterial injury associated with balloon angioplasty that allows penetration of the bacteria into the arterial wall.[43] Whether it is due to a greater degree of endothelial damage, an indwelling foreign body acting as a nidus for infection, or both, is not completely understood. However, there are far more reports of infection following stent placement compared to percutaneous angioplasty alone.

ETIOLOGY

For each infection, several possible vectors of infection exist with no reliable method to determine the actual etiology. Kaviani et. al. report a case of a carotid-cutaneous fistula 20 months after placement of a Precise stent (Cordis Endovascular, New Brunswick, NJ) in the left internal carotid artery.[12] The patient underwent coiling of the left external carotid artery, resection of the left carotid bifurcation, and stent removal and reconstruction of the left internal carotid artery using a saphenous vein interposition graft and pectoralis myocutaneous flap. The authors postulate several potential etiologies: 1) transient bacteremia through the stent causing a superinfection; 2) contamination during the original procedure; 3) erosion of the stent into the dermis with paucity of coverage causing seeding and arteritis secondary to skin flora; and 4) unrecognized pseudoaneurysm at the bifurcation on completion of the original procedure.[12]

The most common scenarios leading to stent infection are contamination during intervention with the stent as a nidus or endothelial injury contributing to contamination, prolonged indwelling catheter from repeat interventions or thrombolysis, and bacteremia from another source of infection (Table 27–2). Giannoukas et. al. reports a case of a 52-year-old male who had stents placed for disabling claudication.[36]

TABLE 27-2. ETIOLOGY OF STENT INFECTION

Etiology of Bare Metal Stent Infection
Bacteremia at or after procedure[8,26,29,38,45]
Stent (foreign body) acting as a nidus for infection[4,28,30]
Recurrent sheath use or prolonged use of sheath[13,16,25]
Access site hematoma[2]
Multiple interventions at the same access site[2,9,18,34,38]
Local thrombolysis with indwelling catheter[34,36,38]
Sheath change over a wire between procedures[13]
Repeat intervention through stented artery[7,32,35]
Septic episode or other infectious source[9,10,13,14,24,27,34,37]
Frequent hemodialysis access punctures[40,41]
Diminished local immune response from drug-eluting stents[21,22]

He presented seven days later with intermittent claudication and was found to have thrombosis. He underwent 30 hours of thrombolysis and underwent placement of two additional stents. One day later, he developed erythema and skin blisters, and was subsequently diagnosed with a *Staphylococcus* infection. He was treated with antibiotics but his stent thrombosed within two days. He eventually underwent surgery and the entire segment of the stented artery was found to have purulence associated with an intramuscular abscess formation. Deitch et. al. reported a case of a 72-year-old woman who underwent percutaneous transluminal renal angioplasty and stenting who developed a methicillin-resistant *Staphylococcus aureus* (MRSA) line infection.[24] This other source of coincidental bacteremia subsequently led to an infected pseudoaneurysm of the renal artery and mycotic aneurysm of the aorta that required complex revascularization.[24]

DIAGNOSIS

Signs and Symptoms

Patients typically present with constitutional symptoms of fever, chills, malaise, pain, and petechiae. Frequently, they will also have symptoms that are specific to the location of their stent including: swelling, pain, and symptoms of arterial occlusion (i.e., claudication, angina, or tissue loss). Kondo et. al. reported on an 84-year-old male who presented four months after a successful left external iliac aneurysm stent for rest pain. He came to the emergency room later with fevers, melena, left lower extremity swelling, and left lower quadrant abdominal pain.[10] A computed tomography (CT) scan demonstrated a pseudoaneurysm at the site of stent placement. The patient underwent emergent operative exploration that revealed a stent fracture that had perforated the colon causing a fistula. Myles et. al. report a case of a 68-year-old male who underwent left subclavian artery stenting for subclavian steal causing angina due to stenosis proximal to a left internal mammary artery to left anterior descending graft.[2] The patient returned to the emergency room within 24 hours with fever, rigors, lethargy, delirium, and a harsh left supraclavicular bruit. CT and angiography revealed a luminal mass at the distal stent margin. The patient recovered without surgery and a prolonged course of intravenous antibiotics. However, more commonly, stent infection is often a diagnosis of exclusion after other sources of bacteremia are exhausted or inconclusive. We reported two cases of stent infections and performed a review the literature. Of 35 cases reported, 26 presented within three weeks of stent implantation.[38] Therefore, close follow-up within three weeks of the procedure and strict instructions to contact a physician should symptoms develop should help eliminate a delay in diagnosis, which is often reported with stent infections.

Imaging Modalities

The most frequently employed modalities to diagnose bare metal stent infections are CT scans, angiography, ultrasonograpy, and tagged white blood cell (WBC) scans. Additional tests may be necessary when addressing specific anatomy. For stent infections based on case reports in the literature, CT scans may show findings of pseudoaneurysm formation, abscess, thrombosis, or perivascular stranding.

Findings for vascular graft infection are similar: 1) thickened graft wall or increased perigraft soft tissue; 2) perigraft fluid; 3) anastomatic pseudoaneurysm; 4) graft occlusion; and 5) gas collection in the graft bed.[47,48] Based on these criteria, the sensitivity is > 90% but the specificity is only around 70–75%. A problem commonly encountered regarding the accuracy of CT scan in diagnosing stent infection is that the radiographic findings may not be apparent when the patient first presents with infectious symptoms. Dosluoglu et. al. and Pruitt et. al. recommend serial imaging to detect late aneurysmal formation.[7,34] In the former, seven initial CT scans did not show any evidence of an infection.[34] Liu et. al. report a case of a *Staphylococcus aureus* septicemia two days following placement of bilateral common iliac artery stents for disabling claudication.[4] The patient presented with right groin pain that radiated to the abdomen, fevers, chills, nausea, and vomiting. A CT done on admission was normal, showing no evidence of arterial restenosis or femoral artery pseudoaneurysm. Ten days later, the symptoms progressed and a repeat CT scan showed an ill-defined streaking adjacent to the aortic bifurcation. The infection failed to resolve with antibiotics alone and another CT scan 10 days later showed a 4 cm enhancing mass adjacent to the aortic bifurcation. Angiography confirmed pseudoaneurysm formation, and the patient underwent resection of an infected aortic bifurcation and right axillobifemoral bypass.[4]

WBC scans are rarely utilized. Dosluoglu et. al. reported on 21 cases of infected stents. Only four patients received WBC scans.[34] Common indications for the use of these scans found in the literature are evaluating epididymitis, bowel ischemia, appendicitis, cholecystitis, occult sepsis, inflammatory bowel disease, osteomyelitis, etc. Many studies exist examining the sensitivity and specificity of WBC scans to detect graft infections, but no studies have been published examining the accuracy of WBC scans for diagnosing bare metal stent infections. Prats et. al. evaluated the utility of WBC scan in 61 patients, 35 with suspected graft infection and 25 controls. They found both the sensitivity and specificity to be 100%.[48] Of note, CT scans were only used in 12 patients, six of whom had graft infections. The WBC scans diagnosed all six, whereas, the CT scan only diagnosed four.[48] Tronco et. al. looked at WBC scan in diagnosing vascular graft infection in 18 patients.[49] They found the sensitivity to be 100% and the specificity to be 50% with early images and 93% with early and late images. The reason for the low specificity is because vascular grafts frequently have false-positive results up to three months postoperatively. Endovascular stent infections tend to present earlier than graft infections, which raises concerns that WBC may have low specificity due to early postoperative false-positives. Liberatore et. al. studied 23 patients after placement of aortic endografts.[50] They found that WBC scintigraphy was unlikely to provide false-positives during the first month postoperatively.

Additional tests may be necessary and helpful when presented with specific anatomy. Leroy et. al. emphasized the need for prompt diagnosis by having a high index of suspicion in patients with unexplained bacteremia and infectious symptoms after cardiac catheterization.[16] He urges cardiologists to perform a catheterization or use transesophageal echo in search of an infected aneurysm early. A delay in diagnosis may have worsened the cardiac function in his patient who ultimately died secondary to a stent infection. Characteristic symptoms of bacteremia and common methods of visualizing arterial anatomy make for an easy diagnosis of stent infections in retrospect, but lack of familiarity and follow-up are the main problems with initially diagnosing stent infections. The absence of a definitive or immediate method to diagnose these infections often leads to a delay in diagnosis that can result in a catastrophic event.

TREATMENT

Antibiotic Therapy

The most common pathogen causing stent infections is *Staphylococcus aureus*. Of 35 reported cases of stent infection, 26 identified *Staphylococcus aureus* as the infecting organism.[38] Four of these were MRSA[24,34,36,37] and four grew another organism in addition to *Staphylococcus aureus*.[9,20,26,29] Other organisms include *Staphylococcus epidermis*,[9,34,35] *Escherichia coli*,[29] beta hemolytic *Streptococcus*,[12,25] *Pseudomonas aeruginosa*,[17] and *Staphylococcus simulans* and *capitis*.[20] These organisms were identified from a combination of operating room wound cultures and blood cultures. Intravenous antibiotics with Gram-positive coverage including first or second generation penicillins or cephalosporins are likely sufficient. Initiating therapy with vancomycin and a broad spectrum agent that covers Gram-positives and negatives such as fourth or fifth generation penicillins or third generation cephalosporins may be prudent until the culture speciates and sensitivities are identified. Treating stent infections with antibiotics alone, either for a lifetime or for a prolonged course similar to that utilized for endocarditis or osteomyelitis, would certainly be less morbid and technically challenging, but likely insufficient. There have been reports, some fatal and some successful, when this approach has been utilized.[2,19,23,25,39-41,46] Myles et. al. reviewed the literature concerning infected stents and found that 13 of 19 cases were treated with operative intervention with a resultant mortality of 31% (four of 13).[2] Of the remaining six cases treated with antibiotics alone, one patient died from septic shock, one required subsequent amputation due to pseudoaneurysm rupture, and two developed pseudoaneurysms while being monitored with serial scans.[2] Four of the 11 reports of stents not treated with surgical intervention were fatalities (Table 27–3). Five of the remaining seven patients developed sequelae of stent thrombosis and aneurysm formation. Therefore, even if no immediate surgical intervention is required, patients may eventually require an operation for complications of stent infection. Close follow-up and serial imaging is necessary.

Delayed Intervention

Almost every case study has a trial where intravenous antibiotics are utilized initially, either because a diagnosis has yet to be made, because all initial imaging was negative, because the patient was too sick to undergo an operation, or because the hope was that the infection would be treated with antibiotics alone (Table 27–4). For Depairine et. al., instability from sepsis prevented an operation initially.[29] Chalmers et. al. noted that delay in referral for definitive surgical intervention was a contributing factor for severity and progression of infectious complications.[28] DeMaioribus et. al. presented a case of septic emboli, arterial necrosis, and acute renal failure after placement of a Palmaz stent (Cordis, Miami Lakes, FL) in the left renal artery for chronic renal insufficiency and a 70% stenosis.[26] The patient ultimately required resection of the left renal artery and kidney with primary aortic closure. Given the morbidity of the procedure to remove infected stents, DeMaioribus et. al. did not advocate mandatory operation over

TABLE 27-3. STENT INFECTIONS SUCCESSFULLY TREATED MEDICALLY

Author	Date	Vessel Location	Organism	Medical Therapy	Complication
Rees[23]	1991	Renal artery	Unknown	Intravenous antibiotics*	Transient sepsis
Quinn[39]	1992	Unknown vein	Unknown	Not available	**Death**
Guest[40]	1995	Right subclavian vein	Staphylococcus aureus	9 weeks of antibiotics	Stent migration and thrombosis
Gordon[25]	1996	Left renal artery	Beta hemolytic Streptococcus	6 weeks intravenous and 6 months oral antibiotics	Pseudoaneurysm formation
Grewe[18]	1999	LAD	Staphylococcus aureus	Unknown	**Death**
Rensing[19]	2000	Obtuse marginal and right coronary artery vein graft	Staphylococcus aureus	6 weeks intravenous antibiotics	Abscess and thrombosed obtuse marginal artery
Naddour[41]	2000	Right inominate vein and right subclavian vein	Staphylococcus aureus	Intravenous antibiotics*	Arm swelling
Myles[2]	2000	Left subclavian artery	Staphylococcus aureus	6 weeks intravenous antibiotics then dicloxacillin indefinitely	Aneurysm formation
Myles[2]	2000	Bilateral CIA and atherectomy of LAD	Staphylococcus aureus	Intravenous antibiotics then oral antibiotics*	Aneurysm formation
Bukhari[27]	2000	Bilateral renal arteries	Unknown	Intravenous antibiotics*	**Death**
Alfonso[22]	2005	Right coronary artery	Staphylococcus aureus	Oral antibiotics switched to intravenous*	**Death**

Abbreviations: CIA = common iliac artery, LAD = left anterior descending
*Time course not given

the use of antibiotics alone, but rather felt every case required surgical evaluation and consideration if antibiotic therapy alone was unsuccessful.[26] Pruitt et. al. reported a case of a 74-year-old female who had undergone PTA and stenting of subclavian and brachiocephalic arteries for digital ischemia. This patient developed a mycotic aneurysm that subsequently ruptured the brachiocephalic artery. No aneurysm was seen on CT scan from the patient's first admission, so she was treated with antibiotics, but a subsequent CT scan showed a 5 cm x 3 cm mycotic pseudoaneurysm.[7] She was taken to the operating room and died during reconstruction attempts after cardiopulmonary bypass was initiated.

Surgical Intervention

Infected endovascular stents pose difficult management problems. Removal of all infected tissue and revascularization may be required. Treatment can be morbid and technically challenging. When possible, the use of autologous tissue is preferred. The use of homografts has recently gained popularity. However, when autologous conduit or homografts are not available, extra-anatomic reconstruction with prosthetic material is often required. Weinberg et. al. reports a case where a right axillo-bifemoral bypass with removal of infected stents was performed for infection of bilateral CIA stents.[30]

From a review of the literature, it is clear that prompt surgical intervention should be considered in all cases (Tables 27–3 to 27–5). Krupski et. al. included mycotic aneurysm, recurrent septic emboli, or persistent sepsis as indications for surgical management.[46] Pruitt et. al. proposed that the development of a pseudoaneurysm is an indication for operation.[7] Principles of operative intervention should include proximal and distal ligation of the infected vessel, removal of the infected artery and stent, irrigation and debridement of the surrounding infected tissue, and revascularization similar to that of infected vascular grafts.[16,17,45] Bouchart et. al. reported on a 38-year-old otherwise healthy male with unstable angina who underwent a short uneventful catheterization and stenting of his circumflex artery. The patient presented four days later with a stent infection diagnosed by CT scan. The patient underwent emergent operative exploration with cardiopulmonary bypass and cold blood cardioplegia, removal of stent, evacuation of purulent pericardial effusion, and ligation of circumflex artery.[17] This case illustrates the magnitude of interventions often required to treat stent infections.

Three of the cases listed in Table 27–4 did not undergo a complete removal of all of the infected stents, and in one case, this led to a fatality.[9] Hoffman et. al. describe a second trip to the operating room requiring complete excision of all infected stents and surrounding tissue.[31] After the debridement, the patient required an aorto-bifemoral bypass for revascularization. In another case, after surgery, the patient deteriorated, necessitating a reoperation for removal of a right common iliac artery stent that was left behind during the first operation.[29] Clearly, repair of the vessel is not sufficient. Removal of the source of infection is paramount. Like any problem, there are exceptions: patients not able to survive an operation; patients with coexisting medical problems that need to be addressed first; or refusal by the patient or surgeon to go to the operating room because of the magnitude of the operation required and high potential for mortality. Scenarios have been reported outside of those mentioned above where nonsurgical management has been successful, but in these individuals, close follow-up is mandatory.

PREVENTION

No consensus is available regarding the prophylactic use of antibiotics for arterial stent placement. Most case reports state that no antibiotics were given or it is not mentioned at all. Only two of the case reports reviewed explicitly discussed the use of prophylactic antibiotics prior to stent deployment.[10,27] Quinn et. al. reported a death from sepsis (one in a series of 19 patients) within 48 hours of stent placement using Gianturco stents (Cook Europe, Denmark) to treat stenosis in hemodialysis access sites.[9] He now advocates the use of prophylactic antibiotics for all stent procedures.

Given the low incidence of stent infection, a clinical trial would not be feasible to answer this question. The main argument against prophylaxis is that due to the low incidence of stent infection, the number needed to treat to prevent infection would be very high. The main argument for prophylaxis is that the complications from an infected stent can be fatal or require extensive surgery to treat. Furthermore, most of these infections occur from contamination at the time of procedure. This concept is not new. A randomized, prospective, double-blind study addressing antibiotic prophylaxis in vascular surgery was performed by Kaiser et. al. in 1978.[51] This showed graft infection in only 4/462 patients (0.87%). Given that no side effects occurred as a result of prophylactic antibiotics, and given the morbidity and mortality of graft infections, the authors recommended prophylaxis. Although the results were not statistically significant, all four infections occurred in the placebo group that did not receive antibiotics.

Some practitioners recommend selective antibiotic prophylaxis in the following instances: for stents in veins of hemodialysis access,[9,40] access site hematoma,[9] repeat arterial puncture,[9,34,36] patients with diabetes,[31] immunosuppressed patients,[31,34] patients with cirrhosis,[31] long catheterization or long indwelling sheaths,[13,34] or when the surgery required to remove the stent would be too morbid due to location.[41] Latham et. al. supported the use of prophylactic antibiotics for stent placement despite no concrete evidence from published studies.[52] Given that there is little harm and cost involved in prophylaxis, contamination typically occurs at the original operation, and surgical repair can be morbid, we recommend the use of prophylactic antibiotics prior to implantation of an endovascular stent.[7,22,24-27,29,30,32,39]

Angiography suite sterility,[53,54] prophylactic antibiotics during subsequent procedures, and patient education after implanting a foreign body are additional areas where health care providers can improve on this problem. Some institutions have developed task forces to determine the optimal environment for combined surgical and interventional procedures.[53] At our institution, we utilize a fully functional angiography suite with state-of-the-art fluoroscopic imaging in the rigid sterile environment of an operating room. Antibiotics should not only be administered at the time of the initial procedure, but also during subsequent procedures where the risk of transient bacteremia exists (i.e., colonoscopy, dental extraction, or repeat arterial access for subsequent procedures).[27,34,40] Although animal studies suggest at three months neointimal formation is accomplished, it is hard to correlate this finding to an older diseased human vessel.[42] Therefore, we recommend prophylaxis similar to patients with artificial valves. It is also prudent to advise patients to carry a card identifying their implants in order to increase awareness of peripheral arterial stents.[7]

TABLE 27-4. STENT INFECTIONS THAT FAILED MEDICAL THERAPY AND UNDERWENT SALVAGE SURGERY

Author	Date	Vessel Location	Organism	Medical Therapy	Surgical Therapy	Mortality
Chalmers[28]	1993	Right CIA	Staphylococcus aureus	Antibiotics and anticoagulation	Axillo-bi-profunda bypass	No
Therasse[9]	1994	Left CIA and right EIA	Staphylococcus aureus and Staphylococcus epidermidis	Broad spectrum antibiotics	Resection left iliac artery and femoral-femoral bypass Stents NOT removed.	Death
Liu[4]	1995	Bilateral CIA	Staphylococcus aureus	Intravenous antibiotics	Resection distal aorta and bilateral CFA with axillo-femoral and femoral-femoral bypass	No
Leroy[16]	1996	LAD	Pseudomonas aeruginosa	Broad spectrum antibiotics	Fatal cardiac arrest during cardiopulmonary bypass	Death
Weinberg[30]	1996	Bilateral CIA	Staphylococcus aureus	Antibiotics	Right axillo-bi-femoral bypass with removal of infected stents	No
Deiparine[29]	1996	Right CIA and Right CFA	Staphylococcus aureus and Escherichia coli	Broad spectrum antibiotics	All right stents and arteries resected EXCEPT right CIA; AKA	No
Hoffman[31]	1997	Right iliac artery	Staphylococcus aureus	Vancomycin	Right EIA ligated, stents NOT removed; AKA	No
DeMaioribus[26]	1998	Left renal artery	Staphylococcus aureus	Vancomycin	Resection renal artery and stent and nephrectomy with primary aortic closure	No
Malek[13]	2000	Left subclavian artery	Staphylococcus aureus	Nafcillin switched to broad spectrum antibiotics	Resection stented subclavian artery and autogenous arterial reconstruction	No

Author	Year	Location	Organism	Treatment	Procedure	Outcome
Dosluoglu[34]	2001	Left CIV	Staphylococcus epidermis	Intravenous antibiotics and anticoagulation	Abscess drainage, stent removal, oversewn iliac vein	No
Dosluoglu[34]	2001	Right EIA and Right CIA	MRSA	Vancomycin	IVC filter, axillo-bi-femoral bypass, small bowel resection, stent removal, and debridement	No
Pruitt[7]	2002	Right subclavian artery and brachiocephalic artery	Staphylococcus aureus	Vancomycin switched to nafcillin	Died in operating room during reconstruction attempts after cardiopulmonary bypass initiated	**Death**
Liu[20]	2003	LAD	Staphylococcus aureus, S. simulans, and S. capitis	Broad spectrum intravenous antibiotics switched to nafcillin for 20 days	Debridement with partial removal of stent. LIMA to LAD graft.	No
Singh[21]	2005	LAD and RCA	Staphylococcus aureus	4 weeks broad spectrum intravenous antibiotics	Resection of aneurysms; revascularization with LIMA and greater saphenous vein grafts	No

Abbreviations: AKA = above knee amputation, ARF = acute renal failure, CFA = common femoral artery, CIA = common iliac artery, CIV = common iliac vein, EIA = external iliac artery, IVC = inferior vena cava, LAD = left anterior descending, LIMA = left internal mammary artery, MRSA = methicillin resistant staphylococcus aureus, RCA = right coronary artery

TABLE 27-5. PRIMARY SURGICAL INTERVENTIONS

Author	Date	Vessel Location	Organism	Surgical Therapy	Mortality
Gunther[15]	1993	Right coronary artery	*Staphylococcus aureus*	Emergent operation for abscess drainage and revascularization	**Death**
Bunt[32]	1997	Left EIA	*Staphylococcus aureus*	AKA	No
Bouchart[17]	1997	Left circumflex artery	*Pseudomonas aeruginosa*	Removal of purulent pericardial effusion, circumflex artery, and stent	No
Deitch[24]	1998	Renal artery	MRSA	Axillo-bi-femoral bypass and aorto-renal bypass with excision of stent and renal aneurysm	No
Muller[33]	1998	Left CIA	*Staphylococcus aureus*	Removal of infected stent, resection of iliac artery, greater saphenous vein grafts for reconstruction, thromboendarterectomy with vein patch, and venous thrombectomy	No
Schachtrupp[8]	1999	Left CIA	*Staphylococcus aureus*	Laparotomy after cardiac arrest with evacuation of hematoma from arterial rupture	**Death**
Giannoukas[36]	1999	Left SFA, left popliteal artery	MRSA	Ligation and removal of left SFA and popliteal arteries, stent removal, abscess drainage, femoral-to-below-knee popliteal bypass with vein	No
Walton[37]	2003	Left SFA	MRSA	Drainage of abscess and PTFE removal. Removal of SFA and stents. Vein bypass.	No

Author	Year	Location	Organism	Treatment	Outcome
Sternbergh[35]	2005	Right CIA	Staphylococcus epidermis	Primary repair of caval fistula, removal infected stents, reconstruction with in situ superficial femoral vein conduit	No
Bates[14]	2005	Left subclavian artery	Staphylococcus aureus	Thromboembolectomy, left upper extremity amputation, and thoracotomy with subclavian stent removal.	**Death** a few weeks later from cardiac complications
Kaviani[12]	2006	Left ICA	Beta hemolytic Streptococcus	Resection of left carotid bifurcation, stent removal, and reconstruction of left ICA using a saphenous vein interposition graft and pectoralis myocutaneous flap	No
Kondo[10]	2007	Left EIA	MRSA	Pseudoaneurysm repair, ligation left CIA, debridement of infected tissue, and femoral-femoral bypass	**Death** a few weeks later from sepsis
Hogg[38]	2007	Left SFA	Staphylococcus aureus	Aorto-bi-iliac bypass with homograft, femoral-to-below-knee popliteal artery bypass with vein	No
Hogg[38]	2007	Bilateral SFA	Pseudomonas aeruginosa	Right femoral-to-anterior tibial artery bypass with vein	No

Abbreviations: AKA = above knee amputation, CIA = common iliac artery, EIA = external iliac artery, ICA = internal carotid artery, MRSA = methicillin resistant Staphylococcus aureus, PTFE = polytetra-fluoroethylene, SFA = superficial femoral artery

CONCLUSION

Infection of bare metal stents may be underestimated due to lack of recognition, underreporting, and widespread application through many different disciplinary specialties. With the increasing number of reports, as well as many cases that likely go undiscovered or unreported, greater awareness by health care personnel who perform endovascular interventions is required. It should not matter who performs PTA and/or stent placement as long as the basic principles of periprocedural sterility are followed. Prophylactic antibiotics should be administered in standard fashion. Patient education and postoperative surveillance should be routine with a high index of suspicion for potential stent infection when a patient presents with any infectious complaint. Medical cards with the type of implanted device should be given to the patient, and patients should be instructed to inform medical personnel of these devices prior to any future procedure that may cause transient bacteremia. Last, prompt surgical attention when a bare metal stent infection is diagnosed is mandatory to prevent further sequelae from the infection including sepsis, limb loss, and death.

REFERENCES

1. Rosamond W, Flegal K, Friday G, et. al. Heart disease and stroke statistics—2007 update: A report from the american heart association statistics committee and stroke statistics subcommittee. *Circulation*. 2007;115:e69–171.
2. Myles O, Thomas WJ, Daniels JT, Aronson N. Infected endovascular stents managed with medical therapy alone. *Catheter Cardiovasc Interv*. 2000;51:471–6.
3. Dworkin LD, Jamerson KA. Is renal artery stenting the correct treatment of renal artery stenosis? Case against angioplasty and stenting of atherosclerotic renal artery stenosis. *Circulation*. 2007;115:271–6;discussion 276.
4. Liu P, Dravid V, Freiman D, et. al. Persistent iliac endarteritis with pseudoaneurysm formation following balloon-expandable stent placement. *Cardiovasc Intervent Radiol*. 1995;18: 39–42.
5. Long AL, Page PE, Raynaud AC, et. al. Percutaneous iliac artery stent: Angiographic long-term follow-up. *Radiology*. 1991;180:771–8.
6. Palmaz JC, Laborde JC, Rivera FJ, et. al. Stenting of the iliac arteries with the palmaz stent: Experience from a multicenter trial. *Cardiovasc Intervent Radiol*. 1992;15:291–7.
7. Pruitt A, Dodson TF, Najibi S, et. al. Distal septic emboli and fatal brachiocephalic artery mycotic pseudoaneurysm as a complication of stenting. *J Vasc Surg*. 2002;36:625–8.
8. Schachtrupp A, Chalabi K, Fischer U, Herse B. Septic endarteritis and fatal iliac wall rupture after endovascular stenting of the common iliac artery. *Cardiovasc Surg*. 1999;7:183–6.
9. Therasse E, Soulez G, Cartier P, et. al. Infection with fatal outcome after endovascular metallic stent placement. *Radiology*. 1994;192:363–5.
10. Kondo Y, Muto A, Ando M, Nishibe T. Late infected pseudoaneurysm formation after uneventful iliac artery stent placement. *Ann Vasc Surg*. 2007;21:222–4.
11. McCready RA, Siderys H, Pittman JN, et. al. Septic complications after cardiac catheterization and percutaneous transluminal coronary angioplasty. *J Vasc Surg*. 1991;14:170–4.
12. Kaviani A, Ouriel K, Kashyap VS. Infected carotid pseudoaneurysm and carotid-cutaneous fistula as a late complication of carotid artery stenting. *J Vasc Surg*. 2006;43:379–82.
13. Malek AM, Higashida RT, Reilly LM, et. al. Subclavian arteritis and pseudoaneurysm formation secondary to stent infection. *Cardiovasc Intervent Radiol*. 2000;23:57–60.
14. Bates MC, Almehmi A. Fatal subclavian stent infection remote from implantation. *Catheter Cardiovasc Interv*. 2005;65:535–9.

15. Gunther HU, Strupp G, Volmar J, et. al. [coronary stent implantation: Infection and abscess with fatal outcome]. *Z Kardiol*. 1993;82:521–5.
16. Leroy O, Martin E, Prat A, et. al. Fatal infection of coronary stent implantation. *Cathet Cardiovasc Diagn*. 1996;39:168–70; discussion 171.
17. Bouchart F, Dubar A, Bessou JP, et. al. Pseudomonas aeruginosa coronary stent infection. *Ann Thorac Surg*. 1997;64:1810–3.
18. Grewe PH, Machraoui A, Deneke T, Muller KM. Suppurative pancarditis: A lethal complication of coronary stent implantation. *Heart*. 1999;81:559.
19. Rensing BJ, van Geuns RJ, Janssen M, et. al. Stentocarditis. *Circulation*. 2000;101:E188–90.
20. Liu JC, Cziperle DJ, Kleinman B, Loeb H. Coronary abscess: A complication of stenting. *Catheter Cardiovasc Interv*. 2003;58:69–71.
21. Singh H, Singh C, Aggarwal N, et. al. Mycotic aneurysm of left anterior descending artery after sirolimus-eluting stent implantation: A case report. *Catheter Cardiovasc Interv*. 2005;65: 282–5.
22. Alfonso F, Moreno R, Vergas J. Fatal infection after rapamycin eluting coronary stent implantation. *Heart*. 2005;91:e51.
23. Rees CR, Palmaz JC, Becker GJ, et. al. Palmaz stent in atherosclerotic stenoses involving the ostia of the renal arteries: Preliminary report of a multicenter study. *Radiology*. 1991;181: 507–14.
24. Deitch JS, Hansen KJ, Regan JD, et. al. Infected renal artery pseudoaneurysm and mycotic aortic aneurysm after percutaneous transluminal renal artery angioplasty and stent placement in a patient with a solitary kidney. *J Vasc Surg*. 1998;28:340–4.
25. Gordon GI, Vogelzang RL, Curry RH, et. al. Endovascular infection after renal artery stent placement. *J Vasc Interv Radiol*. 1996;7:669–72.
26. DeMaioribus CA, Anderson CA, Popham SS, et. al. Mycotic renal artery degeneration and systemic sepsis caused by infected renal artery stent. *J Vasc Surg*. 1998;28:547–50.
27. Bukhari RH, Muck PE, Schlueter FJ, et. al. Bilateral renal artery stent infection and pseudoaneurysm formation. *J Vasc Interv Radiol*. 2000;11:337–41.
28. Chalmers N, Eadington DW, Gandanhamo D, et. al. Case report: Infected false aneurysm at the site of an iliac stent. *Br J Radiol*. 1993;66:946–8.
29. Deiparine MK, Ballard JL, Taylor FC, Chase DR. Endovascular stent infection. *J Vasc Surg*. 1996;23:529–33.
30. Weinberg DJ, Cronin DW, Baker AG, Jr. Infected iliac pseudoaneurysm after uncomplicated percutaneous balloon angioplasty and (palmaz) stent insertion: A case report and literature review. *J Vasc Surg*. 1996;23:162–6.
31. Hoffman AI, Murphy TP. Septic arteritis causing iliac artery rupture and aneurysmal transformation of the distal aorta after iliac artery stent placement. *J Vasc Interv Radiol*. 1997;8:215–9.
32. Bunt TJ, Gill HK, Smith DC, Taylor FC. Infection of a chronically implanted iliac artery stent. *Ann Vasc Surg*. 1997;11:529–32.
33. Muller G, Stockmann H, Markert U, Heise S. [the infected arterial stent]. *Chirurg*. 1998;69:872–6.
34. Dosluoglu HH, Curl GR, Doerr RJ, et. al. Stent-related iliac artery and iliac vein infections: Two unreported presentations and review of the literature. *J Endovasc Ther*. 2001;8:202–9.
35. Sternbergh WC, 3rd, Money SR. Iliac artery stent infection treated with superficial femoral vein. *J Vasc Surg*. 2005;41:348.
36. Giannoukas DD, Tsetis DK, Touloupakis E, et. al. Suppurative bacterial endarteritis after percutaneous transluminal angioplasty, stenting and thrombolysis for femoropopliteal arterial occlusive disease. *Eur J Vasc Endovasc Surg*. 1999;18:455–7.
37. Walton KB, Hudenko K, D'Ayala M, Toursarkissian B. Aneurysmal degeneration of the superficial femoral artery following stenting: An uncommon infectious complication. *Ann Vasc Surg*. 2003;17:445–8.
38. Hogg M, Peterson B, Pearce W, et. al. Bare metal stent infections: Case report and review of the literature. *J Vasc Surg*. 2007;46:813–20.

39. Quinn SF, Schuman ES, Hall L, et. al. Venous stenoses in patients who undergo hemodialysis: Treatment with self-expandable endovascular stents. *Radiology*. 1992;183:499–504.
40. Guest SS, Kirsch CM, Baxter R, et. al. Infection of a subclavian venous stent in a hemodialysis patient. *Am J Kidney Dis*. 1995;26:377–80.
41. Naddour F, Yount RD, Jr., Quintal RE. Successful conservative treatment of an infected central venous stent. *Catheter Cardiovasc Interv*. 2000;51:196–8.
42. Paget DS, Bukhari RH, Zayyat EJ, et. al. Infectibility of endovascular stents following antibiotic prophylaxis or after arterial wall incorporation. *Am J Surg*. 1999;178:219–24.
43. Hearn AT, James KV, Lohr JM, et. al. Endovascular stent infection with delayed bacterial challenge. *Am J Surg*. 1997;174:157–9.
44. Thibodeaux LC, James KV, Lohr JM, et. al. Infection of endovascular stents in a swine model. *Am J Surg*. 1996;172:151–4.
45. Cooper JC, Woods DA, Spencer P, Procter AE. The development of an infected false aneurysm following iliac angioplasty. *Br J Radiol*. 1991;64:759–60.
46. Krupski WC, Pogany A, Effeney DJ. Septic endarteritis after percutaneous transluminal angioplasty. *Surgery*. 1985;98:359–62.
47. Johnson KK, Russ PD, Bair JH, Friefeld GD. Diagnosis of synthetic vascular graft infection: Comparison of ct and gallium scans. *AJR Am J Roentgenol*. 1990;154:405–9.
48. Prats E, Banzo J, Abos MD, et. al. Diagnosis of prosthetic vascular graft infection by technetium-99m-hmpao-labeled leukocytes. *J Nucl Med*. 1994;35:1303–7.
49. Tronco GG, Love C, Rini JN, et. al. Diagnosing prosthetic vascular graft infection with the antigranulocyte antibody 99mtc-fanolesomab. *Nucl Med Commun*. 2007;28:297–300.
50. Liberatore M, Misuraca M, Calandri E, et. al. White blood cell scintigraphy in the diagnosis of infection of endovascular prostheses within the first month after implantation. *Med Sci Monit*. 2006;12:MT5–9.
51. Kaiser AB, Clayson KR, Mulherin JL, Jr, et. al. Antibiotic prophylaxis in vascular surgery. *Ann Surg*. 1978;188:283–9.
52. Latham JA, Irvine A. Infection of endovascular stents: An uncommon but important complication. *Cardiovasc Surg*. 1999;7:179–82.
53. Katzen BT, Becker GJ, Mascioli CA, et. al. Creation of a modified angiography (endovascular) suite for transluminal endograft placement and combined interventional-surgical procedures. *J Vasc Interv Radiol*. 1996;7:161–7.
54. Joffre F, Otal P, Janne d'Othee B. Plea for a "Surgical conscience" In the interventional radiology suite. *Cardiovasc Intervent Radiol*. 1998;21:445–7.

28

Treatment of Atheroembolism with Intra-Arterial Injection of Prostaglandin E1

Juan C. Parodi, M.D. Sheela T. Patel, M.D.
Federico E. Parodi, M.D. Maria G. Uberti, M.D.

The atheromatous embolization syndrome is a common disorder, yet the disease remains underdetected, underdiagnosed, and undertreated. The diagnosis is made postmortem in two-thirds of cases. It may present with a distinct clinical syndrome that is associated with a markedly high morbidity and mortality. Moreover, atheroembolism is a confusing entity to many physicians because it is known by many different names: cholesterol embolization, cholesterol crystal embolization, blue toe syndrome, purple toe syndrome, trash foot, and pseudovasculitis.

Atheroembolism results from distal showering of atheromatous debris from ulcerated or aneurysmatic lesions into the systemic arterial circulation. Typically, the aortas of patients with this syndrome are ulcerated, crystal laden, or lined by friable atheromatous debris. Embolic debris consists of thrombus, platelet fibrin material, and/or cholesterol crystals that dislodge and produce ischemia in various distal arterial beds. It is becoming more common as endovascular procedures grow in indications and candidates. Its protean clinical manifestations are apparent across all specialties, making the differential diagnosis broad and the diagnosis difficult. Atheroembolism has, therefore, been termed the "great masquerader."[1] Symptoms may be absent, go unrecognized, or mimic other diseases. The syndrome can present itself as a spectrum of diseases ranging from an isolated tissue infarction to systemic multiorgan failure. The clinical manifestations depend on the number of organs affected, the composition of the emboli, and quantity of the embolus expelled from the atherosclerotic plaque. The end result is ischemic injury in the skin, kidneys, brain, myocardium, and intestine, but any organ distal to the culprit lesion may be affected. An isolated microembolus of platelets and fibrin can be lysed by the body's own enzymes and remain clinically asymptomatic. As only a minority of patients sustaining cholesterol emboli are recognized clinically, the actual incidence remains uncertain. In the review by Fine et. al. of

221 cases of biopsy-proven cholesterol embolism, a clinical diagnosis or suspicion before histologic diagnosis was reported in only 58 patients (26%).[2] Once atheroembolism has occurred, therapy involves two major strategies: treating the end organ that is the recipient of the embolization, and preventing further embolization. Therefore, it is critical for clinicians to have a high index of suspicion and to recognize the risk factors that precipitate or perpetuate this syndrome.

HISTORICAL PERSPECTIVE

Dahlerup and Fenger were the first to describe the embolization of atheromatous material in their autopsy report of the famous Danish sculptor Bertel Thorvaldsen in 1844. However, Panum, a German pathologist, is usually credited for publishing the first description of the phenomenon in 1862 in a report of a fatal coronary artery occlusion by an atheromatous plaque. Little if any attention was paid to atheroembolism for nearly a century until Flory described an autopsy study of embolization from the aorta to the downstream vessels in 1945. Flory reported a 4.4% incidence of atheroembolism in consecutive autopsy cases. Among 267 consecutive autopsies, he observed nine instances of cholesterol embolization: none in 63 cases in which aortic plaque ulceration was absent, two instances in 147 (1.4%) cases with moderate aortic plaque erosion, and seven instances in 57 (12.8%) in dark cases with severe aortic plaque ulceration. Flory precisely defined cholesterol crystal embolization as the occlusion of arterioles with an external diameter ranging from 55 to 900 micrometers by cholesterol crystals that had dislodged from eroded atheromatous plaques located upstream. Flory tested this hypothesis by dissolving and injecting atherosclerotic plaque into rabbit ear veins and produced analogous embolic lesions in rabbit pulmonary tissue.[3] Since this seminal paper, it has become clear that the risk of atheroembolism is directly related to the severity of aortic atherosclerosis.

In 1952, Venet and Friedfeld were the first to document atheromatous embolization to the lower extremity in a patient undergoing embolectomy for acute femoral artery occlusion.[4] However, it was not until 1959 in the report by Hoye et. al. that cholesterol emboli to the skin of the lower extremity was first documented.[5]

PATHOPHYSIOLOGY

Atherosclerotic plaques consist of a fibrous cap under which are macrophages, necrotic debris, and cholesterol crystals. The plaques at the highest risk of rupture are those with a thin fibrous cap surrounding a large lipid-rich core. The determinants of plaque vulnerability include ratio of lipid core to fibrous cap and a balance between metalloproteinases and their inhibitors. The level of derangement depends on the composition of the emboli and the end-organ response to the embolic atheroma. The initial event may be spontaneous (ie., due to plaque rupture), medication induced (ie, after using thrombolytics or anticoagulation), or most often, following vascular endothelial trauma (either surgical or percutaneous injury). An embolus composed of fibrin and platelet thrombus may be readily lysed by the thrombolytic pathway. When the emboli composition is high in cholesterol, the lightweight and hydrophobic cholesterol crystals travel through the circulation until their passage becomes impeded by small vessels. Cholesterol crystals are generally too small to occlude the artery in which they lodge, but induce an endothelial inflammatory reaction with polymorphonuclear and eosinophilic infiltration. A local inflammatory response secondary to ischemia and reperfusion also initiates a series of events that lead to further tissue damage. Atheroembolism creates a vicious cycle that perpetuates the ischemic process. Activation of leukocytes and complement initiate tissue damage. Platelet activation and release of 5-hydroxy-tryptamine and thromboxane promote intravascular coagulation, which further aggravate the initial insult. Changes in the microcirculation develop progressively during the ischemic period. Cessation of blood flow leads to capillary endothelial cellular edema, which leads to a complete disjunction of endothelial cells. Cellular migration into the extravascular space can be observed. As the duration of ischemia increases, increased vascular permeability and progressive interstitial edema are observed.[6] After two to four weeks, a more chronic inflammatory infiltrate is seen. Cholesterol crystals become embedded in multinuclear giant cells and smooth muscle cells. Endothelial proliferation and fibrous tissue can be found surrounding the crystals, ultimately leading to luminal obliteration and a panarteritis. The crystals are resistant to breakdown by macrophages and have been shown to persist in tissue for up to nine months. Although standard histologic techniques dissolve the birefringent cholesterol crystals, biconvex needle-shaped clefts ("ghosts") remain.

EPIDEMIOLOGY AND INCIDENCE

The atheroembolism syndrome is noted more often in men than women (4:1 ratio) and in whites than African Americans (30:1 ratio).[7] The syndrome may be underdiagnosed secondary to the difficulty of assessing livedo and purple discoloration in dark skin.[8] The typical candidate is a male in his 60s and a smoker, and suffering from various manifestations of atherosclerosis.

The incidence of cholesterol embolism syndrome varies according to population characteristics, diagnostic criteria, and study design. Among unselected series of autopsy studies, the incidence of cholesterol crystal embolism ranges from 0.2% to 2.4%. However, autopsy studies performed in selected populations of patients with atherosclerosis and those who have undergone aortic manipulation have reported a greater prevalence of cholesterol crystal embolism, ranging from 10% to 80%.[9,10] Shah and Leather from the Albany Medical Center Vascular Service found that distal peripheral microembolization comprised 2.5% of the total vascular cases from 1978 to 1995.[11] Fine and colleagues demonstrated that 20% of patients who had atheroembolic events recently had a vascular radiologic procedure.[2] Autopsy studies performed on patients after resection of abdominal aortic aneurysms show evidence of cholesterol emboli in as many as 77%.[10] Estimates of the incidence of atheroembolism after vascular procedures have ranged from 0.15% in clinical studies to 30% in pathologic series.[12,13] The prevalence of cholesterol embolization in the general population is not known, but the Dutch National Pathology Information System estimated frequencies of 6.2 new cases per million inhabitants per year among the general population of the Netherlands and 0.31% of all autopsies per year.[9]

SOURCES OF MICROEMBOLI

The most prevalent source of microemboli causing blue toe syndrome is the aortoiliac segment. In the largest series of atheroembolism, Keen et. al. reported on 100 patients, and found that occlusive aortoiliac disease and small aortic aneurysms were the most common source of atheroemboli. Aortoiliac disease accounted for more than 75% of the cases to the lower extremity and 67% overall.[14]

However, microemboli can originate from any artery with atherosclerotic disease. Stenotic or ulcerated plaque lesions increase the embolization probability. In iatrogenic microembolism, the entire length of the vessel in which the catheter is manipulated becomes a potential source of dislodgement of atheromatous plaque. The use of endovascular stents and angioplasty may cause plaque dislodgement. Care must be taken to minimize manipulation of these lesions during interventions.

Two types of atheroemboli can be distinguished. Macroemboli results from fragmentation of a plaque of sufficient size to occlude arteries more than a millimeter in diameter, resulting in major dysfunction of the organ or typical features of acute peripheral or visceral ischemia. Microemboli result from dislodgement of debris after ulceration and extrusion from the plaque, resulting in the exposure of the soft, friable, highly thrombogenic content of the inner core of the lesion to the arterial flow. This type of atheroembolization is more widespread, lodging in multiple small arteries, arterioles, and microcirculation between 60 to 900 micrometers in diameter producing localized and limited symptoms and signs.

PRECIPITATING FACTORS

The most important risk factor for atheroembolism is established atherosclerosis. Flory was the first person to hypothesize such a relationship between cholesterol crystal embolism and a diseased atherosclerotic aorta.[3] In 1992, Blauth et. al. reported on 46 patient autopsies in which severe atherosclerosis of the ascending aorta was accompanied by evidence of atheroemboli in other vascular beds.[15] Significant risk factors for atheroembolism included peripheral arterial disease, hypertension, older age, and coronary artery disease. Cholesterol embolization may occur spontaneously, but is more common after vascular surgery, endovascular procedures, treatment with anticoagulation, or thrombolytic treatment. In a retrospective analysis of 52 patients with a diagnosis of atheroembolic disease, Scolari and colleagues found that the disease was spontaneous in only 21% of cases.[16] The most common triggering events consist of angioplasty or vascular surgery and long-term anticoagulant therapy. Fibrinolytic therapy is another reported etiology. The atherosclerotic patient may also suffer spontaneous detachment of a plaque, or low grade, clinically silent migration of crystals from the aortic wall. Cross, in a series of 372 necropsies, estimated the incidence of "spontaneous" cholesterol embolization to be 1.9%.[17] This finding underscores the importance of following patients closely after vascular procedures so as not to overlook this potentially catastrophic complication.

Angiography and Catheter Manipulation

Manipulation of the aorta with catheters or guidewires can dislodge atheromatous material from the arterial wall. The entire length of the vessel in which the catheter is manipulated becomes a potential source of dislodgement of atheromatous plaque.

Microembolism is considered to be universal after endovascular procedures. Thompson et. al. quantified lower limb microemboli in 29 patients undergoing conventional and endovascular aneurysm repair by insonation of the superficial femoral artery. Emboli were detected as high-intensity, short-duration signals on the background Doppler trace. The number of emboli were significantly greater in the endovascular group compared with the conventional group.[18] Coronary angiography with angioplasty and stenting is the procedure most commonly inciting atheroembolism. The Cholesterol Embolization Study (CHEST) carried out by investigators in Japan examined prospectively the incidence of cholesterol embolization among patients who underwent cardiac catheterization. They found clinically apparent cholesterol embolism (livedo pattern on the feet, blue toe syndrome, digital gangrene, renal failure) in 1.4% of consecutive 1,786 patients undergoing left heart catheterization with 48% having cutaneous signs and 64% with renal insufficiency.[19] Keeley and Grines showed that in over 50% of 1,000 percutaneous revascularization procedures evaluated, guided catheter placement was associated with scraping off debris from the aorta.[20] Fine and colleagues demonstrated that 20% of patients who had atheroembolic events recently had a vascular radiologic procedure.[2] Baumann and colleagues, in a review of their institution's experience of atheroembolism, revealed that 21% were the result of an invasive radiologic procedure.[21] Sharma et. al. retrospectively reviewed patients with atheroemboli in the territory of aorta and infrainguinal arteries, and found that over 44% of the atheroemboli were iatrogenic.[22] Recent publications have elucidated the importance of atheroembolism in colon ischemia after endovascular abdominal aortic aneurysm repair.[23,24] They identified atheroembolism into the intestinal vascularity related to endovascular maneuvers for aortic aneurysm repair as the main cause for colon ischemia or fatal necrosis. Scolari et. al. retrospectively reported that 15 of 16,223 vascular procedures were complicated with atheroembolism, which was an incidence of 0.09%. In contrast, in 70 age-matched patients with diffuse atherosclerosis, but no history of having undergone endoluminal procedures, the incidence of atheroembolism was only 4.3%.[25] One study evaluating the frequency of atherothrombotic material retrieved during placement of coronary catheters found 0.5% of 7,621 patients to have macroscopically visible atheroembolic debris. None of these patients, however, had clinically apparent atheroembolic disease.[26] In a review of 4,587 cardiac catheterizations, Drost and colleagues found seven cases of clinical cholesterol embolization (0.002%).[12] Colt and associates found eight cases after heart catheterization percutaneous transluminal coronary angioplasty and intra-aortic balloon pump insertion in a total of 3,733 procedures (0.002%).[27] Saklayen and coworkers in a prospective analysis of 267 patients undergoing coronary angiography found the incidence of cholesterol embolism to be less than 2%.[28] Antonucci et. al. reported a 50% incidence of atheroembolism among patients with known atherosclerotic disease and acute renal failure following aortography.[29] Ramirez et. al. reviewed 71 autopsies of patients who died within six months of arteriography, and found that 30% of patients who underwent aortography and 26% of patients who underwent coronary catheterization had evidence of disseminated atheroembolism compared with a 4.3% incidence of spontaneous cholesterol emboli in an age- and disease-matched control group who did not undergo arteriography.[13] Rigid catheters and force of contrast injection increase risk of embolization.

It is impossible to predict the risk of atheroembolism in a patient, but severe peripheral arterial disease, aortic aneurysm, and the finding of protruding mobile atheroma all raise the risk of distal embolization. Advancement and removal of catheters should occur over a guidewire to straighten the catheter and minimize contact with the aortic wall. Brachial and radial access may minimize embolization from the abdominal aorta, but not from the ascending aorta or arch. In a study involving 3,733 procedures, there were no cases of cholesterol embolization after cardiac catheterization when the brachial artery was used.[27]

In a retrospective analysis of 493 patients who underwent a total of 565 aortoiliac stent placements, Lin et. al. found the incidence of atheroembolism to be 1.6%.[30] When embolic protection devices are utilized in stent procedures in the carotid or renal artery, visible atherosclerotic debris appears quite frequently. A lower incidence of atheroembolism has been noted with advancements in the design of catheters, guidewires, balloons, and the advent of emboli-protection devices as well as operator expertise.

Vascular Surgery

The effect of atheroembolism after major vascular surgery was first recognized by Thurlbeck and Castleman in 1957.[10] A 77% incidence of atheroembolism was reported among patients who died after abdominal aortic surgery. Atheromatous embolization either was the cause of death or significantly contributed to it in nearly half of the patients in this series. Vascular surgery procedures may disrupt plaque when the vessel is manipulated, cross-clamped, or incised during surgery. Atheroembolization is also a recognized complication of cardiac surgery. Doty et. al. in a retrospective analysis of 18,402 patients who underwent cardiac surgery found evidence of atheroembolism in 0.2% of patients at autopsy. In 21% of the cases, death was directly attributable to atheroembolism.[31] TEE can identify significant aortic plaque preoperatively. CT may also image the distal ascending aorta and proximal aortic arch. Alteration of the cannulation site and avoidance of aortic manipulation at areas of disease during coronary artery bypass grafting in the patient with such findings may reduce the chance of atheroembolism. When a shaggy aorta is visualized, alternative surgical procedures should be considered to minimize aortic manipulation.

Anticoagulation and Thrombolysis

Both a higher risk of cholesterol embolization with anticoagulation and clinical improvement when anticoagulation was removed have been documented in case reports. Anticoagulation may prevent thrombus formation over unstable atherosclerotic plaque, thus allowing exposed cholesterol crystals to embolize. Another theory is that anticoagulation may initiate the disruption of a complex plaque by causing hemorrhage into it.

However, cholesterol embolization was not seen in patients with documented aortic arch plaque more than 1 mm thick who were treated with warfarin in The French Study of Aortic Plaques in Stroke.[32] Fukumoto et. al. in a prospective evaluation of 25 patients with cholesterol emboli syndrome after cardiac catheterization were unable to show any significant association between the use of anticoagulants and cholesterol embolism.[19] Therefore, the association of anticoagulation with a higher incidence of atheroemboli remains controversial.

Atheromatous emboli have also been associated with thrombolytic therapy. Thombolytic agents act by converting plasminogen to plasmin, which directly degrades fibrin. Theoretically, any therapy that causes the thrombus to undergo lysis may leave atherosclerotic plaque uncovered, thereby putting the patient at risk for embolization.

CLINICAL FEATURES

The syndrome of atheroembolism usually affects elderly males who have multiple risk factors for atherosclerosis. In a prospective study conducted to identify risk factors for cholesterol embolism in patients undergoing cardiac catheterization, Fukumoto confirmed that cholesterol emboli syndrome occurs more commonly in patients with generalized atherosclerosis.[19]

Patients almost always have symptomatic atherosclerosis, manifesting clinically as angina, myocardial infarction, transient ischemic attack (TIA), stroke, renal artery disease, mesenteric ischemia, or claudication. Which organs are involved by cholesterol embolism depends on the locations of the embolic source. Atheroemboli from the ascending aorta and proximal aortic arch usually manifest as central nervous system or retina disease, whereas cholesterol emboli originating from the descending thoracic or abdominal aorta affect the visceral organs and extremities. In general, bilateral lower extremity atheroembolism signifies a source proximal to the aortic bifurcation, and unilateral emboli may originate either proximally or in any artery distal to the aortic bifurcation. Patients with macroemboli arising from a larger atherosclerotic plaque may present with an acutely ischemic limb or renal or mesenteric infarction. Conversely, patients with microemboli may have milder localized signs or a clinical picture that suggests a systemic illness. There may be a temporal delay of up to eight weeks between the inciting event and the appearance of clinical findings, especially for renal failure.

The clinical manifestations of atheroembolism depend on the number of organs affected, the composition of the emboli, the quantity of the embolus expelled from the atherosclerotic plaque, and the body's ability to eliminate the embolus. Nearly every organ system has shown histologic involvement in autopsy studies. Fine et. al. reviewed 221 histologically proven cases. Among 75 cases, clinical diagnosis of gastrointestinal and pancreatic involvement was made in 27%, of renal involvement in 23%, and of spleen, liver, and adrenal involvement in 1%. At autopsy, among 92 cases, the respective figures were 96%, 84%, and 100%, respectively. The frequency of localizations to viscera is roughly proportional to their blood flow. Considering that the renal blood flow represents one-fifth to one-quarter of the cardiac output, it is not surprising that cholesterol embolization ranks among common etiologies of renal disease. Premortem diagnoses were established in 31% of patients, most commonly by biopsy of the muscle, skin, and kidney. Mortality was high at 81%.[2]

Antemortem diagnosis of atheroembolism is difficult and requires a high index of suspicion. Atheroembolization tends to be repetitive. Disseminated atheroembolism can be classified into three major clinical presentations: peripheral syndrome, renal syndrome, and visceral syndrome. The peripheral syndrome associated with atheromatous embolization from the aortoiliac segment was termed "blue toe syndrome" by Karmody and colleagues.[33]

Cutaneous Manifestations

The most common clinical manifestations of atheroembolism involve the skin, with livedo reticularis and blue toe syndrome the most predominant. The appearance of cutaneous signs can be delayed, with 50% of patients in one series showing skin signs of atheroembolism more than 30 days after their procedures or other inciting events.[34] Cutaneous manifestations may be subtle and, therefore, must be looked for specifically.

Livedo reticularis is the most common dermatologic manifestation of atheroembolism, comprising approximately 50% of atheroembolism-related skin lesions. Livedo reticularis is a striking violaceous mottling or discoloration of the skin that occurs in a net-like pattern, most commonly seen on the buttocks, thighs, or legs, but can extend to the trunk and upper extremities. Livedo reticularis is most likely caused by obstruction of small arteries, capillaries, or venules in the deep dermis. Cholesterol crystals may be seen in the dermal blood vessels. Myalgias may precede the livedo reticularis, implying involvement of the small arteries of the lower extremity musculature. A detailed skin examination performed with the patient in both the supine and upright positions is necessary because livedo reticularis is more readily demonstrable in the upright position.[35] Livedo reticularis is, however, not pathognomonic of atheroemboli and may been seen with other diseases.

The blue toe syndrome is characterized by the sudden development of one or more discreet blue or purple areas on the foot or toes that are cool, painful, and tender to touch. Discoloration may also be seen on the sole of the foot. The patient often manifests sluggish capillary refill. Well-demarcated lesions are sometimes accompanied by a more diffuse cyanotic mottling of the surrounding skin. Cyanosis may become more prominent with the legs in a dependent position, and lesions may blanch with moderate pressure. Waxing and waning of cyanosis is typical. Tissue necrosis, ranging from small superficial ulceration to gangrene, may develop. In late presentations, the digits may have developed eschar at the tips. The discoloration may be patchy, and if bilateral, is usually not symmetrical.[36] Repeated episodes can occur and lead to increased tissue damage, whereas extensive showering of atheroemboli gives "trash foot." Classically, this syndrome occurs in the presence of normal, even bounding, peripheral pulses. Thus, the sudden onset of pain and purple discoloration of a toe in the presence of palpable peripheral pulses is known as the three P's of atheroembolism . The recurrent focal nature of the ischemia in this syndrome is most characteristic of embolism. Atheroembolism is the most common cause of blue toe syndrome. Cardiac embolism, hypercoagulability states, vasculitis, calciphylaxis, and corticosteroids also may cause blue toe syndrome. Most emboli to the lower limbs are secondary to lesions in the infrarenal aorta to the distal popliteal arteries. About 60% of emboli originate in the femoropopliteal arteries and 40% from the aortoiliac arteries.

Other skin manifestations are splinter hemorrhages, petechiae, purpura, and raised nodules due to subepidermal inflammation surrounding cholesterol crystals. These nodules are painful, violaceous with a necrotic center, and may mimic a necrotizing vasculitis. Balanitis (necrosis of the penile foreskin, perineal area, and scrotum) has been reported with atheroembolism to the pelvic circulation.

Renal Involvement

The kidney is the most common target organ for atheroembolization. The kidneys are a prime target for cholesterol embolization because of the amount of blood flow and close proximity of the renal arteries to the abdominal aorta, where atheromatous plaque is common. Mayo and Swartz in a review of 402 nephrology consultation charts found that the incidence of clinically detectable atheroembolism is at least 4% of all hospitalized patients examined, representing approximately 5% to 10% of the patients with acute renal failure encountered.[37]

Approximately 50% of atheroembolism cases show renal emboli on necropsy, and renal failure is common. Pathologically, the classic lesion of atheroembolic renal disease is the occlusion of medium-sized arterioles and glomerular capillaries with cholesterol emboli. This leads to ischemic obstruction and an inflammatory reaction within the arterioles. Several days to weeks after the inciting event, an inflammatory infiltration occurs. Later, there is glomerular sclerosis, tubular atrophy, and interstitial fibrosis. The involvement tends to be patchy and, therefore, a renal biopsy specimen may not always show the classic pathologic lesions.

Gradual onset of skin manifestations accompanied by slow but progressive increases in blood urea nitrogen and creatinine over a two- to four-week period following arterial catheterization suggests the diagnosis. The diagnosis is difficult to make because of lack of any constant and specific findings in the usual tests of renal function or urinalysis. The classic triad of this disease include livedo reticularis, acute renal failure, and eosinophilia. Demonstration of cholesterol crystals in renal biopsy specimens is pathognomonic. It is essential to differentiate this from renal failure induced by radiographic contrast.

Atheroembolic renal disease can be categorized into three types: acute, subacute, and chronic renal failure. Acute renal failure occurring within seven days following the inciting event is observed in about one-third of the cases. It is often fulminant, following massive embolization of crystals, and the kidney is seldom if ever the sole organ involved. This multiorgan involvement differentiates cholesterol embolization from early acute renal failure from iodinated contrast media toxicity or that complicating vascular surgery.[38] Oligoanuria appears rapidly, and is accompanied with severe hypertension or the abrupt aggravation of previous hypertension. Flank pain and/or hematuria are uncommon. The subacute subset is deceptive in that renal manifestations appear insidiously weeks or months after the inciting event. It is the most common form. Renal function impairment often develops in a stepwise fashion over the following weeks. Each aggravation follows a triggering event eliciting another shower of crystals such as repeat angiography, vascular surgery, and/or anticoagulation. The chronic subset is frequently asymptomatic and underdiagnosed. It manifests by a slowly progressive form of renal insufficiency with bouts of aggravation.

The renal outcome for patients with atheroembolic renal disease is quite variable. Some progress to end-stage renal failure and hemodialysis. There are some reports of spontaneous recovery of renal function in patients with atheroembolic renal disease.

Gastrointestinal Involvement

The tract is often overlooked as a site of cholesterol embolization. Its rich vascular supply makes it a common target. The most common symptoms are abdominal pain, diarrhea, distention, paralytic ileus, and blood loss. Abdominal pain may be caused by bowel ischemia or by fibrous stricture with bowel obstruction. Bleeding is caused by superficial mucosal ulceration, erosions, and microinfarcts.

Microembolization is a major and probably the predominant factor in the pathogenesis of colon ischemia after endovascular repair of abdominal aortic aneurysm. Interruption of one or both hypogastrics is not a major cause of colon ischemia.[23]

Other areas of the digestive system reported to be involved include pancreas, liver, and gallbladder, presenting as pancreatitis, hepatitis, or cholecystitis. Mucosal punch biopsy specimens from the stomach, duodenum, or colon may be helpful in making the diagnosis. The prognosis of patients with GI involvement tends to be poor. Patients with gasterointestinal (GI) involvement often have a multisystem cholesterol embolization syndrome.

Central Nervous System and Eye Involvement

Cholesterol embolization commonly occurs in the brain and eye. The culprit lesions are located in the ascending aorta, aortic arch, and carotid and vertebral arteries. Patients may experience visual disturbances such as amaurosis fugax. Retinal cholesterol embolization is seen as yellow, highly refractile plaques (Hollenhorst plaques) on ophthalmic fundoscopy.[39] Cerebral cholesterol embolism may manifest as TIA, stroke, confusion, headache, dizziness, or organic brain syndrome. In a retrospective review of 29 patients with autopsy-proven brain cholesterol emboli, encephalopathy was the predominant neurologic finding.[40] It is most likely due to the diffuse and bihemispheric nature of cholesterol embolization. Involvement of the spinal cord has been reported. Atheroembolism is a suggested cause for slowly progressive spinal cord syndromes in the elderly.

Other

Coronary atheroembolism has been reported after strenuous exercise, cardiopulmonary resuscitation, arteriographic procedures, cardiac surgery, and percutaneous transluminal coronary angioplasty (PTCA).

Atheroembolism may simulate a "vasculitis." This is one of the most elusive entities because its diagnosis can only be made with histological examination. The clinical presentation is that of a systemic disease with apparent multiorgan involvement. The presentation may be atypical with fever, weight loss, headaches, intense myalgias, and multiorgan involvement mimicking systemic vasculitides.

DIAGNOSTIC STRATEGIES

The diagnosis of cholesterol embolization syndrome is challenging. The symptoms and signs are nonspecific. A high index of suspicion and a thorough understanding of the various clinical manifestations are needed in order to correctly make the diagnosis antemortem. Part of the difficulty in making this diagnosis relates to the time interval (typically weeks to months) between intervention and disease onset, which tends to obscure the causative link. The diagnosis can often be made on clinical grounds alone, without histological confirmation in a patient who has a precipitating event, acute or subacute renal failure, hypertension that is difficult to control, and evidence of peripheral embolization.

There is no diagnostic serological investigation, and differentiation from a systemic vasculitis can be difficult. Eosinophilia, which was present in 80% of a series of reported cases of renal atheroembolism, might be attributed to the generation of complement factor C5a, which is known to be chemotactic for eosinophils.[41] The eosinophilia tends to be transient. Laboratory markers of inflammation, such as

C-reactive protein, fibrinogen, and erythrocyte sedimentation rate, have been found to be elevated in many patients. A 4.6-fold increase in the risk of atheroembolism was noted in patients with elevated C-reactive protein. This observation is quite consistent with recent data suggesting C-reactive protein (CRP) as a marker of the "inflamed unstable" plaque.[19] Other lab findings include leukocytosis, anemia, thrombocytopenia, and decreased complement levels. Mild proteinuria, microhematuria, and hyaline or granular casts are the most common urinary findings in patients with cholesterol embolization. In addition, these investigators found a significant relationship between C-reactive protein level and cholesterol embolism, indicating an important possible association between systemic inflammation and cholesterol emboli syndrome.

Invasive vascular procedures requiring aortic instrumentation should be avoided because of the potential risk of producing recurrent atheroembolism. Noninvasive imaging modalities such at CTA, MRA, and transesophageal echocardiogram (TEE) can assist in confirming the diagnosis if irregular and shaggy aorta is demonstrated. The following CT findings have been described in patients who suffer spontaneous atheroembolism from an aortic aneurysm (AAA): irregular luminal surface, multiple lumens, heterogeneity of thrombus, calcification within the thrombus, and noncontiguous areas of intraluminal thrombus. Duplex has been particularly useful in detecting embologenic arterial lesions and can be used to quantify the degree of embolic activity.[42,43]

In the absence of obvious clinical clues, a definitive diagnosis may require a tissue biopsy. The highest yield for histologic confirmation is an affected organ. The hallmark of histopathological findings is the demonstration of cholesterol crystals in arterioles of affected organs. These crystals are dissolved during standard tissue fixation techniques, and leave biconvex needle-shaped lacunae ("ghost" crystals) within the blood vessel lumen. The biopsy should be deep and the specimen should be examined in multiple sections.

DIFFERENTIAL DIAGNOSIS

Diseases that should be considered in the differential diagnosis of atheroembolic renal disease are contrast nephropathy, acute tubular necrosis, ischemic injury, necrotizing vasculitis, antiphospholipid syndrome, and multiple myeloma. The urine sediment in atheroembolism is usually benign and shows only microhematuria. By contrast, the urine sediment in patients with acute tubular necrosis often demonstrate pigmented granular casts and renal tubular cells. Atheroembolic renal disease can be differentiated from acute tubular necrosis (ATN) or contrast nephropathy on the basis of the time frame of renal impairment. In contrast nephropathy and ATN, renal failure occurs within 48 to 72 hours after the inciting event, whereas in patient with atheroembolic renal disease, the renal impairment is often delayed for seven to 10 days. Full recovery is the rule for contrast nephropathy and ATN if the precipitating factor is eradicated, but is the exception in atheroembolism. ATN is characterized by normal blood pressures as opposed to the severe hypertension (HTN) present in atheroembolism.

The laboratory evaluation should include blood urea nitrogen and creatinine, chemistry, complete blood count, erythrocyte sedimentation rate, urinalysis with eosinophiluria, and creatine phosphokinase. Following laboratory investigation, an effort should be made to investigate the source of embolization. Patients suspected of having spontaneous distal microembolization should undergo cardiac examination, including electrocardiography, transthoracic echocardiography, and holter monitoring to rule out acute cardiac disease. Ultrasonography is very helpful in identifying the presence of aneurysms. Color Doppler is useful in localizing plaques distal to the inguinal ligament. CT can localize emboli when the source is aortoiliac occlusive disease, a small aortic aneurym, or shaggy abdominal aorta.

In patients with a prosthetic valve, or if the source of the embolism is located in the aortic arch, TEE may be useful. TEE can detect patent foramen ovale that may be responsible for paradoxical emboli causing distal peripheral microembolization.

Biplanar angiography is considered the gold standard in localizing peripheral embolic sources. This mode may demonstrate a small posterior plaque missed by the anterior-posterior view. A definitive diagnosis of atheroembolism can only be made with a tissue diagnosis. There is a high yield from skin or muscle biopsy when the patient manifests cutaneous signs.

MANAGEMENT STRATEGIES FOR ATHEROEMBOLISM

There have been no randomized controlled trials of any therapeutic intervention for patients with cholesterol embolization, and no agent has been strongly correlated with favorable outcomes. The most important aspect of therapy is prevention. Once atheromatous embolization has occurred, therapy is mostly supportive. Avoidance of further inciting events such as aortic manipulation, good control of hypertension and heart failure, and dialysis support is encouraged. Symptomatic care of the end organ where the emboli are located and modification of risk factors are tantamount. The inability to reverse the condition, early diagnosis is crucial.

To locate the source of the embolus requires a systematic and diligent search, and even then, the identified source is not necessarily the actual source. Owing to the high recurrence rate, which ranges from 60% to 90%, patients who are medically fit should undergo an aggressive workup and subsequent elimination or stabilization of the atheroembolic source.

The most common source for peripheral atheroembolism is the aorta, and when bilateral lower extremity involvement occurs without renal or visceral involvement, the infrarenal aorta may be presumed to be the source. Arteriographic findings are not always impressive, and detailed imaging is critical. The goal of therapy is to safely remove the offending atherosclerotic plaque from the arterial blood stream. Balloon angioplasty may stabilize ulcerated atherosclerotic plaques. Stent placement may provide a protective scaffold to help secure these lesions.

MEDICAL THERAPY

Various agents have been used to manage atheroembolism. Medical management described includes heparin, dextran, papaverine, urokinase, aspirin, statins, steroids, and vasodilators. Because atheroembolism resembles a vasculitis, corticosteroids have been used with mixed results. The use of statins, an inhibitor of 3-hydroxy-3-methylglutaryl coenzyme A reductase, has been reported to result in improvement in blue toe syndrome.[44] Statins theoretically stabilize plaques and prevent plaque hemorrhage, thrombosis, and subsequent embolization.[45] Statins stabilize and even obtain regression of atherosclerotic plaques.[46] A prospective study showed that statins ameliorate the renal and patient outcomes in cholesterol embolization.[47] Statins have been reported to be beneficial in the treatment of livedo reticularis, as well as in the treatment of renal and lower limb emboli. In a retrospective analysis of 519 patients with severe thoracic aortic plaque visualized on TEE, multivariate analysis showed that statin use was independently protective against recurrent embolic events (p = .001).[48] It has been proposed that statins stabilize cholesterol-rich aortic atherosclerotic plaques that shower cholesterol emboli. By stabilizing the plaques, the statins may prevent further embolic showers. The prostaglandin analogues appear to be beneficial in the healing of ischemic ulcerations associated with atheroemboli. To improve distal flow, Pardy et. al. reported that the use of prostaglandins E1 and prostacyclin I2 demonstrated prolonged pain relief and promotion of tissue healing.[49] In a small series, Elinav et. al. demonstrated the efficacy of iloprost, a prostocyclin analog, in the treatment of distal peripheral microembolization.[50] Antiplatelet agents such as aspirin, dipyridamole, low-molecular-weight dextran, intra-arterial papaverine, and pentoxifylline help stabilize the source of atheroemboli. Morris-Jones and colleagues described reversal of signs and symptoms in more than 50% of 35 patients treated with aspirin and dipyridamole.[51] Anticoagulation with warfarin does not control atheroembolization and may actually aggravate the condition.[52,53] Moldveen-Geronimus and Merriam suggested that atheroemboli may arise from ulcerated plaques lacking an overlying thrombus covering.[54] Hence, by preventing the formation of a protective thrombus, anticoagulant therapy could aggravate or even initiate the atheroembolic process. Unfortunately, no controlled trials have shown that any of these forms of therapy are of benefit. However, all patients should receive aggressive risk factor modification with an antiplatelet agent, a statin, and an angiotensin-converting enzyme inhibitor.

Prostaglandin Therapy

Prostaglandins (PGs) were discovered in 1930 in seminal fluid by Kurzrock and Lieb. They noted that PGs could stimulate uterine contractions. The name was coined by Von Euler in 1934 because he mistook the substance for a secretory product of the prostate. Prostaglandins are unsaturated fatty acids with a cyclopentane ring that are produced by the metabolism of cell membrane phospholipids proceeding through unstable intermediates. These intermediates are converted to prostaglandins from arachidonic acid in endothelial cells or to thromboxane A2 in platelets by specific enzymes located in these cells. Thromboxane A2 stimulates platelet aggregation and vasoconstriction, which opposes or balances endothelial prostaglandin. There are two naturally occurring prostaglandins: PGE1 (prostin or alprostadil) and PGI2 (or prostacyclin or epoprostenol). In 1973, PGE1 was the first prostaglandin isolated and identified. PGE1 is transported in the bloodstream bound to albumin (81% to 99%). Prostaglandin E1 is best used intra-arterially because one passage through the lung inactivates almost 70% to 90% of the drug.[55] Metabolites are eliminated by the kidneys.

In 1976, Moncada et. al. discovered PGI2 in blood vessel walls that had 40 times more vasodilating and antiplatelet activity than PGE1.[56] PGI2 is not removed by the lungs, but is rapidly hydrolyzed in the circulation to inactive products. PGI2 is chemically unstable and needs to be administered at high pH, which can potentially cause vascular damage. Because the ephemeral nature of PGI2 limits its use clinically, a chemically stable synthetic analog of prostacyclin was developed called iloprost.

Iloprost has a 10-fold higher half-life than PGI2. Novel prostaglandin analogs and formulations have also been developed to improve targeted delivery to ischemic tissues. Esters of prostaglandins can be hydrolyzed in serum and release an active PG over time. Targeted delivery to the vascular wall and areas of neovascularization may be enhanced by lipid encapsulation of the prostaglandin.[57] Lipo-ecraprost is a novel preparation of the PGE1 analog ecraprost in lipid microspheres. Lipid encapsulation allows more rapid infusion of large PG doses, and thus increases tolerability of the therapy and may target the PG to the site of injury.

Prostaglandins potentiates the action of adenyl cyclase in platelets, resulting in an increase in cyclic adenosine monophosphate (cAMP) concentration. The increase in cAMP affects phospholipase activity and cytosolic calcium levels, thereby inactivating platelets and inhibiting platelet aggregation. PGI2 is the most powerful known inhibitor of platelet aggregation. Prostaglandins are powerful vasodilators. The platelet inhibitory and vasodilatory actions of prostaglandins (synthesized in the vascular endothelium) are counterbalanced by the platelet aggregatory and vasoconstrictive effects of thromboxane (synthesized in platelets). Moreover, prostaglandins enhance inherent fibrinolytic potential, increase red blood cell deformability, reduce neutrophil adhesion and chemotaxis to endothelial cells, and has an antiproliferative action on vascular smooth cells. Prostaglandins are also protective of the endothelium by unknown mechanisms.[58] These actions of prostaglandins have stimulated interest in treating cardiac and limb ischemia. Iloprost has been found to inhibit neutrophil migration and activation in cardiac ischemia with a consequential reduction in myocardial infarct size.[59] Simpson et. al. have confirmed in vitro that the production of superoxide by leukocytes is significantly decreased by iloprost.[60] Oxygen-free radicals have been implicated in the injurious effects of ischemia and reperfusion in skeletal muscle. This cytoprotection conferred by prostaglandins has been used to preserve myocardial function. Belkin et. al. found skeletal muscle ischemic injury to be significantly reduced, from 57% to 16%, when pretreated with iloprost.[61]

Prostaglandin synthesis is impaired in atherosclerotic vessels. It has been suggested that treatment with prostaglandin may be a form of replacement therapy for a vasculature depleted of prostaglandin.[62] The mechanisms of anti-ischemic effects of prostaglandins in patients with peripheral arterial disease are probably complex and clearly not limited to a direct vasodilator action. In addition to the known effects on blood flow, viscosity, fibrinolysis, and platelet aggregation, prostaglandins inhibit expression of adhesion molecules (E-selectin, ICAM-1, VCAM-1), release of inflammatory cytokines (TNF alpha, MCP-1), matrix components, and generation and release of growth factors. These actions may contribute to the long-term effects of PGs. Studies suggest that several genes in vascular smooth muscle cells and fibroblasts are modified by prostaglandins at the transcriptional level. The mechanisms of actions of prostaglandins are summarized in Table 28–1.

Therapeutic Uses of Prostaglandins

Prostaglandins have been used extensively in Europe for the treatment of peripheral arterial disease. Two types of prostaglandins are in clinical use: PGE1 and iloprost.[50,63-69] (Table 28–2).

Shortly after PGE1 became available commercially, a brief Scandanavian report described the treatment of four patients with unreconstructible leg ischemia who would otherwise have required amputation.[70] PGE1 was infused into the femoral artery (0.01

TABLE 28-1. EFFECTS OF PROSTAGLANDINS

Vasodilatation

Reduction of platelet adhesiveness and aggregation

Inhibition of proliferation of smooth muscle cells

Increase in red blood cell cell deformability

Inhibition of chemotaxis and activation of white blood cells

Cytoprotection

Promotion of fibrinolysis

Promotion of angiogenesis

Stabilization of endothelial membrane and improvement in endothelial function

---

micrograms/kg/hr) for one to three days. Marked relief of rest pain with significant ulcer healing occurred without the need for subsequent amputation. Because the authors noted some contralateral improvement that suggested a systemic drug effect, they subsequently tested the efficacy of a 72-hour intravenous PGE1 infusion in eight patients. Ulcer healing occurred in 75% and rest pain was relieved in 83% of patients after three weeks follow-up.[71] Pardy et. al. infused PGE1 both intra-arterially and intravenously in patients with severe lower limb ischemia. On the basis of results in four patients, they concluded that intermittent IV infusion of PGE1 at 10 ng/kg/min produced no clinical benefit. Their results also suggested that a patent superficial femoral artery was associated with a better clinical response and a greater rise in temperature following prostaglandin infusion than when the artery was occluded.[49] Sethi et. al. also used intra-arterial infusions of PGE1 in an uncontrolled study of 25 patients with advanced atherosclerosis. After a 72-hour infusion, they claimed significant improvement in the majority of patients using subjective assessment. They also reported reappearance of foot pulses and increased diameter of distal arteries on arteriography.[72] These reports, although uncontrolled, were met with enthusiasm because of the otherwise poor prognosis for limb salvage in patients with surgically unreconstructible disease. The first controlled trial of PGE1 for lower extremity occlusive disease was reported in 1982.[73] Twenty-two patients who had arterial ulcers were randomized to receive PGE1 (20 micrograms given intravenously, seven times each day) or placebo for three days, repeated one month later. Ulcer shapes were determined regularly by stereophotogrammetry. A significant healing effect was found during the first weeks with PGE1 treatment. After two months of follow-up, both placebo and drug-treated groups had a 40% frequency of ulcer healing. The investigators concluded that PGE1 must be given in higher doses, for longer duration, and/or more frequently in order to show a significant long-term benefit. Sakaguchi et. al. conducted a study of intra-arterial PGE1 therapy on 65 patients with ulcers caused by thromboangiitis obliterans. Higher-dose PGE1 infusion (0.15 ng/kg/min) resulted in a significantly higher clinical response rate (68%) than did lower-dose PGE1 (0.05 ng/kg/min, 44% positive response) after a mean infusion time of 24 days.[74] More recently, a multicenter trial of PGE1 administered by a two-hour intravenous infusion daily for an average of 19 days also demonstrated short-term improvement in critical limb ischemia.[68] In a meta-analysis, a decrease in major amputation or death was sustained up to six months after treatment in patients with critical limb ischemia, suggesting that short-term or intermittent administration of prostanoids was not simply the result of vasodilatation and might result in sustained clinical efficacy.[75] Clinical trials of lipo-ecraprost in chronic limb ischemia patients

TABLE 28-2.

Author	Year	Type PG	Route	Dosing	Inclusion criteria	# patients	Study type	Results	Benefit of PG
Nehler MR et. al.[63]	2007	Lipo-ecraporst	IV	60 micrograms w/in 72 hrs of bypass, 5d/wk × 8 wks	Distal bypass	143 Placebo 141 PG	Multicenter randomized 13% placebo	At 6 mos Major amp: 12% PG Mortality: 13% placebo 9% PG Patency: 73% placebo 79% PG	No
Brass EP et. al.[64]	2006	Lipo-ecraporst	IV	60 micrograms 5d/wk × 8 wks	No bypass options	177 placebo 179 PG	Multicenter randomized	At 6 mos Amp: 13% placebo 16% PG Mortality: 5.6% placebo 10.1% PG	
De Donato G et. al.[65]	2006	Iloprost	IA IV	3 micrograms IA intraop, 2.1 - 8.4 micrograms/hr × 6 hrs/d × 4-7 d postop	Distal bypass	151 placebo 149 PG	Multicenter randomized	At 3 mos Mortality + amp: 20% placebo 14% PG Mortality: 10.6% placebo 4.7% PG	

Study	Year	Drug	Route	Dose	Indication	N	Study type	Outcome	Significant
Milio G et. al.[66]	2006	PGE1	IV	2.1 - 8.4 micrograms/hr x 6 hr/d 10d with repeated cycles of 3 mos for 18 mos	Raynaud's phenomenon secondary to systemic sclerosis	30	Prospective		Yes
Milio G et. al.[67]	2005	PGE1	IV	60 micrograms/day x 20 d	Ischemic ulcers	43 placebo 44 PG		Healing: 84% placebo 100% PG	Yes
Elinav E et. al.[50]	2002	Iloprost	IV	Up to 8.4 micrograms/hr x 10-14d, followed by 8hr infusion 3x/wk X 2-3 wks, then 1x/wk	Cholesterol emboli syndrome	4		Ischemic lesions healed	Yes
ICAI Study Group[68]	1999	PGE1	IV	60 micrograms/d x up to 28 days	Chronic critical ischemia	789 placebo 771 PG	Multicenter randomized		Yes (short-term)
Negus D et. al.[69]	1987	PGI2	IA	34 micrograms/hr x 3d	Rest pain, no bypass options	14			Yes

Abbreviations:

IV, intravenous; IA, intra-arterial; Pg, prostaglandin

without revascularization options yielded primarily negative results.[64] However, all these trials were performed using intravenous doses. These studies are limited by the degree to which lip-ecraprost could be delivered to the pedal microcirculation owing to the uncorrected occlusive disease. Nehler et. al. was unable to improve outcomes with intravenous treatment of lipo-ecraprost (60 micrograms/day, five days/week × eight weeks).[63] In another meta-analysis, 634 patients with stage III and IV peripheral arterial disease were analyzed from seven randomized controlled PGE1 studies. At the end of treatment, PGE1 showed a significantly better response (ulcer healing and/or pain reduction) as compared to placebo (48% for PGE1 versus 25% for placebo). The response rate of the pooled treatment groups was 60% for PGE1, 25% for placebo, and 54% for iloprost.[76]

There are several studies that have used prostaglandins for atheroembolism. Gruss et. al. reported on his experience with intravenous PGE1 in patients with post-operative trash foot; there was only one treatment failure among eight patients.[77] Elinav et. al. treated four patients suffering from atheroembolism complicated by painful cutaneous necrotic lesions and renal insufficiency with iloprost. The drug was administered continuously in gradually increasing doses for 10 to 14 days, followed by eight-hour infusions three times a week for three weeks, and thereafter once a week. At one month, his regimen had clearly improved skin lesions, pain, and renal function.[50] Grenader et. al. reported a patient who developed acute renal failure due to cholesterol crystal embolization following percutaneous transluminal angioplasty of a renal artery. Treatment with iloprost for peripheral symptoms of cholesterol emboli resulted in rapid resolution of toe cyanosis, decrease in leg pain, and a significant decrease in serum creatinine. One month after initiation of iloprost therapy, skin signs of cholesterol emboli disappeared and leg pain diminished. Gradually, reduction in serum creatinine was also observed.[78]

In addition to its use in critical limb ischemia and atheroembolism, prostaglandins have also been used for claudication. Recent studies demonstrate that the parenteral administration of PGE1 markedly increases walking distance. The first randomized pilot study showed that a four-week combined course of intravenous PGE1 and intensive physical exercise resulted in a dramatic increase in the pain-free walking distance. Although the increase achieved by exercise alone was 119%, additional administration of PGE1 increased the walking distance by 263%.[79] In a study of 80 patients with intermittent claudication, intravenous AS-103, a PGE1 prodrug with extended half-life, demonstrated modest improvement in maximum and pain-free walking distance. The advantage of AS-103 over prostacyclin is that a bolus injection can be used rather than continuous IV infusion.[80] Inconvenient intravenous dosing of prostaglandins have led to the development of more stable, oral active analogues. Beraprost sodium, the agent used in the study by Mohler et. al., decreases platelet aggregation in vivo with a half-life in serum of 30 to 50 minutes.[81] Two multicenter randomized placebo-controlled trials of beraprost conducted in Europe demonstrated modest efficacy in improved pain-free walking distance.[82,83]

Prostaglandins have also been used in upper limb ischemia. Motz et. al. reported excellent results with intra-arterial iloprost in two women with severe disabling upper limb ischemia due to stabilized chronic thrombus of the brachial and forearm arteries. Arteriography showed occlusion of the brachial arteries, and in one case of the proximal radial and ulnar arteries as well, and very poor distal blood flow. A 24-hour intra-arterial infusion was at a dose 10–40% higher than the maximum recommended for intravenous use. After treatment, there was abundant collateral vessels and rich distal arterial arborization.[84] Treatment of hand or arm ischemia following accidental intraarterial drug injection has been successfully treated with iloprost infusion.[85,86]

Prostaglandins have been shown to have a role in angiogenesis. Implantation of autologous bone marrow mononuclear cells has been shown to augment neovascular formation in ischemic tissues in experimental animals and humans. Otsuka et. al. have demonstrated that therapeutic angiogenesis as stimulated by the implantation of autologous bone marrow cells is enhanced by beraprost sodium in a rabbit made ischemic by surgical resection of the femoral artery.[87] PGE1 has also been shown to stimulate myocardial angiogenesis in humans with chronically ischemic myocardium. Mehrabi et. al. investigated neovascularization in 14 explanted hearts from patients with ischemic cardiomyopathy, who had been bridged to heart transplantation with PGE1, in comparison to 14 hearts from patients who did not receive PGE1 prior to heart transplantation. Their data demonstrated that PGE1 stimulated neoangiogenesis in infarct areas adjacent to viable myocardium via the upregulation of vascular endothelial growth factor (VEGF) expression.[88]

Dosing

For the treatment of peripheral vascular disease, intravenous use predominated due to accessibility and ease. Iloprost has generally been admininstered intravenously as intermittent infusions of < 2 ng/kg/min for five to 12 hours for three to 28 consecutive days. The optimal total dose is not established. Studies have initiated iloprost at 0.5 ng/kg/minute increasing in increments of 0.5 ng/kg/minute until the appearance of mild headache and flushing. Investigators have used intermittent and continuous infusions Tapering the rate of administration is recommended prior to discontinuing the drug. As most of the drug is metabolized during the first passage through the lungs, intra-arterial administration has been shown to result in much higher clinical activity. Schellong et. al. observed that on positron emission tomography, the increase of muscular blood flow by intra-arterial PGE1 averaged 80%. During intravenous PGE1, the muscular blood flow remain unchanged because of metabolism in the lungs.[89]

Adverse Effects

Major side effects of PGE1 and PGI2, namely hypotension and tachycardia, relate to their vasodilating activity that limits the systemic dose of these agents. Patients are highly variable in their ability to tolerate iloprost, but within an individual, adverse reactions are clearly dose-related. Facial flushing and headache are most common with an incidence of approximately 70% followed by nausea in 30% and vomiting in 16%.[90] Abdominal cramping and diarrhea are also frequently reported with an incidence of all gastrointestinal effects becoming more prevalent with higher dosages. These troublesome gastrointestinal reactions can generally be avoided by titrating up to the dosage, which produces flushing and a mild headache. The untoward effects cease very shortly after the infusion is stopped. Less common effects include restlessness, sudden sweating, the appearance of a red line along the infused vein, local erythema, sedation or fatigue, muscular aches or pain/numbness in the limbs, dry mouth, decreased appetite, and wheals. Some develop low-grade temperatures not associated with an infectious source.

Our Experience with PGE1

In 1985, because of the failure of standard treatment of atheromatous embolization, we initiated a study of intra-arterial PGE1 therapy in patients with severe atheroembolism. We have tried corticosteroids in high doses, heparin, local urokinase, papaverine, sodium nitroprusside, nitroglycerin, and sympathectomy, all with poor results. The encouraging results with PGE1 in Buerger's disease induced us to try the drug for atheroembolism.

Once the decision to treat the patient is made, a 3F or 4F size multiperforated catheter is advanced percutaneously from the common femoral artery into the popliteal or brachial artery. In one patient with renal involvement, the catheter was placed in the suprarenal aorta. Mild analgesia is used. Heparin is administered (500 units per hour intravenously) during intra-arterial injection. A dilute solution of prostaglandin E1 (500 to 1500 micrograms, Prostin Pediatric; Upjohn, Kalamazoo, MI) was injected into the artery over a few hours. The total dose varied from 1,000 to 8,000 micrograms of PGE1 and treatment lasted one to five days. This dose is much higher than that used in previous trials and it is our contention that this is necessary to produce significant effects. An increase in skin temperature and capillary refilling was noted (Figure 28–1). The injection is repeated, according to the response, either on the same day or on subsequent days. A total of 25 patients with limb-threatening ischemia of the upper or lower extremities induced by atheroembolism were treated percutaneously. Diagnosis was established clinically using arteriography in all patients and by skin biopsy in selected patients in whom diagnosis was not evident. One patient received a second series of injections one week after the first series.

Criteria for treatment with prostaglandins for atheroembolism included persistent pain resistant to medication, severe ischemia with risk of tissue loss, presence of distal pulses, or positive Doppler signals. Patients with asymptomatic or mild atheroembolism were not included. We considered only those patients suffering from occlusion of small arteries (muscular and dermal).

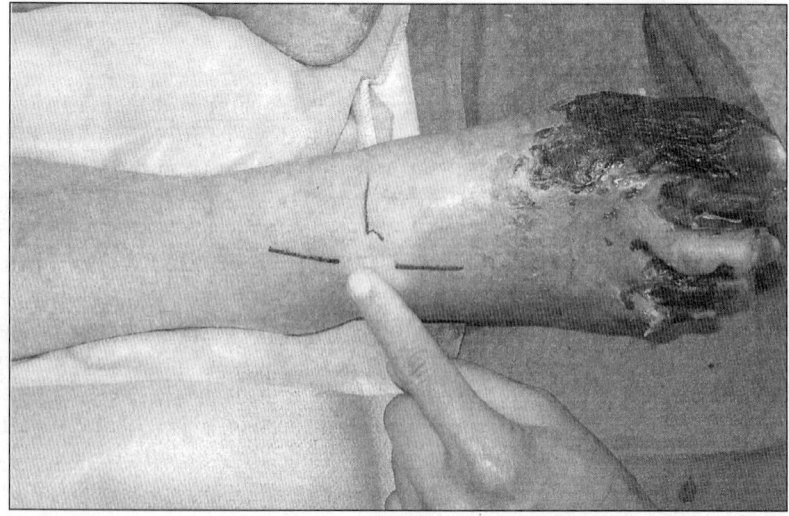

Figure 28-1. Hyperemic response induced by PGE1 infusion in a patient with trash foot.

The sources of atheroemboli included the abdominal aorta, the subclavian artery, the popliteal artery, and the iliac artery. A diagnosis of a patent foramen ovale with aneurysm of the septum was established in one patient. One patient suffered from severe left hand ischemia after several attempts to establish an arterial line in the radial and axillary arteries in the setting of multiple trauma and prolonged hypotension.

Treatment of the source of embolism included open and endovascular abdominal aortic aneurysm repair, aortobifemoral bypass, axillobifemoral bypass with interruption of bilateral external iliac arteries, resection of cervical rib with repair of subclavian artery aneurysm, resection of popliteal aneurysm, and aortic and iliac stenting.

The first patient treated by our group was a 68-year-old patient who underwent resection of an abdominal aortic aneurysm and graft replacement in 1985. After finishing the operation, the surgeon learned that the blood pH was low and the base excess was -20. On examining the extremities, the surgeon found that the left lower extremity was pale, mottled, and cold. Distal pulses, however, were palpable. The patient was complaining of excruciating pain. The diagnosis of massive atheroembolism was made. Intra-arterial PGE1 was injected into the corresponding femoral artery; 250 micrograms of PGE1 injected in the left femoral artery over two hours produced some detectable changes in skin color and temperature. The dose was repeated several times over the next three days. The patient completely recovered without any tissue loss.

In 1992, a 62-year-old patient was admitted to the hospital with multiple, recurrent episodes of atheromatous embolization to the lower extremities. In addition, he had severe unreconstructible coronary artery disease with an ejection fraction of less than 20%. Recent pulmonary edema had been treated successfully. There was no cardiac thrombus found on echocardiogram and no evidence of arrhythmias on Holter monitoring. A small 3.8 cm abdominal aortic aneurysm was found on CT scan with laminated irregular mural thrombus. The distal atheromatous embolization was treated with intermittent treatment with intra-arterial PGE1 injection over four days. The daily dose was 500 micrograms. A marked improvement in the perfusion of distal lower extremities was achieved. Endovascular treatment of the aneurysm was then performed using a tubular dacron graft and two Palmaz stents at the ends.[91] Anuria was reversed within four hours of the procedure. After two weeks, the patient was discharged, completely recovered. The patient survived for nine years. The cause of death was an acute myocardial infarction. Postmortem examination showed a

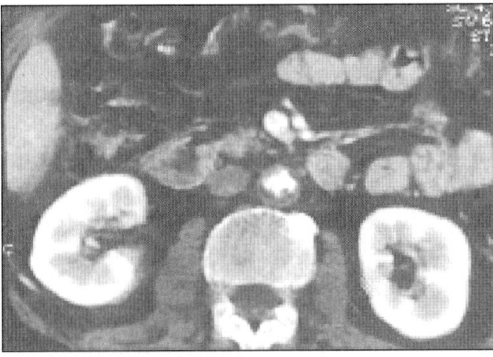 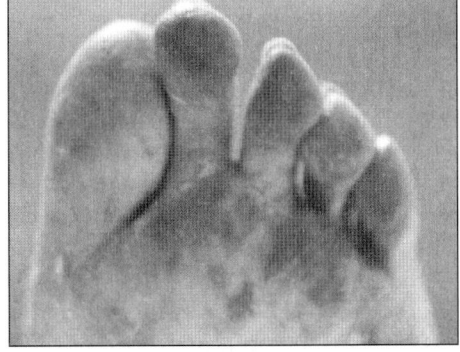

Figure 28-2. CT scan demonstrating a small aneurysm with mural thrombus. This patient presented with massive atheroembolism of the lower extremities.

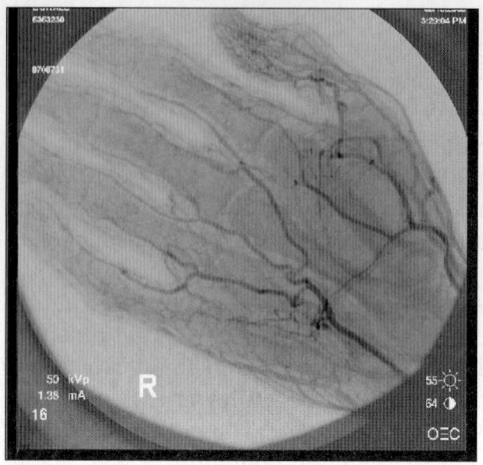 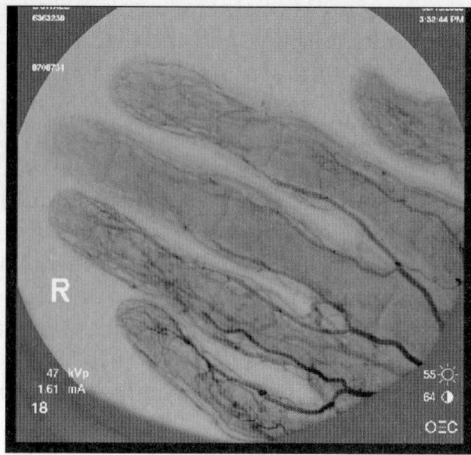

Figure 28-3. Angiogram of the hand before and after PGE1 infusion.

shrunken aneurysm and both ends of the endograft covered by endothelial cells. Focal kidney infarcts were found in both kidneys.

We have also successfully utilized prostaglandins for the treatment of acute upper extremity digital ischemia. (Figures 28–3).

In two cases of massive microembolization caused by endovascular treatment of aneurysms, the intra-arterial injection of PGE1 gave only temporary and partial improvement of perfusion. Both these patients died of multiorgan failure. One patient developed paraparesis from spinal cord emboli. Limb salvage was achieved in 23 patients. Limited toe amputation was needed in two patients. The effect of the drug was evident immediately after the injection when capillary refilling improved, cutaneous temperature increased, and pain subsided. No complications were recorded. In the last nine patients treated, all patients have remained asymptomatic over a follow-up period ranging from two to 134 months. Seven patients have been followed for more than two years.

SURGICAL THERAPY

In the presence of occlusive disease, surgical treatment of spontaneous atheroembolism remains the standard of care. The goal of surgical therapy is to safely remove atherosclerotic plaque from the bloodstream. In surgery, the artery can be clamped proximal and distal to the lesion before manipulating the diseased vessel. Thromboendartectomy or resection and graft replacement have been commonly used. In patients who are too weak for a major surgical intervention, ligation of the external iliac arteries or common femoral arteries followed by an extra-anatomic bypass such as axillobifemoral bypass, have been advocated. The ligation prevents further embolization reaching the legs, although embolization to the kidneys and intestines may still occur. The first report of surgical reconstruction to remove a potential source of cholesterol emboli was by Kazmier et. al. who reported in 1966 on three patients with livedo reticularis and digital infarcts treated by resection of abdominal aortic aneurysms containing ulcerated atheromatous plaques.[92] Two prospective trials reported favorable outcomes with vascular resection of atherosclerotic lesions. However, when the suprarenal aorta was involved, greater mortality rates were observed.[14,21] Some say that surgical elimination of the presumed source of cholesterol embolization should be reserved for patients with lower limb ischemia and infrarenal source of embolization.

ENDOVASCULAR TREATMENT

The endovascular treatment of embolizing lesions include percutaneous atherectomy, balloon angioplasty, and stent implantation. In percutaneous transluminal angioplasty, the intima is cracked and remodeled. Stent placement may provide a protective scaffold to help secure these lesions. Treatment of embolizing abdominal aneurysms with endovascular stents is often considered exceedingly high risk because of the well-founded concern that the unstable plaque or thrombus will dislodge as a result of catheter and wire manipulations before deployment. Lin et. al. in a retrospective study found that recurrent atheroembolism and amputation rates in the surgically treated patients was 0% and 20% in sharp contrast to the outcomes of patients treated with endovascular therapy, whose recurrent atheroembolism and amputation rates were 33% and 66%.[30] Renshaw et. al. reported successful angioplasty with stenting in eight patients with unilateral blue toe syndrome. Symptoms resolved in all eight patients over the ensuing month and there were no recurrences in a mean follow-up of 18.5 months.[93]

Covered stents offer the added advantage of completely excluding the diseased segment, preventing the escape of thrombus or plaque debris. Kumins reported on the successful use of the Wallgraft endoprosthesis in two patients with distal microembolism from common iliac artery disease.[94] Carroccio et. al. reported on endovascular stentgraft repair for abdominal aortic aneurysms in 16 patients presenting with atheromatous embolization syndrome. The 30-day mortality was zero and the aneurysms were successfully excluded in 88%. Resolution of foot ischemia and prevention of further atheromatous embolization was observed in 89% of patients still alive at one year. Six patients died during a mean follow-up of 26 months.[95] Shames et. al. have reported promising results in their treatment of embolizing arterial lesions with stent grafts. None of the eight patients treated with covered stents in their series had atheroembolic complications as a result of the procedure.[96] Likewise, Dougherty et. al. successfully implanted covered stents in two patients with embolizing atheroma in the infrarenal aorta without causing further embolization.[97]

The danger of atheromatous showers in patients with a diffusely atheromatous aorta during an endovascular procedure was addressed by Parodi et. al. This maneuver involves inserting a balloon-tip catheter for occlusion of both common iliac arteries. Antegrade flow is allowed through an iliac-to-femoral arterioarterial shunt connected to an inline filter. Moreover, filter wires are placed in the end-organs and to prevent any antegrade flow of emboli. This novel approach allows the use of endovascular intervention, and limits the possibility of dislodging atheroemboli to the limbs and viscera.[98]

PAIN CONTROL

Pain control is a critical aspect in the management of peripheral cholesterol embolism. The pain associated with lower extremity ischemic and necrotic lesions is generally severe and disproportionate to the amount of tissue involved. Sympathectomy can be used for palliation. The chief effect of lumbar sympathectomy is an increased blood flow through distal cutaneous arteriovenous anastomoses. In some patients, sufficient increase in nutritive flow occurs to permit healing of small superficial ulcers or relief of ischemic rest pain. Adequate arterial flow is essential, and sympathectomy is not of benefit in patients with an ankle to brachial index of less than 0.3. It is used as a palliative measure in patients with severe toe pain or pregangerous lesions who are not fit for major surgery or have inoperable disease. Sympathectomy should be considered as an adjunct to operation to assist digital salvage in patients with pregangerous areas. Lee et. al. demonstrated that adjunctive sympathectomy resulted in improved healing of distal digital ischemic ulcers.[99] Ghilardi et. al. have reported two cases of limb ischemia secondary to cholesterol embolism that were treated with the temporary surgical implantation of spinal cord stimulation devices.[100] They found spinal cord stimulation provided rapid and effective pain control, and rapid resolution of the necrotic lesions within four to six weeks.

OUTCOME

The outcome of patients with cholesterol embolization varies considerably. The natural history of atheroembolism emphasizes a high rate of both recurrent embolic episodes and tissue loss. The clinical syndrome of cholesterol embolization has a poor prognosis, particularly when there is evidence of visceral and renal involvement[2]. Morbidity and mortality in patients with cholesterol emboli syndrome are high. Death most often occurs from cardiovascular causes. Renal failure often progresses to dependence on dialysis. The one-year mortality rate for cholesterol embolization syndrome remains as high as 20% to 90%.[16] Wingo et. al. reviewed 50 reports of anecdotal cases or series of up to 35 patients with blue toe syndrome over the past 35 years. Among 327 patients, arterial reconstruction was carried out in 53% of the limbs. The amputation rate was 14%. There was a 20% mortality rate.[101] The best treatment for atheroembolization is its prevention, avoiding invasive procedures, and detecting potential aortic sources with other noninvasive examinations such at CT, MR, DU, and TEE.

CONCLUSIONS

The key to decreasing atheroembolization is prevention. Judicious use of endovascular therapies is paramount. When iatrogenic atheroembolization does occur, the current treatment regimen depends on keen observations and a prompt diagnostic workup.

Intra-arterial injection of prostaglandins appears to be an effective treatment of severe microembolization when all other treatments have failed. Dramatic response in severe distal ischemia caused by atheroembolism motivated the report of these results because other treatments are usually ineffective. The side effects and complications of prostaglandin therapy are miminal. Surgical or endovascular treatment of the primary source of atheromatous embolization should be performed to prevent recurrence.

REFERENCES

1. Darsee JR. Cholesterol embolism: the great masquerader. *South Med J*. 1979;72:174–80.
2. Fine MJ, Kapoor W, Falanga V. Cholesterol crystal embolization: a review of 221 cases in the English literature. *Angiology*. 1987;38:769–84.
3. Flory CM. Arterial occlusions produced by emboli from eroded aortic atheromatous plaques. *Am J Pathol*. 1945;21:549–65.
4. Venet L, Friedfeld L. Avulsion and embolization of a calcific arterial plaque; femoral embolectomy. *Surgery*. 1952;32:119–22.
5. Hoye SJ, Teitelbaum S, Gore I, Warren R. Atheromatous embolization; a factor in peripheral gangrene. *N Engl J Med*. 1959;261:128–31.
6. Kurose I, Wolf R, Grisham MB, Granger DN. Modulation of ischemia/reperfusion-induced microvascular dysfunction by nitric oxide. *Circ Res*. 1994;74:376–82.
7. Smith MC, Ghose MK, Henry AR. The clinical spectrum of renal cholesterol embolization. *Am J Med*. 1981;71:174–80.
8. Saklayen MG. Atheroembolic renal disease: preferential occurrence in whites only. *Am J Nephrol*. 1989;9:87–8.
9. Moolenaar W, Lamers CB. Cholesterol crystal embolization in the Netherlands. *Arch Intern Med*. 1996;156:653–7.
10. Thurlbeck WM, Castleman B. Atheromatous emboli to the kidney after aortic surgery. *N Engl J Med*. 1957;257:442–7.
11. Shah DJ, Leather RP. Arterioarterial atheromatous microemboli of the lower limb. In: Veith FJ, Hobson RW, William RA, Wilson SE, editors. *Vascular Surgery, 2nd edition*. St. Louis; 1994:397–408.
12. Drost H, Buis B, Haan D, Hillers JA. Cholesterol embolism as a complication of left heart catheterization: report of seven cases. *Br Heart J*. 1984;52:339–42.
13. Ramirez G, O'Neill WM Jr, Lambert R, Bloomer HA. Cholesterol embolization: a complication of angiography. *Arch Intern Med*. 1978;138:1430–2.
14. Keen RR, McCarthy WJ, Shireman PK, et. al. Surgical management of atheroembolization. *J Vasc Surg*. 1995;21:773–80.
15. Blauth CI, Cosgrove DM, Webb BW, et. al. Atheroembolism from the ascending aorta: an emerging problem in cardiac surgery. *J Thorac Cardiovasc Surg*. 1992;103:1104–11.
16. Scolari F, Tardanico R, Zani R, et. al. Cholesterol crystal embolism: a recognizable cause of renal disease. *Am J Kidney Dis*. 2000;36:1089–90.
17. Cross SS. How common is cholesterol embolism? *J Clin Pathol*. 1991;44:859–61.
18. Thompson MM, Smith J, Naylor AR, et. al. Microembolization during endovascular and conventional aneurysm repair. *J Vasc Surg*. 1997;25:179–86.
19. Fukumoto Y, Tsutsui H, Tsuchihashi M, et. al. The incidence and risk factors of cholesterol embolization syndrome: a complication of cardiac catheterization-a prospective study. *J Am Coll Cardiol*. 2003;42:211–6.
20. Keeley EC, Grines CL. Scraping of aortic debris by coronary guiding catheters: a prospective evaluation of 1,000 cases. *J Am Coll Cardiol*. 1998;32:1861–5.
21. Baumann DS, McGraw D, Rubin BG, et. al. An institutional experience with arterial atheroembolism. *Ann Vasc Surg*. 1994;8:258–65.
22. Sharma PV, Babu SC, Shah PM, Nassoura ZE. Changing patterns of atheroembolism. *Cardiovasc Surg*. 1996;4:573–9.
23. Dadian N, Ohki T, Veith FJ, et. al. Overt colon ischemia after endovascular aneurysm repair: the importance of microembolization as an etiology. *J Vasc Surg*. 2001;34:986–96.
24. Sandison AJ, Edmondson RA, Panayiotopoulos YP, et. al. Fatal colonic ischemia after stent graft for aortic aneurysm. *Eur J Vasc Endovasc Surg*. 1997;13:219–20.
25. Scolari F, Bracchi M, Valzorio B, et. al. Cholesterol atheromatous embolism: an increasingly recognized cause of acute renal failure. *Nephrol Dial Tranplant*. 1996;11:1607–12.
26. Eggebrecht H, Oldenburg O, Dirsch O, et. al. Potential embolization by atherosclerotic debris dislodged from aortic wall during cardiac catheterization: histological and clinical findings in 7,621 patients. *Catheter Cardiovasc Interv*. 2000;49:389–94.

27. Colt HG, Begg RJ, Saporito JJ, et. al. Cholesterol emboli after cardiac catheterization: 8 cases and a review of the literature. *Medicine (Baltimore)*. 1988;67:389–400.
28. Saklayen MG, Gupta S, Suryaprasad A, Azmeh W. Incidence of atheroembolic renal failure after coronary angiography: a prospective study. *Angiology*. 1997;48:609–13.
29. Antonucci F, Pizzolitto S, Travaglini M, et. al. Atheroembolic renal disease: clinicopathologic correlations. *Adv Exp Med Biol*. 1989;252:59–64.
30. Lin PH, Bush RL, Conklin BS, et. al. Late complication of aortoiliac stent placement: atheroembolization of the lower extremities. *J Surg Res*. 2002;103:153–9.
31. Doty JR, Wilentz RE, Salazar JD, et. al. Atheroembolism in cardiac surgery. *Ann Thorac Surg*. 2003;75:1221–6.
32. The French Study of aortic plaques in stroke group. Atherosclerotic disease of the aortic arch as a risk factor for recurrent ischemic stroke. *N Engl J Med*. 1996;334:1216–21.
33. Karmody AM, Powers SR, Monaco VJ, Leather RP. "Blue toe" syndrome: an indication for limb salvage surgery. *Arch Surg*. 1976;111:1263–8.
34. Falanga V, Fine MJ, Kapoor WN. The cutaneous manifestations of cholesterol crystal embolization. *Arch Dermatol*. 1986;122:1194–8.
35. Chaudhary K, Wall BM, Rasberry RD. Livedo reticularis: an underutilized diagnostic clue in cholesterol embolization syndrome. *Am J Med Sci*. 2001;321:348–51.
36. Donohue KG, Saap L, Falanga V. Cholesterol crystal embolization: an atherosclerotic disease with frequent and varied cutaneous manifestations. *J Eur Acad Dermatol Venereol*. 2003;17:504–11.
37. Mayo RR, Swartz RD. Redefining the incidence of clinically detectable atheroembolism. *Am J Med*. 1996;100:524–9.
38. Thadhani RI, Camargo CA Jr, Xavier RJ, et. al. Atheroembolic renal failure after invasive procedures: natural history based on 52 histologically proven cases. *Medicine (Baltimore)*. 1995;74:350–8.
39. Gittinger JW Jr, Kershaw GR. Retinal cholesterol emboli in the diagnosis of renal atheroembolism. *Arch Intern Med*. 1998;158:1265–7.
40. Ezzeddine MA, Primavera JM, Rosand J, et. al. Clinical characteristics of pathologically proved cholesterol emboli to the brain. *Neurology*. 2000;54:1681–3.
41. Kasinath BS, Corwin HL, Bidani AK, et. al. Eosinophilia in the diagnosis of atheroembolic renal disease. *Am J Nephrol*. 1987;7:173–7.
42. Nicholls SC, Smith W. Peripheral arterial embolization: Doppler ultrasound scan diagnosis. *J Vasc Surg*. 2000;31:811–4.
43. Al-Hamali S, Baskerville P, Fraser S, et. al. Detection of distal emboli in patients with peripheral arterial stenosis before and after iliac angioplasty: a prospective study. *J Vasc Surg*. 1999;29:345–51.
44. Cabili S, Hochman I, Goor Y. Reversal of gangrenous lesions in the blue toe syndrome with lovastatin: a case report. *Angiology*. 1993;44:821–5.
45. Woolfson RG, Lachmann H. Improvement in renal cholesterol emboli syndrome after simvastatin. *Lancet*. 1998;352:321–2.
46. Corti R, Fuster V, Fayad ZA, et. al. Lipid lowering by simvastatin induces regression of human atherosclerotic lesions: two years' follow-up by high-resolution noninvasive magnetic resonance imaging. *Circulation*. 2002;106:2884–7.
47. Scolari F, Ravani P, Pola A, et. al. Predictors of renal and patient outcomes in atheroembolic renal disease: a prospective study. *J Am Soc Nephrol*. 2003;14:1584–90.
48. Tunick PA, Nayar AC, Goodkin GM, et. al. Effect of treatment on the incidence of stroke and other emboli in 519 patients with severe thoracic aortic plaque. *Am J Cardiol*. 2002;90:1320–5.
49. Pardy BJ, Lewis JD, Eastcott HH. Preliminary experience with prostaglandins E1 and I2 in peripheral vascular disease. *Surgery*. 1980;88:826–32.
50. Elinav E, Chajek-Shaul T, Stern M. Improvement in cholesterol emboli syndrome after iloprost therapy. *BMJ*. 2002;324:268–9.

51. Morris-Jones W, Preston FE, Greaney M, Chatterjee DK. Gangrene of the toes with palpable peripheral pulses. *Ann Surg.* 1981;193:462–6.
52. Bruns FJ, Segel DP, Adler S. Control of cholesterol embolization by discontinuation of anti-coagulant therapy. *Am J Med Sci.* 1978;275:105–8.
53. Hyman BT, Landas SK, Ashman RF, et. al. Warfarin-related purple toes syndrome and cholesterol microembolization. *Am J Med.* 1987;82:1233–7.
54. Moldveen-Geronimus M, Merriam JC Jr. Cholesterol embolization: from pathological curiosity to clinical entity. *Circulation.* 1967;35:946–53.
55. Hammond GL, Cronau LH, Whittaker D, Gillis CN. Fate of prostaglandins E(1) and A(1) in the human pulmonary circulation. *Surgery.* 1977;81:716–22.
56. Moncada S, Gryglewski R, Bunting S, Vane JR. An enzyme isolated from arteries transforms prostaglandin endoperoxides to an unstable substance that inhibits platelet aggregation. *Nature.* 1976;263:663–5.
57. Igarashi R, Takenaga M, Takeuchi J, et. al. Marked hypotensive and blood flow-increasing effects of a new lipo-PGE(1)(lipo-ASO13) due to vascular wall targeting. *J Control Release.* 2001;71:157–64.
58. Marchesi S, Pasqualini L, Lombardini R, et. al. Prostaglandin E1 improves endothelial function in critical limb ischemia. *J Cardiovasc Pharmacol.* 2003;41:249–53.
59. Simpson PJ, Fantone JC, Mickelson JK, et. al. Identification of a time window for therapy to reduce experimental canine myocardial injury: suppression of neutrophil activation during 72 hours of reperfusion. *Circ Res.* 1988;63:1070–9.
60. Simpson PJ, Mitsos SE, Ventura A, et. al. Prostacyclin protects ischemic reperfused myocardium in the dog by inhibition of neutrophil activation. *Am Heart J.* 1987;113:129–37.
61. Belkin M, LaMorte WL, Wright JG, Hobson RW 2nd. The role of leukocytes in the pathophysiology of skeletal muscle ischemic injury. *J Vasc Surg.* 1989;10:14–18.
62. Szczeklik A, Nizankowski R, Skawinski S, et. al. Successful therapy of advanced arteriosclerosis obliterans with prostacyclin. *Lancet.* 1979;1:1111–4.
63. Nehler MR, Brass EP, Anthony R, Dormandy J, et. al. Adjunctive parenteral therapy with lipo-ecraprost, a prostaglandin E1 analog, in patients with critical limb ischemia undergoing distal revascularization does not improve 6-month outcomes. *J Vasc Surg.* 2007;45:953–60.
64. Brass EP, Anthony R, Dormandy J, Hiatt WR, et. al. Parenteral therapy with lipo-ecraprost, a lipid-based formulation of a PGE1 analog, does not alter six-month outcomes in patients with critical leg ischemia. *J Vasc Surg.* 2006;43:752–9.
65. De Donato G, Gussoni G, de Donato G, et. al. The ILAILL study: iloprost as adjuvant to surgery for acute ischemia of lower limbs: a randomized, placebo-controlled, double-blind study by the Italian society for vascular and endovascular surgery. *Ann Surg.* 2006;244:185–93.
66. Milio G, Corrado E, Genova C, et. al. Iloprost treatment in patients with Raynaud's phenomenon secondary to systemic sclerosis and the quality of life: a new therapeutic protocol. Rheumatology (Oxford). 2006;45:999–1004.
67. Milio G, Mina C, Cospite V, et. al. Efficacy of the treatment with prostaglandin E-1 in venous ulcers of the lower limbs. *J Vasc Surg.* 2005;42:304–8.
68. The ICAI Study Group. Prostanoids for chronic critical leg ischemia: a randomized, controlled, open-label trial with prostaglandin E1. *Ann Intern Med.* 1999;130:412–21.
69. Negus D, Irving JD, Friedgood A. Intra-arterial prostacyclin compared to praxilene in the management of severe lower limb ischemia: a double blind trial. *J Cardiovasc Surg.* 1987;28:196–9.
70. Carlson LA, Eriksson I. Femoral artery infusion of prostaglandin E1 in severe peripheral vascular disease. *Lancet.* 1973;1:155–6.
71. Carlson LA, Olsson AG. Intravenous prostaglandin E1 in severe peripheral vascular disease. *Lancet.* 1976;2:810.
72. Sethi GK, Scott SM, Takaro T. Effect of intra-arterial infusion of PGE1 in patients with severe ischemia of lower extremity. *J Cardiovasc Surg.* 1980:21:185–92.

73. Eklund AE, Eriksson G, Olsson AG. A controlled study showing significant short term effect of prostaglandin E1 in healing of ischaemic ulcers of the lower limb in man. *Prostaglandins Leukot Med.* 1982;8:265–71.

74. Sakaguchi S, Kusaba A, Mishima Y, Kamiya K, Nishimura A, et. al. A multi-clinical double blind study with PGE (alpha-cyclodextrin) in patients with ischemic ulcer of the extremities. *Vasa.*. 1978;7:263–6.

75. Dormandy J. Use of the prostacyclin analogue iloprost in the treatment of patients with critical limb ischemia. *Therapie.* 1991;46:319–22.

76. Creutzig A, Lehmacher W, Elze M. Meta-analysis of randomized controlled prostaglandin E1 studies in peripheral arterial occlusive disease stages III and IV. *Vasa.* 2004;33:137–44.

77. Gruss JD. Experience with PGE1 in patients with postoperative trashfoot. *Vasa Suppl.* 1989;28:57–60.

78. Grenader T, Lifschitz M, Shavit L. Iloprost in embolic renal failure. *Mt Sinai J Med.* 2005 ;72: 339–41.

79. Scheffler P, de la Hamette D, Gross J, et. al. Intensive vascular training in stage IIb of peripheral arterial occlusive disease: the additive effects of intravenous prostaglandin E1 or intravenous pentoxifylline during training. *Circulation.* 1994;90:818–22.

80. Belch JJ, Bell PR, Creissen D, et. al. Randomized, double-blind, placebo-controlled study evaluating the efficacy and safety of AS-013, a prostaglandin E1 prodrug, in patients with intermittent claudication. *Circulation.* 1997;95:2298–302.

81. Mohler ER 3rd, Hiatt WR, Olin JW, et. al. Treatment of intermittent claudication with beraprost sodium, an orally active prostaglandin I2 analogue: a double-blinded, randomized, controlled trial. *J Am Coll Cardiol.* 2003;41:1679–86.

82. Lievre M, Azoulay S, Lion L, et. al. A dose-effect study of beraprost sodium in intermittent claudication. *J Cardiovasc Pharmacol.* 1996;27:788–93.

83. Lievre M, Morand S, Besse B, et. al. Oral beraprost sodium, a prostaglandin I2 analogue, for intermittent claudication : a double-blind, randomized, multicenter controlled trial. *Circulation.* 2000;102:426–31.

84. Motz E, Gasparini D, Basadonna P, Ceriello A, Bartoli E. Intra-arterial iloprost for limb ischaemia. *Lancet.* 1995;346:1295.

85. Andreev A, Kavrakov T, Petkov D, Penkov P. Severe acute hand ischemia following an accidental intraarterial drug injection, successfully treated with thrombolysis and intraarterial iloprost infusion. *Angiology.* 1995;46:963–7.

86. Mazzone A, Giani L, Faggioli P, et. al. Cocaine-related peripheral vascular occlusive disease treated with iloprost in addition to anticoagulants and antibiotics. *Clin Toxicol.* 2007;45:65–6.

87. Otsuka H, Akashi H, Murohara T, et. al. The prostacyclin analog beraprost sodium augments the efficacy of therapeutic angiogenesis induced by autologous bone marrow cells. *Ann Vasc Surg.* 2006;20:646–52.

88. Mehrabi MR, Serbecic N, Tamaddon F, et. al. Clinical benefit of prostaglandin E1-treatment of patients with ischemic heart disease: stimulation of therapeutic angiogenesis in vital and infracted myocardium. *Biomed Pharmacother.* 2003;57:173–8.

89. Schellong SM, Burchert W, Boger RM, et. al. Prostaglandin E1 in peripheral vascular disease: a PET study of muscular blood flow. *Scand J Clin Lab Invest.* 1998;58:109–17.

90. Oberender H, Krais T, Schafer M, Belcher G. Clinical benefits of iloprost, a stable prostacyclin (PGI2) analog, in severe peripheral arterial disease (PAD). *Adv Prostaglandin Thromboxane Leukot Res.* 1989;19:311–6.

91. Parodi JC, Palmaz JC, Barone HD. Transfemoral intraluminal graft implantation for abdominal aortic aneurysms. *Ann Vasc Surg.* 1991;5:491–9.

92. Kazmier FJ, Sheps SG, Bernatz PE, Sayre GP. Livedo reticularis and digital infarcts: a syndrome due to cholesterol emboli arisig from atheromatous abdominal aortic aneurysms. *Vasc Dis.* 1966;3:12–24.

93. Renshaw A, McCowen T, Waltke EA, et. al. Angioplasty with stenting is effective in treating blue toe syndrome. *Vasc Endovascular Surg.* 2002;36:155–9.

94. Kumins NH, Owens EL, Oglevie SB, et. al. Early experience using the Wallgraft in the management of distal microembolism from common iliac pathology. *Ann Vasc Surg*. 2002;16:181–6.

95. Carroccio A, Olin JW, Ellozy SH, et. al. The role of aortic stent grafting in the treatment of atheromatous embolization syndrome: results after a mean of 15 months follow-up. *J Vasc Surg*. 2004;40:424–9.

96. Shames ML, Rubin BG, Sanchez LA, et. al. Treatment of embolizing arterial lesions with endoluminally placed stent grafts. *Ann Vasc Surg*. 2002;16:608–12.

97. Dougherty MJ, Calligaro KD. Endovascular treatment of embolization of aortic plaque with covered stents. *J Vasc Surg*. 2002;36:727–31.

98. Parodi JC, Mura RL, Ferreira LM. Safety maneuvers to prevent embolism complicating endovascular aortic repair. *J Vasc Surg*. 2002;36:1076–8.

99. Lee BY, Madden JL, Thoden WR, McCann WJ. Lumbar sympathectomy for toe gangrene: long-term follow-up. *Am J Surg*. 1983;145:398–401.

100. Ghilardi G, Massaro F, Gobatti D, et. al. Temporary spinal cord stimulation for peripheral cholesterol embolism. *J Cardiovasc Surg*. 2002;43:255–8.

101. Wingo JP, Nix WM, Greenfield LJ, Barnes RW. The blue toe syndrome: hemodynamics and therapeutic correlates of outcome. *J Vasc Surg*. 1986;3:475–80.

94. Keeney NH, Cheyne JE, Ochsner SF, et al. Early experience using the V catheter in the management of distal microembolism from common iliac pathology. *Am J Vasc Surg*. 2001:18:?-?

95. Carroccio A, Olin JW, Ellozy SH, et al. The role of aortic stent grafting in the treatment of atheromatous embolization syndrome: results after a mean of 15 months follow-up. *J Vasc Surg*. 2004:10:821-?

96. Shames ML, Rubin BG, Sanchez LA, et al. Treatment of embolizing arterial lesions with endoluminally placed stent grafts. *Ann Vasc Surg*. 2002:16:608-12

97. Dorigo W, Gargiulo M, et al. Endovascular treatment or embolization of aortic plaque with transcatheter. *J Vasc Surg*. 2002:36:227-31

98. Ferrari JC, Mintz GS, et al. Safety maneuvers to prevent embolism complicating intravascular stenting. *J Vasc Surg*. 2001:36:16-?-?

99. Vacek JL, Madrid G, Schneider WR, et al. Lumbar sympathectomy for toe gangrene long-term follow up. *Am J Surg*. 1983:145:598-604

100. Graham LM, Stanley JC, Ushida O, et al. Popular aortic aneurysm and stimulation for peripheral cholesterol embolism. *J Vasc Surg*. 2003. 2003:20:?-?

101. Wingo JP, Nix WM, Greene FL, Barnes RW. The blue toe syndrome: hemodynamics and therapeutic options. *J Vasc Surg*. 1986:37:?-?

29

Inguinal Wound Complications, Lymphatic Leak, Lymphoceles, and Graft Infections

Jonathan B. Towne, M.D.

Access to the common femoral, superficial femoral, and profunda femoris arteries is a mainstay in vascular reconstruction. These vessels often provide outflow for aortoiliac procedures and are universally used to provide inflow for lower extremity bypasses. Incisions in this area can be hazardous given its proximity to the perineum, and the potential for direct contamination from both urine and stool. This part of the body tends to remain moist from lack of hygiene and contact from an overlying pannus in obese patients. Because of this unique anatomy, inguinal wounds have always been problematic in vascular surgery.

WOUND COMPLICATIONS: INCIDENCE

The exact incidence of inguinal wound complications is unknown, but has been reported to be between 1.5% to 12% for prosthetic grafts and 0% to 1.7% for autogenous graft if all time periods are considered.[1,2] Several important risk factors predispose to subsequent graft infection. Wound healing complications such as skin or subcutaneous tissue necrosis, cellulitis, hematoma, or lymphatic leak significantly increases the risk of subsequent graft infection. Local wound complications occur in up to 44% of infrainguinal bypass procedures,[3] and up to a third of graft infection have preceding wound problems. In their study assessing risk factors for primary graft infections, Edwards et. al. identified postoperative wound infection as the primary predisposing factor in 33% of subsequent graft infections.[4] Likewise, Cherry and coworkers reviewed 39 cases of infrainguinal graft infections and found that postoperative wound infection occurred in 28% of cases.[5] The presence of a groin incision greatly increases the risk of both wound and graft infection. In a study of 2,411 consecutive prosthetic arterial reconstructions, 3.5% of 489 femoroperipheral reconstructions developed graft infection, and of note was that graft infection occurred only when a groin incision had been used.[6] Other risk factors for infectious complications include emergency bypass procedures and the need for early reoperation for graft thrombosis or bleeding. In a review of their arterial graft infections, Hoffert et. al. found that 50% of conduit infections had required early reoperation for postoperative hematoma formation, and in Kent's series, infectious complications were associated with emergent operations in 13% of cases.[1,3]

Multiple factors predisposed to wound infections, and relate to specific patient characteristics and to the occurrence of other early postoperative complications. In a review of 126 consecutive patients who underwent in situ vein bypass, Reifsnyder et. al. found that early graft revision (<4 days) and the presence of a lymph leak significantly increased the risk for postoperative wound infection.[7] However, factors such as age, race, diabetes, duration of operation, and presence of gangrene or ulceration did not significantly influence the incidence of infectious complications in that series. Wengrovitz and coworkers retrospectively studied 163 subcutaneous saphenous vein bypasses and found on regression analysis that chronic steroid use, ipsilateral ulceration, and pedal bypasses predicted an increased incidence of wound infection. They also identified female gender, diabetes, use of continuous incisions, and procedures for limb salvage as factors associated with wound complications in their group of patients.[8]

Inguinal wound problems can be divided into three areas: 1) wound healing problems with the groin incision, 2) acute perioperative graft infections, and 3) chronic graft infections. Szilagyi developed an excellent system of classifying inguinal wounds. He graded wounds based on the depth of involvement.[9] We use a modified Szilagyi classification. Grade I only involves the dermis. Grade II infections extend to the subcutaneous tissues but do not invade the graft. Grade III infections directly involve the graft, but not the anastomosis. Grade IV includes infections directly involving the anastomosis but not associated with bacteria or hemorrhage Grade V describes an infected anastomosis with sepsis and bleeding at the time of presentation.

Wound healing complications such as hematoma, lymphocele, or tissue necrosis usually precede deep wound involvement. The timing of infection determines to a large extent how the process will present. Early graft infections will usually present in conjunction with wound infection, and are associated with signs of systemic sepsis including fever, leucocytosis, and bacteriemia.

With Grades I and II wounds involving only the skin and subcutaneous tissue, antibiotic administration and local wound hygiene are sufficient to contain the problem and allow healing. More major complications in terms of Grades III and IV wounds, particularly those resulting from graft exposure, require aggressive wound management to salvage the graft. Critical aspects of treatment of Class III wounds are operative debridement and immediate coverage of the grafts' autogenous tissue. Ouriel et. al. noted delayed coverage of exposed vein grafts until wounds were cleanly granulating, and then covered with full thickness skin grafts or musculocutaneous flaps.[2] Despite these efforts, vein graft rupture was seen. With immediate coverage of grafts, we suffered no leg failures, and although coverage of the graft with muscle is preferable, we think expediting coverage with any autogenous tissue to avoid desiccation and graft exposure prevents subsequent graft rupture.[7] The value of muscle coverage in groin wounds cannot be overemphasized. The muscle myoplasty provides an excellent environment by placing well-vascularized tissue over vascular conduits.

Our initial choice is the sartorius myoplasty followed by gracilis and rectus abdominous myoplasties. Vascular surgeons can perform sartorius myoplasty once the location of blood supply and technique of muscle rotation is understood. The origin of the sartorius from the anterior superior iliac spine is dissected free and transected mobilizing the proximal 8 cm of the muscle. It is important to note that the blood supply to the sartorius muscle primarily branches from the superficial femoral artery, which enters the muscle along its medial edge. In an attempt not to disrupt the blood supply, the muscle is then rotated from lateral to medial, leaving the medial edge intact, flipping the muscle over so its anterior surface becomes the posterior surface. In doing this, an adequate amount of muscle to cover the groin vasculature is available. The mobilized proximal muscle easily reaches under the inguinal ligament to provide coverage of the proximal femoral vessels. The advantage of this rotation technique is that the muscle is not devascularized. This results in an excellent vascularized pedicle that significantly aids in wound healing. Alternate valuable sources of muscle flaps are the gracilis muscle and rectus abdominus muscle. These types of procedures generally require consults with the assistance of plastic surgeons. The effectiveness of muscle flaps has been reported by Graham and colleagues[10] and Tukiainen and associates.[11] Porter and associates reported excellent results with rotational muscle flaps in treating contaminated wounds.[12] They prefer not to use the sartorius muscle because of its segmental arterial supply that is often inadequate after mobilization. Meter and associates also prefer rotational muscle flaps to the Sartorius muscle.[13]

LYMPH LEAKS

A unique aspect of groin wounds is the propensity for development of lymphatic complications due to the rich lymphatic network of the femoral triangle, which are uncommon but potentially serious complications of femoral reconstruction. A review of the Henry Ford Hospital experience by Tyndall et. al. identified 41 lymphatic complications (28 lymphocutaneous fistulas and 13 lymphoceles) in 2,679 arterial reconstructions over a 15-year period, for an incidence of 1.2% per incision.[14] Interestingly, the incidence varied with the type of procedure and whether the procedure was a reoperation. Aortobifemoral bypass for aneurysmal disease in a previously operated groin had the highest incidence (8.1%) of lymphatic complications, followed by an isolated femoral procedure in a previously operated groin (5.3%). The lowest frequency was found in patients undergoing a femoralpopiteal/tibial bypass for the first time (0.5%). Aggressive treatment of lymphatic fistulas provided the best results. There were no wound or graft infections in patients treated with operation.

Drainage from the leg wound, especially the groin, early in the postoperative period is often the result of divided lymphatic vessels that have not sealed. These complications, a common problem in patients who have undergone kidney transplants, are presumably caused by an increase in lymph drainage from placement of the donor kidney in the lower quadrant. The problems caused by a lymph leak were documented in a series of 126 consecutive patients reported by Reifsnyder et. al., who underwent in situ bypasses of the lower extremity.[7] Risk-factor analysis demonstrated that the development of a postoperative lymph leak was significantly related to the subsequent wound infection. Rubin et. al. demonstrated in an animal model that lymphatics contaminated with bacteria resulted in positive blood and graft cultures.[15] Experimentally, transection of lymphatics at the graft site in the presence of a distal infection leads to significantly more graft infections than does lymphatic ligation and exclusion. Lymphatic bacterial transport contributed to the graft infection, both from direct seeding and from transmission of bacteria to the blood, leading to seeding of the graft.

Because of the relationship of the lymph leak with subsequent significant wound infections, these patients should be treated aggressively. Our initial plan is to paint the wound with povidone-iodine (Betadine) and apply a tight compressive dressing. Antibiotics, usually cephalosporins, are given and the patient is placed on bed rest. If the wound continues to drain for more than 72 hours, the patient should be returned to the operating room and the wound explored. The offending lymphatic can often be identified and suture-ligated. A subcutaneous drain, well separated from the arterial prosthesis, is then brought out through a separate stab hole. Placement of the drain allows the skin incision to heal. This technique is generally successful in controlling the wound drainage, and more importantly, prevents secondary infection of the lymphatic cavity.

Resolution of the fistula occurred two and a half times sooner in patients in whom inguinal wounds were re-explored than in those treated conservatively in a study by Roberts et. al.[16] Length of hospital stay, time to resolution, and incidence of wound complications did not vary between those treated operatively or with aspiration, and in those with lymphoceles treated conservatively.

LYMPHOCELES

Patients who develop lymphoceles following groin surgery are followed expectantly. If the lymphoceles increase in size with time, they should be operatively explored and treated as noted above with regard to the leaking wound. Likewise, if they communicate with the groin wound and begin to leak, they should also be explored. Small to moderate size lymphoceles that are away from the incision and do not involve the graft can be followed. Many times, these will resolve slowly over time. Lymphoceles should be treated operatively if they become large or uncomfortable for the patient, or if they distend the groin wound. The injection of isosulfan blue into the foot prior to operation helps to identify the lymphatic channels that feed the lymphocele.[17] The use of duplex ultrasound can clearly identify the lymphocele and determine whether it involves the prosthesis. Lymphoceles that are in close proximity to the vascular prosthesis are best drained surgically in order to prevent any possible secondary infection of the vascular graft. When the lymphocele is well separated from the vascular prosthesis, sclerotherapy using powdered tetracycline can be used. Powdered tetracycline is mixed with sterile saline and injected into the lymphocele, which will often sclerose the lymphocele.[18] Porcellini and associates reported successful treatment of lymphoceles with just leg elevation, limited ambulation, and pressure dressings.[19] They advise against serial aspirations for fear of causing secondary infection. Rotational muscle flaps are also an effective method to deal with lymphatic complications following femoral arterial reconstruction.[20] This treatment should be done when there is concern of coexisting infection and/or exposure of the arterial anastomosis. The most important factor in dealing with lymphatic problems of the groin is prevention, which may be achieved by meticulous dissection with ligation of any lymphatic channels noted during vascular exposure. In particular, if a lymph node is inadvertently bisected during the dissection, both halves should be suture-ligated.

WOUND INFECTION: PROPHYLATIC MEASURES

Preoperatively, patients should undergo a through cleansing of the perineum in the groin. Any fungal infections, if present, should be treated and resolved prior to elective groin incisions. Particularly in obese patients, attention to personal hygiene in the perineum is important to limiting problems with subsequent healing.

Another factor to be considered is patients who have chronic wounds of the lower extremity. These wounds should be cultured and the patient placed on antibiotics specific to the bacteria that are isolated. These bacteria are often present in the lymphatics that drain the groin. Also, if possible, lower extremity infections should be treated and resolved prior to revascularization.

PATHOPHYSIOLOGY

The primary cause of infectious wound or graft complications involves contamination at the time of surgery. Contamination can occur when the graft contacts the skin and from breaks in surgical technique. Emergent operations increase the risk for infectious complications potentially because of lack of attention to sterile technique and possibly due to the immunologic status of the stressed patient. Early reoperation also increases the risk of infection secondary to increased exposure of the graft to potential contamination, and from any retained thrombus or debris that can serve as potent culture media. In addition, factors such as prolonged operative times and extended preoperative hospitalization are thought to contribute to risk of wound and graft infection. Levy et. al. prospectively obtained skin flora cultures on the day of admission, day of surgery, and five days postoperatively in patients undergoing lower extremity revascularization. They demonstrated that patients enter the hospital colonized with slime-producing coagulase-negative staphylococci, and that strains shift from predominantly susceptible to predominately resistant species.[21]

Colonization of native artery can be a source of graft contamination. Macbeth and colleagues cultured arterial specimens and surrounding tissue (as controls) from patients undergoing clean, elective prosthetic arterial reconstructions.[22] Forty-three percent of arterial segments were cultured positive with *Staphylococcus epidermidis* as the most common isolate while all controls were sterile. Correlation of culture data to subsequent suture line disruption in infected grafts at their institution revealed that positive arterial cultures were associated with disruption in 57% of cases, whereas there were no anastomotic disruptions in patients with negative arterial cultures.[14] Durham and associates corroborated this data with a 43% culture positive rate and noted that graft infections occurred only in culture-positive arteries. In addition, they found that positive arterial cultures had no predictive value regarding graft infection at initial operations, but that positive arterial cultures were associated with eventual graft infection in 28% of patients undergoing subsequent vascular reconstructions.[23]

Another potential source of graft infection is from hematogenous or lymphatic seeding from remote sites of infection or colonization. Experiments in dogs have demonstrated intravenous infusion of 10^7 colony-forming units of *Staphylococcus aureus* will produce clinical graft infection in nearly 100% of animals in the early postoperative period.[24] The lymphatic system has also been implicated in the pathogenesis of graft infection originating from a distal septic focus such as an infected ischemic foot ulcer by both hematogenous spread and from direct seeding of the graft. Experimentally, transection of lymphatics at the graft site in the presence of a distal infection leads to significantly more graft infections compared to lymphatic ligation and excision.[25] They concluded that lymphatic bacterial transport contributed to graft infection, both from direct graft seeding and from transmission of bacteria to the blood leading to hematogenous seeding of the graft. The likelihood for a graft to become infected decreases with time due to development of a pseudointimal layer and incorporation within surrounding tissues, but the graft can remain at significant risk for up to a year after implantation. Even years after implantation, the graft can be seeded by bacteremia thought to be due to an incomplete pseudointimal lining. To what extent this mechanism contributes to the pathogenesis of graft infection in humans is unknown, but bacteremia has been associated with such procedures as central venous or bladder catheterization, gastrointestinal endoscopy, dental or genitourinary instrumentation, and in patients harboring remote infections such as pneumonia, endocarditis, and distal foot infections.

Wound healing complications such as hematoma, lymphocele, or tissue necrosis usually precede deeper involvement. Timing of infection determines to a large extent how the process will present. Early graft infections will usually present in conjunction with wound infection, and are associated with signs of systemic sepsis including fever, leukocytosis, and bacteremia. The initial presenting sign of graft infection in up to a quarter of patients is anastomotic disruption with potential exsanguinating hemorrhage.[4] Inguinal wounds are most commonly involved, and the majority of patients presenting with graft infection at the groin present with overt signs of wound sepsis with abscess formation, cellulitis, sinus tract development, or graft exposure.[26] Less commonly, deeper infection may be heralded by distal petechiae from septic microembolization, graft thrombosis, or a pulsatile mass over an anastomotic site. These infections tend to occur within the first weeks of surgery and are generally associated with coagulase-positive staphylococci or virulent Gram-negative organisms.

Wound infection after infrainguinal arterial reconstruction is common and can occur in up to 44% of procedures.[3] Risk factors and classification of wound infection are discussed above and impact on subsequent treatment. Class I and II infections are considered "minor," and generally respond to operative debridement, local wound care, and intravenous antibiotics.[27] Class III wounds with graft exposure are more of a concern and are associated with more conduit complications. Prime management objectives of these wounds are early surgical debridement, drainage of clinically significant fluid collections, and conformation of autogeneous tissue coverage.[28] Ouriel and colleagues managed wounds in 16 patients with exposed autogenous vein grafts with local wound care and delayed autogenous tissue coverage until adequate granulation had developed. They reported hemorrhage or thrombosis in 56% of cases managed in this manner.[2] Alternatively, Reifsnyder and colleagues described their experience with wound complication management with *early* operative debridement, autogenous tissue coverage when indicated, and three times daily dressing changes and parenteral antibiotics in 55 wound infections, 13 of which were graft-threatening. This management protocol resulted in no deaths, no limb loss, and universal graft salvage.[7] There must be a high index of suspicion of graft involvement in any wound infection, and early surgical inspection to rule out graft involvement is required if overt conduit infection is to be avoided.

A distinction needs to be made between exposed vascular conduits that are often secondary to wound healing problems in the groin from conduits that are infected.

The primary indication of infected conduit is bleeding from the suture line. Once we obtain suture line bleeding, usually graft excision and revascularization by remote extra-anatomic bypasses is the best way to salvage the lower extremity and rid the patient of infection. When the conduit is exposed, debridement and coverage with autogenous tissue is necessary.

REFERENCES

1. Hoffert PW, Gensler S, Haimovici H. Infection complicating arterial grafts. *Arch Surg.* 1965;90:427–435.
2. Ouriel K, Geary KJ, Green RM, DeWeese JA. Fate of the exposed saphenous vein graft. *Am J Surg.* 1990;160:148–50.
3. Kent KC, Bartek S, Kuntz KM, et. al. Prospective study of wound complications in continuous infrainguinal incisions after lower limb areterial reconstruction: incidence, risk factors, and cost. *Surgery.* 1996;119:378–83.
4. Edwards WH Jr, Martin RS III, Jenkins JM, Edwards WH Sr. Primary graft infections. *J Vasc Surg.* 1987;6:235–239.
5. Cherry KJ Jr, Roland CF, Pairolero PC, et. al. Infected femorodistal bypass: is graft removal mandatory? *J Vasc Surg.* 1992;15:295–305.
6. Lorentzen JE, Nielsen OM, Arendrup H, et. al. Vascular graft infection: an analysis of sixty-two graft infections in 2411 consecutively implanted synthetic vascular grafts. *Surgery.* 1985;98:81–6.
7. Reifsnyder T, Bandyk D, Seabrook G, et. al. Wound complications of the in situ vein bypass technique. *J Vasc Surg.* 1992;15:843–50.
8. Wengrovitz M, Atnip RG, Gifford RRM, et. al. Wound complications of autogenous subcutaneous infrainguinal ar *J Vasc Surg.* 1990;11:156–63.
9. Szilagyi DE, Smith RF, Elliot JP, Vrandecic MP. Infection in arterial reconstruction with synthetic grafts. *Ann Surg.* 1972;176:321–33.
10. Graham RG, Omotoso PO, Hudson DA. The effectiveness of muscle flaps for treatment of prosthetic graft sepsis. *Plastic Reconstruct Surg.* 2002;109:108–113.
11. Tukiainen E, Bioncuri F, Lep‰ntalo M. Deep infection of intrapopliteal autogenous vein grafts immediate use of muscle flaps in leg salvage. *J Vasc Surg.* 1998;28:611–6
12. Perler BA, Vander Kolk CA, Manson PM, Williams GM. Rotational muscle flaps to treat localized prosthetic graft infection: long-term follow-up. *J Vasc Surg.* 1993;18:358–65.
13. Mixter RC, Turnipseed WD, Smith DJ Jr, et. al. Rotational muscle flaps: a new technique for covering infected vascular grafts. *J Vasc Surg.* 1989;9:472–8.
14. Tyndall SH, Shepard AD, Wilczewski JM, et. al. Groin lymphatic complications after arterial reconstruction. *J Vasc Surg.* 1994,19:858–864.
15. Rubin JR, Malone JM, Goldstone J. The role of lymphatic system in acute arterial prosthetic graft infections. *J Vasc Surg.* 1985;2:92–98.
16. Roberts JR, Walters GK, Zerilman ME, Jones CE. Groin lymphorrhea complicating revascularization involving the femoral vessels. *Am J Surg.* 1991;165:341–344.
17. Stadelmann WK, Tobin G. Successful treatment of 19 consecutive groin lymphoceles with the assistance of intraoperative lymphatic mapping. *Plastic Reconstruct Surg.* 2002;1009(4):1274–80.
18. Cannon L, Walker AJ. Sclerotherapy of a wound lymphocele using tetracycline. *European J Vasc Endovas Surg.* 1997;14(6):505.
19. Porcellini M, Iandoli R, Spinotti F, et. al. Lymphoceles complicating arterial reconstructions of the lower limbs: outpatient conservative management. *J Cardiovascular Surg.* 2002;43 (21):217–21.
20. Shermak MA, Yee K, Wong L, et. al. Surgical management of groin lymphatic complications after arterial bypass surgery. *Plastic Reconstruct Surg.* 2005;115(7):1954–62.

21. Levy MF, Schmitt DD. Edmiston CE, et. al. Sequential analysis of staphylococcal colonization of body surfaces of patients undergoing vascular surgery. *J Clin Microbiol.* 1990;28:
664–64.

22. McBeth GA, Rubin JR, McIntyre KE Jr, et. al. The relevance of arterial wall microbiology to
the treatment of prosthetic graft infections; graft infection vs. arterial infection. *J Vasc Surg.*
1984;1:750–56.

23. Durham JR, Malone, Bernhard VM. The impact of mutiple operations on the importance of
arterial wall cultures. *J Vasc Surg.* 1987;5:160–69.

24. Moore WS. Experimental studies relating to sepsis in prosthetic vascular grafting. In: Duma
RJ, ed. *Infections of Prosthetic Heart Valves and Vascular Grafts.* Baltimore: University Park
Press, 1977:267–85.

25. Rubin JR, Malone JM, Goldstone J. The role of the lymphatic system in acute arterial prosthetic graft infections. *J Vasc Surg.* 1985;2:92–98.

26. Goldstone J, Moore WS. Infection in vascular prostheses: clinical minifestations and surgical
management. *Am J Surg.* 1974;128:225–33.

27. Samson RH, Veith FJ, Janko GS, et. al. A modified classification and approach to the management of infections involving peripheral arterial prosthetic grafts. *J Vasc Surg.* 1988;
8147–53.

28. Gordon IL, Pousti TJ, Stemmer EA, et. al. Inguinal wound fluid collections after vascular
surgery; management by early reoperation. *Southern Med J.* 1995;88:433–36.

30

Soft Tissue Reconstruction of the Groin after Vascular Surgery: Use of the Gracilis Muscle Flap

Gregory A. Dumanian, M.D.

Incisional breakdown of groin wounds is one of the more readily treatable complications of vascular surgery. Scarred or minimally viable local tissue, fluid collections in the surgery site, and the presence of foreign bodies (vascular grafts) colonized with bacteria all lead to a predicable outcome of graft exposure, thrombosis, graft blow-out, and need for further procedures.

This chapter presents a treatment rationale for the patients with incisional groin wounds after vascular surgery. The decision-making process for the need for a soft tissue flap (and specifically which flap to choose) to aid in wound healing will be presented. Finally, a case will be made for *prophylactic flap coverage* at the time of vascular surgery for the most difficult and challenging groins.

GROIN WOUNDS AFTER VASCULAR SURGERY

The reconstructive thought process necessitates an answer to the following questions:

1. What is missing, where is it missing and, therefore, what is critically exposed?
2. What is the chronologic history of the wound?
3. What would be critical not to expose?
4. What is available?

Open groin wounds occur after vascular surgery for numerous reasons familiar to all branches of surgery. Fluid collections including blood and lymph prevent the collapse of soft tissue back into their original locations after vessel dissection. Prosthetic materials, when colonized by bacteria, are difficult for the body to incorporate. The groin incision is difficult to compress with dressings and, therefore, becomes swollen and infection-prone. Patients have multiple procedures in the same area, forcing the surgeon to sew scar-to-scar in order to achieve wound closure. Vascular patients are older and with more co-morbidities than other groups of patients. The motion associated with early patient mobilization (beneficial to the patient) works against initial groin wound healing.

Groin wounds present as missing soft tissues over the inguinal area. Often, not much can be seen. Incisions that are erythematous and weeping slightly purulent material are consistent with an undrained colonized fluid collection over the vascular surgery site. Sometimes, nonviable fat with loose absorbable sutures covers the surgery site, but this tissue cannot provide adequate coverage of vascular suture lines. In the most dramatic presentation, prosthetic grafts and vascular suture lines are present to palpation and visible within the wound. In the first two instances, the tissue that is missing and the structures critically exposed must be imagined and acted on by the reconstructive surgeon. In the third case of exposed prosthetic graft and suture lines, there is nothing left to the imagination, and reconstructive surgery must be performed.

A critical item to assess is whether the critically exposed structures are located above the inguinal crease or not. A knowledge of the vascular procedure performed is important at this juncture. Infected aorto-bifemoral bypass grafts, femoro-femoral bypass grafts, and iliofemoral bypass graft histories point to more superior wounds (and, therefore, soft tissue requirements) than do infected pseudoaneurysms after vascular catheterization procedures and exposed infrainguinal bypass grafts. Exposed critical structures located above the inguinal ligament need be thought of differently than exposed critical structures located solely below the inguinal ligament.

The chronology of the groin wound is important because clinically, the earlier a groin wound is treated, the more successful the outcome. The three examples of wound presentations above roughly correlate to the age of the problem. An erythematous skin closure leaking fluid with prosthetic tissue at its base is at an earlier stage than is visible nonviable fat at the base of a wound over the inguinal triangle. Late presentations of vascular surgery patients with groin wounds to the reconstructive surgeon often involve patients treated with intravenous antibiotics for weeks and who have never had a thoroughly dry inguinal incision. There is no clear distinction between the two time points. A visual clue for chronic infections is the presence of avascular "bursal" tissue around the prosthetic material. Drawing analogies between the treatment of acute and chronic infections from the orthopedic literature, acute infections are easier to treat and often result in healed wounds with preserved vascular bypasses. The salvage of chronic prosthetic infections is poor. Recommendations for chronic inguinal infections include removal of all prosthetic materials.[1] However, even after the removal of prosthetic materials, there still remains tissue loss over the vascular structures of the groin and newly placed suture lines. This soft tissue deficit will need to be addressed in order to achieve wound healing.

Before a final decision is made about the donor site for a soft tissue flap for coverage of vital structures in the groin, the reconstructive surgeon must know the status and location of bypass grafts in the lower abdomen and upper leg. In the vascular surgery patient in a salvage situation, the patient is typically edematous, a bit nutritionally depleted, and with open wounds. The reconstructive surgeon must assume that any new incision made may break down and, therefore, flaps should not be chosen in areas where bypass grafts run. The potential exposure of a prosthetic graft in the donor site of a flap harvest is completely avoidable with proper surgical planning.

The soft tissue available for inguinal wound reconstruction depends on the prior vascular surgery history of the patient, the location of the soft tissue defect, and the status and location of bypass grafts that should be avoided. The success of the procedure and the need to remove any prosthetic material depends on the chronicity of the infection.

ABDOMINAL FLAPS

Numerous soft tissue flaps can reach the groin. Abdominal flaps are defined as those tissues supplied by vascular trees emerging from the external iliac artery and vein. The rectus abdominis and internal oblique pedicled muscle flaps are based on terminal branches off the external iliac artery. The deep inferior epigastric vessel is well known as it courses toward the rectus abdominis muscle, consistent in location, and does not tend to be occluded by atherosclerosis. Use of the rectus abdominis flap can reliably cover wounds above and below the inguinal ligament. However, in cases of donor site wound breakdown, this flap can lead to abdominal hernia formation and open abdominal wounds requiring treatment. This flap is also problematic when there are axillo-femoral or femoro-femoral bypass grafts present, again due to possible wound complications and prosthetic graft exposures in the donor sites. Division of the inguinal ligament for proximal control of the common femoral artery during the prior vascular surgery procedure can lead to division of the deep inferior epigastric vessels, and so this should be investigated with an ultrasound during the surgical planning phase. The internal oblique pedicled muscle flap is based on the deep circumflex iliac artery, which is the last vessel to come off the external iliac artery. This muscle is not compromised by prior ostomies or incisions and, therefore, is a useful alternative to the rectus abdominis muscle.[2] It has an arc of rotation to cover defects above and below the inguinal ligament, but the muscle flap is smaller than the rectus abdominis muscle. Dissection of the muscle often leads to a noticeable bulge in the lower abdominal wall. A final alternative for abdomen-based flaps is use of the contraleral rectus muscle with a long skin paddle extension. Termed the ORAM flap (for oblique rectus abdominis myocutaneous flap), this soft tissue flap easily reaches the opposite groin and can cover wounds both above and below the inguinal ligament.[3,4]

LEG FLAPS

A multitude of flaps arise from the femoral artery system that can reach and cover groin wounds. These flaps have certain advantages and disadvantages in comparison to abdominal flaps. Leg flaps do not run the risk of hernia formation, have lower donor site morbidities and pain, and keep the surgery site localized near the wound. Leg flaps also require the surgeon to work in an inflamed edematous and contaminated field. All things considered, so long as a leg flap is available with patent vessels and adequate size characteristics, it is the preferable option for wound closure in comparison to the abdominal flaps.

The sartorius turnover flap was one of the earliest muscle flaps used for coverage of groin wounds, and is still used successfully in many situations. The sartorius flap has the advantages of being close to the surgical field and easy to dissect.

Unfortunately, the sartorius muscle flap has several disadvantages to its use. The blood supply arises from segmental perforators from the superficial femoral artery, an artery typically involved or even occluded by vascular disease. The added stress of tissue dissection often causes the end of the muscle to be nonviable in vascular surgery patients. Second, the muscle must be dissected free from the anterior superior iliac spine for medialization onto the groin wound. This can lead to injury of the lateral femoral cutaneous nerve, resulting in significant morbidity. The muscle is only two finger breadths in width, and this is enough to cover the femoral artery and vein, but there is little muscle to cover the remainder of the wound. Finally, when transposed medially, the muscle shortens and moves inferiorly, rendering coverage of the common femoral artery difficult and the external iliac artery impossible. Several tricks to adequate mobilization include dissection to the first major vascular pedicle, located 6.5 cm inferior to the anterior superior iliac spine.[5] The muscle flap works best for coverage of the bifurcation of the common femoral artery into superficial and profunda femoral branches.

An excellent muscle flap for closure of groin wounds is the rectus femoris flap.[6] The muscle arises off the deep aspect of the anterior superior iliac spine, and inserts on the patellar tendon mechanism. The muscle is large, and easily covers wounds above and below the inguinal ligament. Most of the muscle can remain viable based on its blood supply from the profunda femoris artery. Seventy percent of the time, the vessel arises off the lateral femoral circumflex artery to enter the deep aspect of the muscle. In the remainder of patients, the vessel arises directly off the profunda femoris artery.[7] The muscle is easy to dissect from surrounding tissues through a straight incision from the groin wound directed toward the patella. The muscle is flipped over on itself to cover the groin vessels, and this bending is facilitated by the thinness of the muscle with increased age and disuse. To many, the importance of this muscle for terminal knee extension is one reason for it not to be used as a first line muscle flap.[8] Second, bypass grafts tunneled anatomically in the subsartorial plane run the risk of exposure within the donor site of the muscle if there is subsequent wound breakdown.

My flap of choice for coverage of groin wounds is the pedicled gracilis flap. Like the rectus femoris flap and unlike the sartorius flap, the gracilis muscle is supplied by the profunda femoris artery, and is typically patent despite vascular disease. This major pedicle supplying the muscle typically will keep the entire muscle viable after transfer, up to the area where the muscle becomes tendinous (where the minor pedicle off the superficial femoral artery enters the muscle). The muscle typically is unscarred, no matter what the previous surgical history of the thigh has been. Bypass grafts are rarely tunneled in this area, and so a breakdown of the donor site skin incision will not cause a second equally large problem. Transfer of the gracilis muscle does not result in any functional loss to the leg.[9] Finally, with the proper maneuvers, the muscle easily covers almost any size groin wound, both above and below the inguinal ligament.

SURGICAL ANATOMY AND TECHNIQUE

A thorough and aggressive debridement of the groin wound is performed with the knowledge that anything exposed will soon receive coverage. If this is a prophylactic placement of a flap at the time of vascular surgery, the flap can be elevated while other incisions are being closed.

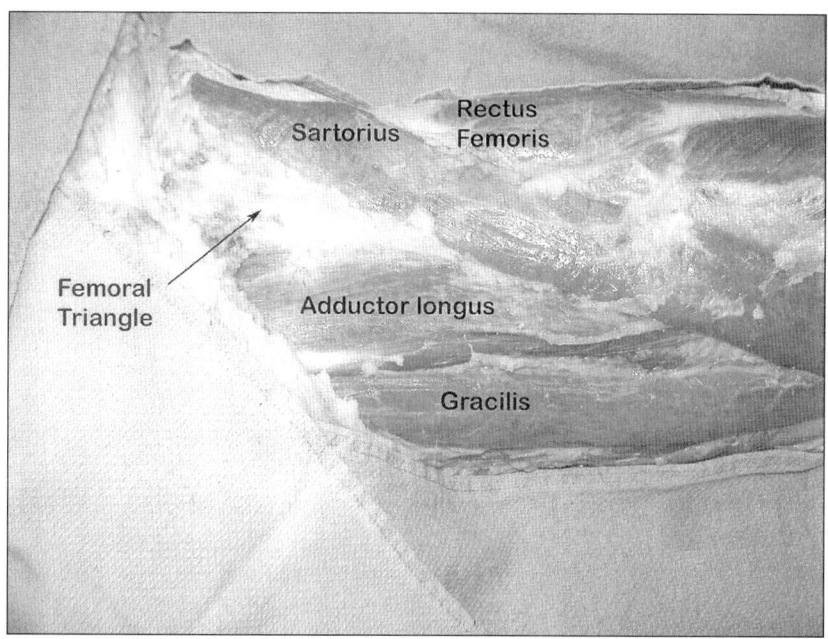

Figure 30-1. Cadaver dissection of left thigh showing the inguinal triangle and thigh muscles commonly used as flaps for groin coverage.

The gracilis muscle is identified as the medial-most and most superficial of the thigh adductors. The standard saphenous vein harvest incision will typically be 1-2 cm from the anterior edge of the muscle. A previous saphenous vein incision would be re-opened to locate the gracilis muscle. Otherwise, a 15 cm incision is made on the medial-most aspect of the thigh all the way to the groin crease. This is typically not connected with the groin incision to help preserve skin vascularity.

There are three helpful tips used to confirm the identity of the gracilis muscle (Figure 30–1). The muscle is triangular in shape whereas the other thigh muscles are rectangles. No superficial sensory nerves should be encountered over the muscle. Finally, the fascia surrounding the muscle is not adherent, allowing the dissecting finger to easily slide up and down the muscle. The adductor fascia is much more adherent and resists this finger "slide."

On opening the fascia in the proximal one-third of the muscle, a constant skin perforator emerges from the muscle. As this skin perforator is the continuation of the major vascular vessel as it travels through the muscle, it is a landmark for later in the dissection of the pedicle location. The muscle is then dissected on its superficial surface inferiorly to the level where the tendon fibers appear. The muscle is transected at this level, and a dissection on the deep aspect of the muscle begun. The pedicle enters the deep aspect of the muscle 10 cm inferior to the pubic tubercle. Elevating the adductor longus widely from deep fascial attachments helps to better see and locate the gracilis vascular pedicle (Figure 30–2). After identification of the pedicle, the muscle is divided off the pubic tubercle.

The key to dissection of the gracilis flap is to realize that the adductor longus muscle is dissected away from the gracilis, rather than to dissect the gracilis muscle free

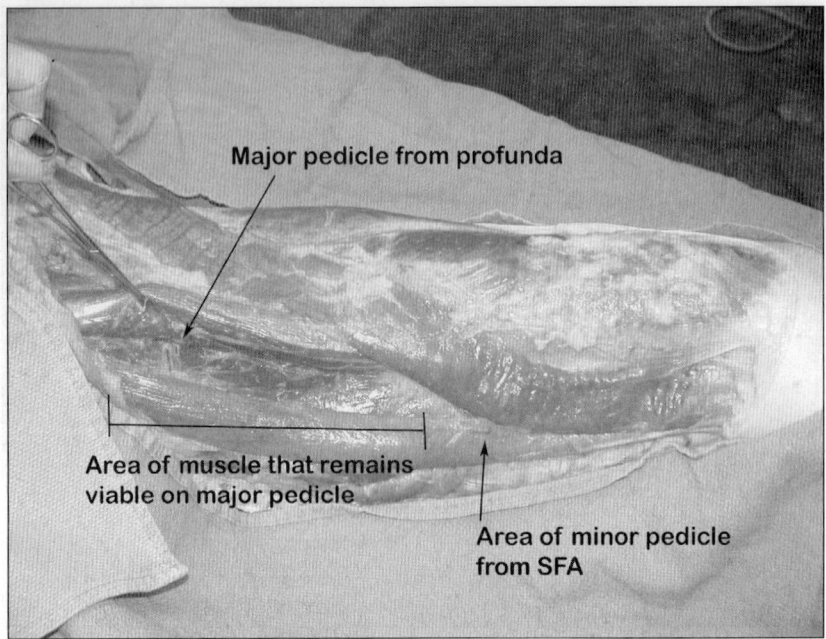

Figure 30-2. Demonstration of the vascular pedicle to the gracilis muscle that arises from the profunda femoris artery. The proximal two-thirds of the muscle can be transferred on just the dominant vascular pedicle.

from surrounding tissues. With the gracilis in place still attached by soft tissues to the adductor magnus, the traction is applied to elevate the adductor longus from the gracilis muscle. In two areas, small blood vessels emerge from the gracilis pedicle to enter the adductor, and these vessels are divided carefully between vascular vessel clips. The space between the adductor longus and sartorius is opened bluntly to reach the same vascular pedicle to the gracilis from a lateral direction. A space is now developed underneath the adductor longus and the vascular pedicle is now clearly viewed in its entirety (Figure 30–3). Finally, the remainder of the soft tissue elements holding the gracilis and its vascular pedicle are dissected from the adductor magnus, and the muscle flap is passed into the area of the femoral triangle (Figure 30–4).[10] The 180-degree twist of the pedicle does not seem to hurt the blood flow, but the patency of the vessels is confirmed by Doppler inspection of the flap. The donor site is closed over two drains. The groin area tends to have impressive lymphatic leaks in these inflamed reoperative cases. I tend to inset the muscle to surrounding soft tissues with absorbable sutures over a drain, and to simply place a moist dressing on the flap. This allows for a daily inspection of the wound and soft tissues. This wound can be treated over the subsequent week with a skin graft or a subatmospheric pressure dressing.

A typical patient is demonstrated in Figures 30–5-8. An obese diabetic female with an infrainguinal vascular reconstruction has a nonhealing groin wound (Figure 30–5). After radical debridement of the wound, a gracilis flap was harvested (Figure 30–6) and transposed under the adductor longus to reach the femoral triangle (Figure 30–7). The muscle flap easily fills the space of the wound, and the end is even draped back on itself (Figure 30–8). The skin wound went on to close by secondary intention.

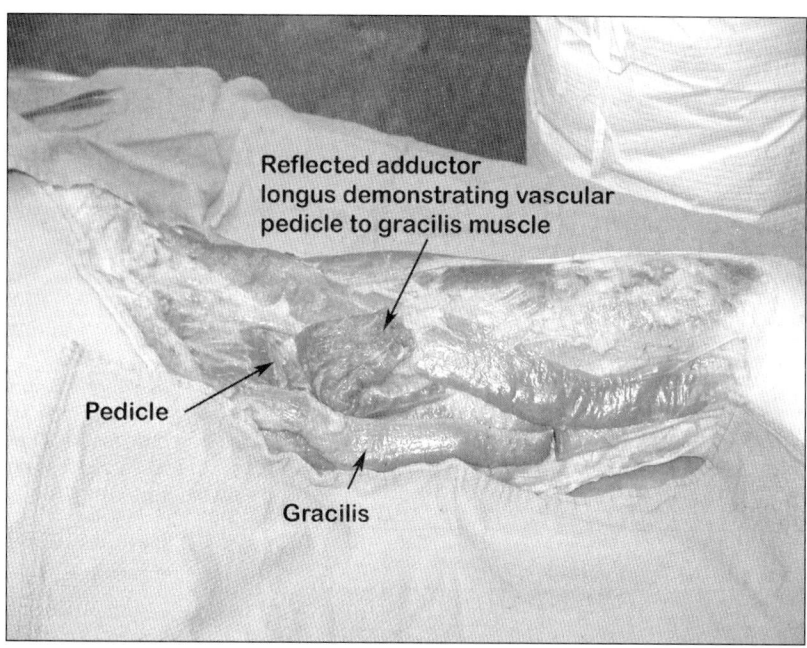

Figure 30-3. The adductor longus has been divided to better demonstrate the path of the vascular pedicle to the gracilis muscle. This is *not* done in the coverage of groin wounds with the gracilis flap.

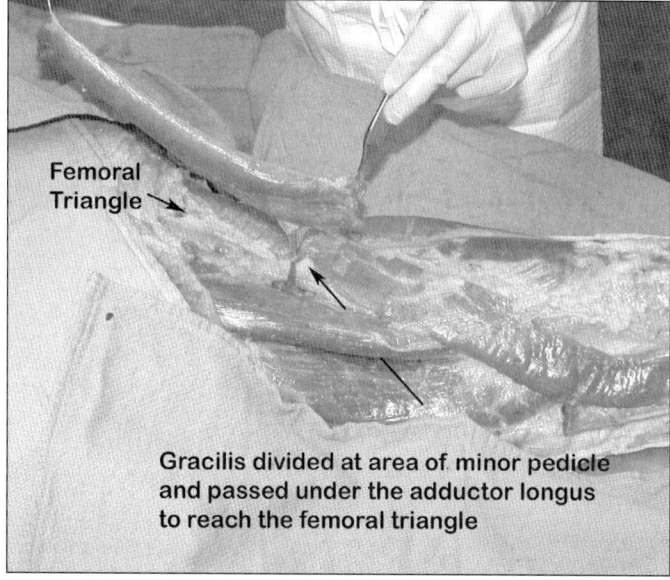

Figure 30-4. The gracilis muscle is passed underneath the adductor longus to reach the femoral triangle. Note the ability of the muscle to cover the tissues above the inguinal ligament.

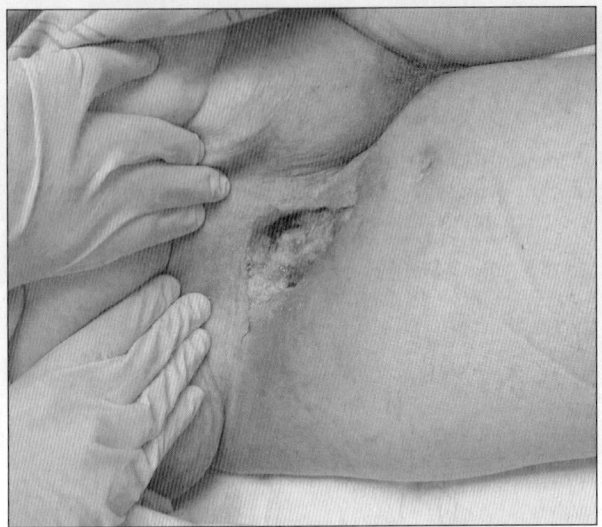

Figure 30-5. Nonhealing right groin wound with necrotic tissue at the base in a diabetic obese female. She had undergone a below-knee femoral-popliteal bypass with vein graft. The vein graft is tunneled subsartorially.

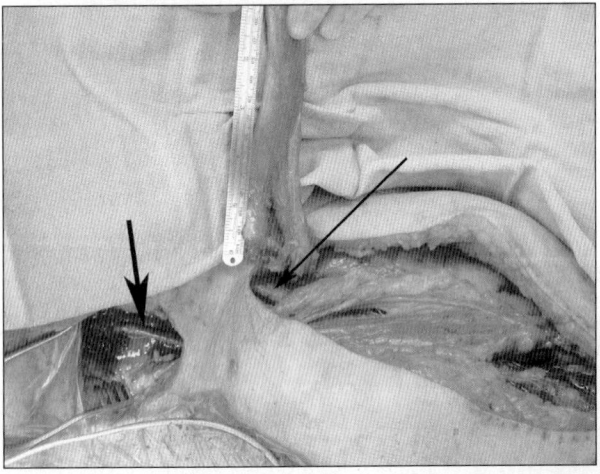

Figure 30-6. The gracilis flap is harvested through a second incision on the medial leg. The large arrow demonstrates the intact vein graft. The thinner arrow shows the location of the adductor longus.

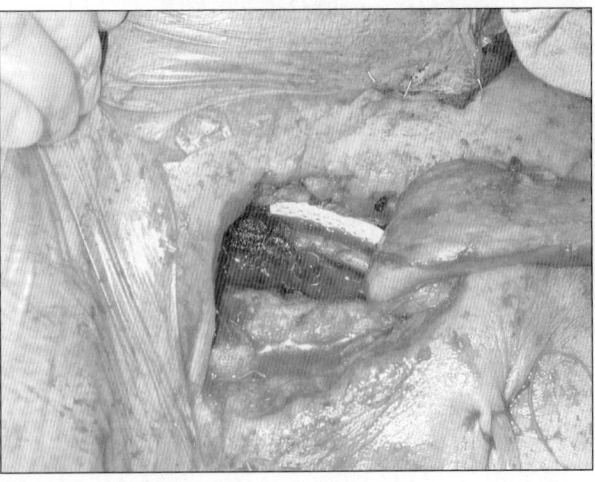

Figure 30-7. The gracilis muscle has been transposed into the femoral triangle. A drain is seen adjacent to the vein graft. Note that the skin opening has not been enlarged to transpose the flap into the defect because most of the work was done through the medial thigh incision.

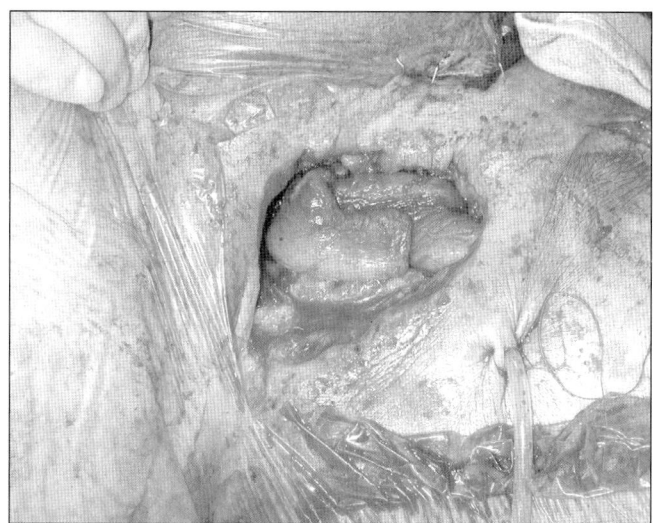

Figure 30-8. The gracilis muscle fills the groin wound, and redundant flap is draped over onto itself.

RESULTS

Several years ago, the results of use of this flap were documented from Northwestern Memorial Hospital.[11] Eighteen patients received 20 flaps for coverage of infected groin wounds. Twelve of 14 patients with exposed prosthetic reconstructions had salvages of their vascular surgery. Autogenous reconstructions and exposed femoral vessels all uniformly did well. All 18 patients grew out organisms from the groin wound, with seven polymicrobial infections. Two flaps were lost, one partial loss perhaps due to tension on the pedicle, and one total loss in delayed fashion due to acute thrombosis of the external iliac artery. Seven of the patients died within 28 months of their surgery, demonstrating the fragility of this patient population.

DISCUSSION

The gracilis flap has demonstrated an equal ability to heal wounds of the femoral triangle in comparison to other soft tissue flaps, and we present our rationale for its use. In our experience, it is the preferred method to achieve wound closure. It can close higher and larger wounds than a sartorius flap. It has less donor site problems than the rectus femoris flap. It has a predictable blood supply despite preexisting vascular disease. Donor site skin breakdown of the gracilis muscle harvest is easily treated with dressings and exposes no critical structures.

One issue is when to do this flap prophylactically to improve the soft tissues of the groin at the time of a vascular surgery procedure. There are no hard and fast rules, and much depends on the assessment of the soft tissues by the vascular surgeon. Close cooperation and ease of communication between the vascular and plastic surgery services facilitates performance of these flaps on a moment's notice. Our general recommendations for prophylactic flaps include the multiply operated groin with stiff soft tissues, prior radiation to the groin for cancer treatment, pseudoaneurysms that push local soft tissue away from the vessels, and prior infection in the area. A final group in whom prophylactic reconstructions are helpful are those patients with "high profile" prosthetic reconstructions. Patients who have undergone axillo-femoral and femoro-femoral bypasses have one groin with twice as much prosthetic material as the other side. In cases where it is difficult for the soft tissues to cover the high profile of the prosthetic vascular material, prophylactic gracilis flap coverage is useful.

REFERENCES

1. Darouiche RO. Infections associated with surgical implants. *NEJM*. 2004;350:1422–1429.
2. Ramasastry SS, Futrell JW. Surgical anatomy of the internal oblique muscle: a practical approach. *Am Surg*. 1987;53:278–81.
3. Ramasastry SS, Liang MD, Hurwitz DJ. Surgical management of difficult wounds of the groin. *Surg Gynecol Obstet*. 1989;169:418–22.
4. Lee MJ, Dumanian GA. The oblique rectus abdominis musculocutaneous flap: revisited clinical applications. *Plast Reconstr Surg*. 2004;114:367–73.
5. Wu LC, Djohan RS, Liu TS, et al. Proximal vascular pedicle preservation for sartorius muscle flap transposition. *Plast Reconstr Surg*. 2006;117:253–8.
6. Alkon JD, Smith A, Losee JE, et al. Management of complex groin wounds: preferred use of the rectus femoris muscle flap. *Plast Reconstr Surg*. 2005;115:776–83.
7. Koshima I, Moriguchi T, Soeda S, et al. Free rectus femoris muscle transfer for one-stage reconstruction of established facial paralysis. *Plast Reconstr Surg*. 1994;94:421–25.
8. Kozlowski JM, Dumanian GA, Fine NA, Cohn EB. Utility of the "Mutton-Chop" flap for reconstruction of large defects involving the lower abdominal wall and groin. *Contemp Urol*. 1997;9:85–96.
9. Zukowski M, Lord J, Ash K, et al. The gracilis free flap revisited: a review of 25 cases of transfer to traumatic extremity wounds. *Ann Plast Surg*. 1998;40:141–4.
10. Hasen KV, Gallegos ML, Tepper RE, Dumanian GA. An extended approach for the vascular pedicle of the gracilis muscle flap: An anatomic and clinical study. *Plast Reconstr Surg*. 2003;111:2203–2208.
11. Morasch MD, Sam AD, Kibbe MR, et al. Early results with use of gracilis muscle flap coverage of infected groin wounds after vascular surgery. *J Vasc Surg*. 2004;39:1277–1283.

Emerging Biotechnology Techniques for Treatment of Limb Ischemia

31

The Use of Stem Cells in the Treatment of Inoperable Limb Ischemia

William H. Pearce, M.D., Richard Burt, M.D., and Brian Peterson, M.D.

Peripheral arterial disease (PAD) of the lower extremity is an important clinical problem causing claudication, ischemic rest pain, foot ulcers, and gangrene.[1-5] It is estimated that as many as 10 million Americans are affected by this disease.[6] The prevalence of lower extremity arterial disease may range from as low as 0.1% to as high as 13% of the population. The difference in these numbers depends on whether PAD is defined by clinical symptoms or the use of the ankle-brachial index (ABI).[7-11] For the majority of patients, PAD remains stable over five years. However, between 15% and 25% of patients will progress to require either revascularization or amputation.[12] When critical limb ischemia occurs, patients require some method of revascularization to avoid amputation. The gold standard, autogenous vein bypass, is being replaced by endovascular procedures. These endovascular procedures including recannalization and stenting have surprisingly good results. However, for a small portion of patients, the anatomy is not suitable for revascularization, either surgically or by endovascular techniques. In these patients, there are no distal targets for reconstruction. In addition, an autogenous bypass is not possible because of prior utilization of the saphenous vein and a prosthetic is used. The long-term patency of prosthetic bypasses to tibial vessels is disappointingly low. Alternative methods of revascularization are needed. Here, cell-based therapy may be a promising option.

There is very little data on the natural history of critical limb ischemia (CLI). It is estimated that the amputation rate in patients with CLI ranges between 30% and 70% at one year. Spontaneous improvement occurs in 5%, but the mechanism for improvement is unknown.[13-14] Clearly, patients with minor gangrene or ulcer may heal with conservative therapy. The medical therapy for CLI has been suggested using either pentoxifylline or cilostazol. Intravenous pentoxifylline has been associated with lessened pain scores in patients with CLI; however, the benefit is shortlived.[15-16] Cilostazol has not been used or studied in patients with CLI. Another drug, Iloprost, has been studied and has been proven not to be an effective therapy to reduce the risk of amputation.[17-18]

Unfortunately, despite the efforts of vascular surgeons, the rate of amputation in the United States has been unchanged over the past 10 years.[19] Thus, gene therapy and cell-based therapies may offer an option to amputations in patients with CLI.

Revascularization of ischemic tissue may occur by two separate mechanisms: angiogenesis and vasculogenesis. Angiogenesis is the process in which capillaries sprout from mature or existing capillaries. Angiogenesis follows an orderly process in which endothelial cells migrate into the ischemic tissue to form capillaries. The process is regulated by cytokines released in the ischemic tissue. Another process is vasculogenesis where blood vessels are formed. Vasculogenesis was originally thought to occur only in embryos. However, recent studies have demonstrated that circulating stem cells participate in the revascularization of ischemic tissue (vascular endothelial growth factor [VEGF] or basic fibroblast growth factor ([βFGF] and others). Vasculogenesis is the in-situ formation of blood vessels from stem cell progeny. In addition, circulating stem cells have been implicated in a wide variety of processes including atherosclerosis, arterial repair, and the vasculopathy following cardiac transplantation.[20-22]

GENE THERAPY AND GROWTH FACTORS FOR CHRONIC LIMB ISCHEMIA

Angiogenesis is a complex biologic process involving multiple growth factors at differing times. In an attempt to create new vessel growth in patients with endstage PAD and chronic limb ischemia, Isner used naked DNA plasmids, encoding for either VEGF or bFGF.[23-27] These genes were injected into the lower extremity. Using a single dose of phVEGF165 DNA plasmid, Isner treated 10 patients with critical limb ischemia. Gene expression was documented by a rise in serum VEGF. Improvement in limb perfusion occurred in seven patients as measured by an increase in ABI and by an increase in collateral vessels seen by angiography. Ischemic ulcers also improved and healed in four of seven patients.[23] Transient lower extremity edema was a common side effect. In another trial of 22 patients, ischemic symptoms improved particularly with peripheral neuropathies. Nerve conduction studies improved following gene therapy.[24] In patients with Beurger's disease, gene therapy avoided amputation in five of seven patients.[25] Enthusiasm for VEGF gene therapy has waned because of the potential for remote tumor growth and the short duration of expression. More recently, Comerota evaluated the safety of increasing and repeated doses of intramuscular injections of naked plasmid DNA encoding fibroblast growth factor (FGF) type 1 in 51 patients with CLI.[28] The side effects were minor and included injection site pain and edema. There was significant reduction of ischemic rest pain and enhanced healing of foot ulcers. Also, there was a significant increase in the ABIs and transcutaneous oxygen (TCO_2) levels. However, the authors commented that the duration of the effect of gene therapy was unknown. Recombinant fibrob-last growth factor (rFGF) has been studied in patients with claudication. A prospective randomized trial of intra-arterial infusion of rFGF showed improvement in peak walking time.[29] There were no significant side effects. Long-term outcomes are not known.

STEM CELLS AND VASCULOGENESIS

In the developing embryos, the early vasculature is comprised of angioblasts encircling hematopoietic stem cells. The spatial relationship of these cells is determined by cell surface antigens including FLK-1, TIE-2, and CD34. The cells differentiate to form blood vessels and blood products. Human stem cells from peripheral blood can differentiate into endothelial cells. Asahara et al. isolated CD34$^+$ cells from human peripheral blood and plated them on fibronectin plates.[30] Cocultures with CD34− cells yielded tube-like cellular networks and blood island-like cell clusters similar to those seen in vessel development. In animal experiments, they found that injecting peripheral blood of an overexpressing (β-galactosidase animal into an ischemic hind limb of a nontransgenic animal of the same breed, that (β-galactosidase expression was found in the ischemic limb. Furthermore, these cells were associated with neovascularity and increased collateralization. The use of embryonic stem cells is different from adult stem cells. Direct injection of embryonic stem cells may produce teratomas or graft versus host disease. However, embryonic stem cells may be used if they are terminally differentiated by cytokines into EPCs. Adult stem cells, unlike embryonic cells, have a predetermined lineage (i.e., neural, gut, skin, muscle, liver, hematopoietic, and alveolar). Therefore, to use adult stem cells for vasculogenesis, hematopoietic, and in particular hematopoietic stem cells destined to be EPC, must be selected. These cells include CD34+, AC133+, or CD34−, AC 133+, or CD34+ AC133−.

The first successful stem cell transplant for PVD was reported by Tateishi-Yuyama et al in 2002.[31] This prospective pilot study evaluated 47 patients with severe peripheral vascular disease and ischemic rest pain. Twenty-five patients with unilateral ischemia received intramuscular injections of bone marrow-derived mononuclear cells including endothelial progenitor cells (EPCs). Intramuscular injections were made in a 3 cm × 3 cm grid. Saline was injected to the less ischemic limb. A second group of patients with bilateral leg ischemia were injected with either bone marrow-derived mononuclear cells or peripheral mononuclear cells as the control. In both groups (A and B), there was a significant improvement in patients injected with the bone-marrowed derived cells. The ABIs, TCO$_2$ tension, and pain-free walking times were all improved. The effect was sustained at 24 weeks. Bone marrow cells were aspirated under general anesthesia. Blood was studied for serum levels of VEGF, _FGF, tumor necrosis factor-alpha, Interleukin-β, Interleukin-6, and CD34 cell numbers at baseline, 12 hours, 24 hours, and 48 hours. The only significant rise from baseline was that of Interleukin-6. Rest pain resolved in 16 of 24 patients in Group B. Angiography in these patients demonstrated an increase in collateral blood supply in 27 of 45. There were no local inflammatory reactions or other adverse systemic events.

In a second study by Huang et al.[32], peripheral blood stem cells (PBSCs) were injected in the calf muscles in five patients with CLI (32). The patients received recombinant granulocytes colony stimulating factor (rhG-CSF, 600 mg/day subcutaneously for five consecutive days). On the fifth day, the PBSCs were collected from the peripheral blood using a version 4 blood cell separator and injected into the lower extremity. In these five patients, there was improvement in pain score, skin temperature, healing of ulcers, and pain-free walking. There were no significant adverse events including myocardial infarction, liver dysfunction, or kidney failure.

Northwestern Stem Cell Experience

With both FDA and IRB approval, we have started a stem cell transplant program for peripheral vascular disease. For the development of peripheral angiogenesis, hematopoietic stem cells—particularly CD34 and AC133—are important. Since AC133+ cells are considered to be more permanent markers for endothelial cell precursors, this subgroup of PBSCs was chosen for our program.[33] The primary end point of our study is the safety and efficacy of using PBSCs, AC133+ harvest, purification, and intramuscular calf injections. Eligibility for patients entering the study included the following.

1. Atherosclerotic ischemic peripheral vascular disease with rest pain defined as pain that occurs at night or at rest that involves the foot and/or ischemic lower extremity ulcers, due to infrainguinal arterial disease. Ulcers must be present for at least 14 days with no improvement with standard wound care.
2. Ankle-brachial index (ABI) < 0.4, toe brachial index < 0.3, and flat or minimally pulsatile doppler on two conservative examinations, at least one week apart.
3. No surgical or endovascular options for revascularization (e.g., prior vascular reconstruction, inability to locate a suitable vein for grafting, or diffuse multi-segment disease without distal target).
4. Age > 18 years old.

The following studies were obtained at baseline and at two weeks, three weeks, four weeks, eight weeks, 12 weeks, 24 weeks, and 52 months postinjection: ABI, TBI, lower extremity arterial blood flow (LEAF), pain assessments, magnetic resonance imaging/magnetic resonance parameter, and SF-36. If ulcers are present, the ulcers will be measured (area) and compared at each time point. All patients entering the study will undergo cardiac testing and evaluation by cardiology.

The patients receive G-CSF at 100 mg/kg for four days. At day 4, the ACC133+ HSC are harvested using the CliniMACS cell separator (Miltenyi Biotec, Inc. Auburn, CA). Complications associated with G-CSF vary with the protocols being used. With our protocol, the complications are generally mild. Ninety percent of patients will experience some side effects, the most common of which include bone pain, headaches, body fatigue, and occasional nausea and vomiting. Of particular concern are patients with systemic atherosclerosis. As stated earlier, these patients undergo preoperative cardiac evaluation consisting of dipyridamole thallium stress testing and cardiology consultation. Sludging of white cells may produce an acute coronary syndrome. The patients are heparinized during the period of marked leukocytosis. During mobilization, the patients' EKG and troponin levels are followed.

The intramuscular injections in the lower extremity are based on distribution of the arterial disease and from duplex imaging. Our patients have had intact circulation to the knee without tibial or pedal vessels. Therefore, the injections are made either in the calf or the foot. Duplex imaging is used to determine the depth of the muscle groups from the skin surface and the location of muscle compartments (i.e., gastrocnemius, soleus, anterior, and lateral compartment). The depth of the injection ranges from 2.5 cm to 3 cm. Two to five million cells are injected at each location (2 cm x 2 cm grid) for a total of between 40 and 100 million cells (Figure 31–1). The procedure has been well tolerated under local anesthesia and there have been no significant inflammatory complications as a result of the injections.

EXCLUSION CRITERIA

1. Recent lower extremity angioplasty or surgical bypass
2. Severe comorbidity limiting one-year survival of patients
3. Positive serology for Hepatitis B or C or HIV
4. Poorly controlled diabetes mellitus, HbAIC greater than 6.5%, and/or proliferative retinopathy

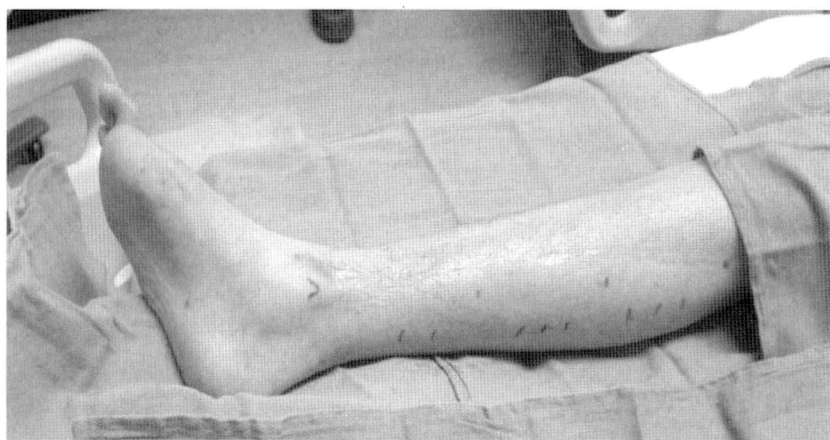

Figure 31-1. The location for stem cell injection is marked on the calf. The medial malleolous is identified and 10 cm marks are made to the tibial plateau. At each of these locations, the depth of the muscle group is determined using duplex ultrasound scanning. Similarly, on the lateral aspect of the leg from the lateral malleolous at 10 cm increments, the depth of muscles is also determined. Then at 2 cm increments, stem cells are implanted at the predetermined depth.

5. Extensive gangrene or sepsis
6. Nonambulatory patient
7. Evidence of malignancy

To date, we have transplanted three patients with severe endstage arterial disease. The first was a 78-year-old African American female with ischemic rest pain and early gangrenous changes. In this patient, the stem cells were transplanted two weeks following stem cell harvest. During this interval, the ischemic disease progressed. The stem cell transplant was performed but did not reverse the ischemic change, and the patient required amputation. The patient did not suffer any ill effect from the stem cell transplant. There was no myocardial infarction, leg edema, or rise in serum creatinine level. The amputated leg demonstrated clusters of hematopoietic stem cells within the muscle and was viable (Figure 31–2). This experience led us to believe that patients with progressive rest pain would not be good candidates for this procedure since vasculogenesis will probably take several months to occur.

Our second patient was a 26-year-old male with Buerger's disease who had undergone a femoral to dorsalis pedis bypass graft six months prior. The dorsalis pedis bypass graft failed, leaving the patient's foot ischemic. The ABI was 0.3 with moderate to severe claudication and no rest pain. The patient underwent a stem cell transplant. At 12 weeks post implant, the patient reported that his walking time had increased with no recurrence of ischemic rest pain or gangrene in the foot.

The third patient was a 52-year-old female who had extensive emboli to her forefoot three years prior. Since that time, the patient has had ischemic symptoms in the forefoot. Stem cell transplant was performed in the foot. The patient is now one month postoperative and doing well without complications. None of our patients have experienced an adverse event. Based on this experience, we are broadening the inclusion criteria to accept patients who have short distance claudication (18 minutes peak walking time using the Gardner protocol).

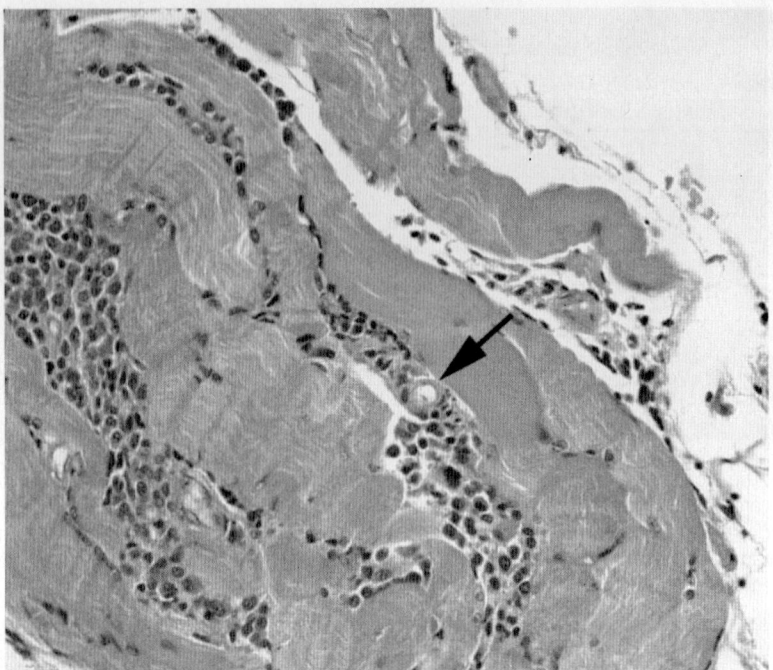

Figure 31-2. Photomicrograph demonstrating striated muscles with clusters of AC133+ cells. Note the early formation of a capillary (arrow).

COMMENTS

Stem cell-based therapy offers many advantages over gene therapy for CLI. Transplant stem cells are a renewable source of multiple cytokines and growth factors. Autologous adult stem cells are not rejected and do not form teratomas. The intramuscular injections are well tolerated without local or systemic effects. Gene therapy, on the other hand, has several potential drawbacks. First, whether one uses adenoviral vectors or naked plasmid DNA, there is only transient expression of the growth factors required. Plasmid DNA can be injected multiple times but the transfection rate is low. On the other hand, adenovirus-based gene therapy improves the rate of transfection but is limited to a one-time injection because of an inflammatory response to the viral proteins. Also, since only one gene can be injected, selection of the appropriate gene for the development of a blood vessel is mandatory. Unfortunately, blood vessel growth is a complicated, orchestrated event requiring multiple growth factors and cytokines, both spatially and in time. This early experience at Northwestern is only preliminary but does demonstrate the safety of the technique. However, the efficacy and durability of stem cell transplants in patients with lower extremity ischemia is yet to be determined.

ACKNOWLEDGEMENTS

Michael Havens, M.D., Resident, Pathology, Northwestern Memorial Hospital, provided the microphotographs of the pathology samples.

REFERENCES

1. Kannel WB. The demographics of claudication and aging of the American population. *Vasc Med.* 1996;1:60–64.
2. Coni N, Tennison B, Troup M. Prevalence of lower extremity arterial disease among elderly people in the community. *Br J Geri Pract.* 1992;42:149–152.
3. Bowlin SJ, McDalie JH, Flocke SA, et al. Epidemiology of intermittent claudication in middle-aged men. *Am J Epidemiol.* 1994;140:418–430.
4. Kannel WB, McGee DL. Update on some epidemiologic features of intermittent claudication: The Framingham Study. *J Am Geriatr Soc.* 1985;33:13–18.
5. Criqui MH, Langer RD, Fronek H, et al. Mortality over a period of 10 years in patients with peripheral arterial disease. *N Eng J Med.* 1992;326:381–386.
6. Nehler MR, McDermott MM, Treat-Jacobsen D, et al. Functional outcomes and quality of life in peripheral arterial disease: current status. *Vasc Med.* 2003;8:115–126.
7. Fowkes FG, Housley E, Cawood EH, et al. Edinburgh artery study: prevalence of asymptomatic and symptomatic peripheral arterial disease in the general population. *Int J Epidemiol.* 1991;20:384–392.
8. Stoffers HE, Rinkens PE, Kester AD, et al. The prevalence of asymptomatic and unrecognized peripheral arterial occlusive disease. *Int J Epidemiol.* 1996;25:282–290.
9. Golomb B, Criqui M, Budens W. Epidemiology. In: Creager M, ed. *Management of Peripheral Arterial Disease.* London: ReMEDICA Publishing; 2000:1–18.
10. Ness J, Aronow WS. Prevalence of coexistence of coronary artery disease, ischemic stroke, and peripheral arterial disease in older persons, mean age 80 years, in an academic hospital-based geriatrics practice. *J Am Geriatr Soc.* 1999;47:1255–1266.
11. Hiatt WR, Marshall JA, Baxter J, et al. Diagnostic methods for peripheral arterial disease in the San Luis Valley Diabetes Study. *J Clin Epidemiol.* 1990;43:597–606.
12. Anonymous. Critical limb ischaemia: Management and outcome report of a national survey. The Vascular Surgical Society of Great Britain and Ireland. *Eur J Vasc and Endovasc Surg.* 1995;10:108–113.
13. The ICAI group. The study group of crticial chronic ischemia of the lower extremities. Long-term mortality and its predictors in patients with critical leg ischaemia. *Eur J Vasc Endovasc Surg.* 1999;12:154–161.
14. Dormandy JA, Rutherford RB. Management of peripheral arterial disease (PAD). TASC Working Group. TransAtlantic Inter-Society Concensus (TASC). *J Vasc Surg.* 2000;31: S1–S296.
15. The European Study Group. Intravenous pentoxifylline for the treatment of chronic critical limb ischaemia. *Eur J Vasc Endovasc Surg.* 1995;9:426–436.
16. Norwegian Pentoxifylline Multicenter Trial Group. Efficacy and clinical tolerance of parenteral pentoxifylline in the treatment of critical limb ischemia. A placebo controlled multicenter study. *Int Angiol.* 1996;15:75–80.
17. Schuler JJ, Flanigan DP, Holcroft JW, et al. Efficacy of prostaglandin E1 in the treatment of lower extremity ischemic ulcers secondary to peripheral vascular occlusive disease. Results of a prospective randomized, double-blind, multicenter clinical trial. *J Vasc Surg.* 1984;71: 506–508.
18. Cronenwett JL, Zelenock GB, Whitehouse WM, et al. Prostacyclin treatment of ischemic ulcers and rest pain in unreconstructable peripheral arterial occlusive disease. *Surgery.* 1986; 100:369–375.
19. Feinglass J, Brown JL, LoSasso A, et al. Rates of lower extremity amputation and arterial reconstruction in the United States, 1979-1996. *Am J Publ Health.* 1999:89:1222–1227
20. Shintani S, Murohara T, Ikeda H, et al. Mobilization of endothelial progenitor cells in patients with acute myocardial infarction. *Circulation.* 2001;103:2776–2779.
21. Sata M, Saiura A, Kunisato A, et al. Hematopoietic stem cells differentiate into vascular cells that participate in the pathogenesis of atherosclerosis. *Nat Med.* 2002;8:403–409.

22. Simper D, Wang S, Deb A, et al. Endothelial progenitor cells are decreased in blood of cardiac allograft patients with vasculopathy and endothelial cells of noncardiac origin are enriched in transplant atherosclerosis. *Circulation*. 2003;107:143–149.

23. Isner JM. Arterial gene transfer of naked DNA for therapeutic angiogenesis: early clinical results. *Adv Drug Deliv Rev*. 1998;30:185–197.

24. Isner JM, Pieczek A, Schainfeld R, et al. Clinical evidence of angiogenesis after arterial gene transfer of ph VEGF165 in patients with ischaemic limb. *Lancet*. 1996;348:370–374.

25. Isner JM, Baumgartner I, Rach G, et al. Treatment of thromboangitis obliteran (Buerger's disease) by intramuscular gene transfer of vascular endothelial growth factor: preliminary clinical results. *J Vasc Surg*. 1998:28:964–73.

26. Baumgartner I, Pieczek A, Manor O, et al. Constitutive expression of ph VEGF165 after intramuscular gene transfer promotes collateral vessel development in patients with critical limb ischemia. *Circulation*. 1998;97:1114:23.

27. Isner JM, Walsh K, Symes J, et al. Arterial gene therapy for therapeutic angiogenesis in patients with peripheral artery disease. *Circulation*. 1995;91:2687–92.

28. Comerota AJ, Throm RC, Miller KA, et al. Naked plasmid DNA encoding fibroblast growth factor type 1 for the treatment of end-stage unreconstructable lower extremity ischemia: Preliminary results of a phase I trial. *J Vasc Surg*. 2002;35:930–6.

29. Lederman RJ, Mendelsohn FO, Anderson RD, et al. TRAFFIC Investigators. Therapeutic angiogenesis with recombinant fibroblast growth factor-2 for intermittent claudication (the TRAFFIC study): a randomised trial. *Lancet*. 359:2053–8, 2002

30. Asahara T, Murohara T, Sullivan A, et al. Isolation of putative progenitor endothelial cells for angiogenesis. *Science*. 1997;275:964–967.

31. Tateishi-Yuyama E, Matsubara H, Murohara T et al. Therapeutic Angiogenesis using Cell Transplantation (TACT) Study Investigators. Therapeutic angiogenesis for patients with limb ischaemia by autologous transplantation of bone-marrow cells: a pilot study and a randomised controlled trial. *Lancet*. 2002;360:427–35.

32. Huang PP, Li SZ, Han MZ et al. Autologous transplantation of peripheral blood stem cells as an effective therapeutic approach for severe arteriosclerosis obliterans of lower extremities. *Thromb Haemost*. 2004;91:606–609.

33. Burt R. Pearce W. Luo K et al. Hematopoietic stem cell transplantation for cardiac and peripheral vascular disease. *Bone Marrow Transplantation*. 2003;32 Suppl 1:S29–31.

32

Nitric Oxide-based Therapies in Vascular Disease

Muneera Kapadia, M.D., Samer F. Najjar, M.D. and Melina R. Kibbe, M.D., R.V.T.

Atherosclerosis is a leading cause of morbidity and mortality in all developed nations. Most commonly, it affects patients in the form of coronary artery disease and peripheral vascular disease. Current therapeutic modalities for arterial atherosclerosis consist of balloon angioplasty and stenting, arterial bypass grafting, or surgical endarterectomy. Unfortunately, the long-term durability of these procedures is limited due to the development of neointimal hyperplasia (NIH) and subsequent arterial stenosis/restenosis. Nitric oxide (NO) has been shown to protect the vasculature and limit the formation of NIH in animal models of arterial injury and vein bypass grafting. Here, we discuss the pathophysiology of NIH, the role of NO in the vasculature, and current NO-based therapies aimed at limiting the development of NIH.

NITRIC OXIDE AND NITRIC OXIDE SYNTHASE

NO was originally described as endothelium-derived relaxing factor by Furchgott and Zawadzki in 1980.[1] NO is a highly diffusible molecule that has a half life of seconds. It is quickly bound by hemoglobin and converted to inactive end products, nitrite, and nitrate. NO is normally synthesized by a family of NO synthase (NOS) enzymes. The three different isoforms include endothelial NOS (eNOS), neuronal NOS (nNOS), and inducible NOS (iNOS). All three enzymes are similar in that they produce NO through oxidation of one of the nitrogens of L-arginine in the presence of molecular oxygen.[2-3] However, eNOS and nNOS are constitutively expressed, and NO production via eNOS and nNOS is regulated by intracellular calcium fluxes through calmodulin binding.[3] In contrast, iNOS is transcriptionally regulated and is produced in response to cellular stress.[3] When induced, iNOS can produce 100–1,000 times the NO compared with its constitutive counterparts.[4]

DEVELOPMENT OF NEOINTIMAL HYPERPLASIA FOLLOWING ARTERIAL INJURY

In order to understand the roles of NO and NOS in the vasculature, a brief overview of the events that occur following arterial injury is required. Injury to the arterial wall, such as balloon angioplasty, leads to endothelial cell denudation and exposure of the underlying vascular smooth muscle cells (VSMC) to the circulating blood elements.[5-6] Platelets quickly aggregate and adhere to the site of injury within seconds.[7] Leukocyte chemotaxis then occurs, which is followed by secretion of many cytokines and growth factors.[8] Basic fibroblast growth factor (bFGF) is responsible for initial smooth muscle cell proliferation.[9] Platelet-derived growth factor is mainly responsible for the migration of VSMC from the media to the intima.[10] Transforming growth factor-β stimulates interstitial collagen gene expressed from VSMC, leading to extracellular matrix deposition.[11]

Smooth muscle cell proliferation begins as early as 24 hours following injury and continues for several weeks.[6] In order for VSMC to migrate from the media to the intima, the extracellular matrix must undergo some degradation as it stands as a barrier to migration. Plasminogen activators—proteases that lyse clots and activate matrix-degrading enzymes—and matrix metalloprotinases—that degrade collagen and elastin—are upregulated following injury.[12-13] The degradation of the extracellular matrix allows VSMC to migrate to the intima between one and three days following the injury, where they continue to proliferate for several weeks. Concurrently, endothelial regeneration begins through the stimulation of bFGF within 24 hours of injury.[14] There is also a marked upregulation of the genes that encode for extracellular matrix proteins such as collagen and elastin.[11,15] Deposition of the extracellular matrix is a significant component of the vascular remodeling that occurs after injury. As an end result of this complex process, intimal thickening occurs at the site of injury, thus encroachment on the arterial lumen.

DEVELOPMENT OF NEOINTIMAL HYPERPLASIA FOLLOWING VEIN AND PROSTHETIC BYPASS GRAFTING

The molecular cascade that leads to NIH following arterial injury occurs in a similar manner following vein and prosthetic bypass grafting. However, there are some distinct differences. In vein bypass grafting, the vein is subjected to cyclical, high pressure, and stretching.[16] This serves as a constant source of injury and trigger for the development of neointimal hyperplasia. Furthermore, vein grafts undergo extensive medial remodeling through the entire length of the graft as well as during the life of the graft, in addition to the NIH that develops. In contrast, prosthetic bypass grafts develop NIH predominately at the distal anastamosis. This is thought to occur mainly as a result of the compliance mismatch between the artery and the prosthetic material.[17-18] Additionally, the prosthetic material lacks an endothelial cell layer and its various biologic properties, which temper the development of NIH.

BENEFICIAL ROLE OF NO IN THE VASCULATURE

NO has been shown to possess many different vasoprotective properties including inhibition of platelet aggregation, inhibition of leukocyte adherence, inhibition of VSMC proliferation and migration, stimulation of VSMC apoptosis, and stimulation of endothelial cell growth (Figure 32–1).[4,19-25] NO is also a potent vasodilator. By stimulating soluble guanylate cyclase and leading to increased cyclic guanosine monophosphate (cGMP) release, NO regulates basal vasomotor tone.[26] These properties of NO serve to maintain vascular homeostasis by affecting all the key components in the arterial injury response.

Inhibition of Platelet Aggregation

Nitric oxide acts through several mechanisms to protect vasculature. One of the initial observations was the capacity of NO to prevent platelet adherence and aggregation. Arterial injury results in the exposure of collagen to circulating blood elements, causing platelets to aggregate at the site of injury.[7] Injury also results in the upregulation of iNOS in VSMC in the arterial wall. In 1987, Radomski et al. showed that the adhesion of unstimulated and thrombin-stimulated platelets, washed and labeled with indium-111, to bovine endothelial cells was lower in the presence of bradykinin or exogenous nitric oxide.[19] The inhibitory action of both bradykinin and exogenous nitric oxide was abolished by hemoglobin and was potentiated by superoxide dismutase. This data suggested that the effect of bradykinin is mediated by the release of nitric oxide from the endothelial cells, and that nitric oxide release contributes to the nonadhesive properties of vascular endothelium.[19]

In 1996, Yan et al. showed that this upregulation of iNOS in vivo not only prevented the adherence of platelets to the injured site but also preserved blood flow.[27] These investigators injured rat carotid arteries with a balloon catheter and exposed vessels to the NOS inhibitor L-NAME. L-NAME administration resulted in a threefold increase in[111] In-labeled platelets to the site of injury and a 24% reduction of blood flow. Because the injury resulted in the endothelial denudation with loss of eNOS, it was concluded that the upregulation of iNOS represents a protective mechanism against platelet adherence that compensates for the loss of the endothelium.

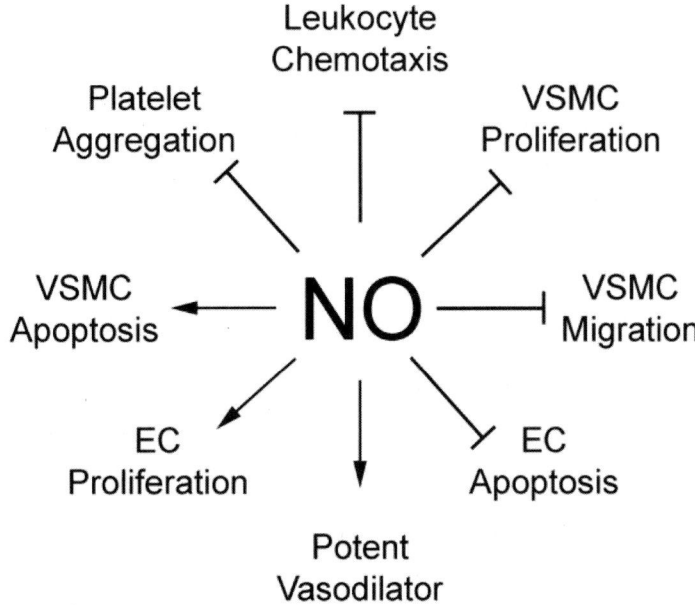

Figure 32-1. Vasoprotective effects of nitric oxide.

Inhibition of Leukocyte Chemotaxis

Following arterial injury, leukocytes accumulate at that site and produce several growth factors and cytokines.[8] This, in turn, stimulates VSMC proliferation and migration. NO has been shown to inhibit the leukocyte chemotatic response and hence negatively effect the downstream events. In 1991, Kubes et al. infused cat mesenteric preparations with inhibitors of NO production and observed single venules by intravital video microscopy.[20] Both NG-monomethyl-L-arginine (L-NMMA) and NG- nitro-L-arginine methyl ester (L-NAME), NOS inhibitors, increased leukocyte adherence more than 15-fold. To specifically evaluate the role of iNOS in the leukocyte–endothelium interaction, iNOS knockout mice were studied.[28] The authors demonstrated that the number of rolling and adherent leukocytes in the cremasteric postcapillary venules and liver postsinusoidal venules of iNOS-deficient mice were significantly greater compared to the wild-type mice. These results suggest that NO produced following iNOS upregulation may function as a homeostatic regulator of leukocyte recruitment and may play an important role in vascular inflammation.

Inhibition of VSMC Proliferation

In 1989, Garg et al. demonstrated that NO could inhibit rat aortic smooth muscle cell (RASMC) proliferation.[22] They administered the NO donors sodium nitroprusside (SNP), S-nitroso-N-acetylpenicillamine (SNAP), and isosorbide dinitrite exogenously to RASMC in culture. A dose-dependent inhibition of RASMC proliferation was demonstrated.

Since these early studies, much research has investigated how NO inhibits VSMC proliferation. One mechanism is through the induction of a G0/G1 cell cycle arrest, preventing cells from entering the synthesis phase of the cell cycle and undergoing proliferation. Ishida et al. in 1997 demonstrated that SNAP induced a G0/G1 cell cycle arrest that was associated with inhibition of VSMC proliferation.[29] Sarkar et al. treated cultured RASMC with SNAP and S-nitrosoglutathione, and observed a 50% decrease in the cells in the G2/M and S phases of the cell cycle and a corresponding increase in the cells in G0/G1.[30] This cell cycle arrest was reversible on withdrawal of the NO donors. We and others found that NO induced a G0/G1 cell cycle arrest in association with the upregulation of the cyclin-dependent kinase inhibitor (CDKI) p21.[21,30] p21 is known to inhibit progress of the cell cycle at various stages. In addition, NO has been shown to increase the expression of another CDKI p27, as well as alter the expression of cyclin A and decrease the activity of cyclin dependent kinase 2 (CDK2).[30-31]

Inhibition of VSMC Migration

A key step in the formation of neointimal hyperplasia following arterial injury is the migration of VSMC from the media to the intima. NO has also been shown to retard this process. In 1995, Dubey et al. showed that SNP and SNAP could inhibit angiotensin II-induced VSMC migration by 60%.[32] To determine if NO produced from iNOS would inhibit this migratory process, they stimulated iNOS expression using IL-1β and showed that NO produced from iNOS upregulation could also inhibit migration of the RASMC by 60%. Sarkar et al. demonstrated that three other NO donors, namely diethylamine NONO-ate, spermine NONOate, and S-nitrosoglutathione, all exhibited concentration-dependent inhibition of both the number of VSMC migrating and the maximal distance migrated following wounding of a confluent culture of RASMC.[33] This inhibition was reversible on removal of the NO donors.

Stimulation of VSMC Apoptosis

Apoptosis of VSMC has an important role in the prevention of neointimal hyperplasia. While the regulation of VSMC apoptosis is not fully understood, NO has been shown to induce VSMC apoptosis. In 1998, Iwashina et al. transfected rat and human VSMC with an iNOS cDNA-expressing construct.[24] The authors found that overexpression of iNOS led to decreased DNA production and increased apoptosis in VSMC. This was quantified using internucleosomal DNA fragmentation by agarose gel electrophoresis, positive staining for TdT-mediated dUTP biotin end-nick labeling, and appearance of hypodiploid cells by flow cytometry analysis. When the NOS inhibitor L-NMMA was administered to iNOS cDNA transfected VSMC, apoptosis was markedly suppressed.

Stimulation of EC Proliferation

NO has also been shown to affect endothelial cells during the injury response. Some evidence indicates that NO stimulates the growth of endothelial cells (EC). One example comes from studies examining angiogenesis, a process that requires the stimulation of proliferation and migration of endothelial cells. In 1994, Ziche et al. evaluated the effects of NO donors and endogenous NO on the angiogenesis process.[34] They monitored the angiogenic response in rabbit corneas and found that sodium nitroprusside (SNP) potentiated angiogenesis and this was inhibited by L-NAME. By examining coronary endothelial cells in culture, they found that NO-generating compounds produced a dose-dependent increase in endothelial cell proliferation. Endogenous production of NO following stimulation of the coronary endothelial cells with substance P also resulted in increased EC proliferation and migration. This response was prevented by pretreatment with NOS inhibitors. In 1997, Tzeng et al. demonstrated yet another beneficial effect of NO on endothelial cells.[25] Overexpression of iNOS using an adenoviral vector increased endothelial proliferation and suppressed apoptosis. This data suggests that NO production favors healing of the injured vasculature by stimulating endothelial proliferation and rapid coverage of the injured site. Following arterial injury, once the injured site has undergone reendothelialization, the stimulus for platelet adherence and leukocyte chemotaxis is removed. Thus, the subsequent cascade of cytokine and growth factor release that leads to the development of neointimal hyperplasia is no longer present.

NO PREVENTS NEOINTIMAL HYPERPLASIA

Inhalational NO

While NO has been shown to inhibit individual components of the arterial injury response, it has also been shown to prevent the development of NIH as a whole. Several NO-based therapies have been studied in the animal model with regard to preventing NIH. In 1996, Lee et al. examined the effects of inhalational NO on NIH following balloon-induced injury of the adult rat carotid artery.[35] There was a 43% reduction in the intima/media ratio in rats that were exposed to inhalational NO for two weeks as compared to control rats breathing room air. However, to achieve this inhibition, the rats needed to continuously breathe NO for 14 days: inhaling NO for the first seven days after injury followed by seven days of airbreathing did not inhibit neointimal formation at 14 days. In addition, it is unlikely that NO reaches the carotid artery injury site despite the high concentration. Rich et al. (Inhaled nitric oxide: Dose response and the effects of blood in the isolated rat lung. *J Appl Physiol.* 1993;75:1278–1284) measured the concentration of NO in the effluent of isolated perfused rat lungs ventilated with 1,000 ppm NO; they observed that if the lungs were perfused with whole blood, NO was undetectable in the effluent due to its rapid inactivation of NO by hemoglobin. Therefore, it is unlikely that NO absorbed into the pulmonary circulation decreases neointimal formation at the site of carotid injury via a direct effect.

Administration of NO-Donors Systemically

Groves et al. used the oral NO donor molsidomine in a porcine carotid angioplasty model.[36] There was a 32% reduction in the NIH at 21 days. However, this was only in circumstances when the internal elastic lamina remained intact following the angioplasty. In arteries where disruption of the internal elastic lamina had occurred, there was diminished VSMC proliferation, and there was no difference in NIH between molsidomine and placebo. It was felt that the antiproliferative effects of orallyadministered nitric oxide were possibly overwhelmed when injury was severe and, therefore, not associated with a reduction in intimal thickening.

NO-donors have even been administered to patients intravenously and orally, and demonstrated a beneficial effect. The ACCORD study showed that in patients undergoing angioplasty, intravenous administration of the NO-donor linsidomine followed by oral molsidomine for six months was associated with a modest improvement in immediate angiographic results, which was sustained at a six-month angiographic follow-up (minimal lumen diameter 1.54 mm versus 1.38 mm, $P = 0.007$).[37]

Administration of L-Arginine Systemically

In 1993, McNamara et al. administered the nitric oxide precursor L-arginine to rabbits from two days prior to two weeks following catheter-induced injury to the rabbit thoracic aorta.[38] Animals receiving L-arginine displayed 39% less NIH compared to control untreated animals. This reduction in NIH was reversed by coadministration of L-NAME. Similar results have been achieved by other groups. Chen et al. administered L-arginine in the drinking water of Sprague-Dawley rats that underwent balloon denudation on the left common carotid artery.[39] L-arginine-treated animals showed a 65% reduction of the intima/media area ratio and a 26% reduction of the intimal cell proliferation compared with control animals. These data indicate that oral administration of L-arginine significantly reduced intimal hyperplasia of balloon-injured arteries without any detectable toxicity.

NOS Gene Therapy

In 1995, von der Leyen delivered eNOS complexed with the HVJ to rat carotid arteries following injury and demonstrated a 70% reduction in the neointima/media area ratio.[40] Chen et al. seeded VSMC expressing eNOS via retroviral transfection onto the luminal surface of balloon-injured rat carotid arteries and inhibited neointimal formation by 37% at two weeks postinjury.[41] Other studies have similarly shown that adenoviral delivery of eNOS to balloon-injured rat and porcine arteries can limit intimal hyperplasia for up to 4 weeks.[41-43]

Shears et al. in1998 demonstrated that adenoviral delivery of human iNOS (AdiNOS) to the rat carotid artery following injury resulted in a 96.7% inhibition of intimal thickening using just 2×106 plaque-forming units (pfu)/artery.[44] This protective effect was reversed by the continuous administration of an iNOS selective inhibitor L-N6-(1-iminoethyl)-lysine. Delivery to a more clinically relevant model, the pig iliac artery injury model, resulted in a 51.8% reduction in the intima/media area ratio using 5×108 pfu/artery.[45] Kibbe et al. performed AdiNOS gene transfer in a porcine model of vein bypass grafting.[46] The internal jugular vein was infected with the adenoviral vector after it was harvested and the IJ vein was then transposed into the carotid artery. The AdiNOS treated veins showed a 30% decrease in the intimal/medial area ratio at 21 days as compared to controls.

Local Application of NO-Donors

Marks et al investigated the effects of a locally delivered polythiolated form of bovine serum albumin (pS-BSA) modified to carry several S-nitrosothiol groups (pS-NO- BSA) on neointimal responses in an animal model of vascular injury.[47] Locally delivered S-NO-BSA bound preferentially to denuded rabbit femoral vessels producing a 26-fold increase in local concentration compared with uninjured vessels ($P = 0.029$). pS-NO-BSA significantly reduced the intimal/medial ratio (77% decrease, $P = 0.038$). pS-NO-BSA treatment also inhibited platelet deposition ($P = 0.031$) after denuding injury. Therefore, local administration of a stable protein S-nitrosothiol inhibits intimal proliferation and platelet deposition after vascular arterial balloon injury.

NO Polymers

An alternative strategy that has clinical therapeutic potential may be to use local application of NO through biocompatible gels and polymers. In the past five years, there has been a significant advance in polymeric and nonpolymeric based approaches to deliver NO to the vasculature. West's group has been evaluating NO releasing photopolymerized polyethylene glycol hydrogels on the inhibition of VSMC proliferation.[48] Kaul et al. delivered (Z)-1-(N-[3-Aminopropyl]-N-[4-(3-aminopropylammoniobutyl)])diazen-1-ium-1,2-diolate (SPER/NO) in a polylactic-polyglycolic acid polymer matrix to the external surface of injured rat ileofemoral arteries and inhibited neointimal hyperplasia by ~75% at 14 days.[49] Chaux et al. delivered SPER/NO in a biodegradable polymer to the external surface of vein grafts in hypercholesterolemic rabbits and found a 41% reduction in vein graft hyperplasia at 28 days.[50] Kown et al. used L-arginine polymer to treat vein grafts.[51] They demonstrated increased NO levels and decreased NIH in the vein bypass of rabbit carotid arteries. The intima/media ratio also reflected both length- and concentration-dependent inhibition of NIH. Other examples of polymer- and nonpolymeric-based delivery of NO-donors to the vasculature include a hydrogel-coated angioplasty balloon to deliver molsidomine and a pleuronic gel with the NO donor S-ni-troso-N-acetylpenicillamine (SNAP).[52-53]

Limitations of NO-Based Therapies

All of the discussed therapies have been effective in the animal models to prevent the development of neointimal hyperplasia following arterial injury or vein bypass grafting. However, each of these therapies has some limitations as far as clinical applicability due to systemic side effects, safety concerns, inability to concentrate the NO at the site of interest, short-half life of the NO-donor, a complicated delivery scheme, or potential toxic metabolites of the NO-donor. For example, when NO is administered systemically, it can have undesirable side effects such as vasodilation, hypotension, headaches, and increased bleeding complications. This precludes delivering a concentrated dose to the site of injury with systemic methods. Gene therapy with viral vectors is associated with theoretic concerns of malignant transformation. Additionally, this form of therapy has been associated with inflammation secondary to the introduction of foreign viral DNA. Some NO-donors pose a potential hazard based on the final breakdown products. For example, SPER/NO dissociates into NO and spermine, the latter of which has its own biological properties that are deleterious to the vasculature. Spermine is a small organic polycation involved in numerous diverse biological processes. It has been shown to bind DNA and RNA and cause DNA condensation and aggregation.[54] It has also been shown to play a role in spermatogenesis, skin physiology, promotion of tumorigenesis, and organ hypertrophy, as well as neuronal protection.[55] All of these shortcomings have led our group to develop NO-based therapies that minimize these risks, yet capitalize on the beneficial aspects of NO.

OUR APPROACH

Our goal is to develop a pharmacological NO-based therapy that has clinical utility to prevent the development of NIH following vein and prosthetic bypass grafting and surgical endarterectomy. To that end, we have developed a biocompatible NO-eluting gel that can be applied to the adventitia at the site of vascular injury or bypass grafting to prevent the development of NIH. Our future directions involve developing a polymer cross-linked spontaneous NO-eluting PTFE graft that will prevent the development of neointimal hyperplasia. The benefits of these forms of therapy are numerous. First, a pharmacologic approach utilizing a drug applied locally at the site of injury avoids systemic effects of NO-release such as hypotension. Second, local application at the site of injury allows the effect of the NO-gel to be concentrated at one location. A similar argument can be made for the NO-releasing PTFE. Third, safety concerns of gene therapy are eliminated. Fourth, the duration of NO-release can be tailored for individual need. For example, following arterial injury, NO-release may only be necessary for a few days or weeks, whereas with bypass grafting, the insult at the distal anastomosis is ongoing and the therapeutic need for NO-release may last months to years.

NO-Eluting Gels

Diazeniumdiolates, often referred to as NONOates, are chemical species containing the [N(O)NO]-functional group, that have unique characteristics that make them suitable choices to use in models of vascular injury (Figure 32–2). The advantages of diazeniumdiolates over other NO-donors include known predictable rates of NO-release, rates of NO generation over a wide range, spontaneity of NO generation, and tunable generation of NO redox forms.[56-57] Two diazeniumdiolate NO-donors have been specifically chosen for this study: disodium 1-[(2-carboxylato)pyrrolidin-1-yl]diazen-1-ium-1,2-diolate (PROLI/NO) and diazeniumdiolated poly(acrylonitrile) (PAN/NO). PROLI/NO is a water-soluble ultrafast NO generator and releases 2 moles of NO per mole of compound.[58] PAN/NO is a

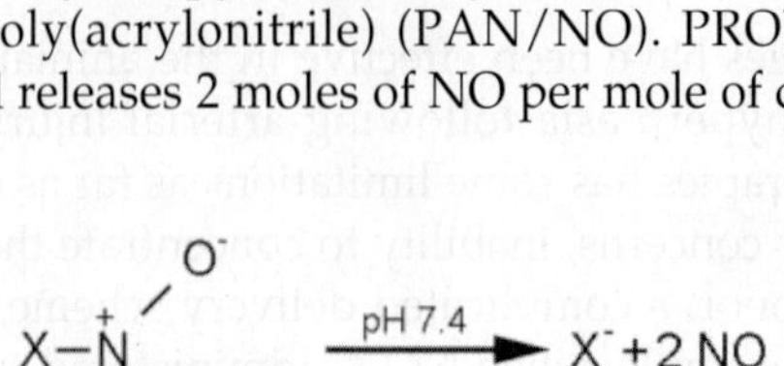

$$X-N_{\diagdown N-O}^{\diagup O^-} \xrightarrow{pH\ 7.4} X^- + 2\ NO$$

Figure 32-2. The release of nitric oxide from diazeniumdiolates.

particulate material based on polyacrylonitrile (PAN) that has a much longer half life compared to PROLI/NO, on the order of many days (Larry Keefer, Ph.D.—personal communication). It is difficult to estimate the amount of NO release from PAN/NO since it is a polymer in which only the outer nitrile groups contained in the chain react with NO to form diazeniumdiolates, but we know comparatively that PAN/NO releases very high concentrations of NO. A benefit of both of these NO-donors is that in contrast to many other diazeniumdiolates, the corresponding N-nitroso derivative, is considered noncarcinogenic. These are important considerations because some NO-donors have biologically active metabolites. A NO-donor with no other biological activities is preferred, as this would constitute an obvious advantage for potential clinical applications.

In order for diazeniumdiolates to release NO, they must react with hydrogen ions in the medium to which they are exposed.[56] If the NO-donor is blended with materials lacking hydrogen ions, the duration of NO-release will be extended greatly. Poloxamer 407, also known as Pleuronic® F127, is composed of polyethylene-polypropylene glycol, which is also relatively free of hydrogen ions. Therefore, we predict that Poloxamer 407 will extend the NO-release profile of the NO-donors. Poloxamer 407 also possesses unique reverse-phase gelatin properties in that it is liquid at 4°C but forms a gel at 37°C, making it an ideal material for external application to an artery or bypass graft.

Adult male Sprague-Dawley rats were anesthetized and the left common, external, and internal carotid arteries were dissected; proximal and distal control was obtained with microclips. Following a transverse arteriotomy on the external carotid artery, a 2 Fr. embolectomy catheter was inserted into the common carotid artery through the external carotid artery, and the common carotid artery was injured by inflating the balloon to 5 atmospheres of pressure for five minutes. Following injury, the catheter was removed, the external carotid artery was ligated, and flow restored to the common and internal carotid arteries. The NO-eluting gels (PAN/NO or PROLI/NO) or the control saline-gel were applied to the external surface of the injured common carotid artery. The neck wound was closed. At two weeks, the animals were euthanized and the carotid arteries were removed following in situ perfusion-fixation. As seen in Figures 32–3 and 32–4, preliminary studies show near complete inhibition of neointimal hyperplasia with both the PAN/NO (Figure 32–3C) and PROLI/NO (Figure 32–3D) gels, compared to the arteries that underwent injury alone (Figure 32–3A) or injury with application of the saline gel (Figure 32–3B) (Intima/Media area ratio: Injury 1.02β0.04; Injury+saline gel 1.09β0.06; Injury+PAN/NO 0.28β0.04*; Injury+PROLI/NO 0.32β0.07*; *$P < 0.001$ versus injury or injury+saline gel). No foreign body reaction was observed in the neck wounds at the time of harvest. Thus, it appears from this preliminary data that both of these gels have clinical potential to dramatically inhibit the development of neointimal hyperplasia following vascular injury.

Future Directions

Autogenous vein is often not available for bypass grafting due to prior harvesting or is of poor quality, necessitating the use of a prosthetic conduit in one-third of patients.[59] Prosthetic bypass conduits have significantly lower patency rates compared to autogenous vein grafts.[60-63] The majority of prosthetic graft failures are due to compliance mismatch between the prosthetic material and the native artery, and lack of EC coverage of the PTFE grafts, both of which causes neointimal hyperplasia to develop more aggressively at the distal anastomosis.[17-18,64] We hypothesize that a novel releasing polymer cross-linked

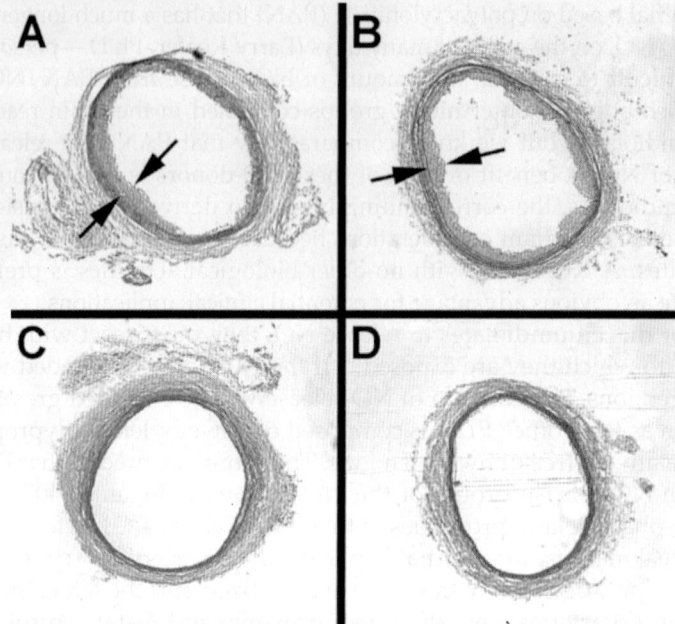

Figure 32-3. Cross-sectional view of H&E stained rat carotid arteries that have undergone **A.** balloon injury alone or balloon injury followed by application of **B.** saline gel, **C.** PAN/NO gel, or **D.** PROLI/NO gel.

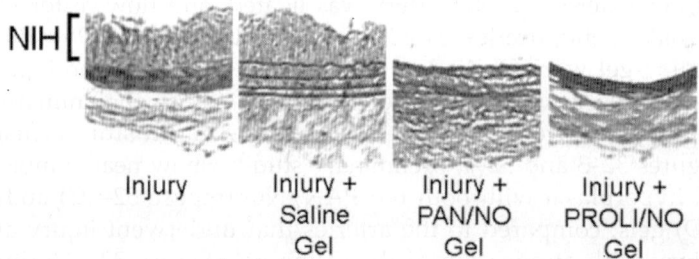

Figure 32-4. Cross-sectional view of a section of H&E stained rat carotid artery demonstrating the development of neointimal hyperplasia (NIH) following balloon injury and external application of therapeutic NO-releasing gels.

NO-eluting PTFE graft would reduce the development of NIH and increases graft patency compared to conventional PTFE grafts. As NO can prevent the development of NIH at sites of arterial injury, this form of NO therapy will have a significant impact on prosthetic graft patency rates. In addition, the steady release of NO from the entire length of the graft over a long time period will have a greater effect on VSMC proliferation at the distal anastomosis compared to the proximal anastomosis. We also predict that NO will have an impact on the endothelialization of PTFE grafts, given the stimulatory effects NO has on EC proliferation and migration. The latter would have a beneficial effect on both the thrombogenicity of the graft and the development of neointimal hyperplasia. Therefore, we are currently developing a spontaneous NO-releasing PTFE graft that releases NO over extended periods of time in a stable manner through polymer cross-linking of the PTFE material. We anticipate that this form of therapy will have tremendous clinical applicability in the future.

CONCLUSION

NO-based therapies have tremendous potential to have a significant impact on the development of NIH following arterial injury or vascular bypass grafting in the clinical arena. In this chapter, we described the mechanisms by which NO is able to have such a profound effect in the vasculature, include the ability of NO to inhibit platelet aggregation, inhibit leukocyte adherence, inhibit VSMC proliferation and migration, stimulate VSMC apoptosis, and stimulate endothelial cell growth. Furthermore, the benefits of NO-based therapy in various animal models of arterial injury and bypass grafting were discussed. Overall, we believe that NO-based pharmacological approaches will be advantageous as the NO gel can be applied locally at the site of injury, concentrated, and the half life of NO release can be tailored. Furthermore, this form of therapy is safe and free from side effects. Our promising preliminary data support this notion. Through further research, our hope is that this form of therapy will eventually make it to the clinical arena for vascular surgery.

REFERENCES

1. Furchgott RF, Zawadzki JV. The obligatory role of endothelial cells in the relaxation of arterial smooth muscle by acetylcholine. *Nature.* 1980;288:373–376.
2. Bredt DS, Snyder SH. Nitric oxide: a physiologic messenger molecule. *Ann Rev Biochem.* 1994;63:175–95:175–195.
3. Forstermann U, Closs EI, Pollock JS, et al. Nitric oxide synthase isozymes. Characterization, purification, molecular cloning, and functions. *Hypertension.* 1994;23:1121–1131.
4. Guo JP, Panday MM, Consigny PM, Lefer AM. Mechanisms of vascular preservation by a novel NO donor following rat carotid artery intimal injury. *Am J Physiol.* 1995;269: H1122–H1131.
5. Clowes AW, Reidy MA, Clowes MM. Mechanisms of stenosis after arterial injury. *Lab Invest.* 1983;49:208–215.
6. Clowes AW, Reidy MA, Clowes MM. Kinetics of cellular proliferation after arterial injury. I. Smooth muscle growth in the absence of endothelium. *Lab Invest.* 1983;49:327–333.
7. Fingerle J, Johnson R, Clowes AW, et al. Role of platelets in smooth muscle cell proliferation and migration after vascular injury in rat carotid artery. *Proc Natl Acad Sci USA.* 1989;86: 8412–8416.
8. Davies MG, Hagen PO. Pathobiology of intimal hyperplasia. *Br J Surg.* 1994;81:1254–1269.
9. Lindner V, Lappi DA, Baird A, et al. Role of basic fibroblast growth factor in vascular lesion formation. *Circ Res.* 1991;68:106–113.
10. Kullo IJ, Mozes G, Schwartz RS, et al. Enhanced endothelium-dependent relaxations after gene transfer of recombinant endothelial nitric oxide synthase to rabbit carotid arteries. *Hypertension.* 1997;30:314–320.
11. Majesky MW, Lindner V, Twardzik DR, et al. Production of transforming growth factor beta 1 during repair of arterial injury. *J Clin Invest.* 1991;88:904–910.
12. Bendeck MP, Zempo N, Clowes AW, et al. Smooth muscle cell migration and matrix metalloproteinase expression after arterial injury in the rat. *Circ Res.* 1994;75:539–545.
13. Hasenstab D, Forough R, Clowes AW. Plasminogen activator inhibitor type 1 and tissue inhibitor of metalloproteinases-2 increase after arterial injury in rats. *Circ Res.* 1997;80: 490–496.
14. Lindner V, Majack RA, Reidy MA. Basic fibroblast growth factor stimulates endothelial regrowth and proliferation in denuded arteries. *J Clin Invest.* 1990;85:2004–2008.
15. Nabel EG, Shum L, Pompili VJ, et al. Direct transfer of transforming growth factor beta 1 gene into arteries stimulates fibrocellular hyperplasia. *Proc Natl Acad Sci USA.* 1993;90: 10759–10763.

16. Shuhaiber JH, Evans AN, Massad MG, Geha AS. Mechanisms and future directions for prevention of vein graft failure in coronary bypass surgery. *Eur J Cardiothorac Surg.* 2002;22: 387–396.

17. Rahlf G, Urban P, Bohle RM. Morphology of healing in vascular prostheses. *Thorac Cardiovasc Surg.* 1986;34:43–48.

18. Clowes AW, Kirkman TR, Clowes MM. Mechanisms of arterial graft failure. II. Chronic endothelial and smooth muscle cell proliferation in healing polytetrafluoroethylene prostheses. *J Vasc Surg.* 1986;3:877–884.

19. Radomski MW, Palmer RM, Moncada S. Endogenous nitric oxide inhibits human platelet adhesion to vascular endothelium. *Lancet.* 1987;2:1057–1058.

20. Kubes P, Suzuki M, Granger DN. Nitric oxide: an endogenous modulator of leukocyte adhesion. *Proc Natl Acad Sci USA.* 1991;88:4651–4655.

21. Kibbe MR, Li J, Nie S, Watkins SC, et al. Inducible nitric oxide synthase (iNOS) expression upregulates p21 and inhibits vascular smooth muscle cell proliferation through p42/44 mi-togen-activated protein kinase activation and independent of p53 and cyclic guanosine monophosphate [In Process Citation]. *J Vasc Surg.* 2000;31:1214–1228.

22. Garg UC, Hassid A. Nitric oxide-generating vasodilators and 8-bromo-cyclic guanosine monophosphate inhibit mitogenesis and proliferation of cultured rat vascular smooth muscle cells. *J Clin Invest.* 1989;83:1774–1777.

23. Nishio E, Fukushima K, Shiozaki M, Watanabe Y. Nitric oxide donor SNAP induces apoptosis in smooth muscle cells through cGMP-independent mechanism. *Biochem Biophys Res Commun.* 1996;221:163–168.

24. Iwashina M, Shichiri M, Marumo F, Hirata Y. Transfection of inducible nitric oxide synthase gene causes apoptosis in vascular smooth muscle cells. *Circulation.* 1998;98:1212–1218.

25. Tzeng E, Kim YM, Pitt BR, Lizonova A, et al. Adenoviral transfer of the inducible nitric oxide synthase gene blocks endothelial cell apoptosis. *Surgery.* 1997;122:255–263.

26. Ignarro LJ, Buga GM, Wood KS, Byrns RE, Chaudhuri G. Endothelium-derived relaxing factor produced and released from artery and vein is nitric oxide. *Proc Natl Acad Sci USA.* 1987;84:9265–9269.

27. Yan ZQ, Yokota T, Zhang W, Hansson GK. Expression of inducible nitric oxide synthase inhibits platelet adhesion and restores blood flow in the injured artery. *Circ Res.* 1996; 79:38–44.

28. Hickey MJ, Sharkey KA, Sihota EG, et al. Inducible nitric oxide synthase-deficient mice have enhanced leukocyte- endothelium interactions in endotoxemia. *FASEB J.* 1997;11: 955–964.

29. Ishida A, Sasaguri T, Kosaka C, et al. Induction of the cyclin-dependent kinase inhibitor p21(Sdi1/Cip1/Waf1) by nitric oxide-generating vasodilator in vascular smooth muscle cells. *J Biol Chem.* 1997;272:10050–10057.

30. Sarkar R, Gordon D, Stanley JC, Webb RC. Cell cycle effects of nitric oxide on vascular smooth muscle cells. *Am J Physiol.* 1997;272:H1810–H1818.

31. Tanner FC, Meier P, Greutert H, et al. Nitric oxide modulates expression of cell cycle regulatory proteins: a cytostatic strategy for inhibition of human vascular smooth muscle cell proliferation. *Circulation.* 2000;101:1982–1989.

32. Dubey RK, Jackson EK, Luscher TF. Nitric oxide inhibits angiotensin II-induced migration of rat aortic smooth muscle cell. Role of cyclic-nucleotides and angiotensin1 receptors. *J Clin Invest.* 1995;96:141–149.

33. Sarkar R, Meinberg EG, Stanley JC, et al. Nitric oxide reversibly inhibits the migration of cultured vascular smooth muscle cells. *Circ Res.* 1996;78:225–230.

34. Ziche M, Morbidelli L, Masini E, et al. Nitric oxide mediates angiogenesis in vivo and endothelial cell growth and migration in vitro promoted by substance P. *J Clin Invest.* 1994; 94:2036–2044.

35. Lee JS, Adrie C, Jacob HJ, et al. Chronic inhalation of nitric oxide inhibits neointimal formation after balloon-induced arterial injury. *Circ Res.* 1996;78:337–342.

36. Groves PH, Banning AP, Penny WJ, et al. The effects of exogenous nitric oxide on smooth muscle cell proliferation following porcine carotid angioplasty. *Cardiovasc Res.* 1995;30: 87–96.
37. Lablanche JM, Grollier G, Lusson JR, et al. Effect of the direct nitric oxide donors linsidomine and molsidomine on angiographic restenosis after coronary balloon angioplasty. The ACCORD Study. Angioplastic Coronaire Corvasal Diltiazem. *Circulation.* 1997;95:83–89.
38. McNamara DB, Bedi B, Aurora H, et al. L-arginine inhibits balloon catheter-induced intimal hyperplasia. *Biochem Biophys Res Commun.* 1993;193:291–296.
39. Chen C, Mattar SG, Lumsden AB. Oral administration of L-arginine reduces intimal hyperplasia in balloon-injured rat carotid arteries. *J Surg Res.* 1999;82:17–23.
40. von der Leyden, Gibbons GH, Morishita R, et al. Gene therapy inhibiting neointimal vascular lesion: in vivo transfer of endothelial cell nitric oxide synthase gene. *Proc Natl Acad Sci USA.* 1995;92:1137–1141.
41. Chen L, Daum G, Forough R, et al. Overexpression of human endothelial nitric oxide synthase in rat vascular smooth muscle cells and in balloon-injured carotid artery. *Circ Research.* 1998;82:862–870.
42. Janssens S, Flaherty D, Nong Z, et al. Human endothelial nitric oxide synthase gene transfer inhibits vascular smooth muscle cell proliferation and neointima formation after balloon injury in rats. *Circulation.* 1998;97:1274–1281.
43. Varenne O, Pislaru S, Gillijns H, et al. Local adenovirus-mediated transfer of human endothelial nitric oxide synthase reduces luminal narrowing after coronary angioplasty in pigs. *Circulation.* 1998;98:919–926.
44. Shears LL, Kibbe MR, Murdock AD, et al. Efficient inhibition of intimal hyperplasia by ade-novirus-mediated inducible nitric oxide synthase gene transfer to rats and pigs in vivo. *J Am Coll Surg.* 1998;187:295–306.
45. Shears LL, Kibbe MR, Murdock AD, et al. Efficient inhibition of intimal hyperplasia by adenovirus-mediated inducible nitric oxide synthase gene transfer to rats and pigs in vivo. *J Am Coll Surg.* 1998;187:295–306.
46. Kibbe MR, Tzeng E, Gleixner SL, et al. Adenovirus-mediated gene transfer of human inducible nitric oxide synthase in porcine vein grafts inhibits intimal hyperplasia. *J Vasc Surg.* 2001;34:156–165.
47. Marks DS, Vita JA, Folts JD, et al. Inhibition of neointimal proliferation in rabbits after vascular injury by a single treatment with a protein adduct of nitric oxide. *J Clin Invest.* 1995; 96:2630–2638.
48. Bohl KS, West JL. Nitric oxide-generating polymers reduce platelet adhesion and smooth muscle cell proliferation. *Biomaterials.* 2000;21:2273–2278.
49. Kaul S, Cercek B, Rengstrom J, et al. Polymeric-based perivascular delivery of a nitric oxide donor inhibits intimal thickening after balloon denudation arterial injury: role of nuclear factor-kappaB. *J Am Coll Cardiol.* 2000;35:493–501.
50. Chaux A, Ruan XM, Fishbein MC,et al. Perivascular delivery of a nitric oxide donor inhibits neointimal hyperplasia in vein grafts implanted in the arterial circulation. *J Thorac Cardiovasc Surg.* 1998;115:604–612.
51. Kown MH, Yamaguchi A, Jahncke CL, et al. L-arginine polymers inhibit the development of vein graft neointimal hyperplasia. *J Thorac Cardiovasc Surg.* 2001;121:971–980.
52. Rolland PH, Mekkaoui C, Palassi M, et al. Efficacy of local molsidomine delivery from a hydrogel-coated angioplasty balloon catheter in the atherosclerotic porcine model. *Cardiovasc Intervent Radiol.* 2003;26:65–72.
53. Fulton GJ, Davies MG, Barber L, et al. Local effects of nitric oxide supplementation and suppression in the development of intimal hyperplasia in experimental vein grafts. *Eur J Vasc Endovasc Surg.* 1998;15:279–289.
54. Ouameur AA, Tajmir-Riahi HA. Structural Analysis of DNA Interactions with Biogenic Polyamines and Cobalt(III) hexamine Studied by Fourier Transform Infrared and Capillary Electrophoresis. *J Biol Chem.* 2004;279:42041–42054.

55. Janne J, Alhonen L, Pietila M, Keinanen TA. Genetic approaches to the cellular functions of polyamines in mammals. *Eur J Biochem.* 2004;271:877–894.
56. Hrabie JA, Keefer LK. Chemistry of the nitric oxide-releasing diazeniumdiolate ("nitrosohydroxylamine") functional group and its oxygen-substituted derivatives. *Chem Rev.* 2002;102:1135–1154.
57. Fitzhugh AL, Keefer LK. Diazeniumdiolates: pro- and antioxidant applications of the "NONOates" *Free Radic Biol Med.* 2000;28:1463–1469.
58. Keefer LK. Progress toward clinical application of the nitric oxide-releasing diazeniumdiolates. *Annu Rev Pharmacol Toxicol.* 2003;43:585–607.
59. Sayers RD, Raptis S, Berce M, Miller JH. Long-term results of femorotibial bypass with vein or polytetrafluoroethylene. *Br J Surg.* 1998;85:934–938.
60. Stonebridge PA, Prescott RJ, Ruckley CV. Randomized trial comparing infrainguinal polytetrafluoroethylene bypass grafting with and without vein interposition cuff at the distal anastomosis. The Joint Vascular Research Group. *J Vasc Surg.* 1997;26:543–550.
61. Weyand M, Kerber S, Schmid C, et al. Coronary artery bypass grafting with an expanded polytetrafluoroethylene graft. *Ann Thorac Surg.* 1999;67:1240–1244.
62. Biancari F, Railo M, Lundin J, et al. Redo bypass surgery to the infrapopliteal arteries for critical leg ischaemia. *Eur J Vasc Endovasc Surg.* 2001;21:137–142.
63. Eagleton MJ, Ouriel K, Shortell C, Green RM. Femoral-infrapopliteal bypass with prosthetic grafts. *Surgery.* 1999;126:759–764.
64. Tiwari A, Salacinski H, Seifalian AM, Hamilton G. New prostheses for use in bypass grafts with special emphasis on polyurethanes. *Cardiovasc Surg.* 2002;10:191–197.

33

Bioengineered Arteries

Jeffrey A. Caves and Elliot L. Chaikof, M.D., Ph.D.

As we enter the 21st century, atherosclerosis remains a serious source of morbidity and death despite advances in preventive measures and pharmacological therapeutics. Nearly 700,000 vascular surgical procedures are performed annually in the United States, along with several hundred thousand peripheral and coronary angioplasties.[1] Prosthetic bypass grafts, and more recently, arterial stents and other endovascular prostheses, have been utilized in association with these reconstructive procedures. Although large diameter vascular grafts (> 6 mm internal diameter) have been successfully developed from polymers such as polytetrafluoroethylene and polyethylene terephthalate, the fabrication of a durable small diameter prosthesis (< 6 mm internal diameter) remains unsolved. Furthermore, while prosthetic bypass grafting can be performed in the infrainguinal position with reasonable short-term success, within five years, 30% to 60% of these grafts will fail.[2-5] Several bioengineering strategies for vascular graft design have evolved that are currently areas of critical research.

BIOHYBRID VASCULAR GRAFTS

It is recognized that the adverse events leading to the failure of many vascular prostheses are related to maladaptive biological reactions at the blood-material and tissue-material interface. In response to these problems, researchers have endeavored to design an arterial prosthesis through the mimicry of some or all of the characteristics of the arterial wall. For example, several investigators have sought to develop a functional endothelial lining on the luminal surface of a *synthetic vascular prosthesis*, either by the transplantation of endothelial cells onto the prosthetic surface prior to graft implantation or by promoting the in situ regeneration of an endothelial intimal lining.[6-9] While promising results have been reported with cell transplantation, the success of this approach continues to be limited by problems related to cell sourcing, attachment and retention of endothelial cells onto the graft surface, and the time frame required for the formation of a complete intimal lining.[10] In addition, there remains a propensity for transplanted endothelial cells to develop a procoagulant and/or proinflammatory phenotype.[11] Likewise, strategies based on the coating of a prosthetic surface with matrix proteins or integrin-selective peptide sequences that promote the growth of host endothelial cells onto the graft surface have been unable to overcome the capacity of these same substrates to activate platelets and the coagulation cascade. Furthermore, vascular grafts made from nonbiodegradable *synthetic* polymeric materials remain at risk for bacterial colonization and subsequent graft infection and, in addition, are capable of promoting a low-level, chronic inflammatory response that may contribute to the development of neointimal hyperplasia.[12] Finally, a "compliance mismatch" that characteristically exists between a prosthetic graft and the host artery may also lead to neointimal hyperplasia and late graft failure.[13-14] Thus, the inherent limitations of a biohybrid prosthesis that consists, in part, of nonbiological elements have motivated many investigators to develop arterial constructs that are comprised exclusively of biological components.

TISSUE ENGINEERED CONSTRUCTS: CELL-ASSISTED ASSEMBLY OF MATRIX PROTEINS

In 1986, Weinberg and Bell[15] generated an arterial construct consisting of a cell populated collagen gel. Significantly, *cell-mediated* development and alignment of the surrounding collagen matrix enhanced the mechanical integrity of the construct. However, even when reinforced with a Dacron mesh, this model did not display sufficient tensile strength necessary for in vivo applications. Subsequent to this report, efforts have been directed at improving the mechanical characteristics of collagen gel-based constructs, either by increasing collagen concentration, reducing endogenous proteolytic enzyme activity, or through the introduction of techniques that promote cell-assisted matrix protein assembly and crosslinking.[16-19] Both endogenous crosslinking processes and methods to control cell alignment, including mechanical conditioning, have been investigated.[20-21] Despite these efforts, the reassembly of *exogenous*, native structural proteins into an ECM of physiological density and organization has not been achieved. In contrast, recent investigations have demonstrated that a mechanically robust multilayered arterial equivalent can be generated from cell driven assembly of *secreted endogenous* matrix proteins. In this regard, L'Heureux and colleagues[22-23] observed that following prolonged culture in medium containing ascorbic acid, cellular sheets composed of smooth muscle cells or fibroblasts, could be rolled around a mandrel in sequential layers to construct a tubular vessel. Rupture strengths exceeding 2000 mm Hg were observed. Alternatively, Nikalson and coworkers seeded tubular biodegradable polyglycolic acid (PGA) scaffolds with bovine smooth muscle cells, cultured and mechanically conditioned the constructs for eight weeks in a bioreactor, and seeded endothelial cells in the vessel lumen. The resulting conduits were composed largely of an endogenous collagen matrix and had burst strengths over 2000 mm Hg. Grafts derived from autologous cells displayed adequate patency at four weeks in a swine model.[24] Several similar technologies have been developed and recently reviewed.[25]

Shin'oka and coworkers have employed a related strategy to demonstrate feasibility in the reconstruction of the pulmonary artery. In this clinical study, the authors seeded autologous cells, either cultured from vein harvests or from bone marrow aspirates, onto synthetic biodegradable scaffolds. Tubular and flat-sheet constructs were typically implanted to repair the pulmonary artery in young patients with congenital defects. Postoperative angiography demonstrated the repairs were consistently open to flow without constriction or dilation, although little is known with respect to the nature of the resulting engineered tissues.[26-27] Notwithstanding these promising results, important limitations remain associated with tissue engineering strategies that are based on cell-assisted matrix protein assembly. Specifically, cellular constructs require months of incubation before vessels are suitable for implantation in the arterial system; cell differentiation and proliferation must be assessed and controlled; there are significant immunologic challenges related to the use of allogeneic cells; and though elastin fiber formation has occasionally been observed, the compliance of these constructs is much less than that of a native blood vessel.

DECELLULARIZED ALLO- AND XENOGENEIC TISSUE ARTERIAL SUBSTITUTES

As an alternative to cell-based constructs, *acellular* allo- and xenogeneic blood vessels have been investigated as vascular conduits, including human umbilical vein[28-30] and bovine carotid artery.[31-32] The existing concept has been to produce a structure with: (1) inherent *resistance to degeneration* conferred by maximal preservation of structural proteins and their three dimensional organization; (2) *low potential for host inflammatory attack* because of extraction of antigenic cellular proteins; and (3) *low thrombogenicity* due to the maintenance of the subendothelial basement membrane as the flow surface. Approaches to generate an acellular vascular conduit typically include the initial removal of cellular contents by enzymatic and/or detergent extraction processes so as to reduce tissue antigenicity and the likelihood of later calcification.[33-34] In all cases, the remaining acellular matrix is chemically crosslinked, most often by glutaraldehyde, principally to enhance stability and to further reduce tissue immunogenicity. Nevertheless, biodegradation, with progressive dilatation and aneurysm formation, remain persistent problems such that the placement of a surrounding Dacron mesh remains a fabrication requirement. Furthermore, most reports document that at least 30% of glutaraldehyde-treated bovine carotid artery and human umbilical vein grafts will fail within one year when placed in the femoral-popliteal position.[29,32,35] These disappointing patency rates and the suboptimal handling conditions of these thick-walled grafts have induced most clinical centers to limit their use as arterial substitutes.

Recent investigations have also demonstrated that xenogenic tissue that is of nonvascular origin can be processed into an acellular tubular prosthesis. For example, following the treatment of porcine small intestine submucosa by mechanical and chemical extraction procedures, a 100-μm thick sheet of cell-free collagen is generated that can be used to form a vascular graft [36-37] In a rabbit carotid artery interposition model, infiltration with smooth muscle and endothelial cells was observed over a three-month period and all grafts remained patent.[38] Significantly, these studies confirm that native protein fiber networks, derived from allogeneic or xenogeneic tissues of vascular or nonvascular origin, can be used to fabricate an arterial substitute. Nonetheless, recognized drawbacks continue to dampen enthusiasm for this approach including tissue heterogeneity, incomplete cell extraction, the generation of ill-defined chemical crosslinks, progressive biodegradation, and the potential risk of viral transmission from animal tissue. In addition, the inability to tailor matrix composition and content, fiber size and architecture, or other features that may influence 3-D hierarchical tissue structure significantly limit the capacity to rationally design an allogeneic or xenogeneic tissue prosthesis with precisely defined mechanical and biological properties.

FUTURE DIRECTIONS IN ARTERIAL BIOENGINEERING

Bioengineers continue to explore a wide range of strategies related to biohybrid conduits, tissue engineered constructs, and decellularized tissues. In spite of the acknowledged drawbacks of sustained tissue-biomaterial interactions, considerable industrial development has focused on alternative nondegradable, synthetic materials for biohybrid conduits. In particular, new polyurethanes (PUs) displaying improved elasticity, compliance, biocompatibility, and biostability may offer improved patency rates.[39]

The tissue engineering approach with cell-assisted assembly of exogenous and endogenous matrix proteins has generated intriguing preliminary results; however, extended culture times will likely result in high manufacturing costs, variability, and risk of contamination. In addition to cost concerns, the use of autologous cells in this approach may not be feasible for many patients unable to wait weeks to months for the culturing and conditioning of a custom biological construct. Rather than depending on cell-assisted matrix assembly, alternative strategies seek to directly fabricate compliant, resilient, matrix-mimetic protein scaffolding at a reasonable cost. To this end, several groups have endeavored to create protein materials and scaffolding that mimic the collagen and elastin architecture of native ECM. Collagen is readily purified from a variety of tissues, but the highly stable, crosslinked fiber networks of native elastin resist common purification techniques. Some investigators have focused on more robust purification schemes to process insoluble native elastin.[40] while others have engineered recombinant proteins polymers comprised of selected amino acid repeat sequences from native elastin.[41-43] The electrospinning approach, in which tens of kilovolts of static electrical potential are used to spin dry nano-fibrous mats from concentrated polymer solutions, has been used to form collagen and elastin-mimetic materials into dense nanofiber scaffolds.[44-46] The generation of extracellular matrix protein fiber scaffolding, of physiologic density and with a degree of nanofiber alignment, thus seems feasible. Challenges remaining in this area of research include improved cellular infiltration or seeding in electrospun scaffolding, and the application of electrospinning technologies that are less toxic and circumvent the destruction of aspects of native protein structure.[47]

As an alternative to direct fabrication of protein scaffolds, investigators are also exploring improved biodegradable scaffolds to prompt endogenous ECM production. In arterial tissue engineering, these materials may reduce the culture period required with PGA or native structural proteins while enhancing the compliance and elasticity of both the synthetic polymers and the resulting soft tissues. For example, cells have been seeded in fibrin gels, which stimulate the production of more dense, aligned ECM.[48-49] Alternatively, Shum-Tim et al.[50] reported that a multilayer aortic construct could be generated seven days after implantation of a cell seeded scaffold in lamb animal model. The inner layer, a nonwoven mesh of PGA fibers seeded with mixed autologous cells, provided an environment for cell attachment and growth, while the outer layers consisted of nonporous polyhydroxyoctanoate (PHO). Outer PHO degraded more slowly than PGA, sealing the conduit and contributing mechanical support as new ECM developed in the PGA layer. Polyhydroxyoctanoate is a member of the large polyhydroxyalkanoate (PHA) class of natural polyesters; advances in the removal of endotoxin and other contaminants may further enhance the applicability of these polymers in tissue engineering.[51-52] Several additional classes of biodegradable synthetic polymers are under analysis. Polymer engineers generally seek to access and control a wide array of biodegradation rates and mechanical properties while ensuring the biocompatibility of both the polymer and its degradation products.

A range of equally critical enabling technologies are evolving that relate to expanding options for cell sourcing including stem and progenitor cells and improving immune acceptance. For example, engineered telomerase expression in human vascular cells has successfully extended cell lifespan and furthered the development of bioengineered arteries for older male patients from an autologous cells source.[53] Stem cells, differentiated into endothelial cells and endothelial progenitor cells, are also promising cell sources.[54-55] However, for efficient "off-the-shelf" delivery, allogeneic cell sources are preferred and immune acceptance strategies will remain a limiting factor.[56]

Significant progress toward a bioengineered vessel has been made over the past 20 years. However, substantial challenges remain before the goal of achieving a non-thrombogenic, mechanically resilient small diameter vascular prosthesis capable of remodeling and repair, is in hand. A global strategy addressing the development of scaffold and cellular technologies, and their integration into a device that is feasible to manufacture and distribute, will be required.

REFERENCES

1. Graves E. Detailed diagnoses and procedures, National Hospital Discharge Survey, 1992. *Vital Health Stat*. 1994;13:1–281.
2. Rutherford R, Jones D, Bergentz S, et al. Factors affecting the patency of infrainguinal bypass. *J Vasc Surg*. 1988;8:236–246.
3. Veith FJ, Gupta SK, Ascer E, et al. Six-year prospective multicenter randomized comparison of autologous saphenous vein and expanded polytetrafluoroethylene grafts in infrainguinal arterial reconstructions. *J Vasc Surg*. 1986;3:104–114.
4. Whittemore AD, Kent KC, Donaldson MC,et al. What is the proper role of polytetrafluoroethylene grafts in infrainguinal reconstruction? *J Vasc Surg*. 1989;10:299–305.
5. Hunink MG, Wong JB, Donaldson MC, et al. Patency results of percutaneous and surgical revascularization for femoropopliteal arterial disease. *Med Decis Making*. 1994;14:71–81.
6. Herring MB, Dilley R, Jersild RA, Jr, et al. Seeding arterial prostheses with vascular endothelium. The nature of the lining. *Ann Surg*. 1979;190:84–90.
7. Clagett GP, Burkel WE, Sharefkin JB, et al. Platelet reactivity in vivo in dogs with arterial prostheses seeded with endothelial cells. *Circulation*. 1984;69:632–639.
8. Greisler HP, Gosselin C, Ren D, et al. Biointeractive polymers and tissue engineered blood vessels. *Biomaterials*. 1996;17:329–336.
9. Meinhart JG, Deutsch M, Fischlein T, et al. Clinical autologous in vitro endothelialization of 153 infrainguinal ePTFE grafts. *Ann Thorac Surg*. 2001;71:S327–331.
10. Zilla P, Deutsch M, Meinhart J. Endothelial cell transplantation. *Semin Vasc Surg*. 1999;12:52–63.
11. Hedeman Joosten PP, Verhagen HJ, Heijnen-Snyder GJ, et al. Thrombogenesis of different cell types seeded on vascular grafts and studied under blood-flow conditions. *J Vasc Surg*. 1998;28:1094–1103.
12. Anderson J. Inflammatory reaction: the nemesis of implants. In: *Tissue engineering of vascular prosthetic grafts*. Zilla P, Greisler H, eds. ?? : R.G. Landes; 1999.
13. Ballyk PD, Walsh C, Butany J, Ojha M. Compliance mismatch may promote graft-artery intimal hyperplasia by altering suture-line stresses. *J Biomech*. 1998;31:229–237.
14. Salacinski HJ, Goldner S, Giudiceandrea A, et al. The mechanical behavior of vascular grafts: a review. *J Biomater Appl*. 2001;15:241–278.
15. Weinberg CB, Bell E. A blood vessel model constructed from collagen and cultured vascular cells. *Science*. 1986;231:397–400.
16. Hirai J, Matsuda T. Self-organized, tubular hybrid vascular tissue composed of vascular cells and collagen for low-pressure-loaded venous system. *Cell Transplant*. 1995;4:597–608.

17. Hirai J, Matsuda T. Venous reconstruction using hybrid vascular tissue composed of vascular cells and collagen: tissue regeneration process. *Cell Transplant*. 1996;5:93–105.
18. Barocas VH, Girton TS, Tranquillo RT. Engineered alignment in media equivalents: magnetic prealignment and mandrel compaction. *J Biomech Eng*. 1998;120:660–666.
19. Girton TS, Oegema TR, Grassl ED,et al. Mechanisms of stiffening and strengthening in media-equivalents fabricated using glycation. *J Biomech Eng*. 2000;122:216–223.
20. Hirai J, Kanda K, Oka T, Matsuda T. Highly oriented, tubular hybrid vascular tissue for a low pressure circulatory system. *Asaio J*. 1994;40:M383–388.
21. Seliktar D, Black RA, Vito RP, Nerem RM. Dynamic mechanical conditioning of collagen-gel blood vessel constructs induces remodeling in vitro. *Ann Biomed Eng*. 2000;28:351–362.
22. L'Heureux N, Paquet S, Labbe R, et al. A completely biological tissue-engineered human blood vessel. *Faseb J*. 1998;12:47–56.
23. L'Heureux N, Stoclet JC, Auger FA, et al. Human tissue-engineered vascular media: a new model for pharmacological studies of contractile responses. *Faseb J*. 2001;15:515–524.
24. Niklason L, Gao J, Abbott W, Hirschi K, Houser S, Marini R, Langer R. Functional arteries grown in vitro. *Science* 1999;284:486–493.
25. Kakisis J, Liapis C, Breuer C, Sumpio B. Artificial blood vessel: the holy grail of peripheral vasular surgery. *J Vasc Surg*. 2005;41:349–354.
26. Shin'oka T, Imai Y, Ikada Y. Transplantation of a tissue-engineered pulmonary artery. *N Engl J Med*. 2001;344:??.
27. Matsumura G, Hibino N, Ikada Y,et al. Successful application of tissue engineered vascular autografts: clinical experience. *Biomaterials*. 2003;24:2303–2308.
28. Wengerter K, Dardik H. Biological vascular grafts. *Semin Vasc Surg*. 1999;12:46–51.
29. Sciacca V, Walter G, Becker HM. Biogenic grafts in arterial surgery—long-term results (I. The homologous vein—II. The modified heterologous bovine carotid artery—III. The human umbilical vein). *Thorac Cardiovasc Surg*. 1984;32:157–164.
30. Dardik H. The second decade of experience with the umbilical vein graft for lower-limb revascularization. *Cardiovasc Surg*. 1995;3:265–269.
31. Rosenburg N, Martinez A, Sawyer P, et al. Tanned collagen arterial prosthesis of bovine carotid origin in man. Preliminary studies of enzyme-treated heterografts. *Ann Surg*. 1966; 164:247–256.
32. Hurt AV, Batello-Cruz M, Skipper BJ, et al. Bovine carotid artery heterografts versus polytetrafluoroethylene grafts. A prospective, randomized study. *Am J Surg*. 1983;146:844–847.
33. Schmidt CE, Baier JM. Acellular vascular tissues: natural biomaterials for tissue repair and tissue engineering. *Biomaterials*. 2000;21:2215–2231.
34. Courtman DW, Errett BF, Wilson GJ. The role of crosslinking in modification of the immune response elicited against xenogenic vascular acellular matrices. *J Biomed Mater Res*. 2001;55:576–586.
35. Holdsworth RJ, Naidu S, Gervaz P, McCollum PT. Glutaraldehyde-tanned bovine carotid artery graft for infrainguinal vascular reconstruction: 5-year follow-up. *Eur J Vasc Endovasc Surg*. 1997;14:208–211.
36. Badylak SF, Lantz GC, Coffey A, Geddes LA. Small intestinal submucosa as a large diameter vascular graft in the dog. *J Surg Res*. 1989;47:74–80.
37. Marshall SE, Tweedt SM, Greene CH, et al. An alternative to synthetic aortic grafts using jejunum. *J Invest Surg*. 2000;13:333–341.
38. Huynh T, Abraham G, Murray J, et al. Remodeling of an acellular collagen graft into a physiologically responsive neovessel. *Nat Biotechnol*. 1999;17:1083–1086.
39. Xue L, Greisler HP. Biomaterials in the development and future of vascular grafts. *J Vasc Surg*. 2003;37:472–480.
40. Daamen W, Hafmans T, Veerkamp J, van Vroonhoven TJ. Comparison of five procedures for the purification of insoluble elastin. *Biomaterials*. 2001;22:1997–2005.
41. Cappello J, Crissman J, Dorman M, et al. Genetic engineering of structural protein polymers. *Biotechnol Prog*. 1990;6:198–202.
42. McGrath KP, Tirrell DA, Kawai M, et al. Chemical and biosynthetic approaches to the production of novel polypeptide materials. *Biotechnol Prog*. 1990;6:188–192.

43. Nagapudi K, Brinkman WT, Thomas BS, et al. Viscoelastic and mechanical behavior of recombinant protein elastomers. *Biomaterials*. 2005;26:4695–4706.

44. Huang L, Nagapudi K, Apkarian RP, Chaikof EL. Engineered collagen-PEO nanofibers and fabrics. *J Biomater Sci Polym Ed*. 2001;12:979–993.

45. Huang L, Apkarian RP, Chaikof EL. High-resolution analysis of engineered type I collagen nanofibers by electron microscopy. *Scanning*. 2001;23:372–375.

46. Huang L, McMillan R, Apkarian RP,et al. Generation of synthetic elastin-mimetic small diameter fiber and fiber networks. *Macromolecules*. 2000;33:2989–2997.

47. Stankus JJ, Guan J, Wagner WR. Fabrication of biodegradable elastomeric scaffolds with sub-micron morphologies. *J Biomed Mater Res A*. 2004;70:603–614.

48. Ye Q, Zund G, Benedikt P, Jockenhoevel S, et al. Fibrin gel as a three dimensional matrix in cardiovascular tissue engineering. *Eur J Cardiothorac Surg*. 2000;17:587–591.

49. Grassl ED, Oegema TR, Tranquillo RT. A fibrin-based arterial media equivalent. *J Biomed Mater Res A*. 2003;66:550–561.

50. Shum-Tim D, Stock U, Hrkach J, et al. Tissue engineering of autologous aorta using a new biodegradable polymer. *Ann Thorac Surg*. 1999;68:2298–2304; discussion 2305.

51. Williams SF, Martin DP, Horowitz DM, Peoples OP. PHA applications: addressing the price performance issue: I. Tissue engineering. *Int J Biol Macromol*. 1999;25:111–121.

52. Chen GQ, Wu Q. The application of polyhydroxyalkanoates as tissue engineering materials. *Biomaterials*. 2005.

53. Poh M, Boyer M, Solan A, et al. Blood vessels engineered from human cells. *Lancet*. 2005; 365:2122–2124.

54. Levenberg S, Golub JS, Amit M, et al. Endothelial cells derived from human embryonic stem cells. *Proc Natl Acad Sci USA*. 2002;99:4391–4396.

55. Kaushal S, Amiel GE, Guleserian KJ, et al. Functional small-diameter neovessels created using endothelial progenitor cells expanded ex vivo. *Nat Med*. 2001;7:1035–1040.

56. Nerem RM, Ensley A. The tissue engineering of blood vessels and the heart. *Am J Transplantation*. 2004;4:36–42.

34

Modified Prosthetic Vascular Conduits

Muneera R. Kapadia, M.D., Daniel A. Popowich, M.D., and Melina R. Kibbe, M.D., R.V.T.

Over 71 million Americans are afflicted by cardiovascular disease. Atherosclerosis in the form of peripheral artery disease (PAD) affects approximately eight million Americans, which includes 12% to 20% of individuals over the age of 65.[1] Approximately 20% of patients with PAD have typical symptoms of lower extremity claudication, rest pain, ulceration or gangrene, and another one-third have atypical exertional symptoms.[2] Persons with PAD have impaired function and quality of life, even if they do not report symptoms and experience decline in lower extremity function over time. Thus, PAD represents a significant source of morbidity and mortality.

Several options exist for treating atherosclerotic lesions including percutaneous transluminal angioplasty (PTA) with and without stenting, endarterectomy (EA), and bypass grafting. For lower extremity disease, bypass conduit options include vein or prosthetic material. When possible, vein graft is the conduit of choice because it has superior patency rates. Unfortunately, in at least 30% of patients, these vein grafts are not available because of poor quality or prior use for cardiac or peripheral bypass procedures.[3] This chapter will discuss the outcome of prosthetic bypass grafting, the etiology of prosthetic bypass graft failure, and therapeutic strategies in clinical use and under investigation to modify prosthetic bypass conduits to achieve improved patency with less morbidity and limb loss.

PROSTHETIC BYPASS GRAFTING

When vein is not available, it is necessary to use an alternative conduit (Table 34–1). The two most common prosthetic graft materials used today are polyethylene terephthalate, or dacron, and polytetrafluorethylene (PTFE). Dacron was developed in Great Britain in 1941 by two chemists, Whinfield and Dickinson. However, it was in 1952 when Dr. DeBakey had heard that a Columbia University scientist had used Vinyon-N

TABLE 34-1. PERIPHERAL GRAFTS CURRENTLY COMMERCIALLY AVAILABLE

Material	Company	Product Name	Product Information	Product Uses
Expanded Polytetrafluoroethylene (ePTFE) [-(CF$_2$-CF$_2$)-]n	Braun	VascuGraft®	ePTFE	Peripheral bypass/Hemodialysis access
	W.L. Gore	Gore-Tex®	ePTFE	Peripheral bypass/Hemodialysis access
		Gore-Tex® Stretch	Stretch ePTFE	Peripheral bypass/Hemodialysis access
		Gore-Tex® Intering	Unibody radially supported ePTFE	Peripheral bypass/Hemodialysis access
		Gore-Tex® Propaten	Heparin-coated ePTFE	Peripheral bypass
	Bard	Impra®	ePTFE	Peripheral bypass/Hemodialysis access
		Impra® Carboflo®	Carbon-coated ePTFE	Hemodialysis access
		Venaflo™	Carbon-coated and cuffed ePTFE	Hemodialysis access
		Distaflo®	Carbon-coated and cuffed ePTFE	Peripheral bypass below knee
		Dynaflo™	Carbon-coated and cuffed ePTFE.	Peripheral bypass above knee
	Boston Scientific	Exxcel™ ePTFE	Peripheral bypass/Hemodialysis access	
	Angiotech/Edwards Life Sciences	Lifespan®	ePTFE	Peripheral bypass/Hemodialysis access
	Atrium	Advanta™	ePTFE	Peripheral bypass/Hemodialysis access
		Flixine™	ePTFE laminated with biomaterial film.	
	Vascutek	Maxiflo™	Unsealed ePTFE	Peripheral bypass/Hemodialysis access
		SealPTFE™	Gelatin sealed ePTFE	Peripheral bypass/Hemodialysis access
		Taperflo™	Gelatin sealed and tapered	Peripheral bypass/Hemodialysis access
		Rapidax™	Trilaminar self-sealing ePTFE	Hemodialysis access 24 hours after placement

Material	Manufacturer	Product	Description	Application
Poly(ethylene terephthalate) Dacron [O-C=-C6H6-O-C= O-CH2CH2]n	Braun	SilverGraft®	`Knitted double velour, Gelatine impregnated. Antimicrobial	Peripheral bypass with anti-infective protection
		Protegraft®	Knitted double velour	Peripheral bypass
		UniGraft®	Woven or knitted double velour, Gelatine impregnated	Peripheral bypass
	InterVascular	InterGard™	Collagen coated knitted polyester	Peripheral bypass
		InterGard™ Heparin	Heparin-coated knitted polyester antibacterial	Peripheral bypass
		InterGard® Silver	Collagen-impregnated knitted double velour	Peripheral bypass with anti-infective protection
	Boston Scientific	Hemashield Gold™		Peripheral bypass
		Microvel(r)	Gel-impregnated	Peripheral bypass
	Atrium	Ultramax™	Gelatin-sealed, knitted,	Peripheral bypass
	Vascutek	Fluoropassiv™	Fluoropolymer coated	Peripheral and ax-bifemoral bypass
		Gelseal™	Gelatin-impregnated, knitted	Peripheral and ax-bifemoral bypass
		Gelsoft™	Gelatin-impregnated, knitted	Peripheral bypass
		Gelsoft™ Plus	Gelatin-impregnated, knitted, dilation resistant	Peripheral bypass
Polyurethane [-NH-O=C-O-R-]n	Thoratec	Vectra®	Composed of a Thoralon® trilayer (polyetherurethaneurea and a siloxane)	Hemodialysis access 24 hours after placement
	LeMaitre	Expedia®	Polycarbonate urethane inner composition, Heparin impregnated	Hemodialysis access 24 hours after placement

cloth to create aortic grafts. Since Vinyon-N was not yet commercially available, DeBakey went to the store looking for nylon, the closest material to Vinyon-N. The store did not have nylon but had the new material called dacron. He made the first dacron tube graft for aortic reconstruction on his wife's sewing machine that year. Currently, dacron is most commonly used for aortic replacement and large diameter lower extremity bypass surgery.

PTFE was developed by DuPont researcher, Dr. Roy Plunkett, in 1938, and it was first marketed under the Teflon® trademark (DuPont) in 1945. It is virtually inert to all chemicals and is considered one of the slipperiest materials in existence; these qualities have made it useful in several applications including nonstick cookware, stain repellent, and textile products. Researchers at W. L. Gore developed expanded PTFE (ePTFE), which was much more compliant and porous compared to its nonexpanded counterpart. Soon, ePTFE found a new market. The first report of ePTFE used as a lower extremity bypass conduit was in 1976.[4] Today, ePTFE is the most commonly used graft for lower extremity and arteriovenous bypass grafting.[5]

It has been well established that prosthetic grafts are inferior when compared to vein bypass grafts. This was shown by Veith et al. in a multicenter prospective trial that examined four-year patency rates for vein and ePTFE bypass grafts.[6] According to this study, primary patency rates at four years for ePTFE grafts to the infrapopliteal artery were 12% +/− 7% versus saphenous vein grafts that have patency rates of 49% +/− 10%.

In high-pressure systems like the aorta, stiffer and stronger polymeric grafts such as dacron and ePTFE are ideal. However, in smaller diameter conducting vessels, radial compliance is more important than strength for use as a vascular conduit. In an attempt to meet this requirement, polyurethane (PU), which has the highest elasticity amongst existing polymers, has been developed into vascular grafts. Despite this promising property, two properties have limited the clinical application of virtually all polyurethane vascular grafts: poor biostability and loss of compliance postimplantation. In fact, a clinical trial using PU grafts for below-knee bypasses was aborted midway due to overwhelming graft occlusion caused by degradation in grafts that were left in for extended periods of time.[7]

There have been multiple attempts to improve the biostability of polyurethane grafts, and many have been tested in animal and human trials. For example, Seifalian and coworkers developed a compliant poly(carbonate-urea)urethane vascular graft, MyoLink™ (Cardiotech). Studies showed that it possessed a compliance profile similar to human arteries and it was more resistant to biodegradation than earlier versions of PU grafts.[8] The MyoLink™ graft is currently undergoing a multicenter clinical trial in Europe for use in hemodialysis access grafts and peripheral bypass grafts. Currently, the only PU graft available for use in the United States for vascular surgical procedures is the Vectra® graft (Thoratec), which is FDA-approved for hemodialysis access.

SURGICAL MODIFICATIONS OF PROSTHETIC VASCULAR GRAFTS

Because of the lower patency rates observed with prosthetic bypass grafting, surgical approaches have been developed to improve graft outcomes. These modifications are largely intended to decrease the compliance mismatch between the prosthetic graft and the native artery. They include vein cuffs, vein patches, vein boots, and arteriovenous fistulae (AVF) at the distal anastomosis (Figure 34–1). Stonebridge et al. conducted a

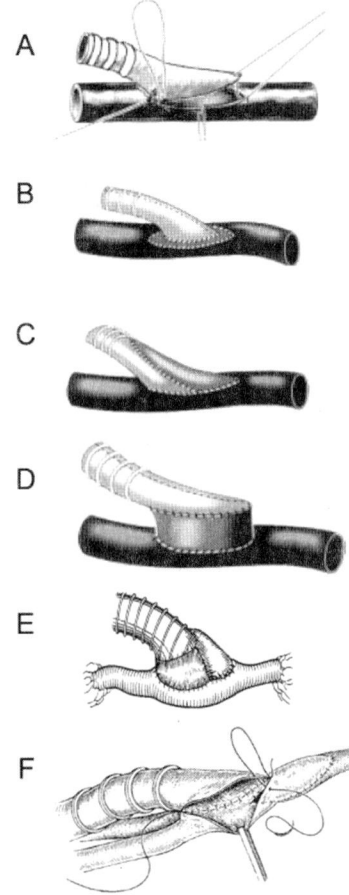

Figure 34-1. Surgical techniques for prosthetic graft modifications at the distal anastomosis. **(A)** Standard end-to-side anastomosis. **(B)** Linton patch. **(C)** Taylor patch. **(D)** Miller cuff. **(E)** Saint Mary boot. **(F)** Arteriovenous fistula. With permission from Trubel W, Schima H, Czerny M, Perktold K, Schimek MG, Polterauer P. Experimental comparison of four methods of end-to-side anastomosis with expanded polytetrafluoroethylene. *British Journal of Surgery*. 2004;91:159–167; and Ascer E, Gennaro M, Pollina RM et al. Complementary distal arteriovenous fistula and deep vein interposition: A five-year experience with a new technique to improve infrapopliteal prosthetic bypass patency. *Journal of Vascular Surgery*. 1996;24:134–143.

prospective randomized trial to examine the efficacy of Miller vein cuffs in improving lower extremity ePTFE graft patency.[9] Vein cuffs did not improve patency rates in bypasses to the above-knee popliteal artery. However cuffed below-knee popliteal artery grafts had a 45% three-year patency rate versus a 19% patency rate in uncuffed grafts (p = 0.018).[10]

Similarly, the use of vein patches such as those described by Taylor and Linton at the distal anastomosis, yields better long-term patency rates versus prosthetic material alone.[11] While there have been no randomized prospective trials to date, several retrospective reviews have demonstrated improved patency of vein-patched ePTFE over ePTFE alone when used for below-knee bypasses. One such review was performed by Taylor himself who reported a five-year primary patency of 54% for 83 infrapopliteal ePTFE grafts using his vein patch modification.[11] While there is no control arm to this study, previously reported patency rates with ePTFE alone are significantly worse.

Dairaku and coworkers reviewed 145 patients who had undergone either above- or below-knee bypasses using autologous vein, unmodified ePTFE, and Linton-patch modified ePTFE.[12] For the above-knee bypasses, they found no statistical difference in one- and three-year patency rates among the three groups. However, the cumulative patency rates of one, three, and five years after below-knee bypasses were 93%, 75%, and 75% for the autologous vein group ($n = 30$); 74%, 52%, and 42% for the unmodified ePTFE group ($n = 37$); and a 93%, 93%, and 93% for the Linton patch modified ePTFE group ($n = 16$). They speculated that the improved results over unmodified ePTFE bypass grafts were due to improved compliance mismatch between the prosthetic graft and the targeted native artery. A potential limitation of the study was the small number of Linton patch modified ePTFE grafts used compared to the autologous vein and ePTFE groups.

Syrek et al. retrospectively analyzed outcomes of patients with AVF modifications of ePTFE grafts, originally described by Enrico Ascer, versus ePTFE alone to the infrapopliteal arteries.[13] The AVF is created by first mobilizing an adjacent vein and transecting it. The vein is then anastomosed to the artery in an end-to-side fashion. A veinotomy is created near the arteriovenous fistula and the ePTFE is anastomosed, creating the AVF modification at the distal anastomosis (Figure 34–1F). The authors found that two-year patency rates were significantly better for grafts with the AVF modification (23% versus 5% for the ePTFE grafts alone, $P<0.05$). In spite of these surgical improvements, patency rates remain dismal, especially when the distal outflow is at or below the level of the popliteal artery.

CHEMICAL AND BIOLOGICAL MODIFICATIONS OF PROSTHETIC VASCULAR GRAFTS

Because of the poor patency of prosthetic bypass grafts to distal popliteal or infrapopliteal vessels, several researchers have focused efforts on modifying currently available prosthetic materials to improve clinical outcomes. These approaches will be discussed in this section (Table 34–2).

Graft Coatings

One approach for improving long-term graft outcome is the use of coatings to decrease thombogenicity and neointimal hyperplasia. One such strategy is the use of

TABLE 34-2. TYPES OF GRAFT MODIFICATIONS

Coatings	Protein Modifications	Endothelial Cell Seeding	Nitric Oxide Modifications
Carbon	Heparin	One-stage	Diazeniumdiolates
Silicone	Hirudin	Two-stage	S-nitrosothiols
Phospholipid polymers	FGF		
	TPA		
	Peptides		
	Rapamycin		
	Paclitaxel		

carbon-impregnated ePTFE grafts. Carbon is highly biocompatible and has been used in other applications to reduce thrombogenicity. The Impra® Carboflo® graft (Bard), a carbon-modified ePTFE vascular graft, was evaluated in a prospective randomized multicenter trial compared to standard ePTFE.[14] All bypasses were to the anterior tibial artery, and a vein patch or cuff was used in each case. At 36 months, the primary patency and limb salvage rates for the carbon and standard ePTFE groups were not statistically different (33% and 30%, 67% and 58%, respectively).

An alternative material has recently been described for use in small diameter (2.5–3.5 mm) bypass grafting: the Aria™ graft (Thoratec) is composed of three layers of Thoralon®.[15] Thoralon® is a proprietary polyetherurethaneurea (PEUU) blended with a siloxane-based surface modifying additive (SMA) during fabrication. After fabrication, siloxane migrates to the surface and reduces surface free energy as well as platelet activation and adhesion, thereby providing thromboresistance. This biomaterial is successfully being used for the thromboresistant blood-contacting surfaces of an FDA-approved ventricular assist device. This graft has demonstrated its biocompatibility and durability in sheep in both peripheral access and coronary artery bypass grafting.[15] Furthermore, it has been successfully implanted into 27 patients in Canada and Europe with no serious device-related injuries.[15] Based on these results, a prospective randomized controlled clinical study, called the AEGIS/Canada (AlternativE Graft Investigational Study) trial using the Aria™ graft for coronary artery bypass grafting, is underway.

Several polymer-based vascular graft coatings have undergone preliminary testing. Karrer et al. coated ePTFE with polypropylene sulfide (PPS)-polyethylene glycol (PEG) and tested these grafts in a porcine extracorporeal femoro-femoral arteriovenous shunt.[16] Grafts were perfused for three and nine minutes with and without heparin. Scanning electron microscopy was used to quantify cellular and microthrombi deposition and the PPS-PEG coated ePTFE showed decreased thrombogenicity when used in combination with heparin. Yoneyama et al. used the phospholipid polymer 2-methacryloyloxyethyl phosphorylcholine (MPC) and polyurethane to form a 2 mm vascular graft.[17] These grafts were anastomosed to rabbit carotid arteries and harvested at eight weeks. Neither thrombus nor neointimal formation was observed. While these and other polymeric applications to vascular grafts are in their preliminary stages, they certainly have potential to improve long-term vascular bypass graft outcomes.

Protein Modifications

In the last few years, several commercially available grafts have used heparin coating technologies to improve graft patency. One such product is a heparin-bonded dacron (HBD) graft called InterGard™ Heparin (InterVascular). In a prospective multicenter randomized trial, Devine et al. examined the outcomes of HBD versus ePTFE grafts in 209 patients that required femoropopliteal bypasses.[18] This included both above-knee ($n = 179$) and below-knee ($n = 30$) popliteal arteries as the distal target. The minimum follow-up time for each patient was five years. Primary patency was significantly better at one and three years for the HBD grafts (70% and 54%) as compared to the ePTFE grafts (56% and 44%, $p<0.044$). However, at five years, this difference was no longer significant: HBD 54% versus ePTFE 35% ($p<0.055$). Overall limb salvage rates were higher with the HBD grafts (86%) compared to ePTFE grafts (74%, $p<0.025$). The authors remarked that because previous studies showed no difference between ePTFE and dacron, the initial improvement in primary patency for HBD grafts may be because of the heparin bonding.

Bosiers et al. conducted a prospective nonrandomized clinical study to examine a heparin bonded ePTFE graft that used the Carmeda® BioActive Surface (CBAS™) modification (GORE-TEX® PROPATEN, W. L. Gore).[19] This product has been available for clinical use in Europe since 2002. The CBAS™ technology involves covalent endpoint linkage to retain heparin on the device surface. This study included 86 patients who underwent a total of 99 bypasses—55 above-knee and 44 below-knee procedures—of which 21 were femorocrural procedures. The overall one-year primary patency rate was 82%. Patency by location was 84% for above-knee, 81% for below-knee, and 74% for femorocrural bypass grafts. While there is no control arm in this study, when compared to a meta-analysis of about 40 studies of nonheparincoated ePTFE graft bypasses to the infrapopliteal arteries conducted by Albers et al., the pooled one-year primary patency rates were reported to be 59%.[20] This suggests better outcomes with the heparin-bonded CBAS™-ePTFE graft; however, longer term patency data are needed, preferably as a prospective randomized controlled trial.

Battaglia et al. conducted a retrospective review comparing the ePTFE grafts modified with the CBAS™ heparin technology against saphenous vein used for infragenicular bypasses.[21] In the CBAS™-ePTFE group, eight of 37 grafts thrombosed whereas in the vein bypass group, seven of 37 grafts occluded. While the results seem comparable, the authors are careful to note that the vein bypass group had more significant disease and a higher graft thrombosis risk. Their conclusions did state, however, that the heparin-bonded grafts represent a valid prosthetic alternative when vein is not available. While there are clearly impressive results with these heparin-bonded grafts, one big drawback remains the risk of heparin-induced thrombocytopenia that can result in lethal outcomes.

Another anticoagulant under investigation for modification of ePTFE grafts is hirudin in combination with iloprost. Hirudin is a direct thrombin antagonist; iloprost is an inhibitor of platelet aggregation and it promotes vasodilation. Heise and colleagues used these two drugs along with polyethelene glycol (PEG) as the delivery mechanism to coat 4 mm ePTFE grafts. As the PEG is hydrolyzed, there is a slow, continuous release of drug over several weeks to months.[22] The control grafts included untreated ePTFE and grafts coated with polylactide polymer alone. Femoropopliteal arterial bypasses were conducted in pigs and the endpoint was six weeks. Flow rates were measured via ultrasonography at the time of graft implantation and just prior to sacrifice. The PEG-hirudin/iloprost group maintained nearly equivalent flow rates at six weeks as compared to baseline, whereas the two control groups had markedly reduced flow. Furthermore, neointimal hyperplasia developed at the distal anastomosis in these grafts with low flow states. The PEG-hirudin/iloprost grafts were noted to have the least amount of neointimal hyperplasia.

The antithrombotic agent, tissue plasminogen activator (tPA), which degrades fibrin complexes (a major component of thrombus), has been used in the treatment of graft thrombosis. In 1989, Harvey et al. demonstrated that tPA could be bound to vascular prostheses using tridodecylmethylammonium to act as a slow-release drug delivery system with enzymatic activity against thrombus formation.[23] Greco et al. implanted 1 mm tPA-iloprost modified ePTFE grafts into rat aortas.[24] The rats were sacrificed at one week and grafts were harvested. In the control ePTFE group, only four of 10 grafts were patent; however, in the tPA-iloprost group, nine of 10 were patent ($p<0.03$). While these results were initially promising, there was a high mortality in the experimental group, which raises concerns for drug safety.

More recently, Yu et al. transfected vascular smooth muscle cells with vector plasmids containing genes for tPA.[25] These smooth muscle cells were seeded onto fibronectin-coated ePTFE grafts and cultured for one day in medium. The resultant grafts were then implanted into infrarenal rabbit aortas. The animals were sacrificed at 30 and 100 day time points, and the grafts were then analyzed for thrombus formation and neointimal hyperplasia. At 30 days, grafts seeded with tPA-transfected smooth muscle cells were nearly thrombus-free compared to control grafts; however, at 100 days, these grafts had more neointimal hyperplasia than controls, likely secondary to smooth muscle cell proliferation of the implanted cells.

Fibroblast growth factor (FGF)-modified ePTFE grafts have been studied in animal models. In 1992, Greisler et al. pretreated ePTFE grafts with ^{125}I-labeled FGF-1/fibrin glue (FG) mixtures with heparin through pressure perfusion.[26] The resulting grafts were interposed into the infrarenal aorta of rabbits and procured at multiple time points to check residual radioactivity. At one week and 30 days, 13.4% and 3.8% radioactivity remained, respectively. Next, the grafts were used for aortoiliac bypass grafting in a canine model. The authors found that FGF-1/FG promoted endothelialization, which was not seen in control groups.

Another protein that has been applied to vascular grafts and studied in vivo is P15. P15 is a cell-binding peptide that was first discovered as the cell adhesion domain within type 1 collagen. The rationale for its use was that by coating P-15 onto the surface of vascular grafts, it would promote the adhesion of endothelial cells and result in a more biomimetic graft. Li and colleagues were able to covalently bind P15 onto ePTFE grafts through an atmospheric plasma coating method.[27] In vitro studies showed that P15 coated grafts effectively promoted the adhesion and proliferation of endothelial cells (700% more than uncoated grafts) and to a lesser extent, smooth muscle cells (100% more than uncoated grafts). They then tested these grafts in vivo using a sheep model. They implanted two P-15 ePTFE coated grafts and one ePTFE graft into two different sheep (total of six grafts). The grafts were implanted as arterial venous shunts between the femoral artery and femoral vein and the common carotid artery and the ipsilateral jugular vein. One animal was sacrificed at 14 days and the other at 28 days. At the end of the study, all of the grafts were patent, although the P-15 coated grafts showed a higher degree of endothelialization in the graft lumen and significantly less neointimal hyperplasia at the venous anastomosis.

Rapamycin-eluting stents have been used in coronary interventions and have been shown to reduce the incidence of restenosis.[28] Cagiannos et al. coated 6 mm ePTFE for 1 cm at each end of the graft with rapamycin and used a porcine iliac artery bypass model to examine efficacy.[29] Animals were sacrificed at four weeks and the authors found a statistically significant reduction in percent of cross-sectional narrowing in the rapamycin group versus untreated and adhesive-treated ePTFE grafts (28.5% and 16.2%, respectively, $p = 0.007$). While these results are promising, there are no long-term studies to demonstrate durability of effect, nor have there been any clinical data to demonstrate efficacy in human subjects.

Similar to rapamycin, paclitaxel has been shown to prevent restenosis when used in coronary stenting.[30] Recently, Lee et al. examined paclitaxel-coated ePTFE grafts using a porcine model for arteriovenous grafting; this involved creation of a bypass from the common carotid artery to external jugular vein.[31] The pigs were sacrificed at six weeks and cross-sections of the venous anastomoses of the grafts were analyzed. While the hemodynamics are not exactly the same as in the arterial bypass situation, the authors found that the mean percent of luminal stenosis in the paclitaxel-coated ePTFE graft was 10.4% compared to the control ePTFE graft that was 60.5% ($p<0.05$).

Endothelial Cell Seeding

Endothelial cells secrete a variety of substances that inhibit both thrombosis and neointimal hyperplasia. They are critical for homeostasis and maintenance of vascular integrity in the circulation. It is because of these vasoprotective properties that researchers have attempted to modify prosthetic grafts by seeding endothelial cells onto the luminal surface of grafts. There are two types of seeding techniques: two-stage and one-stage procedures.

Two-stage seeding techniques involve procuring vein or artery from the patient, harvesting endothelial cells from these vessels, and allowing them to expand in culture for approximately four weeks before seeding them on the graft. The graft is then implanted in the patient. This technique has had positive outcomes in clinical trials. Magometschnigg et al. harvested venous endothelial cells, seeded them onto ePTFE, and used the grafts for crural reconstruction.[32] They showed a 30-day graft patency of 92% compared to 53% in the control ePTFE group. Deutsch et al. reported their results with this procedure for infrainguinal (both above- and below-knee popliteal) bypass in a two-phase study.[33] Phase 1 involved 27 endothelial cell seeded ePTFE grafts and 17 unseeded ePTFE grafts. The nine-year patency rate was significantly better for the experimental group (65% versus 16%, $p = 0.002$). Phase 2 did not have a control arm, but of the 86 endothelial cell lined ePTFE grafts, 68% were patent at five years. While the two-stage procedures clearly have impressive results, there are also significant limitations. Because of the four-week cell culture delay, these grafts cannot be used in an emergency situation. The process of seeding is labor-intensive, costly, and carries the risk of infection. Additionally, endothelial cell growth in culture requires several growth factors that may cause unwanted effects once the cells are seeded and the graft is implanted.

One-stage procedures involve isolating endothelial cells from venipuncture or fat sources such as subcutaneous fat or omentum. The advantage of the one-stage procedure is that the entire procedure, including harvesting and seeding the endothelial cells, can be completed during the time of one surgical procedure. Herring et al. first successfully introduced the concept of single-stage seeding in 1978 using a canine model.[34] Subsequently, their group reported clinical results in which venous endothelial cells were seeded on preclotted grafts, but results were mostly disappointing. In this randomized multicenter prospective trial, seeded femoropopliteal grafts were compared to saphenous vein grafts.[35] The 30-month patency rates were 38% and 92%, respectively ($p = 0.006$). The failure of the seeded grafts was due to anastomotic hyperplasia. Other suggested reasons for failure included low endothelial cell seeding density, lack of endothelial cell attachment, and lower propensity for endothelialization as compared to the canine model.

Other sources for seeding have included microvascular endothelial cells derived from fatty tissue such as subcutaneous fat or omentum. The advantages of these cells include ease of obtaining them in large quantities and the lack of required cell culture. However, results with seeding of these cells have also been disappointing in clinical trials. Meerbaum et al. showed patency rates of seeded vascular grafts of 19% at 36 months in peripheral reconstructions.[36] Williams et al. also conducted seeding with microvascular endothelial cells and showed a four-year patency rate of 55%; however, this study only included 11 patients, four of whom died secondary to unrelated causes in the course of the study.[37] There are no major clinical trials to date.

Nitric Oxide Modifications

An area of current and active focus for prosthetic graft modification is nitric oxide (NO). Nitric oxide is normally constitutively produced from endothelial cells and is vital in the regulation of vascular tone, prevention of platelet aggregation, adhesion and activation, and inhibition of vascular smooth muscle cell proliferation and migration.[38] All of these properties contribute to the thromboresistant surface of endothelial cells and maintenance of a healthy vasculature.

Because of the vasoprotective properties of NO, several investigators have utilized NO-based approaches to modify prosthetic bypass grafts in order to reduce the thrombogenicity of the grafts and prevent the development of neointimal hyperplasia long term. The overall goal of utilizing a NO-based approach is to reproduce the same thromboresistive moiety observed with normal endothelial cells in prosthetic vascular grafts by producing NO. The vast majority of research has focused on the use two classes of NO donors: diazenumdiolates and S-nitrosothiols (Figure 34–2). These compounds are doped within or grafted to polymers to create materials that release NO for a wide range of time periods.

Diazeniumdilates.   Diazeniumdiolates are NO donors that are formed by the reaction of secondary amine structures with two moles of NO under high pressures.[39] They generate bioactive NO in physiologic fluids (37°F, pH 7.4) spontaneously (i.e., without metabolism or redox activation), with reliable half-lives ranging from two seconds to 20 hours depending on the ionic structure.[40] Multiple researchers have shown that diazeniumdiolates can be dispersed into, coated upon, or covalently bound to multiple synthetic polymers, which then could be used to create NO-eluting vascular grafts. This allows the delivery of NO locally to the injured endothelium without any systemic release of NO, which could cause undesirable adverse effects.

Smith and colleagues were the first to use diazeniumdiolates as NO donors in polymers and then to incorporate those polymers into vascular grafts.[41] They dipped 4 mm ePTFE grafts into a freshly prepared solution of poly-(ethylenimine) (PEI) and a cross-linking agent such that the cross-linked PEI chains became intimately interwoven with

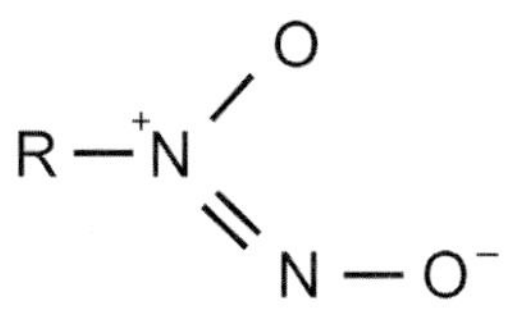

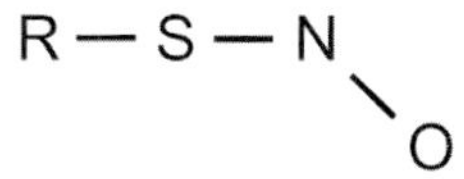

Figure 34-2. Generic structures of two nitric oxide donors. **(A)** Diazeniumdiolates, and **(B)** S-nitrosothiol.

the graft. The dipped grafts were then exposed to NO to create diazeniumdiolate groups on the PEI. These grafts were shown to produce NO for several weeks in vitro, and they exhibited decreased platelet deposition and vascular smooth muscle cell proliferation compared to untreated grafts. These grafts were then inserted as arteriovenous shunts into baboons for one hour, and analysis showed that there was significantly less platelet deposition on the NO-releasing vascular grafts compared to untreated grafts. Although this technique initially looked promising, the coating process changed the architecture of the graft, which may create long-term biocompatibility complications secondary to compliance mismatch.

Pulfer et al. speculated that the incorporation of polymeric diazeniumdiolate PEI/NO microspheres into the pores of an ePTFE (GORE-TEX®) would allow for the spontaneous release of the NO similar to the prior study without a resulting change in the graft architecture.[42] They were able to show that the grafts retained the same physical properties, even after the addition of the microspheres, and that the grafts released NO in vitro for greater than 150 hours (Figure 34–3).

Another method of incorporating NO donors into vascular grafts without altering their mechanical properties is to coat the inside lining with a NO-eluting polymer that would not alter the architecture of the graft material. Zhang et al. created diazeniumdiolated silica nanoparticles and embedded them into hydrophobic matrixes that were then used to coat the inside of tubing used for extracorporeal venovenous circuits in a rabbit model.[43] They found that the NO release was substantial, and that there was much less platelet consumption and activation when compared to controls when blood was run through the circuit for four hours.

Although these studies provided an efficient method for delivering NO, it was subsequently shown that some of the diazeniumdiolate polymers used in these studies can leach out of the polymer matrixes and form measurable levels of nitrosamines, a

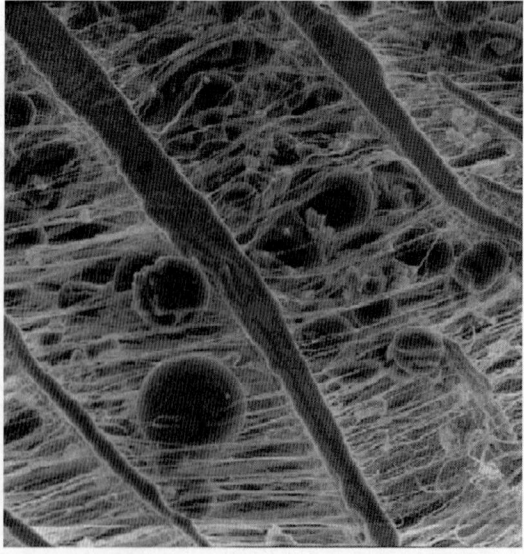

Figure 34-3. Scanning electron microscopy of the PEI/NO microspeheres embedded within the ePTFE graft. With permission from Pulfer SK, Ott D, Smith DJ. Incorporation of nitric oxide-releasing crosslinked polyethyleneimine microspheres into vascular grafts. *Journal of Biomedical Materials Research* 1997; 37:182–189.

well-known class of carcinogens. To address this issue, Batchelor and colleagues reported the preparation of a more lipophilic discrete diazeniumdiolate species that was resistant to leaching because it was covalently bound to the backbone of the polyurethane.[44] They coated polyurethane vascular grafts (Vectra®) with this new diazeniumdiolate that was dispersed in a polyvinyl (PVC) matrix. These grafts were then implanted in sheep as arteriovenous shunts connecting the common carotid artery to the ipsilateral jugular vein. Results showed that the NO-coated grafts were patent at three weeks and had a mean luminal thrombus free surface area of 95% whereas the controls grafts had all occluded. They concluded that not only did these coated grafts release a biologically significant amount of NO to improve graft patency, but also that the potentially carcinogenic byproducts that previously had leached out into the systemic circulation remained confined to the polymer matrix.

In a subsequent study using this same sheep model, Fleser et al. dip-coated 5 mm PU grafts (Vectra®) with multiple layers of a PVC film containing a diazeniumdiolate.[45] A total of 12 grafts were then implanted as arteriovenous grafts into sheep connecting the common carotid artery to the ipsilateral jugular vein. The grafts were left in place for a total of three weeks. Results showed that all three uncoated grafts had occluded, two of the sham-coated grafts had occluded, and only one of the NO-releasing grafts had occluded. Although they were able to show that there was a significant reduction in surface thrombus accumulation in the NO-releasing grafts compared to sham-coated and uncoated grafts, they did not observe a statistically significant improvement in patency.

Recent studies have been conducted to create NO-producing polyurethanes by covalently binding a diazeniumdiolate donor into the polyurethane backbone. Using this approach, there is no need for reaction additives and leaching of undesired byproducts is avoided. Jun and coworkers showed that NO production by these polyurethane films occurred for approximately two months under physiologic conditions in vitro, and mechanical properties of the material were suitable for vascular graft applications.[46] Platelet adhesion to these grafts was greatly diminished (Figure 34–4). Furthermore, endothelial cell growth was stimulated across the polyurethane graft while vascular smooth muscle cell growth was inhibited. To date, there are no published in vivo studies utilizing these grafts.

S-nitrosothiols.   The second class of NO donors that has been utilized in developing NO-releasing polymers are S-nitrosothiols. S-nitrosothiols are thought to serve as a reservoir and transporter of NO within biological systems. S-nitrosothiols are present in the circulating blood and also found within cells. They release NO by three known

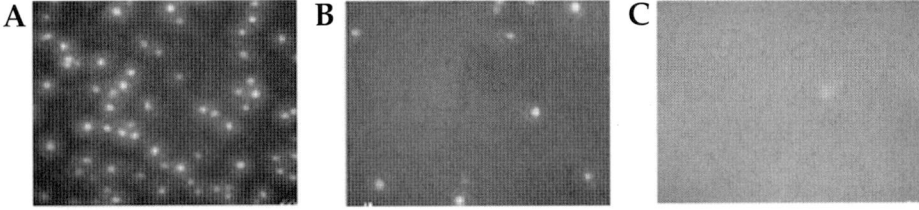

Figure 34-4. Digital images of platelet adhesion to **(A)** collagen I film alone, **(B)** polyurethane graft, and **(C)** polyurethane-NO graft. With permission from Jun HW, Taite LJ, West JL. Nitric oxide-producing polyurethanes. *Biomacromolecules* 2005; 6:838–844.

mechanisms: copper ion mediated decomposition, direct reaction with ascorbate, and homeolytic cleavage of the S-NO bond by light.

Several polymers have been developed with the S-nitrosothiol covalently linked to the polymer in order to prevent leaching of the donor or reaction by-products. Bohl and West created NO-releasing hydrogels that showed decreased smooth muscle cell proliferation and decreased platelet adhesion on collagen-coated slides.[47] They speculated that these materials could be used to coat the outside of a vessel wall and vascular graft to provide local and sustained NO delivery following vascular injury.

An exciting property of S-nitrosothiols is their ability to release NO when exposed to visible light. This provides the opportunity to control the timing of the release of NO. To test this property, Frost et al. blended the NO donor, S-nitroso-N-acetylpenicillamine (SNAP) that was covalently attached to fumed silica particles into the center layer of a tri-layer of silicone rubber (SR) and polyurethane (PU) films.[48] They demonstrated that SNAP, when blended into a SR matrix, but not PU, released NO only in the presence of light and not when exposed to physiologic solution (i.e., blood). They concluded that this represented an external on/off trigger to the temporal and spatial release of NO, and that this material had the potential application of making extracorporeal tubing or other intravascular devices that would be more biocompatible.

The main limitation to using polymers loaded with either diazeniumdiolate or S-nitrosothiol NO donors is the finite reservoir of NO that exist within these materials, thus limiting the duration of NO generation/release that could impact their utility for coating more permanent types of implants such as vascular bypass grafts. It would be more desirable if it were possible to create a graft that continuously released NO indefinitely. New materials are being developed that rely on S-nitrosothiols and/or nitrate that already circulate in blood as the source of NO. Duan and Lewis immobilized L-cysteine on dacron and PU surfaces. This yields a free thiol group that can undergo an NO exchange reaction with endogenous S-nitrosothiols.[49] The resulting relatively unstable S-nitrosocysteine decomposes to locally release NO. The potential advantage of this type of material is the essentially unlimited source of NO that could be generated locally when in contact with circulating blood. Oh and colleagues developed a biomimetic lipophilic copper complex that is able to reduce S-nitrosothiols and nitrite to NO under physiologic conditions.[50] The complex was doped into PVC and PU films and catalytically generated NO in the presence of a reducing agent capable of cycling Cu (II) to Cu (I) (i.e., ascorbic acid, cysteine, or glutathione) in vitro.

CONCLUSION

Standard prosthetic grafts used for peripheral vascular bypass grafting have considerable limitations with respect to patency. Because so many patients require bypass grafting with prosthetic conduits, it is imperative to develop good alternatives to vein bypass grafting. Currently available modified prosthetic grafts have shown improvements in outcome. However, the work of several researchers shows significant promise for even better bypass graft materials. The upcoming years will likely prove to be an exciting time for both investigators and vascular surgeons alike, as new methods and materials are employed in an effort to improve patient care.

REFERENCES

1. Thom T. Heart disease and stroke statistics - 2006 update: A report from the American Heart Association Statistics Committee and Stroke Statistics Subcommittee (vol 113, pg e85, 2006). *Circulation*. 2006;113:E696.
2. McDermott MM, Mehta S, Greenland P. Exertional leg symptoms other than intermittent claudication are common in peripheral arterial disease. *Arch Intern Med*. 1999;159:387–392.
3. Greenwald SE, Berry CL. Improving vascular grafts: the importance of mechanical and haemodynamic properties. *J Pathol*. 2000;190:292–299.
4. Campbell CD, Brooks DH, Webster MW, Bahnson HT. Use of Expanded Microporous Polytetrafluoroethylene for Limb Salvage - Preliminary-Report. *Surgery*. 1976;79:485–491.
5. Kannan RY, Salacinski HJ, Butler PE, et al. Current status of prosthetic bypass grafts: A review. *J Biomed Mater Res B Appl Biomater*. 2005;74B:570–581.
6. Veith FJ, Gupta SK, Ascer E, et al. Six-year prospective multicenter randomized comparison of autologous saphenous vein and expanded polytetrafluoroethylene grafts in infrainguinal arterial reconstructions. *J Vasc Surg*. 1986;3:104–114.
7. Zhang Z, Marois Y, Guidoin RG, et al. Vascugraft(R) polyurethane arterial prosthesis as femoro-popliteal and femoro-peroneal bypasses in humans: Pathological, structural and chemical analyses of four excised grafts. *Biomaterials*. 1997;18:113–124.
8. Seifalian AM, Salacinski HJ, Tiwari A, et al. In vivo biostability of a poly(carbonate-urea)urethane graft. *Biomaterials*. 2003;24:2549–2557.
9. Stonebridge PA, Prescott RJ, Ruckley CV. Randomized trial comparing infrainguinal polytetrafluoroethylene bypass grafting with and without vein interposition cuff at the distal anastomosis. *J Vasc Surg*. 1997;26:543–550.
10. Griffiths GD, Nagy J, Black D, Stonebridge PA. Randomized clinical trial of distal anastomotic interposition vein cuff in infrainguinal polytetrafluoroethylene bypass grafting. *Br J Surg*. 2004;91:560–562.
11. Taylor RS, Loh A, Mcfarland RJ, et al. Improved Technique for Polytetrafluoroethylene Bypass-Grafting - Long-Term Results Using Anastomotic Vein Patches. *Br J Surg*. 1992;79: 348–354.
12. Dairaku K, Fujioka K, Yamashita A, et al. Experimental and clinical studies investigating the efficacy of distal anastomosis with patch plasty in bypass operations with expanded polytetrafluoroethylene grafts. *Surg Today*. 2003;33:349–353.
13. Syrek JR, Calligaro KD, Dougherty MJ, et al. Do distal arteriovenous fistulae improve patency rates of prosthetic infrapopliteal arterial bypasses? *Ann Vasc Surg*. 1998;12:148–152.
14. Kapfer X, Meichelboeck W, Groegler FM. Comparison of Carbon-impregnated and Standard ePTFE Prostheses in Extra-anatomical Anterior Tibial Artery Bypass: A Prospective Randomized Multicenter Study. *Eur J Vasc Endovasc Surg*. 2006;Aug; 32(2): 155–68.
15. Farrar DJ. Development of a prosthetic coronary artery bypass graft. *Heart Surg Forum*. 2000;3:36–40.
16. Karrer L, Duwe J, Zisch AH, et al. PPS-PEG surface coating to reduce thrombogenicity of small diameter ePTFE vascular grafts. *Int J Artif Organs*. 2005;28:993–1002.
17. Yoneyama T, Sugihara K, Ishihara K, et al. The vascular prosthesis without pseudointima prepared by anti thrombogenic phospholipid polymer. *Biomaterials*. 2002;23:1455–1459.
18. Devine C, McCollum C. Heparin-bonded Dacron or polytetrafluorethylene for femoropopliteal bypass: Five-year results of a prospective randomized multicenter clinical trial. *J Vasc Surg*. 2004;40:924–931.
19. Bosiers M, Deloose K, Verbist J, et al. Heparin-bonded expanded polytetrafluoroethylene vascular graft for femoropopliteal and femorocrural bypass grafting: 1-year results. *J Vasc Surg*. 2006;43:313–318.
20. Albers M, Battistella VM, Romiti M, et al. Meta-analysis of polytetrafluoroethylene bypass grafts to infrapopliteal arteries. *J Vasc Surg*. 2003;37:1263–1269.

21. Battaglia G, Tringale R, Monaca V. Retrospective comparison of a heparin bonded ePTFE graft and saphenous vein for infragenicular bypass: implications for standard treatment protocol. *J Cardiovasc Surg.* 2006;47:41–47.

22. Heise M, Schmidmaier G, Husmann I, et al. PEG-hirudin/iloprost Coating of Small Diameter ePTFE Grafts Effectively Prevents Pseudointima and Intimal Hyperplasia Development. *Eur J Vasc Endovasc Surg.* 2006;May 5; [Epub ahead of print].

23. Harvey RA, Kim HC, Pincus J, et al. Binding of Tissue Plasminogen-Activator to Vascular Grafts. *Thromb Haemost.* 1989;61:131–136.

24. Greco RS, Kim HC, Donetz AP, Harvey RA. Patency of A Small Vessel Prosthesis Bonded to Tissue-Plasminogen Activator and Iloprost. *Ann Vasc Surg.* 1995;9:140–145.

25. Yu H, Dai WD, Yang Z, et al. Neointimal hyperplasia on a cell-seeded polytetrafluoroethylene graft is promoted by transfer of tissue plasminogen activator gene and inhibited by transfer of nitric oxide synthase gene. *J Vasc Surg.* 2005;41:122–129.

26. Greisler HP, Cziperle DJ, Kim DU, et al. Enhanced Endothelialization of Expanded Polytetrafluoroethylene Grafts by Fibroblast Growth-Factor Type-1 Pretreatment. *Surgery.* 1992;112:244–255.

27. Li C, Hill A, Imran M. In vitro and in vivo studies of ePTFE vascular grafts treated with P15 peptide. *J Biomater Sci-Polym Ed.* 2005;16:875–891.

28. Morice M, Serruys PW, Sousa JE, et al. A randomized comparison of a sirolimus-eluting stent with a standard stent for coronary revascularization. *N Engl J Med.* 2002;346: 1773–1780.

29. Cagiannos C, Abul-Khoudoud OR, DeRijk W, et al. Rapamycin-coated expanded polytetrafluoroethylene bypass grafts exhibit decreased anastomotic neointimal hyperplasia in a porcine model. *J Vasc Surg.* 2005;42:980–987.

30. Grube E, Silber S, Hauptmann KE, et al. Six- and twelve-month results from a randomized, double-blind trial on a slow-release paclitaxel-eluting stent for de novo coronary lesions. *Circulation.* 2003;107:38–42.

31. Lee B.H., Nam HY, Kwon T., et al. Paclitaxel-coated expanded polytetrafluoroethylene haemodialysis grafts inhibit neointimal hyperplasia in porcine model of graft stenosis. *Nephrol Dial Transplant.* 2006 Sep;21(9):2432–8. (Epub 2006 Mar 22)

32. Magometschnigg H, Kadletz M, Vodrazka M, et al. Prospective Clinical-Study with Invitro Endothelial-Cell Lining of Expanded Polytetrafluoroethylene Grafts in Crural Repeat Reconstruction. *J Vasc Surg.* 1992;15:527–535.

33. Deutsch M, Meinhart J, Fischlein T, et al. Clinical autologous in vitro endothelialization of infrainguinal ePTFE grafts in 100 patients: A 9-year experience. *Surgery.* 1999;126:847–855.

34. Herring M, Gardner A, Glover J. Single-Staged Technique for Seeding Vascular Grafts with Autogenous Endothelium. *Surgery.* 1978;84:498–504.

35. Herring M, Smith J, Dalsing M, et al. Endothelial Seeding of Polytetrafluoroethylene Femoral Popliteal Bypasses - the Failure of Low-Density Seeding to Improve Patency. *J Vasc Surg.* 1994;20:650–655.

36. Meerbaum SO, Sharp WV, Schmidt SP. Lower extremity revascularization with polytetrafluoroethykebe grafts seeded with microvascular endothelial cells. In: Zilla P., Fasol R, Callow P (eds). *Applied Cardiovascular Biology.* Basel: Karger; 1992:107–119.

37. Williams SK. Human clincal trials of microvascular endothelial cell sodding. In: Zilla P, Greisler HP (eds). *Tissue Engineering of Vascular Prosthetic Grafts.* Austin, TX: R.G. Landes; 1999:143–147.

38. Kibbe M, Billiar T, Tzeng E. Inducible nitric oxide synthase and vascular injury. *Cardiovasc Res.* 1999;43:650–657.

39. Hrabie JA, Keefer LK. Chemistry of the nitric oxide-releasing diazeniumdiolate ("nitrosohydroxylamine") functional group and its oxygen-substituted derivatives. *Chem Rev.* 2002;102:1135–1154.

40. Hrabie JA, Keefer LK. Chemistry of the nitric oxide-releasing diazeniumdiolate ("nitrosohydroxylamine") functional group and its oxygen-substituted derivatives. *Chem Rev.* 2002;102:1135–1154.

41. Smith DJ, Chakravarthy D, Pulfer S, et al. Nitric oxide-releasing polymers containing the [N(O)NO](−) group. *J Med Chem*. 1996;39:1148–1156.
42. Pulfer SK, Ott D, Smith DJ. Incorporation of nitric oxide-releasing crosslinked polyethyleneimine microspheres into vascular grafts. *J Biomedic Mater Res*. 1997;37:182–189.
43. Zhang HP, Annich GM, Miskulin J, et al. Nitric oxide-releasing fumed silica particles: Synthesis, characterization, and biomedical application. *J Am Chem Soc*. 2003;125:5015–5024.
44. Batchelor MM, Reoma SL, Fleser PS, et al. More lipophilic dialkyldiamine-based diazeniumdiolates: Synthesis, characterization, and application in preparing thromboresistant nitric oxide release polymeric coatings. *J Med Chem*. 2003;46:5153–5161.
45. Fleser PS, Nuthakki VK, Malinzak LE, et al. Nitric oxide-releasing biopolymers inhibit thrombus formation in a sheep model of artcriovenous bridge grafts. *J Vasc Surg*. 2004;40:803–811.
46. Jun HW, Taite LJ, West JL. Nitric oxide-producing polyurethanes. *Biomacromolecules*. 2005;6:838–844.
47. Bohl KS, West JL. Nitric oxide-generating polymers reduce platelet adhesion and smooth muscle cell proliferation. *Biomaterials*. 2000;21:2273–2278.
48. Frost MC, Meyerhoff ME. Fabrication and in vivo evaluation of nitric oxide-releasing electrochemical oxygen-sensing catheters. *Methods Enzymol*. 2004; 381:704–715.
49. Gappa-Fahlenkamp H, Duan X, Lewis RS. Analysis of immobilized L-cysteine on polymers. *J Biomed Materic Res* Part A. 2004;71A:519–527.
50. Oh BK, Meyerhoff ME. Catalytic generation of nitric oxide from nitrite at the interface of polymeric films doped with lipophilic Cu(Il)-complex: a potential route to the preparation of thromboresistant coatings. *Biomaterials*. 2004;25:283–293.

Arterial Trauma

35

The Intraoperative Consult

John J. Ricotta, M.D.

One of the least discussed and potentially most problematic issues facing a vascular surgeon is the appropriate approach to requests for intraoperative consultation. While such situations are infrequent, they arise with some regularity, and by definition, all are unanticipated. The clinical scenarios are usually stressful with potentially negative patient outcome and significant risk of practitioner liability. As vascular surgery has emerged as a distinct specialty and fewer general surgeons are comfortable dealing with vascular complications, the frequency of such consultation will increase. It is worthwhile, then, to reflect on appropriate conduct of intraoperative consultation in order to develop a plan for dealing with these situations as they arise. The question will be broken down into several components: management of the acute medical situation, postoperative clinical responsibilities, postoperative ethical responsibilities, medical-legal considerations, and documentation and billing issues.

MANAGEMENT OF THE ACUTE MEDICAL SITUATION

Intraoperative consultation is by its very nature unplanned. Consultations for evaluation of unanticipated pathology identified during the course of operation (e.g., aortic aneurysm found unexpectedly during laparotomy), which do not require immediate treatment, will not be discussed here. Consultation may be requested from any surgical specialty. Reasons for consultation can be grouped into three broad categories: bleeding, ischemia, and more recently, complications associated with catheter placement or removal. These scenarios all share some common features that are worthy of consideration.

First, the surgeon requesting consultation is often flustered, frustrated, and/or embarrassed. These emotions stem from the fact that either an unanticipated event has occurred in the course of a planned operation, or the surgeon has found himself or herself unable to deal with an emergency situation. The surgeon's emotional state often transfers to the operating room team, who may be equally unsettled. Second, the consultant usually has less than complete information on which to base his or her clinical judgments. There is often inadequate time to review the chart to completely appreciate the medical comorbidities. The details of the patient's baseline vascular condition are often either unknown or unreliable. The majority of patients will not have had a focused vascular evaluation, and in many instances, the degree of vascular disease will be unknown or underestimated. Third, the consultant is often called away from some other clinical activity either in or outside the operating room. Finally, the situation often has the potential to impact either life or limb. A series of suggestions will allow you to address these common issues and to meet the challenges they may present.

As a consultant, you should make arrangements to get to the operating room in question as quickly as possible. If some delay is required, notify the consulting surgeon, and if possible, suggest or even arrange for an alternate consultant. Whenever a delay is anticipated, you should communicate this directly to the surgeon, attending anesthesiologist, or circulating nurse as the situation allows. The surgeon requesting assistance should have a clear idea of when to expect consultation, and even what to do in the interim.

If you are engaged in another procedure in or out of the operating room, ensure the safety of your own patient and appropriate supervision of the patient before leaving. This is sometimes overlooked in the heat of the moment. It may require calling one of your partners to take over your own case. Once you arrive at the room in question, maintain a calm and supportive demeanor toward the consulting surgeon and the operating room staff. Assess the situation and get as complete an understanding of it as you can before you scrub into the operation. This allows you time to develop a rudimentary plan while at the scrub sink, and provides a break between your initial interaction with the operating room team and your entrance into the procedure. Try to anticipate any instrumentation and technology you will require for your participation in the case. Vascular or endovascular instruments, and even a vascular scrub team if necessary, can be marshalled while you are scrubbing. If you anticipate requiring help from another trained vascular surgeon, a vascular fellow, or a general surgery resident, you should make sure that they have been called at this stage. The need for these adjuncts should be identified as early as possible and communicated to the circulating nurse before you scrub whenever possible.

When you join the operating team, make it clear that you are taking responsibility for the conduct of the case until the vascular issues are resolved. This action requires diplomacy and may be difficult in some instances, but it is essential. The team and the surgeon will usually welcome a transfer of responsibility, and this is the easiest way to restore the equanimity so essential to the conduct of a successful operation. The level of assistance the primary surgeon can provide will vary according to his or her training, and will determine whether or not you need to bring help with you. Remember that you will be held responsible for the outcome of any vascular intervention; thus, it is important that you control the decisions and conduct of all operations relative to the vascular issue in question. Communicate not only with the primary surgeon but also with the anesthesiologist to assess the patient's overall condition.

It is important to remember the principles of damage control, particularly in the setting of significant hemorrhage. Many patients have already had a significant anesthetic exposure and may be cold, coagulopathic, or hemodynamically unstable. Furthermore, major vascular reconstruction and its potential complications have not been discussed with the patient or family members. In these circumstances, priorities of life and limb take precedence over definitive vascular repair and even completion of the initially planned operation. Decisions on vascular control versus repair will be driven by the amount of blood loss, degree of contamination, and the degree of residual ischemia without complete revascularization. When vascular reconstruction is required, prosthetic conduits should be used whenever possible. These have the advantage of ready access and associated reduction in operative time. If contamination exists, ligation and extra-anatomic bypass will usually permit the use of prosthetics as a safe alternative. In cases where prosthetics are contraindicated, consider the use of nonautogenous biologic materials if they are available. When encountered, venous injuries should be ligated whenever possible or controlled with packing. Getting the patient off the table alive is the first priority. Damage control will also permit a more thorough evaluation using computed tomography, magnetic resonance imaging, or catheter angiography to plan definitive therapy at a later date.

Before you leave the operating room, discuss the future plan of care with the primary surgeon and define your role in this process. A significant issue may be that surgeon's desire to continue with the original operation after the vascular problem is managed. In cases where the operation cannot be suspended (e.g., organ transplantation), this approach is acceptable, but whenever possible, the primary operation should be truncated. This approach requires discussion with the primary surgeon who may initially be resistant to it. However, the surgeon can usually be convinced that it is in the best interest of the patient as well as himself or herself to stabilize the situation and regroup. It is generally unwise to leave the operating room without establishing how the remainder of the procedure will be conducted. Unless this action is taken, you may find that the patient and primary surgeon are still in the operating room, and potentially in trouble, several hours after you left, assuming that all was well. Continuation of the primary procedure may place the patient in danger and leave you open to liability. If you do leave the operating room before the operation is concluded, which is often the case, be sure to check back at regular intervals to make sure that things are proceeding as planned prior to your departure. At this time, it is also important to define with the primary surgeon how your role in the procedure will be explained to the patient and the patient's family, and what follow-up care you will be providing.

Whenever possible, you and the primary surgeon should get together to discuss the operation, complications encountered, and your role in treatment with both the patient and the patient's family. This team communication is often overlooked because the consultant has a desire to get on with the tasks of his or her day, and does not wish to go out and meet the family alone for the first time to bring them news of a complication. However, it is crucial that the family and patient understand your participation in the patient's care, and that they are given a clear, unambiguous description of the events that led to your involvement. In addition, such patients have the right to know what your future role in their care will be, and how they can contact you should they have further questions related to your procedure, or require further care. These topics are all best covered in a meeting with the family involving both surgeons. Occasionally, consultants feel that they can minimize their involvement in a case, particularly one with potential liability, by "keeping a low profile" and avoiding contact with the patient or family members as much as possible. This is never the case. You will be listed, if nowhere else, in the operative log. Should any litigation result, your name will be readily available to the plaintiff and any attorneys. It is best to approach the patient and family members as if you were the primary surgeon.

POSTOPERATIVE CLINICAL RESPONSIBILITIES

Some of the postoperative clinical responsibilities have been discussed above. Bear in mind that, as a consultant, you have established a relationship with the patient by virtue of your participation in the patient's operating room care. It is important that you visit such patients postoperatively, identify your role in their care, and provide them with an opportunity for appropriate follow-up. Specific questions about the procedure are best addressed by the primary surgeon; however, it is completely appropriate for patients to receive follow-up visits from you during their hospital stay, and to have a mechanism for outpatient follow-up as dictated by the clinical situation. Ongoing care as an outpatient may not be required. However, a means to contact you after discharge should be provided to the patient, both for medical and legal reasons.

POSTOPERATIVE ETHICAL RESPONSIBILITIES

A potentially difficult situation arises when you feel that the primary surgeon was negligent in managing the patient. In these cases, your first responsibility is to make sure the patient receives adequate postoperative care. This can be done by establishing a relationship with the patient that allows him or her access to your services during the follow-up period. Your availability should be presented to patients as an opportunity for follow-up in the context of the care you provided for them, not a solicitation from you to become their primary surgeon. In addition, during your postoperative discussion with the patient, you must be clear in describing your role in his or her ongoing care in order to minimize the chance that you will be asked to "second guess" the primary surgeon and that surgeon's care of the patient.

Responsibilities of the consultant in the event of malpractice litigation will be discussed later. These issues are difficult and must be handled individually, but your responsibility as a physician to protect the patient's well-being is the paramount consideration. There may be a separate issue concerning your responsibility to the medical staff of the institution involved if you believe that the primary surgeon did not meet the standard of care. This is a very unusual occurrence, and a single approach to managing it cannot be advocated. However, there are some guidelines that seem reasonable. If you believe that the surgeon undertook a procedure outside his or her sphere of competence, the ideal approach is a direct discussion with the surgeon after a few days have passed. If this approach is not fruitful, a discussion with the surgeon's administrative superior within the surgical department would be the next step. There is rarely an easy resolution in such situations, and private conversation with the surgeon combined with an offer of future assistance will provide the most constructive outcome.

Concerns of gross negligence or evidence that the surgeon was operating while incapacitated need to be brought to the attention of the hospital medical director. Such allegations must be based on fact rather than opinion since they can have severe consequences for the physician in question. However, if the circumstances are undeniable, your professional obligation is clear. You may expose yourself to liability and sanctions by failing to report behavior that may negatively impact patient safety.

MEDICAL-LEGAL CONSIDERATIONS

Vulnerability to malpractice actions is a major concern for any surgeon providing intraoperative consultation since most of these consultations result from unanticipated complications, and are often associated with prolonged convalescence and less than optimal results. This alone increases the likelihood that situations where an intraoperative consultation is required will have an increased rate of litigation. However, concern for increased liability cannot override your ethical obligation to come to the aid of a patient, or a colleague, in need of your expertise. It is important to remember that in the setting of an intraoperative consultation, a "doctor-patient relationship" exists between you and the patient, even though you have never had a discussion with this patient or his or her family members prior to your operative intervention. Liability is best minimized by thorough discussion with the family and patient after the fact, full disclosure of events, and the cultivation (rather than avoidance) of the doctor-patient relationship that does indeed exist.

As in most medical-legal matters, accurate documentation, as discussed above, is crucial. Your liability can be limited to the area of expertise for which you were called as a consultant. This is an important matter when a vascular surgeon is called by a general surgeon, or is caring for a patient who develops subsequent or concurrent general surgical problems. Consultants should be clear in the record on what issues they are providing opinion and management, and should document discussions with other services on topics of mutual interest. The recommendations, described above, to establish a mechanism for the patient to receive ongoing vascular care will help establish a positive relationship with the patient and focus your involvement in the case. The ethical obligations you have to your patient and the hospital have been discussed above. Fulfilling these obligations is not only a professional obligation, but also is the best way to minimize your liability should a legal action ensue.

Should legal action occur, the chance that you will be named as a defendant is significant. An accurate and truthful description of events is crucial in such circumstances, and this is facilitated by accurate documentation in the record. It is important for you to have your own counsel in these circumstances, to protect your own interests, and to separate them from the interests of other physicians or institutions. However, it is not professionally appropriate to deflect blame and liability from yourself by blaming others, be they physicians, hospital employees, or residents. Whenever possible, focus your opinions and testimony on your actions in the case. Avoid serving as a supernumerary "expert witness" for the plaintiff during either deposition or trial.

DOCUMENTATION AND BILLING ISSUES

It is important to document your role as a consultant both in the medical record and through an operative report. A note in the medical record should be completed at the end of your intraoperative involvement. It should include all of the elements discussed above, including the reasons for consultation, relevant elements of the patient's history and examination that were known to you at the time the consultation was performed, your operative findings, and your plan for future care. The note should document the conversations you had with the primary surgeon, with specific mention of the plan for completion of the current operation, and any details of future care that have been decided on. Each time the patient is seen in follow-up, a progress note should appear in the chart focused on the relevant vascular findings. When the patient is beyond the acute vascular issue and no longer requires close vascular follow-up, a note should be written outlining the plan for outpatient follow-up and a mechanism for the patient to obtain a postoperative appointment (or a note stating that no further follow-up is needed). A separate operative report should be dictated outlining your role in the operating room and the procedure performed.

Appropriate bills should be submitted for all services rendered. A bill can be submitted for any intraoperative vascular procedures, without a modifier, as long as a separate and distinct operative note is dictated. Again, the note should contain the reason for consultation and a brief description of the findings and procedures performed. Billing for subsequent inpatient and outpatient services will be governed by the same rules that pertain to any other procedures, including restrictions on billing for services covered through a global payment.

CONCLUSION

Intraoperative consultation is an important part of everyday surgical care. It should facilitate optimal patient care. At some point in our professional careers, we will all seek such consultation. The consultant in these circumstances must place patient safety above all other considerations. Diplomatic and constructive participation in the operating room in a calm fashion is crucial to securing short-term success. The surgical team should focus its efforts on addressing the immediate situation that necessitated consultation. Effective, clear communication with the surgeon requesting consultation, both during and after the procedure, is the responsibility of the consultant.

A doctor-patient relationship is established by virtue of the intraoperative consultation. This relationship imposes a series of obligations on the consulting surgeon, including postoperative interaction with the patient and his or her family as well as the potential of providing postoperative care. The consultant should also assume the same responsibilities of chart documentation that are associated with any doctor-patient interaction. Liability is often an issue in these cases, which usually result from an unanticipated, and perhaps, untoward event. The consultant will best protect himself or herself from liability by good communication with physicians and patient, provision of ongoing care to the patient as appropriate, and accurate, complete documentation of the consultant role in the medical record.

36

Iatrogenic Intra-Abdominal and Pelvic Vascular Injuries

Kenneth J. Cherry, Jr., M.D.

Iatrogenic injuries to abdominal and pelvic arteries and veins are serious, often life-threatening, complications for patients, and pose major challenges for vascular surgeons. Iatrogenic vascular injuries are encountered with conventional open surgical techniques, laparoscopic surgery, and with endovascular catheter-based therapies. Most commonly, they involve the arterial system, although venous injuries are not uncommon and are arguably more difficult to treat.[1] When bleeding ensues in a closed space such as the brachial sheath or a confined space such that overlying the lumbosacral plexus, neurologic complications can accompany the vascular injury. The true incidence of iatrogenic trauma to the aorta and its branches and to the inferior vena cava and its tributaries is not known, and is probably much higher than is reported in the literature. It is understandably unappealing for surgeons to catalogue their complications in peer review journals. Whereas vascular surgeons will report their consultative emergency practice, they are unlikely to list injuries to their own patients either for publication or under separate operative coding if those injuries are successfully repaired swiftly and without sequelae. Thus, it is not a topic easy to tabulate, being dependent on operative dictation and coding for recovery, chart review, and the surgeon's willingness to analyze the data.

The relative incidence of iatrogenic trauma in relationship to noniatrogenic sharp and blunt vascular trauma varies widely from country to country and institution to institution. At Baylor in Houston, one of the premier trauma centers in the country, only .7% of injuries in a huge experience involving 5,760 vascular injuries were iatrogenic, reflecting that institution's vast emergency room practice.[2] The Mayo Clinic has entirely different demographics from Houston, is in a semi-rural setting, and by and large has an elective referral practice. Of 713 vascular injuries seen over a 17-year period, 75% were iatrogenic.[1] In Europe, despite its relatively small geographic size, the incidence of iatrogenic vascular injuries varies widely from country to country, often reflecting the religious or ethnic strife current at a particular time.[3-5]

The etiologies of in-hospital vascular trauma are essentially three: 1) conventional open surgery; 2) laparoscopic surgery; and 3) catheter-based procedures. These are more frequent than in years past as a result of the marked increase in endovascular diagnostic and—mainly—therapeutic interventions. A discussion of such arterial and venous trauma may be based on etiology or on arterial versus venous locations. For simplicity, this chapter will address separately intra-abdominal arterial trauma and that of the venous side of the circulation.

Serious injury incurred during performance of what was planned to be a relatively minor case requires more than technical help from the vascular surgeon. If bleeding can be controlled by digital pressure, the surgeon should allow the anesthesiologist time to correct fluid losses and the blood bank to provide type-specific blood. As a matter of course, the vascular surgeon should have a vascular pan brought into the room so that the retractors, clamps, and other instruments peculiar to our specialty are on hand. Appropriate suture material is also a necessity that might have to be imported. If at all possible, an assistant skilled in vascular operations should be called in also.

IATROGENIC INTRA-ABDOMINAL AND PELVIC ARTERY TRAUMA

It is most fitting for this topic to be presented here at Northwestern. Three fairly well known surgeons here, John Bergan, Richard Dean, and James Yao, wrote about "Vascular Injuries in Pelvic Cancer Surgery" in 1975, published in *Gynecology*.[6] In that article, they listed the major problems encountered by the vascular surgeon: laceration, through-and-through penetration, destruction of the wall, division of the vessel, intimal disruption, subadventitial hematoma, and arterial spasm. They also described the chronic sequelae of these injuries, pseudoaneurysm, and A-V fistulas.

Bergen, Dean, and Yao described extra-anatomic arterial (i.e., femoral-femoral) bypass reconstructions for isolated injuries of the iliac arteries, especially if consequent to colon resections. They also recommended extra-anatomic venous reconstruction (i.e., Palma-Dale) procedures for iliac venous trauma including thrombotic occlusion. Since that publication, the relative contribution of laparoscopic and cathter injuries has, as a matter of evolution, increased.

Catheter-based injury to the vasculature is almost entirely arterial, resulting from diagnostic and therapeutic interventions. Venous injuries are usually in the form of A-V fistulas. Most catheter trauma is to the access vessel, be that femoral or brachial. With the expanding and maturing role of endovascular therapy, injury to the iliac arteries primarily, but to the aorta and all its intra-abdominal branches, is not infrequently encountered. Occlusion, dissection, and rupture have been and will continue to be encountered. As skill with stents and endografts increases, and as indications for placement expand, these problems are more frequently resolved in an endovascular fashion than in the past. These solutions include even the endovascular correction of hemorrhage if the patient can be kept stable to allow the time necessary for deployment of covered stents. Unstable patients are usually converted to conventional operation to allow rapid control of ruptured vessels. Dissections are well handled by deployment of stent grafts.

If open operation is necessary, rapid control of the affected vessels is obviously paramount. With control, the options of in-line or extra-anatomic repair can be considered and standard operative techniques employed. Primary repairs, as in all trauma, require tension-free anastomoses or nonstenosing lateral repair. If necessary, prosthetic graft replacement is performed. It is rare with these catheter-based injuries that there is contamination from the bowel, and as a consequence, autogenous tissue is seldom needed.

Laparoscopic injury to the aorta and its branches has been recognized for the last two decades and more.[7-9] These injuries might occur doing gynecologic, urologic, colorectal, and general surgical procedures. Laparoscopic arterial injury usually involves the aortic bifurcation, common iliac arteries, external iliac arteries, and hypogastric arteries, essentially in that order. These injuries are made with either the needle or trocar. Insufficient insufflation of the peritoneal cavity, failure to place the patient in Trendelenburg, 90% angulation of the device insertion, failure to rotate the trocar, previous operation, inappropriate physical force, obesity, extreme thinness, and other factors have all been recognized as contributing to these complications.[9]

Once recognized, iatrogenic laparoscopic arterial injury must be repaired openly. Bleeding might not always be evident, however. Blood loss may be obscured by folds of the mesentery or bowel, and may present as an expanding hematoma rather than frank hemorrhage later in the procedure, or it might be diagnosed after the fact by an unexpected fall in hemoglobin or hematocrit. Although not technically intra-abdominal, abdominal wall trauma with epigastric artery injury can be quite serious.[8]

It is probable that iatrogenic laparoscopic injury is underreported.[8] Despite that, the true incidence is probably low. Geers and Holden reviewed their community experience with 2,201 laparoscopic procedures performed during a three-year period and found only three major vascular injuries for an incidence of .14%.[9]

Usually, lateral repair, or resection of the injured site, and mobilization of the arterial segments and end-to-end reconstruction can be performed. Repair under tension is to be avoided. If reconstruction must be performed, graft choices, of course, are dependent on whether the GI tract or other parenchyma have been entered. If the vascular surgeon determines that graft reconstruction is necessary, even in the face of contamination, alternatives to PTFE and polyester include spiral vein grafts, panel vein grafts, saphenous vein grafts, superficial femoral vein, and rifampin-soaked polyester grafts. If the latter are used, the reconstructed area should be wrapped in omentum or other autogenous tissue for the full length and entire circumference of the graft. Injuries of the iliac system complicated by contamination with bowel contents are well-handled by femoral-femoral prosthetic graft reconstruction following closure of the abdomen, and reprepping and draping of the patient with an entirely new setup. Care must be taken to keep the tract of the femoral-femoral reconstruction separate from the abdominal incision with normal tissue planes interposed between the two, depending on the incision chosen. This may be a difficult requisite to meet satisfactorily if a low mid-line incision has been used by the primary service.

Of most interest and complexity to vascular surgeons are injuries made during open operations. Although some authors have maintained that iatrogenic arterial trauma presents less often with hemorrhage and with less incidence of associated injuries,[10] that has not been the experience at the Mayo Clinic.[1] In our review, the most challenging patients are those with both arterial and venous injuries incurred during complex resection of retroperitoneal tumors. These operations include internal pelvectomies as well as resection of tumors deep in the pelvic retroperitoneum. Such resections often require both anterior and posterior approaches, and the iliac venous confluences and iliac artery bifurcations are especially prone to injury, often during the posterior approach when vision is limited. Injuries to both arterial and venous systems are of particular note and occurred in 20% of our patients. The open operations most often complicated by iatrogenic vascular trauma include neurosurgical/orthopedic spine reconstructions, orthopedic hip nailing or replacement, orthopedic internal pelvectomies, general surgical operations especially for cancer or chronic pancreatitis, colorectal operations, gynecologic procedures, and urologic operations.

Pancreatico-biliary surgery is a worrisome etiology with an incidence of hemorrhage reported in up to 4% of certain complex cases primarily involving chronic pancreatitis.[11] In a review from the Indiana University Medical Center of over 2,500 pancreatico-biliary operations, there was a .56% incidence of vascular injury.[12] In those 14 patients, six had injury to two or more vessels. The incidence of aberrant or variant vascular anatomy ranges from 25–50% in this area of the upper abdominal aorta with a replaced right hepatic artery being the most frequently encountered variation.[13] If present, its course posterior to the pancreatic head may contribute to problems. Vascular complications are more frequent in this area, not only because of this variant anatomy but also because of inflammation surrounding tumor masses and blurred tissue planes related to previous operation, radiation therapy, and the frank involvement of the portal triad or celiac and superior mesenteric arteries in the tumor process or chronic inflammatory process. Exposure here may well be problematic, notably so if injury occurs early in the operation before planes are developed and spaces exposed. For that reason, Schirmer and colleagues recommended wide dissection prior to addressing the arterial supply of the specimen.[14] Temporary supraceliac aortic clamping to control bleeding might be necessary and has been performed. In our hands, that has been a beneficial maneuver. It must be of short—less than 20 minutes—duration to avoid ischemic complications. The usual ability to sacrifice the proper hepatic artery safely might not be practicable as the pancreatico-duodenal arcade and other collateral vessels are either involved in the tumor process, have undergone previous resection, or are to be resected. Thus, it is probably best to reconstruct arteries here in the upper abdomen if there is any doubt at all about parenchymal viability. This imperative includes reconstruction of the hepatic artery even in the face of an open portal vein. The hepatic artery delivers 25% of the liver's blood supply but over 50% of its oxygen.[14]

Some injuries relate to prior vascular surgery. We have seen one patient undergoing a hysterectomy for cancer in whom the initial incision bisected a known and mapped femoral-femoral prosthetic graft. Unfortunately, we were not involved until the uterine mucosa had been exposed in the presence of the two transected, clamped graft ends. The resultant graft infection was successfully treated, albeit over a prolonged period.

Particular injuries in the abdomen and pelvis related to certain operations such as lumbar disc surgery are in part predictable because of anatomic relationships. The proximity of the aortic bifurcation and the L4-5 disc space, the known incidence of aberrant arteries in the upper abdomen, and the relationship of the femoral head to the iliac and femoral vessels all predict certain patterns and frequency of injuries.[15]

IATROGENIC VENOUS INJURIES OF THE ABDOMEN AND PELVIS

Venous injuries of the abdomen and pelvis are, if anything, more lethal than arterial injuries.[1] Predictable control is not as easily attained, and attempts at clamp control might and often do aggravate the situation with further tearing of the vessel. This is well-known in the surgical management of ruptured abdominal aortic aneurysms. Injury to the inferior vena cava or left renal vein has long been recognized as one of the major contributors to increased morbidity and mortality. Further, venous walls do not have the tensile strength of their arterial counterparts, and repair itself in the face of suboptimal exposure may worsen rather than alleviate the situation. Tears in the left renal vein, for instance, can extend into the hilum and necessitate venous ligation at the hilum, resulting in either decreased renal function or nephrectomy. All vascular surgeons with experience in aortic surgery have had the chastening experience of injury to the lumbar or adrenal veins, seemingly minor at first but defying rapid adequate exposure and ligation, especially in large or obese patients. Iliac veins, and most especially the hypogastric vein, are notoriously difficult to control in large patients and/or those with deep pelvises, previous operation, or radiation changes. Digital control at the site of injury or proximal and distal compression with sponge sticks is preferred to clamp control in the great majority of cases. If the site of injury is small enough and well exposed and defined, an Allis clamp is a particularly useful instrument in controlling venous blood loss and holding the cut edges securely together to allow lateral repair. Mattress sutures of fine Prolene are placed on either side of the clamp and the laceration closed. Unfortunately, the vascular surgeon is seldom called for such easily managed, localized trauma.

Trauma to the portal vein itself or the portal venous system presents formidable problems.[16] The portal vein supplies 75% of the liver's blood flow.[14] Despite that, in extreme cases when exsanguination is the only alternative, ligation may be necessary. It is a far preferable practice, however, as it is with hepatic artery injury, to reconstruct the vein. If the abdomen is contaminated, vein grafts, internal iliac artery, or other autogenous conduits should be employed. It is vitally important that the portal system not be stenosed by the repair. Postoperative portal or mesenteric venous thrombosis may be asymptomatic but is more likely to be fatal with necrosis of the bowel or unremitting portal hypertension. Injury to the splenic vein should necessitate splenectomy to prevent left-sided portal hypertension.

As with arterial injuries, laparoscopic injuries most often involve the iliac confluences and the inferior vena cava. In all but the most extreme of situations, the inferior vena cava should be repaired. Spiral or panel vein grafts might be necessary if there is bacterial contamination. Although not as predictable as arterial repair, inferior vena cava repair with 18 or 20 mm diameter segments of ringed PTFE works well as the grafts are usually of short length only. If prosthetics must be used in a contaminated field, an omental or other autogenous wrap should be created around the graft for its full length and circumference. Injuries of the hypogastric vein are ligated; its location deep in the pelvis often makes that simple goal one that is difficult to achieve.

Oderich et al recently reviewed iatrogenic operative injuries of the abdominal and pelvic veins at the Mayo Clinic.[1] Of the 713 patients seen over the 17-year period ending December 31, 2001, 367 experienced catheter-related iatrogenic trauma (52%) and 166 sustained iatrogenic operative trauma (23%). Thus, iatrogenic trauma accounted for 75% of the vascular trauma seen at that institution. Of those 713 patients, 40 (5.6%) had 44 injuries of the abdominal or pelvic veins. The iliac veins were involved in 30 patients (68%). The order of frequency was external, common, and internal iliac vein. Perioperative mortality was 18% with seven deaths. All of those operative deaths were related to the venous injury and included exsanguinating hemorrhage, multisystem organ failure, and pulmonary embolism. Multisystem organ failure was obviously a sequelae of massive blood loss and a complicated hospital course.

In that series of iatrogenic venous injuries, 12 of the 40 patients injured were undergoing a general surgical procedure, nine a colorectal operation, eight an orthopedic procedure, six gynecologic, and three urologic procedures. Sixty-five percent of patients were undergoing an operation for cancer, and hostile or disturbed anatomy was reported in 63%. There were eight associated arterial injuries (20%) and three ureteral injuries (7.5%). We found the associated arterial and venous injuries especially problematic. Delay in seeking help was one of the major contributors to the high mortality and morbidity seen in these patients. For 37% of these patients, the primary service attempted repair for a lengthy, unknown period before calling the vascular surgery consultant. Mean estimated blood loss in these patients was 3900 ml, mean length of stay was 41 days (ranging from two to 280 days), and major morbidity occurred in 70% of the patients. Mortality was 18%. All of these facts underscore the devastating nature of these injuries. As stated previously, 68% percent of the injuries were to the iliac veins. There were nine portal vein injuries, six inferior vena cava injuries, and one left renal vein injury. Sixty-five percent of the patients were undergoing resection for cancer, either primary or recurrent. The surgical field was clean-contaminated in 50% of the patients, and contaminated or dirty in another 13%, further complicating the repair of the venous injury.

CONCLUSION

Iatrogenic injury to the intra-abdominal arterial and venous circulation is a very serious complication and can raise the morbidity and mortality of the planned operation immensely. The two areas of greatest concern to the vascular surgeon and of greatest difficulty in treating are the two extremes of the abdomen: 1) the upper abdomen involving the portal triad, the celiac artery, and the superior mesenteric artery, and 2) the pelvis, involving both arterial but primarily venous injuries.

REFERENCES

1. Oderich GS, Panneton JM, Jofer J, et al. Iatrogenic operative injuries of abdominal and pelvic veins: a potentially lethal complication. *J Vasc Surg.* 2004;39 (5):931–936.
2. Mattox KL, Feliciano, DV, Burch J, et al. Five thousand seven hundred sixty cardiovascular injuries in 4459 patients. *Ann Surg.* 1989;209(6):698–705.
3. Lazarides MK, Tsoupanos SS, Georgopoulos SE, et al. Incidence and patterns of iatrogenic arterial injuries: A decade's experience. *J Cardiovasc Surg.* 1998;39(3):281–285.
4. Fingerhut A, Leppaniemi AK, Androulakis GA, et al. The European experience with vascular injuries. In *Vascular Trauma: Complex and Challenging Injuries, Part II: Surgical Clinics of North America 2002.* February;82(1):175–188.
5. Pedrini L, Stella A, Curti T, et al. Iatrogenic vascular lesions. Pathogenesis and treatment: an 18 year review. *Int Angiol.* 199;10(4):233–237.
6. Bergan JJ, Dean RH, Yao JST. Vascular injuries in pelvic cancer surgery. *Am J Obstet Gynecol.* 1976 March;124(6);562–566.
7. Mills JL, Wiedeman JE, Robison JG, et al. Minimizing mortality and morbidity from iatrogenic arterial injuries: the need for early recognition and prompt repair. *J Vasc Surg.* 1986;4(1):22–27.
8. Nordestgaard AG, Bodily KC, Osborne RW Jr, et al. Major vascular injuries during laparoscopic procedures. *Am J Surg.* 1995;169:543–545.

 9. Geers J and Holden C. Major vascular injury as a complication of laparoscopic surgery: a report of three cases and review of the literature. *Amer Surg*. 1996 May;62(5):377–379.
10. Lazarides MK, Arvanitis DP, Liatas AC. Iatrogenic and noniatrogenic arterial trauma: a comparative study. *Eur J Surg*. 1991;157:17–20.
11. Gall FP, Muhe E, Gwohardt C. Results of partial and total pancreaticoduodenectomy in 117 patients with chronic pancreatitis. *World J Surg*. 1981;5:269–275.
12. Cikrit DF, Dalsing MC, Sawchuk AP, et al. Vascular injuries during pancreatobiliary surgery. *Am Surg*. 1993;59(10):692–697.
13. Braasch JW, Gray BN. Technique of radical pancreatico-duodenectomy with consideration of hepatic arterial relationships. *Surg Clin North Am*. 1976;56:631–647.
14. Schirmer WJ, Rossi RL, Hughes KS, et al. Common operative problems in hepatobiliary surgery. *Surg Clin North Am*. 1991;71:1363–1389.
15. Nehler MR, Taylor LM, Porter JM. Iatrogenic vascular trauma. *Sem Vasc Sur*. 1998 ; 11(4):283–293.
16. Graham JM, Mattox KL, Beall AC Jr. Portal venous system injuries. *J Trauma*. 1978; 18 (6):419–422.

37

Acute Arterial Complications of Total Hip and Knee Arthroplasty

Matthew J. Dougherty, M.D. and
Keith D. Calligaro, M.D.

In the last two decades, there have been significant improvements in technology and technique of total joint replacement. Like atherosclerotic vascular disease, degenerative joint disease and osteoarthritis share the demographic of an aging population. This has led to spectacular growth in the number of patients undergoing joint replacement. Despite the expected prevalence of atherosclerotic vascular disease among this population, total hip arthroplasty (THA) and total knee arthroplasty (TKA) are rarely associated with acute arterial injury and limb-threatening ischemia. The infrequent nature of these complications may make their diagnosis and treatment challenging for vascular specialists unfamiliar with their management as evidenced by high rates of limb loss (approximately 70%) and other morbidity in previous reports.[1-5] Critical factors in management include early recognition of the injury, appropriate use of diagnostic imaging, and effective technique for treating the injury. The infrequency of such injuries also makes it difficult to glean management guidance from published data. Our group has previously addressed treatment of a smaller series of patients who developed ischemic complications following TKA,[5,6] and we recently reported the largest single-center experience addressing the diagnosis and management of acute ischemic and hemorrhagic arterial complications associated with THA and TKA on a high volume orthopedic service.[7] It is this experience that informs the basis for our approach to arterial injuries in the setting of total joint replacement to be outlined in this chapter.

PREOPERATIVE ASSESSMENT

The majority of arterial complications occurring with total joint replacement are ischemic rather than hemorrhagic in nature, accounting for about two-thirds of the total[7,8] (Table 37–1). We have found a high prevalence of preexisting atherosclerosis in

TABLE 37-1. ACUTE ARTERIAL COMPLICATIONS ASSOCIATED WITH TOTAL KNEE (TKA) AND TOTAL HIP ARTHROPLASTY (THA): TYPE AND TIMING OF COMPLICATION

	Recognized same day (SD) as orthopedic procedure*	Recognized postoperative (PO) days 1–5**	Total
Acute ischemia only	9	9	18
Bleeding only	4	0	4
Arterial transection—both ischemia and bleeding	5	0	5
Arterial pseudoaneurysm	0	5	5
Total	18	14	32

*Same day = less than six hours after the orthopedic procedure

**Postoperative days 1–5 = minimum of 24 hours following the orthopedic procedure

With Permission: Calligaro KD, Dougherty MJ, Ryan S, et al., Acute arterial complications associated with total hip and knee arthroplasty. *J Vasc Surg.* 2003;38:1170–1177.

patients who develop ischemic complications after THA and TKA. Given this, we have previously addressed the role of preoperative vascular evaluation prior to total joint replacement. With an overall arterial complication rate of only 0.13% of 23,199 joint replacements performed at Pennsylvania Hospital between 1989 and 2002,[7] it clearly would not be cost-effective to recommend preoperative vascular laboratory evaluation for all TKA and THA patients (Table 37–2). Intermittent claudication is an insensitive indicator of arterial disease in this cohort of patients with limited ambulation due to joint disease. Certainly, any patient with preexisting critical limb ischemia (ischemic rest pain, nonhealing ulcer, prior lower extremity bypass) should undergo vascular laboratory testing and evaluation by a vascular specialist prior to orthopedic surgery. We recommend liberal use of the vascular laboratory for patients with nonpalpable pedal pulses, utilizing segmental Doppler pressures and pulse volume recordings in preference to duplex ultrasonography. While the vast majority of patients with moderate arterial insufficiency (ankle-brachial index [ABI] >.50) can undergo TKA and THA

TABLE 37-2. ACUTE ARTERIAL COMPLICATIONS ASSOCIATED WITH TOTAL KNEE (TKA) AND TOTAL HIP ARTHROPLASTY (THA): CORRELATION WITH FIRST-TIME AND RE-DO JOINT REPLACEMENTS

	Acute Arterial Complications			
	TKA (#)/complications (#) (%)	THA (#)/complications (#) (%)	Total (%)	p value**
TOTAL	24/13,618 = 0.17%	8/9,581 = 0.08%	32/23,199 = 0.13%	0.0609
1st TIME	18/11,953 = 0.15%	7/7,812 = 0.09%	25/19,765 = 0.13%	0.2383
RE-DO	6/1,665 = 0.36%	1/1,769 = 0.06%	7/3,434 = 0.20%	0.0485
p value*	0.0112	0.6636	0.2596	

*Comparing horizontal values.

**Comparizing vertical values.

With Permission: Calligaro KD, Dougherty MJ, Ryan S, et al., Acute arterial complications associated with total hip and knee arthroplasty. *J Vasc Surg.* 2003;38:1170–1177.

without incident, having an objective baseline examination can prove useful if vascular concerns arise in the perioperative period.

For patients with more significant arterial insufficiency, preoperative arteriography should be considered. We generally recommend this for patients with ABI < .40. The rationale is to define potential reconstruction options should the need arise emergently after joint replacement. Preoperative duplex vein mapping to define conduit source is also appropriate in this setting.

In the small subset of patients with indications for lower extremity revascularization in addition to their need for joint replacement, an individualized approach is optimal. Revascularization prior to TKA or THA may be appropriate in some, though the subsequent risk of graft manipulation and occlusion with the orthopedic procedure should be considered.

OPERATIVE ASPECTS

Arterial complications with TKA and THA can be classified as hemorrhagic, ischemic, or both (Table 37–2). Mechanisms of injury are variable. In our experience, there was a trend toward a higher incidence of arterial injury for TKA compared to THA (0.17% versus 0.08%, p = 0.0609).[7] In our cohort, revision surgery carried a higher risk than primary surgery for TKA (0.36% versus 0.15%, respectively; p = 0.0112), and others have reported this as well[8] (Table 37–2). Though we could not demonstrate a similar higher risk to redo hip replacement, this was observed in a report based on a survey of orthopedists in the United Kingdom where two-thirds of vascular injuries were observed in revision surgery.[9] The difficulty with optimizing diagnosis and management of such injuries was illustrated by the fact that the injury incidence in the UK report was only one injury per 14 years of consultant practice. Poor outcomes were indeed noted in these patients.

For THA, retractor injuries to the iliofemoral segment are probably the most common mechanism of injury, causing dissection or thrombosis, while drilling injuries more commonly cause bleeding complications.

The mechanism of arterial injury in TKA varies. The role of the commonly used thigh tourniquet remains unclear. Most TKA procedures are performed with a thigh tourniquet inflated to 250–350 mmHg. In our series, a single patient had a dissection at the mid-portion of the superficial femoral artery, remote from the location of the arthroplasty but corresponding to the location of the tourniquet. However, tourniquets have in recent years been routinely used by vascular surgeons to avoid arterial clamping, and despite the severe atherosclerosis present in vascular patients, the tourniquet itself does not seem to cause problems. We do recommend that tourniquets be avoided in patients with functioning bypass grafts having TKA, and in patients with significant preexisting occlusive disease, heparin should be utilized if a tourniquet is applied.

The most common mode of injury during TKA appears to be from excessive traction on the popliteal artery at the joint line. In a study utilizing 50 cadavers, Ninomaya and colleagues performed intraoperative arteriography while performing TKA, and noted the relationship of the vessel to commonly used retraction maneuvers and manipulations.[10] The majority of injuries appeared to relate to use of a posterior retractor and to hyperextension of the knee that splays the artery over the femoral condyle. The authors suggest that the posterior retractor be confined to the medial half of the joint to avoid injuring the popliteal artery, and the avoidance of excessive hyperextension.

Dissection with thrombosis is the most common mechanism for arterial injuries associated with ischemia, but we have also observed complete popliteal transection, which may also cause hemorrhage. Another mechanism for development of ischemia may be from loss of collateral circulation in patients with preexisting arterial occlusions.

For hemorrhagic injuries with TKA, side branch avulsions of popliteal branches as a result of hyperflexion and hyperextension can occur. These may present as pseudoaneurysms in the postoperative period, and become clinically evident due to popliteal vein compression causing severe edema or popliteal nerve neuropathy. Popliteal arterial laceration or transection is more likely to present acutely with hematoma and compartment syndrome.

DIAGNOSIS

Aside from popliteal pseudoaneurysms, bleeding complications tend to present quickly and dramatically. In contrast, ischemic complications may be more difficult to recognize. Excluding polpliteal pseudoaneurysms, in our review, all 14 other bleeding complications (five of whom had associated ischemia) were recognized on the day of surgery, while half (9 of 18) of ischemic complications were not diagnosed until one to five days after surgery. Though none lost limbs, the patients with later ischemic diagnosis were more likely to require fasciotomy and have residual neurological deficits.[7] The challenge in recognizing significant ischemia is multifactorial. Pain is a poorly predictive symptom in this setting, and joint pain often masks or overwhelms more typical ischemic rest pain. Epidural analgesia is frequently utilized in these patients, which may not only mask ischemic pain but may produce sensory and motor defects of the lower extremity. The neurological signs of advanced ischemia are often mistakenly ascribed to the epidural anesthesia and analgesia, delaying recognition of arterial compromise. Pulse examination is notoriously subjective and unreliable in caregivers not primarily treating vascular disease. Postoperative edema and the utilization of bulky dressings and elastic wraps also confound reliable pulse assessment. Additionally, patients with preexisting arterial disease, who are considerably more likely to develop ischemic complications, may have absent pedal pulses at baseline. We now favor routine Doppler interrogation of the pedal vessels after joint replacement as this is a far more sensitive indicator of severe ischemia than pulse examination. However, Doppler assessment is not applied routinely in most orthopedic settings.

When ischemia is suspected, diagnostic evaluation is tailored to the severity and duration of the ischemia. Simple Doppler evaluation with ankle-brachial indices (ABI) may be sufficient to establish the diagnosis. When ischemia is severe (ABI < .30, neurologic deficit), a clinical conundrum in the past has been whether to obtain diagnostic arteriography. While generally valuable in patients with preexisting atherosclerotic occlusive disease, with acute ischemia there is usually thrombosis, which may mask causative lesions. Collateralization may be poor such that opacification of viable target vessels for distal bypass may not be possible. Significant delays in recognition of ischemia often make the added delay of diagnostic arteriography unappealing. With good quality digital subtraction fluoroscopy now available in many operating rooms, the issue of preoperative arteriography may be moot. Planning for revascularization procedures can be readily accomplished at the time of exploration in this setting.

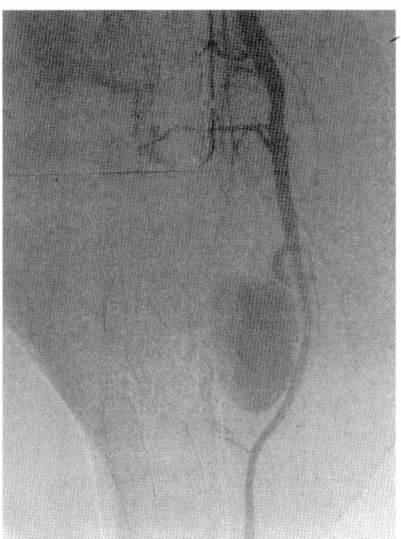

Figure 37-1. Popliteal fossa pseudoaneurysm, likely secondary to genicular artery avulsion from joint manipulation.

For acute hemorrhage, diagnostic studies are rarely appropriate as immediate and direct exposure of the injured vessel is paramount. For pseudoaneurysm, duplex ultrasound plays a valuable role. In our experience with five such patients, all were initially diagnosed by color duplex obtained for swelling and pain with suspicion of deep vein thrombosis. Arteriography demonstrates the exact location and nature of the pseudoaneurysm (Figure 37–1), and may discriminate which lesions may be amenable to endovascular treatment.

TREATMENT

Treatment strategies depend on the presentation of the arterial complication. For intraoperative arterial bleeding, access and exposure are primary issues. The exposures utilized for THA and TKA are not favorable exposures for the iliofemoral or popliteal arterial segments, but in most cases, the vessels can be accessed through the orthopedic incisions and repaired primarily. Exceptions include drill injuries that may be remote from the incision, and require separate incisions and sometimes repositioning.

For pseudoaneurysms, which we have observed only at the popliteal level, there are several treatment options. In most cases, these present with symptoms secondary to pressure on neighboring structures such as the popliteal vein or nerve. For this reason, we most often have preferred a surgical approach. With the patient in the prone position, an S-shaped incision extending from the medial supragenicular popliteal fossa to the lateral aspect below the joint provides good access. Most pseudoaneursysms represent avulsion injuries of genicular branches, which can be suture ligated, while the pseudoaneurysm cavity is evacuated. If compressive symptoms are not severe, endovascular treatment is attractive. We have utilized this approach in a single patient (Figure 37–2). Catheter access was obtained via a femoral approach, and thrombin was then injected into the pseudoaneursysm sac. Direct injection with

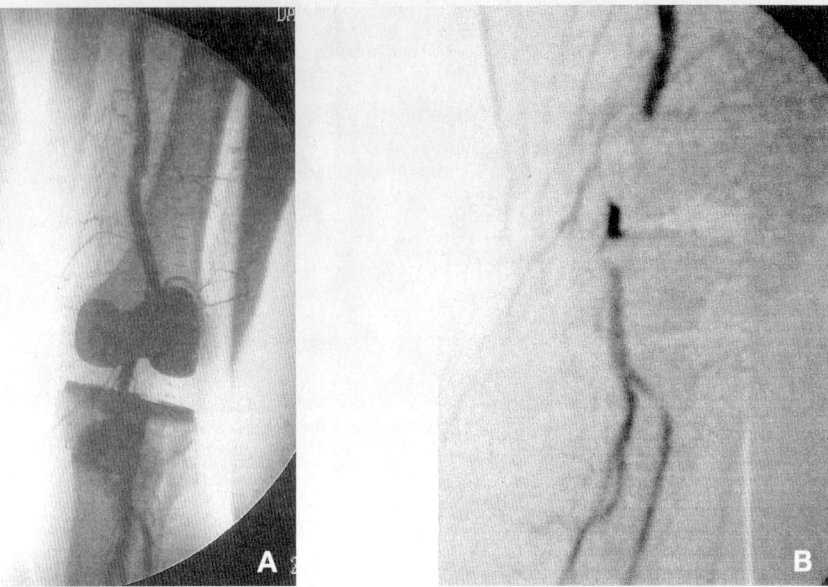

Figure 37-2. **A.** popliteal pseudoaneurysm. **B.** after endovascular thrombin injection.

ultrasound guidance is another alternative. While residual hematoma will eventually be resorbed, the confined space of the popliteal fossa makes compressive neuropathy a significant risk, so this approach should be avoided in the setting of neuropathic symptoms. Likewise, significant popliteal vein compression associated with severe edema is a relative indication for open surgical repair.

For ischemic complications, tenets of optimal management include prompt revascularization when ischemia is severe, utilizing fasciotomy when reperfusion risk is significant; complete revascularization in the setting of preexisting occlusive disease; and arteriographic confirmation of a successful arterial intervention.

As previously noted, we are more frequently utilizing arteriography in the operating room rather than preoperative imaging. For THAs with absent femoral pulse, the femoral artery is explored and gently thrombectomized under fluoroscopic guidance, and aortofemoral and infrainguinal arteriography is then performed. We prefer to treat iliac arterial dissections with endovascular stents, but we have performed iliofemoral and femorofemoral prosthetic graft reconstruction when necessary.

For ischemia associated with TKA, both groins and legs are prepped and draped. The femoral artery is accessed percutaneously, preferably in an antegrade fashion on the affected side, and subtraction arteriography is performed. Typically, occlusion of the popliteal segment is noted with variable reconstitution of more distal vessels. If minimal chronic occlusive disease is noted, the femoral artery is exposed and thrombectomy performed, inflating the Fogarty balloon with contrast for direct fluoroscopic visualization. Once all thrombus is extracted, arteriography is repeated. In a minority of cases (28% in our series), no lesion, or a trivial intimal abnormality, will be noted.[7] These patients are treated with antiplatelet therapy. In the majority, significant abnormalities remain. Our preference is to perform bypass to suitable outflow arteries distal to the area of acute thrombosis. This will most often mandate bypass to the crural level, which should be done with autogenous material. The contralateral saphenous vein is our first choice for conduit, but we will not hesitate to use ipsilateral vein in preference to prosthetic grafts, despite theoretical concerns about the risk of deep venous thrombosis and the need for superficial collateral venous outflow in this group.

Bypass grafts are usually reversed, and tunneled subcutaneously to avoid the orthopedic incision. Completion angiography is always performed. Limbs with profound and prolonged ischemia are treated with four-compartment fasciotomy through medial and lateral incisions. If there is significant muscle bulging, skin wounds are not closed. If skin is closed, close postoperative monitoring is critical as severe edema is common, and if any neurovascular compromise develops, skin clips are then removed. Patients are treated with antiplatelet therapy and receive low-intensity warfarin therapy as per the orthopedic protocol.

With this approach, we have observed no limb loss as compared with amputaion rates of 14 to 70 % in other series.[2-5, 8] We believe suboptimal results reported elsewhere may reflect overreliance on thrombectomy alone without completion imaging. Three-quarters of our patients required complex revascularization, most often to the tibioperoneal level, to achieve success.

Despite generally good outcomes, even within our high-volume joint replacement center, ischemia is often recognized late. Preoperative identification of patients at higher risk, with increased vigilance in this subgroup, will hopefully reduce delays in vascular intervention and subsequent morbidity.

REFERENCES

1. Fortune WP. Complications of total and partial arthroplasty in the knee. In: Epps CH, ed. *Complications in orthopedic surgery.* Philadelphia: JB Lippincott; 198: 949–977.
2. McAuley CE, Steed DL, Webster MW. Arterial complications of total knee replacement. *Arch Surg.* 1984;119:960–962.
3. Rush JH, Vidovich JD, Johnson MA. Arterial complications of total knee replacement: The Australian experience. *J Bone Joint Surg Br.* 1987;69:400–402
4. Zahrani HA, Cuschieri RJ. Vascular complications after total knee replacement. *J Cardiovasc Surg.* 1989;30:951–952
5. Calligaro KD, DeLaurentis DA, Booth RE, et al. Acute arterial thrombosis associated with total knee arthroplasty. *J Vasc Surg.* 1994;20:927–932
6. DeLaurentis DA, Levistsky KA, Booth RE, et al. Arterial and ischemic aspects of total knee arthroplasty. *Am J Surg.* 1992;164:237–40
7. Calligaro KD, Dougherty MJ, Ryan S, et al. Acute arterial complications associated with total hip and knee arthroplasty. *J Vasc Surg.* 2003;38:1170–1177
8. Wilson JS, Miranda A, Johnson Bl, et al. Vascular injuries associated with elective orthopedic procedures. *Ann Vasc Surg.* 2003;17:641–644
9. Sharma DK, Kumar N, Mishra V, et al. Vascular injuries in total hip replacement arthroplasty: a review of the problem. *Am J Orthop.* 2003;32:487–491.
10. Ninomiya JT, Dean JC, Goldberg VM. Injury to the popliteal artery and its anatomic location in total knee arthroplasty. *J Arthroplasty.* 1999;14: 803–809.

38

Lower Extremity Vascular Injury in Children Younger than 13 Years of Age

Michael C. Dalsing, M.D., Michelle E. Sohn, M.D.,
Dolores F. Cikrit, M.D., Alan P. Sawchuk, M.D.,
Shoab Shafique, M.D., Ryan Nachreiner, M.D.,
and Michael Murphy, M.D.

Childhood lower extremity vascular injury is an uncommon occurrence in the experience of most vascular surgeons. As a consequence, familiarity with the clinical presentation, the best methods to confirm the diagnosis, and the appropriate management strategy for any given situation can be lacking. It is hoped that a review of the experience gained in our institution, in addition to a review of pertinent literature, may help to close this informational gap.

PREVALENCE/ETIOLOGY

One large multicenter experience reports that pediatric vascular trauma accounts for only about 1% of all pediatric trauma admissions, confirming the fact that many vascular surgeons may not see a significant number of these patients during their careers.[1] In addition, the etiology of pediatric vascular trauma changes with the age of the patient. Iatrogenic injuries are most common during the first two years of life, while the vast majority of older child and adolescent will experience penetrating injuries, and up to 38% of cases reported in the young or middle aged child will be due to blunt truama.[1-21] It is interesting that one study of low birth weight neonates (< 1500 grams) and normal weight neonates (>1500 grams) admitted to the neonatal ICU reported a limb ischemia risk of 2/335 (0.6%) and 7/2563 (0.3%), respectively, over a seven-year period.[10] This is a select population of neonates with a high risk of iatrogenic injury, yet the incidence is quite low. Lower extremity arterial injury accounts for only 30% of reported pediatric vascular trauma cases and blunt injuries appear to be concentrated in the lower limbs.[1] Seventy percent of blunt impact vascular trauma is reported to occur in the lower extremity.[1] Our own experience found blunt injuries to be the most common etiology (50% of cases).[11] Our patients were young to middle aged children (average age 6.8 years) from a tertiary care facility with injuries limited to the lower extremity, a finding quite consistent with prior experiences noted in the literature for this age group.

The actual mechanism by which vascular injury is inflicted on children encompasses the scope of experiences the child meets as maturing. Penetrating injuries are caused by bullets, knives, or falls onto sharp objects.[1-3,5,8,9,12-14,16,17] One unusual agent found in our study and noted by others are the blades of a small water craft propellor.[5,11,15] Blunt injuries result from a variety of mechanisms in this age group but bicycle-related injuries, falls, and collisions with moving objects (autos) are quite frequent with more than 100 cases reported per year from one active pediatric trauma center and confirmed by various surgical series.[1,3,7,8,11,12,14,17-20] Iatrogenic injuries are generally access and catheter placement related, or much less commonly, surgical in nature.[1-6,10,11,14,21]

The most common vessel to be injured in the lower extremity of this age group is the femoral artery, the popliteal artery, and the tibial vessels in descending order of frequency.[2,3,6,9,11,13,14,16,19-21] The iliac artery may certainly be involved as an extension of a common femoral artery injury, introducing the need to consider the retroperitoneum in some childhood vascular injuries. The femoral vein is the most common venous injury in the lower extremity of children.[3,6,13,19] This anatomic location of injury will vary, depending on the mechanism of injury, age, and factors specific to a particular reporting institution. In our series, one common femoral, two superficial femoral, and three popliteal artery injuries were observed.[11]

PRESENTATION

A careful physical examination and history of the injury is valuable and often must be obtained from the parents or a responsible adult present. Particular attention should be given to understanding the type and extent of trauma experienced (e.g. fall with specification of height, speed of car if pedestrian-auto trauma, and so forth). The child should be fully examined with careful attention given to potential entry and exit sites in the case of penetrating trauma. Inspection for bony deformity, the location of hematoma formation, swelling, bleeding, and any other signs of external trauma must be made. Palpation of pulses proximal and distal in the extremity is mandatory. As in the adult patient, hard or soft signs of vascular injury can be observed.[22,23] Some hard signs of vascular injury (i.e., bleeding) can be quite evident and, therefore, the need for further vascular care obvious. However, other "hard signs" of adult vascular trauma may be difficult to discern in the neonate and young child who lack sophisticated communication skills. The surgeon may have a difficult time making the proper diagnosis of distal ischemia or nerve damage, diagnoses that rely so heavily on the patient's perception and verbalization of pain or diminished or absent sensation. The soft signs of vascular injury may be especially difficult to determine and, therefore, a high index of suspicion for vascular injury must be maintained. In fact, in my experience and others, active bleeding is the sole impetus for immediate operation in the very young.[11,24]

TABLE 38-1. HARD AND SOFT SIGNS OF VASCULAR INJURY (ADULT VS. NEONATE/INFANT/CHILD)

Adult	
Hard Signs	Soft Signs
Expanding hematoma	Nonexpanding hematoma
Active arterial bleeding	Hypotension
Absent pulse	Peripheral nerve deficit
Distal ischemia	History of bleeding
Bruit/thrill over wound	
Neonate/Child	
Expanding hematoma	Nonexpanding hematoma
Active arterial bleeding	Hypotension
	Peripheral nerve deficit
	History of bleeding
	Bruit/thrill over wound
	Absent pulse
	Distal ischemia

Since the hard and soft signs of vascular injury in adults often denote no need for further diagnostics and a direct trip to the operating room, I believe the hard and soft signs of vascular injury must be changed somewhat in the neonate and infant as shown in Table 38–1. One cannot ignore the soft signs of vascular injury in the neonate and child, but in some cases, medical therapy or even observation may be the more prudent course of action.

Children have been observed to experience an intense vasospastic response to injury or trauma of any sort. Angiography alone can induce significant vasospasm.[25] However, it is usually transient in the normothermic child and should spontaneously resolve with return of distal pulses in one hour (in 80% of cases), and certainly within a few hours.[6,21,25] Those without return of pulses have experienced a vascular thrombosis. This is true even after fracture reduction where one author suggests that all should be normal within 10 minutes in the well-perfused and warm child.[17] The physician should never assume that an abnormal pulse examination is due to spasm unless there is a rapid return of distal pulses following a short observation period.

As in the adult, when limb ischemia is of concern, the absence of significant sensory impairment and skin mottling in the presence of good capillary refill, whether or not a femoral pulse and/or distal doppler signal (recordable ABI) is present, suggests a threatened limb but of an urgent rather than emergent nature (Rutherford's class I, IIa).[11,14,20,21,26] The alternative suggests a more eminent limb-threatening ischemia (Rutherford's class IIb, III).[26]

An abnormal physical examination provides evidence of a high likelihood that vascular injury is present. In one study, 10 of 10 patients found to have positive findings on angiography had abnormalities on physical examination.[16] Only four of 77 children (5%) had physical findings suggestive of injury, but none was found on angiographic evaluation. An overall sensitivity of 100% and specificity of 95% for physical examination is demonstrated. The presence of symptoms increased the positive predictive value from 33% to 67% without affecting the accuracy. Injuries potentially hidden to the physical examination are intimal flaps, pseudoaneurysms, segmental narrowings, or arteriovenous fistula that may or may not place the limb in jeopardy in the near term, at least in the adult patient and likely in the child as well.[22,27,28]

The ankle-brachial index (ABI) is an integral and useful adjunct to the physical examination. An ABI of less than 0.9 is suggestive of potential vascular injury in adults as well as children over two years of age.[11,20,21,27,29] In the adult[27] and some pediatric literature,[16] an ABI of < 1.00 is considered abnormal following potential vascular injury, indicating the need for further investigation. In the very young (< two years if age), a lower ABI may be normal. Investigators in Israel have studied a large cohort of healthy infants younger than two years of age and found a mean ABI of 0.88 +/− 0.11 in newborns.[29] There is normalization of the ABI values such that all have an ABI over 0.9 at one year of age. They concluded that lower reference values should be applied to determine the presence of limb ischemia in neonates and infants. We have generally used an ABI of < 0.9 to trigger further study in infants and children as well as neonates, but certainly a lower ABI in neonates (> 0.8) could be tolerated with the information provided by Katz et al.[29] In addition to physical signs and symptoms of vascular injury, the use of an abnormal ABI should result in further investigations for arterial injury.

The insidious presentation of blunt vascular trauma, overshadowed by associated injuries or simply missed, is well recognized.[1] Blunt trauma around the knee joint is notorious for missed vascular injury, potentially leading to a nonfunctioning limb or amputation.[1,8,19,20] One review suggests that about 3% of long bone fractures have associated arterial injury, often with associated nerve and/or soft tissue injury, a finding support by the pediatric literature, adding another dimension of complexity to the care of these children.[1,6-8,17,24]

Irrespective of the mechanism of the extremity vascular injury, a delay in diagnosis must be avoided to avert disability or amputation.[1,9,11,14,30] The combination of physical findings, the mechanism of injury (i.e., knee dislocation), and the ABI will drive the need for confirmatory diagnostic studies.

CONFIRMATORY DIAGNOSTIC STUDIES

Findings on physical examination or concerns of the surgeon based on a high index of suspicion can be further evaluated by color flow duplex imaging. This confirmatory study is particularly useful in children due to its noninvasive nature.[10,11,27] It can detect intraluminal defects that are even difficult to identify with other diagnostic modalities. Even in adults, the accuracy of duplex imaging is highly operator-dependent, but under optimal circumstances, the sensitivity and specificity for determining vascular injury has approached 95+% and 97+%, respectively.[31,32] The necessity for trained proficient technicians and reading physicians is stressed since poorer results have been reported.[33,34]

Obtaining an angiogram in an injured child is reserved for specific indications in view of the increased risk of thrombotic complications, especially in children younger than five years of age.[35,36] One study has reported a thromboembolic complication rate of 37% in the pediatric population who required a cardiac catheterization.[37] The use of smaller catheters introduced percutaneously and the use of systemically administered heparin (1 mg/kg) has decreased but not eliminated this risk (2% to 10%).[35,38,39] Lin et al. found that only 0.02 % (36) of 1,674 diagnostic and therapeutic catheterizations required open operative intervention.[40] Evans et al. studied 92 children for arterial trauma and advocates liberal use of angiography.[9] Six patients had a poor functional outcome, four of which had a delay in diagnosis and had injuries adjacent to the joints. Their conclusion was that angiography would have detected the unrecognized injury, which would have averted an unfortunate outcome. Others investigating children with blunt injuries have found angiography useful but only in the setting of clinical deterioration.[19] Blunt injury isolated to the knee in the adult population has a high incidence of angiographically identified vascular injury (20+%), generally identified by an abnormal physical examination. Therefore, routine angiography in the absence of physical findings is not recommended.[27,41] Certainly, erring toward further diagnostic evaluation in cases where a good examination is not possible may be reasonable due to the high likelihood of injury in these cases. In the case of penetrating injuries, Reichard and colleagues evaluated 87 pediatric trauma patients over a five-year period.[16] Twenty-four children received angiography, 12 for hard signs of vascular injury, and of these, eight (67%) were found to have a vascular injury. An additional 12 children were studied for proximity only and none had a vascular injury. This study suggests that proximity of injury alone is not an indication for angiography in children.[16] Such conclusions reflect similar findings in the adult population.[42,43] Meagher and colleagues state that angiography is seldom used while Richardson et al. and Fayiga et al. find selective use more advantageous.[2,3,7] No patient in our series underwent diagnostic angiography who was younger than seven years of age.[11] We believe selective angiography is the best approach when duplex imaging is difficult to interpret or not available. Situations in which angiography is best applied are injuries with multiple wounds (e.g., shotgun wounds), crush injury with extensive soft tissue damage, and fractures or dislocations near joints, especially when pulses do not rapidly return following reduction.

As the technologic advancement of computerized tomographic angiography and magnetic resonance angiography (MRA) reach maturity, each will likely replace standard angiography in many instances including evaluation of traumatic arterial injuries in the extremities.[44] This will take place in the pediatric population as well, but only certain centers have developed these modalities sufficiently to evaluate the adult, and presently, hard data to determine sensitivity and specificity or accuracy in the diagnosis of pediatric vascular extremity injuries is lacking. We had one instance in which MRA was not sufficiently sensitive to determine the distal runoff vessels and, therefore, angiography was performed.[11]

MANAGEMENT

Neonates and Infants

Neonates and infants younger than two years of age who experience lower extremity vascular injury are unique in that their lower extremity arteries are very small, prone to intense vasospasm, and collaterals seem to develop rapidly. The presentation is often not as eminent limb-threatening ischemia but rather as a less threatening event (lack of sensory impairment, good capillary refill, the absence of skin mottling, and generally with audible distal doppler signals although not always).[14,21] As in adults, these children have viable limbs (Rutherford class I, IIa)[26] and can be treated medically, at least initially. Flanigan and his colleagues have demonstrated that systemic heparinization to therapeutic levels in addition to good symptomatic care (e.g., warming of the child, protecting the extremity from further trauma, and the like) will result in return of a normal ABI in 93% of cases while observation alone has this result in only 63% of cases ($p< 0.10$)[21] The price to pay for this minimally invasive therapy is a near tripling of the risk of limb length discrepancy when compared to surgical intervention (23% vs. 9%) but still with less than a fourth of children affected. A consensus statement on this topic recommends the use of heparin anticoagulation for children affected with femoral artery or even more proximal thrombosis if life-threatening (renal or mesenteric ischemia) or eminent limb-threatening ischemia is not a factor.[45] The recommended method of administration of unfractionated heparin was an initial bolus of 75–100 units/kilogram with an infusion dependent on age: for the < two-month-old, 28 units/kilogram/hour, while children slightly older require only 20 units/kilogram/hour. Older children mimic adults since the average dose is 18 units/kilogram/hour. Futhermore, these authors recommend the use of thrombolytics only in the 30% who do not respond to systemic heparin anticoagulation, and in dosages that can be found in the article.[45] Savena and colleagues found that heparin alone allowed return of pulses, improved skin temperature and/or normalized capillary refill in 66% of children affected with postcardiac catheterization limb ischemia, with the remaining being effectively treated with streptokinase.[39] Wang and his colleagues demonstrated 97% complete lysis in acute thrombosis of less than two weeks' duration with the use of tissue plasminogen activator (TPA) and with lower starting doses than currently recommended: 0.06 mg/kg/ hour in neonates and 0.03 mg/kg/hour in nonneonates.[46] The degree of tissue ischemia in this study was difficult to determine. Weiner et al. used recombinant TPA to treat arterial thrombosis in neonates (< 44 weeks postconceptional age) with four of seven demonstrating complete resolution of clot and symptoms, but two had serious bleeding.[47] The risk of bleeding was a major factor in not recommending thrombolysis more aggressively in initial treatment by the American College of Chest Physicians (ACCP).[45] Others have confirmed findings similar to Flanigan and his associates with or without the addition of thrombolytic agents.[10,14,48,49] Some investigators report limb salvage with medical therapy, even in the face of severe limb ischemia in these very young patients.[4,14] Only after failure of all medical interventions, except when aortic thrombosis threatens ischemic bowel or renal failure, does the ACCP document suggest surgical intervention.[45] Although somewhat out of the scope of this review, transverse aortic thrombectomy may be required in such cases with the potential for a 75% complete recovery, at least in one series.[50] Others agree that this is an important option in such children.[21] Truly, there are challenges to surgical intervention in neonates and young children. The small vessel size and intense vasospasm may not allow passage of a 2 French Fogarty embolectomy catheter past the common femoral artery, and makes repair challenging. Current practice does not reflect the very poor results noted by Smith and Green during a time when neither systemic heparin anticoagulation nor the use of prolene suture for vascular repair was standard practice.[4] Review of the literature confirms that most surgeons only recommend operation when limb-threatening ischemia is clearly present. Therefore, the results reported in surgical series should be interpreted with this is mind. A limited surgical thrombectomy with or without patch is often successful in salvaging a limb unresponsive or past the point of medical interventions.[3-5,10,11,21,51] Chaikof noted a return of palpable pulses in only about 50% of cases in his series, even though all limbs were salvaged. This was an impressive result since all had mottling, coolness, and no doppler signals on presentation.[51] He cautioned that one should not expect complete restoration of distal pulses when open thrombectomy is required.

Guzzetta has reported that the saphenous vein is often too small to use as a bypass conduit in infants less than 10 kilograms in weight.[17] Recent case reports have used the great saphenous vein (GSV) to perform both arterial and venous bypasses in neonates and children up to two years of age with the aid of microvascular techniques.[52,53] Even with the advent of microvascular techniques, most vascular surgeons are cautious when recommending open operations on infants due to the potential for inflicting additional trauma to the patient. I personally have experienced a few cases, prior to our recent report, where open intervention was not successful, and have experienced first-hand the difficulty in keeping very small arteries open after surgery. However, when required, the surgeon should feel that there is at least an opportunity to help the young patient with surgical intervention.

Arterial injuries with apparent bleeding, or symptomatic false aneurysm or arteriovenous fistula, do require repair in many cases on clinical grounds alone.[11,24,40,48] Although often not discussed specifically for the small child, less invasive and/or more conservative methods of treating relatively benign pseudoaneurysm or AVF may not be unreasonable.[27,54]

Children Two to 13 Years of Age

The vascular surgeons in our institution aggressively attempt vascular repair for limb salvage unless the child's life is at risk. In our experience, we are consulted only when vascular repair is eminent due to severe ischemia or active bleeding. This is the case in many other surgical series.[2-9,12,17,19,20] In one case, a child was seen after a delay in establishing the presence of a popliteal pseudoaneurysm with occlusion and an ABI of 0.6. Surgery was undertaken to resolve claudication symptoms, repair the large pseudoaneurysm, and to avert any problem with limb length discrepancy.[11] Similarly, arteriovenous fistula and/or pseudoaneurysms are repaired (open or less invasively) if symptomatic with the possibility that a period of observation may be the best therapy in some circumstances.[27,40,54]

The more difficult situation exits when there is apparent vascular injury; but conservative therapy is a reasonable choice based on the presence of distal doppler signals, good capillary refill, and the absence of skin mottling. Many vascular surgeons have made the decision to operate on older children (> six years of age) to prevent potential sequelae (limb length discrepancy) with the knowledge that immediate results are often quite acceptable.[5,11,14] However, those preschool children (≤ six years of age) and certainly those under 12.5 kg may not do as well with surgical repair.[14,16] In select cases, some surgeons have decided to observe the patient with plans for delayed repair if required. Reichard et al. are observing two two-year-old patients with popliteal injury but adequate distal flow with the anticipation of repair when the children are older.[16] Having observed excellent clinical improvement in such patients when placed on heparin anticoagulation, Lazarides and colleagues consider the age group from 2.5 to 6 a grey zone regarding the decision to operate, and operation is not recommended for those under 2.5 years of age.[14] He believes that a delayed vascular repair or bone-lengthening techniques may provide a more opportune surgical intervention for these small children. Furthermore, vascular injury does not always result in limb length discrepancy (23% when not repaired vs. 9% with surgical repair).[21] The ABI may or may not inversely correlate with the severity of limb length discrepancy.[21,36] While some investigators have noted no improvement in limb length discrepancy with delayed vascular repair,[5] there is growing evidence that it will help to correct limb length discrepancy to some degree.[36,55] In reality, the decision to operate rests on the degree of ischemia (will the limb survive), the general condition of the child (associated medical or trauma issues), the risk of the intervention (vessel size, presence of adequate conduit, and so on), and last, for concerns of limb length discrepancy.

Care of the child in the operating suite must follow established trauma protocols in addition to recognizing specific requirements for the lower extremity vascular injury. In the absence of confounding events, our approach is as follows. Both lower extremities are included in the sterile field so that the contralateral saphenous vein is available as required. Vascular exposure mimics that familiar to the surgeon for the conduct of adult surgery. Careful dissection of the vessels for proximal and distal control is performed under loupe magnification. Venous collaterals are meticulously preserved to ensure adequate outflow. The children are given heparin to obtain systemic anticoagulation (75–100 units/kg), papaverine is judiciously injected within the graft and distal vasculature as well as liberally applied externally, and all operations are performed under at least 3.5 loupe magnification. When available, an activated clotting time (ACT) is maintained at 1.5 to 2 times the normal baseline value. The use of vessel loops and/or soft coronary bulldog clamps for vascular control is standard care. On some occasions, the major axial vein has been repaired to control bleeding and/or maintain the outflow tract. The recommendation is to repair the vein first, generally by lateral repair, but with bypass if required.[3,6,13,19,53] Technical aspects are much like that described subsequently for an arterial repair. Small diameter (2 or 3 Fr.) Fogarty embolectomy catheters are used in the setting of acute thrombosis to clear the proximal and distal vascular beds of clot. A tension-free primary repair can be accomplished if sufficient length of the artery exits. A tension-free repair is required. Pseudoaneurysm, arteriovenous fistula repair, and very localized intimal flaps may require only simple suture repair or arterial patching. When required, our experience and others suggests that the saphenous vein is an excellent conduit for repair of vascular injuries for children within this age group, whether used as a patch or long bypass conduit (Figure 38–1).[6,7,9,11,30,40,55] The great saphenous vein is preferentially harvested from the opposite extremity to limit additional venous insult to the traumatized limb. The dissection is meticulous so as not to manipulate the conduit excessively or induce excessive vasospasm. Side branches of the vein are tied and removal of the vein carried out as would be accomplished in the adult patient. Operative repair involves resection or bypass of all damaged segments and interposition of the reversed vein graft as an arterial conduit. The anastomoses are spatulated to a length of at least two times the diameter of the vessel being repaired where possible. In most cases, the method of repair was interrupted by 7, 8, or 9 "O" prolene suture technique. In older, nearly full-grown children, a running suture technique may be appropriate and more expeditious. Dilation through the near completed anastomosis provided a method to relieve vasospasm and to confirm a widely patent repair. Unless mandated by bleeding concerns, heparin given during the operation is not reversed and systemic anticoagulation is not provided postoperatively. Intraoperative angiography may be obtained prior to or after repair if required. In general, return of distal pulses with normalized ABI following repair obviates the need for postprocedural angiography.

If other life-threatening injuries precludes immediate vascular reconstruction, one might consider intra-arterial shunting as a temporary measure to establish distal perfusion while more pressing interventions must be completed.[17,20,27] There are some technical difficulties associated with shunt insertion in the infant, but it has been done.[53] In addition, four-compartment fasciotomy should be considered in the setting

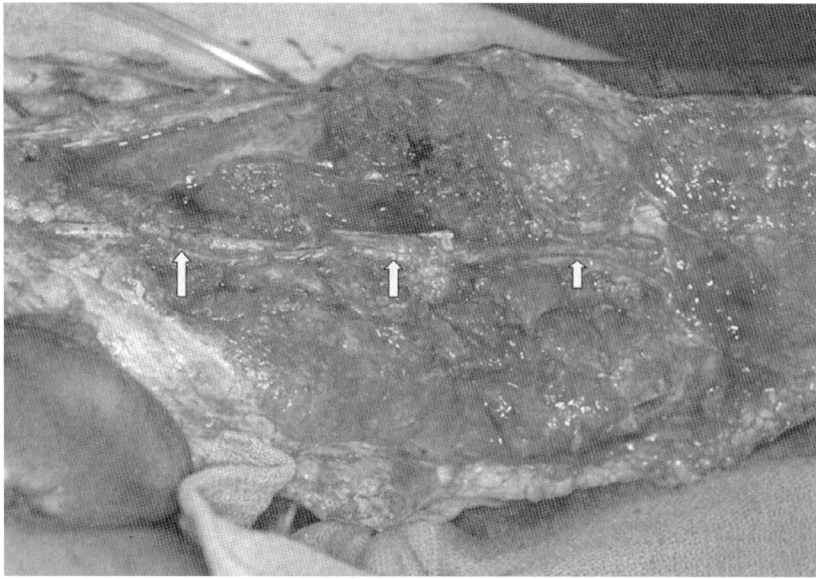

Figure 38-1. This is an intraoperative photograph of a long length greater saphenous vein by pass graft (arrows) required to repair a damaged superficial femoral artery.

of severe ischemia present for four to six hours, concurrent artery and vein injury, severe soft tissue injury, and/or elevated intramuscular compartment pressures (>30mmHg).[1,2,6,11,19,20,30] If reperfusion is a concern, all medical maneuvers used in adults must be utilized.

RESULTS

In the very young, supportive care and the use of systemic anticoagulation with heparin appears to provide the best management in most cases, and certainly performs better than observation alone.[21] One can expect return of near normal distal perfusion in 70% to 90% of neonates and infants so managed for moderate and even severe lower extremity ischemia.[14,21,39,45] Thrombolysis will often resolve symptoms in the remainder.[39,45] In the rare event that conservative measures fail, thrombectomy with or without patch angioplasty or even a lengthy vein bypass may be attempted with success.[3-5,10,21,51-53] The repair of localized arteriovenous fistula, pseudoaneurysms, and intimal lesions without thrombosis are reported to do well with microsurgical repair.[10]

The potential for limb length discrepancy and/or a poor functional outcome poses challenges for the vascular surgeon who must also deal with the anatomic and physiologic limitations of the child (older than two years of age) with limb ischemia. Some data reassuring the vascular surgeon that success is likely if the operation is preformed in a timely fashion and with proper technique would make this challenge less daunting.

The most difficult situation arises when a long length of artery is damaged. Our surgeons have faced this situation several times and have opted for the use of the small diameter, long-length reverse saphenous vein conduit. The major concerns when using such long conduits was the risk of occlusion and/or aneurysmal degeneration over time. Our personal experience would suggest excellent results if the operation is performed in a timely fashion.[11] One external jugular vein bypass failed as a result of a delay in diagnosis, extensive distal thrombosis, and muscle ischemia that eventually necessitated an above-knee amputation (AKA). The remaining three reverse GSV bypass grafts are patent (ABI > 1.0, $n = 3$) without stenosis or dilation by duplex evaluation ($n = 2$) after a mean 37.7 months (21–49 months). In two cases, the bypass was performed since no other conduit was available to span the distance required. The Guzzetta series specifically mentions three such repairs undertaken for blunt trauma and describes the use of saphenous vein in penetrating trauma.[17] Furthermore, he mentions that the distal saphenous vein is sufficiently large in children greater than 10 kg to use as a free graft. A child with propeller injury to the thigh required the use of distal saphenous vein because it was the only graft of sufficient length available. The graft remains patent without dilation at four years follow-up.

The remaining patient presented late with claudication and pseudoaneurysm after a minor bicycle accident, and required a significant length of conduit for reconstruction. A similar presentation of delayed pseudoaneurysm formation following minor blunt trauma to the popliteal fossa has been reported and was successfully repaired with a vein bypass graft.[56]

Most experienced vascular surgeons faced with a severely damaged femoral or popliteal artery will use reverse GSV without hesitation. Most have not reported problems with occlusions or aneurysmal degeneration, but precise data are hard to gather from the few reports with limited patients stretched over many years of reporting. In addition to the risk of a possible occlusion, there are concerns that these veins would dilate over time, much as has been described in renal artery reconstructions.[57,58] Fayiga et al., de Virgilio et al., and Evans et al. describe 1, 16, and 14 reverse vein bypass grafts for lower limb vascular reconstructions with no mention of dilation.[6,7,9] The follow-up was short or difficult to discern. Reed and his colleagues have performed four GSV bypass grafts to reconstruct the popliteal artery for blunt and penetrating trauma with no limb loss for a follow-up of 10–42 months.[30] The mean follow-up was not mentioned and no evaluation for graft dilation was mentioned, but palpable pulses, normal sequential pressures, and normal waveforms were obtained at postoperative office visits. Richardson commented, in a reply to questions, that his group has noted no reverse GSV bypass dilation in their series of seven cases.[2] A recent study by the University of Michigan group has the longest follow-up of lower abdominal/lower extremity autogenous saphenous vein bypass grafts in the literature.[55] Only one patient was on operated for lower extremity trauma and required a popliteal-to-popliteal artery bypass graft. However, also mentioned was a femoropopliteal and poplitealposterior tibial artery bypass. Only one of these grafts demonstrated mild, progression dilation at 23.7 years of follow-up, but only reached 48% dilation (50% was considered aneurysmal). The other two bypasses demonstrated no dilation at 11.8 and 26.1 years after implant. Based on all reviewed pediatric cases with long-term follow-up, there appears to be little risk of significant aneurysmal dilation or occlusion of arterial lower extremity saphenous vein bypasses.

The risk of limb loss, even with vascular repair, is a real possibility in children with lower extremity vascular injury since repair is often performed only as a last resort. Studies in the literature reporting on the operative repair of children generally consistent with ages two to 13 report an amputation rate of 0% to 33%, depending on which patients are included in the review.[10,11,14,19-21] The vascular injury per se does not appear to the major determinant of limb loss since judicious and meticulous repair is most often successful. Rather, a delay in diagnosis and/or associated injuries may have the most significant impact on the results.[1,9,11,14,30] Two of our three patients with blunt trauma to the popliteal region did experience significant limb ischemia from a delay in diagnosis. An aggressive attempt to salvage a limb in one of these patients was successful but with persistent nerve damage and muscle loss. The other patient required a primary BKA. A missed diagnosis of popliteal artery injury, blunt or penetrating, is important since the experience of Reed and colleagues demonstrated minimal limb loss when unequivocal physical findings allow prompt diagnosis and repair.[30] The final delay in diagnosis resulted from an iatrogenic event and required an AKA shortly after attempted bypass graft failure. In one series of pediatric arterial injury, four of six patients with a poor functional outcome (67%) had a delay in diagnosis.[9] King and Wise confirmed this impression for both penetrating and blunt injuries, especially around the knee.[1] Irrespective of the etiology causing the extremity artery injury, a delay in diagnosis is of major concern and often has dire consequences.[1,9,11,14,30]

Furthermore, there are data to suggest that associated nerve, bone, and soft tissue injury, in conjunction with a vascular injury when taken together, are essential determinants of limb salvage in adults and may have an impact in children as well.[2,12,20,59] The Mangled Extremity Severity Score (MESS) scores the skeletal/soft tissue injury (1–4), limb ischemia (1–3 with doubling if ischemia > six hours), shock (1–3), and age (1–3) with a score of >7 suggestive of an assurance that amputation will be required. In 36 injuried children, the MESS had predictive accuracy of 93%.[60]

In general, a 0% operative mortality is reported in children undergoing operative repair for a lower extremity vascular injury.[3,6,10,12,14,19,20] An overall mortality of 10% - 15% has been reported in some series but always due to associated injuries.[2,4,11,21] The only mortality in our series was the result of a fall from a porch with resultant severe head injury; this case was also the only case requiring primary amputation without attempt at reconstruction.[11] This patient is one of the 1.6% of deaths resulting from accidental falls in children, all due to intracranial trauma.[61]

CONCLUSIONS

The conclusion of this paper is summarized in Figure 38–2, being cognizant of special anatomic and physiologic responses of neonates and children to vascular trauma, including the response to an open intervention. Active bleeding needs to be addressed at any age with the most expeditious and simple repair possible. Arteriovenous fistula and pseudoaneurysms require a period of observation if minor in nature and, therefore, likely to resolve, but simple repair with or without patch angioplasty if symptomatic and/or fail to resolve. A confirmatory duplex evaluation usually provides a clue to the nature of the problem. Although the literature on the vascular treatment of childhood lower limb ischemia is not abundant and is generally combined with upper extremity vascular trauma, some general concepts can be gained. In general, none of the articles specifically define the degree of limb ischemia by Rutherford's classification, but this classification does provide a framework under which to suggest treatment based on my best interpretation of the data provided in the pertinent articles mentioned previously. A delay in the diagnosis of acute limb ischemia in the young child occurs, jeopardizes the ability to salvage the limb, and must be guarded against by a high index of suspicion, especially in particular trauma situations. Class I and IIa

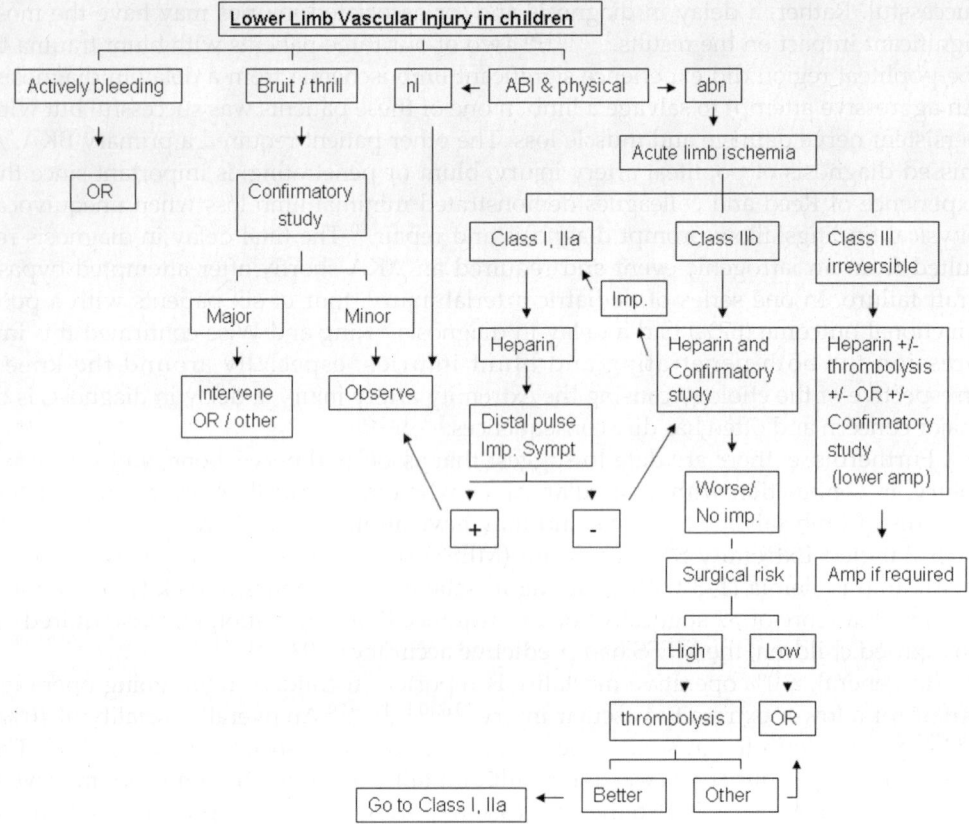

Figure 38-2. Algorithm for care of neonate/infant/child with vascular trauma. OR = operating room, nl=normal, ABI = ankle-brachial index, abn = abnormal, Class I-III refers the Rutherford classification.[29]   Imp = improved, sympt = sympt.

are limbs with acute limb ischemia but without eminent risk of limb loss. The use of heparin anticoagulation to allow collateral enlargement and recruitment is warranted in all cases. In many neonates and young children (< six years of age), heparinizaion alone will generally result in the return of distal pulses in the majority of cases. Up to one-third may development limb length discrepancy but the inherent risks of operation on these very small vessels may well warrant a conservative approach. If ischemia worsens, further diagnositic study confirms the clinical impression and helps plan more aggressive interventions. Duplex imaging, if available, may be effective, but in some situations, angiography may still be useful. In the very young, most physicians will move to thrombolytic therapy even with the risk of significant bleeding. In all age groups, advancement to eminent limb-threatening ischemia warrants an attempt at surgical salvage. The simpler the operation, the more likely the success, but even bypass using reverse saphenous vein can be successful. In the older child, open operation may be less risky than thrombolysis and, therefore, offered early in treatment. It may provide an opportunity to prevent later problems with limb length discrepancy. The surgeon must make it clear to the parents and patient (as appropriate) that open operation is more difficult the younger the child, and may not be successful regardless of the age. Faced with a severely ischemic limb, however, it may be the best and only approach available. Fasciotomy should be employed liberally when considered. A limb that seems unsalvageable (Class III) in the adult may do better in the neonate/ child than initially thought. Prolonged heparin therapy, thrombolysis, or even surgical intervention to provide a longer limb prior to demarcation is often attempted and may be successful. At demarcation or for signs of sepsis, amputation is appropriate.

Operations for trauma with a delay in presentation (claudication, pseudoaneurysm, and the like) have passed the phase of acute ischemia and required repair based on the risk of operation verses continued observation. The older the child, the less technically demanding the operation, and the more realistic the chance of success. Most current literature would suggest that over the age of six, even surgical bypass with reverse greater saphenous vein is often successful without a significant risk of aneurysmal degeneration or graft failure on long-term follow-up.

REFERENCES

1. King DR, Wise WE. Vascular Injuries. In: Buntain WL (ed). *Management of Pediatric Trauma*. Philadelphia: W.B. Saunders Company; 1995:265–276.
2. Richardson JD, Fallat M, Nagaraj HS, Groff DB, Flint LM. Arterial injuries in children. *Arch Surg*. 1981;116:685–690.
3. Meagher DP Jr., Defore WW, Mattox KL, Harberg FJ. Vascular trauma in infants and children. *J Trauma*. 1979;19(7):532–536.
4. Smith C, Green RM. Pediatric vascular injuries. *Surgery*. 1981;90(1):20–31.
5. Whitehouse WM Jr, Coran AG, Stanley JC, et al. Pediatric Vascular Trauma. *Arch Surg*. 1976;111:1269–1275.
6. de Virgilio C, Mercado PD, Arnell T, et al. Noniatrogenic pediatric vascular trauma: a ten-year experience at a level I trauma center. *Am Surg*. 1997;63(9):781–784.
7. Fayiga YJ, Valentine RJ, Myers SI, et al. Blunt pediatric vascular trauma: Analysis of forty-one consecutive patients undergoing operative intervention. *J Vasc Surg*. 1994;20:419–425.
8. Navarre JR, Cardillo PJ, Gorman JF, et al. Vascular Trauma in Children and Adolescents. *Am J Surg*. 1982;143:229–231.
9. Evans WE, King DR, Hayes JP. Arterial Trauma in Children: Diagnosis and Management. *Ann Vasc Surg*. 1988;2(3):268–270.
10. Gamba P, Tchaprassian Z, Verlato F, et al. Iatrogenic vascular lesions in extremely low birth weight and low birth weight neonates. *J Vasc Surg*. 1997;26(4):643–646.
11. Dalsing MC, Cikrit DF, Sawchuk AP. Open surgical repair of children less than 13 years old with lower extremity vascular injury. *J Vasc Surg*. 2005;41(6):983–987.
12. Harris L, Hordines J. Major Vascular Injuries in the Pediatric Population. *Ann Vasc Surg*. 2003;17(3):266–269.
13. Schnitzer JJ, Fitzgerald D. Peripheral Vascular Injuries From Plastic Bullets in Children. *Surg Gynecol Obstet*. 1993;176:172–174.
14. Lazarides MK, Georgiadis GS, Papas TT, et al. Operative and nonoperative management of children aged 13 years or younger with arterial trauma of the extremities. *J Vasc Surg*. 2006;43(1):72–76.
15. Beierle EA, Chen MK, Langham MR, et al. Small Watercraft Injuries in Children. *Am Surg*. 2002;68(6):535–538.
16. Reichard KW, Hall JR, Meller JL, et al. Arteriography in the evaluation of penetrating pediatric extremity injuries. *J Ped Surg*. 1994;29(1):19–22.
17. Guzzetta PC. Vascular Trauma. In: Eichelberger MR (ed). *Pediatric Trauma: Prevention, Acute Care, Rehabilitation*. St Louis: Mosby Year Book; 1993:326–331.
18. Brown RL, Koepplinger ME, Mehlman CT, et al. All-Terrain Vehicle and Bicycle Crashes in Children: Epidemiology and Comparison of Injury. *J Ped Surg*. 2002;37(3):375–380.

19. Friedman RJ, Jupiter JB. Vascular Injuries and Closed Extremity Fractures in Children. *Clin Orthop Relat Res*. 1984;188:112–119.
20. Rozycki GS, Tremblay LN, Feliciano DV, McClelland WB. Blunt Vascular Trauma in the Extremity: Diagnosis, Management, and Outcome. *J Trauma*. 2003;55(5):814–824.
21. Flanigan DP, Keifer TJ, Schuler JJ, et al. Experience with Iatrogenic Pediatric Vascular Injuries. *Ann Surg*. 1982;198(4):430–442.
22. Frykberg ER, Crump JM, Dennis JW, et al. Nonoperative observation of clinically occult arterial injuries: A prospective evaluation. *Surgery*. 1991;109:85–96.
23. Fryberg ER, Feliciano DV. Arteriography: Are we in proximity to an answer yet? *J Truama*. 1992;32:551–554, (editorial).
24. Mill RP, Robbs JV. Paediatric arterial injury: management options at the time of injury. *JR Coll Surg Edinb*. 1991;36:13–17.
25. Frachen EA Jr., Girod D, Sequeira FW, et al. Femoral artery spasm in children: Catheter size is the principal cause. *AJR*. 1982;138:295–298.
26. Rutherford RB, Baker JD, Ernst C, et al. Recommended standards for reports dealing with lower extremity ischemia: Revised version. *J Vasc Surg*. 1997;26:517–538.
27. Rowe VL, Yellin AE, Weaver FA. Vascular Injuries in the Extremities. In: RB Rutherford (ed). *Vascular Surgery: 6th Edition*. Elsevier, Saunders: Philadelphia, Pennsylvania; 2005: 1044–1058.
28. Itani KM, Rothenburg SS, Brandt ML, et al. Energency center angioigraphy in the evaluation of suspected peripheral vascular injuries in children. *J Pediatr Surg*. 1993; 28(5): 677–680.
29. Katz S, Globerman A, Avitzour M, Dolfin T. The Ankle-Brachial Index in Normal Neomates and Infants is Significantly Lower than in Older Children and Adults. *J Ped Surg*. 1997;32(2): 269–271.
30. Reed MK, Lowry PA, Myers SI. Successful repair of pediatric popliteal artery trauma. *Am J Surg*. 1990;160(3):287–290.
31. Bynoe RP, Miles WS, Bell RM, et al. Noninvasive diagnosis of vascular trauma by duplex ultrasonography. *J Vasc Surg*.1991:14: 346–352.
32. Fry WR, Smith RS, Sayers DV, et al. The success of duplex ultrasonographic scanning in diagnosis of extremity vascular proximity trauma. *Arch Surg*. 1993;128:1368–1372
33. Schwartz M, Weaver FA, Yellin AE, et al. The utility of color-flow Doppler examination in penetrating extremity trauma. *Am Surg*. 1993;59:375–378.
34. Gagne PJ, Cone JB, McFarland D, et al. Proximity penetrating extremity trauma: The role of duplex ultrasound in the detection of occult vascular injuries. *J Trauma*. 1995;38:1157–1163.
35. Freed MD, Keane JF, Rosenthal A. The use of heparinization to prevent arterial thrombosis after percutaneous cardiac catherization in children. *Circulation*. 1974;50:565–569.
36. Taylor LM, Troutman R, Feliciano P, et al. Late complications after femoral artery catheterization in children less than five years of age. *J Vasc Surg*. 1990;11:297–306.
37. McMillan I, Nurie JA. Vascular injury following cardiac catheterization. *Br J Surg*. 1984;71: 832–835.
38. Rubenson A, Jacobsson B, Sorensen SE. Treatment and sequelae of angiographic complications in children. *J Pediatr Surg*. 1982;14:154–157.
39. Saxena A, Gupta R, Kumar Rk, Wasir HS. Predictors of Arterial Thrombosis after Diagnostic Cardiac Catheterization in Infants and Children Randomized to Two Heparin Dosages. *Cathet Cardiovasc Diagn*. 1997;41:400–403.
40. Lin Ph, Dodson TF, Bush RL, et al. Surgical intervention for complications caused by femoral artery catherization in pediatric patients. *J Vasc Surg*. 2001;34:1071–1078.
41. Abou-Sayed H, Berger DL. Blunt Lower-Extremity Trauma and Popliteal Artery Injuries: Revisiting the Case for Selective Anteriography. *Arch Surg*. 2002;137(5):585–589.
42. Gomez GA, Kries DJ Jr., Ratner L, et al. Suspected vascular trauma of the extremities: The role of arteriography in proximity injuries. *J Trauma*. 1986;26:1005–1008.
43. Weaver FA, Yellin AE, Bauer M et al. Is arterial proximity a valid indication for arteriography in penetrating extremity trauma? A prospective analysis. *Arch Surg*. 1990;125:1256–1260.

44. Busquets AR, Acosta JA, Colon E, et al. Helical Computed Tomographic Angiography for the Diagnosis of Traumatic Arterial Injuries of the Extremities. *J Trauma*. 2004;56(3):625–628.
45. Monagle P, Chan A, Massicotte P, et al. Antithrombotic Therapy in Children: The Seventh ACCP Conference on Antithrombotic Therapy. *Chest*. 2004;126:645S–687S.
46. Wang M, Hays T, Balasa V, et al. Low-dose Tissue Plasminogen Activator Thrombolysis in Children. *J Pediatr Hematol Oncol*. 2003;25(5):379–386.
47. Weiner GM, Castle VP, DiPietro MA, Faix RG. Successful Treatment of Neonatal Arterial Thrombosis with Recombinant Tissue Plasminogen Activator. *J Pediatr*. 1998;133(1):133–136.
48. Gamba PG, Pettenazzo A, Kalapurackal M, et al. Primary occlusion of the iliac and femoral artery in two newborn infants: efficacy of medical treatment. *J Pediatr Surg*. 1993;28:735–737.
49. Dorfman GS, Cronan JJ. Postcatheterization femoral artery injuries: is there a role for non-surgical treatment? *Radiology*. 1991;178:629–630.
50. O'Neil JA, Neblett WW, Born ML. Management of major thrombotic complications of umbilical artery catheters. *J Pediatr Surg*. 1981;16:972–978.
51. Chaikof EL. Dodson TF. Salam AA. et al. Acute arterial thrombosis in the very young. *J Vasc Surg*. 1992;16(3):428–435.
52. LaQuaglia MP, Upton J, May JW Jr. Microvascular reconstruction of major arteries in neonates and small children. *J Pediatr Surg*. 1991;26(9):1136–1140.
53. Nicholas RM, Boston VE, Small J, Graham HK. Limb Salvage After Bony and Vascular Gunshot Injuries in a Five-Week Old Infant. *J Bone Joint Surg Br*. 1995;77–B(3):439–441, 1995.
54. Brawley JG, Modrall JG. Traumatic Arteriovenous Fistula. In: Rutherford RB (ed). *Vascular Surgery: 6th Edition*. Elsevier, Saunders: Philadelphia, Pennsylvania; 2005:1619–1626.
55. Cardneau JD, Henke PK, Upchurch GR, Wakefield TW, Graham LM, Jacobs LA, Greenfield LJ, Coran AG, Stanley JC. Efficacy and durability of autogenous saphenous vein conduits for lower extremity arterial reconstructions in preadolescent children. *J Vasc Surg*. 2001; 34:34–40.
56. Votapka T, Backer CL, Mavroudis C. Giant Popliteal False Aneurysm in an 8-year-old child. *J Ped Surg*. 1993;28(12):1594–1596.
57. Stanley JC, Ernst CB, Fry WJ. Fate of 100 aortorenal vein grafts: characteristics of late graft expansion, aneurysmal dilatation, and stenosis. *Surgery*. 1973;74:931–944.
58. O'Neil JA Jr. Long-term outcome with surgical treatment of renovascular hypertension. *J Pediatr Surg*. 1998;33:106–111.
59. Whitman, Gr, McCroskey BL, Moore EE, et al. Traumatic popliteal and trifurcation vascular injuries: Determinants of functional limb salvage. *Am J Surg*. 1987;154:681–684.
60. Fagelman MF, Epps HR, Rang, M. Mangled extremity severity score in children. *J Pediatr Orthop*. 2002;22:182–184.
61. Wang MY, Kim KA, Griffith PM, et al. Injuries from falls in the pediatric population: an analysis of 729 cases. *J Pediatr Surg*. 2001;36(10):1528–1534.

39

Popliteal Trauma

Rao Gutta M.D., Marshall E. Benjamin M.D., and William R. Flinn M.D.

Prior to the modern era, major vascular injury in the popliteal fossa was associated with a significant rate of limb loss. Debakey and Simeone[1] reported the first large study of vascular injuries treated during World War II and observed a 75% amputation rate with vessel ligation. During the Korean conflict, surgeons began routine repair of popliteal vascular injuries and amputation rates decreased to 32.4%.[2] The landmark Vietnam Vascular Registry[3] observed a further reduction in amputation rates to 13%–16% after treatment of wartime popliteal artery injuries. The leadership provided by military surgeons, both in the realm of vascular reconstruction and musculoskeletal preservation, has led to a continued decline in these amputation rates in the practice of civilian trauma and vascular surgeons today. Modern OR suites are equipped with arteriographic imaging capabilities that provide an optimal environment for prompt, accurate diagnosis and treatment of these injuries. Contemporary amputation rates now range from as low as 1% for penetrating injuries to 6% after popliteal injuries due to blunt trauma.[4-5]

PROGNOSTIC FACTORS AFFECTING LIMB SALVAGE

The aggressive management of popliteal vascular injuries with early, accurate diagnosis and effective techniques for limb revascularization has led to significantly improved limb salvage. However, several key prognostic factors associated with these injuries still have a significant impact on the success of treatment in these cases. The severity of limb ischemia and most importantly, its duration, are among the most critical factors. The lower leg has limited collateral circulation (particularly in normal young people) and trauma victims can rapidly develop critical limb ischemia when their injuries result in acute popliteal artery occlusion. The duration of limb ischemia also has a significant impact on limb salvage. Several studies have documented that ischemia times > eight hours result in increased amputation rates.[6-9] For trauma cases, ischemia time "in the field" can be an uncontrolled variable, so prompt diagnosis and treatment after presentation becomes even more critical. It has also been shown that patients who present with more severe ischemia have worse outcomes that those with moderate ischemia (Wagner). The mechanism of injury also has been shown to have an effect on limb salvage. Not surprisingly, penetrating injuries of the popliteal artery due to stab wounds have a superior outcome compared to high-velocity gunshot wounds with their more destructive potential. Following blunt trauma, popliteal artery injury due to knee dislocation can be challenging when these cases are not addressed in a timely fashion. However, at present, cases of modern vehicular trauma to the extremities, where popliteal vascular injuries are combined with extensive skeletal and neuromuscular injuries, are by far the most challenging for the surgical team.

CLINICAL EVALUATION

Little controversy exists regarding the management of patients with "hard" signs of major vascular injury: (1) active bleeding or a rapidly expanding hematoma, or (2) profound limb ischemia. The latter is characterized by absent pedal pulses as well as absent pedal doppler signals, and is often associated with significant neuromotor dysfunction. Further diagnostic evaluation (Figure 39–1) and treatment for all these cases should be carried out in the operating room.

In patients with suspected vascular injury in whom these hard signs are absent, a standard comprehensive vascular examination should be performed. Pulse palpation

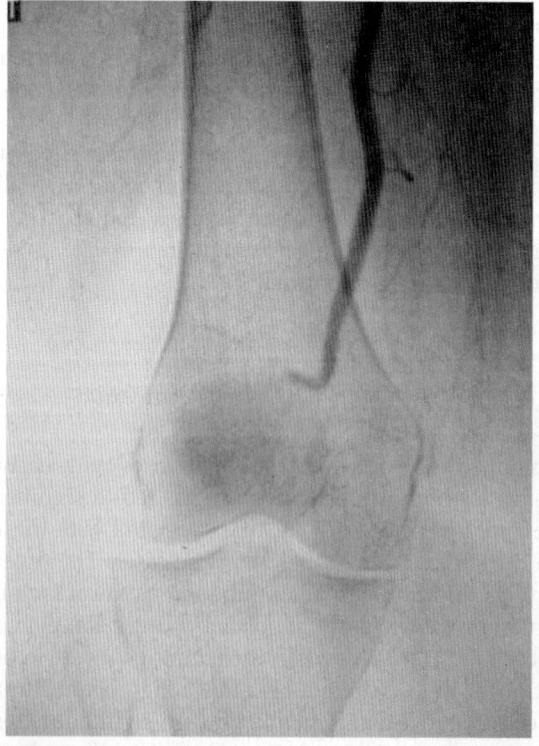

Figure 39-1. A patient presented with critical limb ischemia following an MVA with obvious instability of the knee joint. Intraoperative arteriogram revealed popliteal artery occlusion. The obvious displacement of the distal vessel was due to transaction of the vessel.

should be routinely accompanied by a doppler exam of pedal pulses and measurement of ankle/brachial index (ABI) should be performed in all cases. The ABI provides objective, quantitative, and reproducible documentation of distal arterial perfusion at the time of presentation, and also serves as a reference point for cases that require serial examinations. Neuromotor dysfunction alone may be an unreliable sign of either the presence or severity of ischemia, and must be evaluated based on the nature of the trauma (e.g., blunt versus penetrating). Direct nerve injury may produce lower limb paralysis, or it may be due to compartmental hypertension unrelated to ischemia.

Ankle/Brachial Index

A significant reduction of the ABI following extremity trauma (when the ABI can be performed reliably) indicates the presence of significant arterial injury and warrants further diagnostic evaluation. Schwartz et. al. found that pulse deficits and an ankle/brachial index of <1.0 were significant predictors of popliteal injury in patients following penetrating extremity trauma, with a sensitivity and specificity of 86% and 33%, respectively.[10] Klienberg et al. found that among patients with posterior knee dislocations, those with an ABI > 0.8 had no angiographic evidence of popliteal artery injury, while 48% of patients with ABI < 0.8 had angiographic evidence of popliteal artery injury.[11] ABI measurements may be inaccurate in diabetics, and can be abnormally low in the presence of shock states, but in cases of suspected popliteal vascular injury, patients with an ABI <0.8 should undergo further diagnostic evaluation including duplex ultrasound scanning (when appropriate) or arteriography.

Duplex Ultrasound Scanning

Duplex ultrasound scanning combines B-mode ultrasound imaging of vascular structures with pulsed-doppler spectral flow analysis. Color assignment to the diagnostic display (color-flow duplex) is based on direction and velocity of flow. This unique combination can provide high-resolution real-time imaging of the vessel wall and detection of significant flow disturbances. In this setting (is this a trauma report?), duplex ultrasound has achieved a sensitivity and specificity of 90% and 99%, respectively.[12] In some cases, intimal injuries that produce a minimal reduction in ABI can be identified (Figure 39–2). Color-flow duplex scanning may also be ideal for identifying the presence of a pseudoaneurysm (Figure 39–3) and distinguish it from a benign hematoma. Ultrasound studies can be performed sequentially without risk to follow patients when nonsurgical management is elected. With increasing technological sophistication of portable ultrasound units (which are used routinely in many trauma units for abdominal exams), more sophisticated vascular exams with these lap-top sized scanners may also become routine. One of the obvious limitations of duplex ultrasound exams in popliteal trauma is direct access to the area of possible injury that may be significantly compromised by associated musculoskeletal injury. Compared to arterigrophy alone, duplex scanning also enables visualization and evaluation of the femoral and popliteal veins.

Arteriography

Arteriography remains the most direct technique for accurate identification of vascular injuries and for planning repair of those injuries. Routine arteriography for all "proximity injuries" is, of course, outdated. Routine arteriography for blunt injury to the popliteal fossa (i.e., secondary to posterior knee dislocation) also has low yield, diagnosing arterial injury

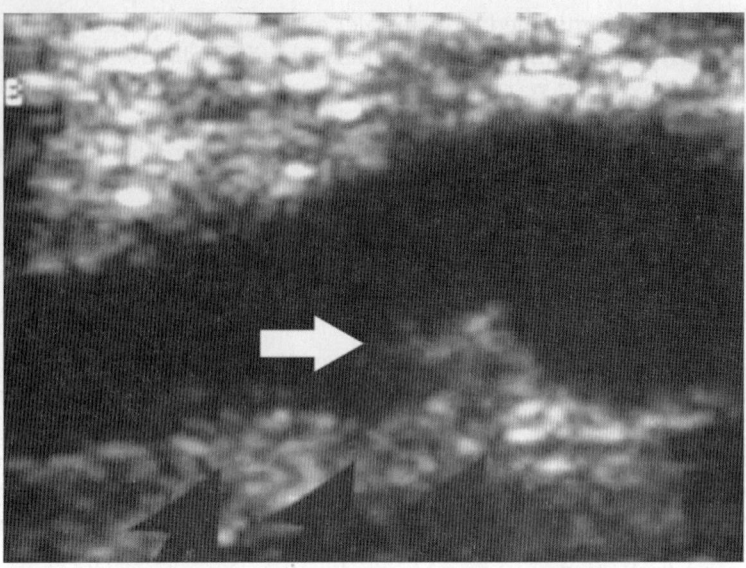

Figure 39-2. A. Duplex ultrasound scan reveals an intimal flap (arrow) in the vessel. The ABI (0.9) was minimally reduced, but elective exploration and repair was elected.

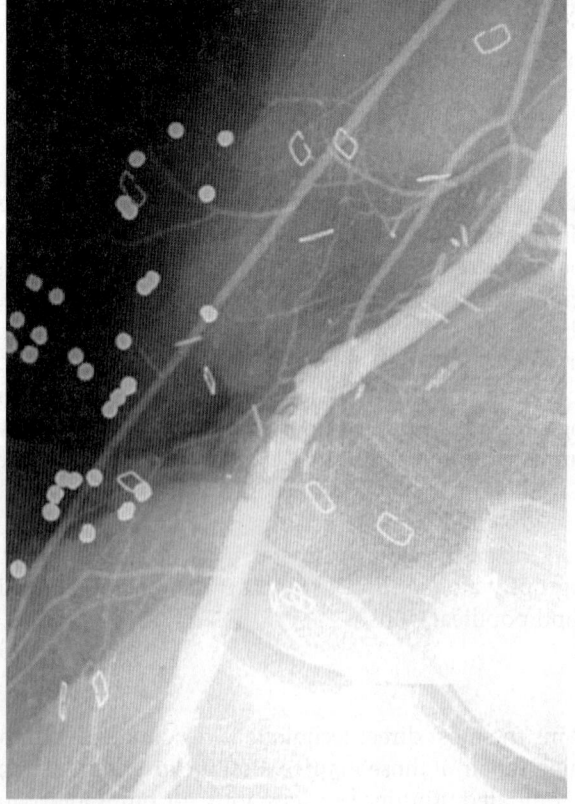

Figure 39-2. B. Arteriogram confirming duplex finding of an intimal flap.

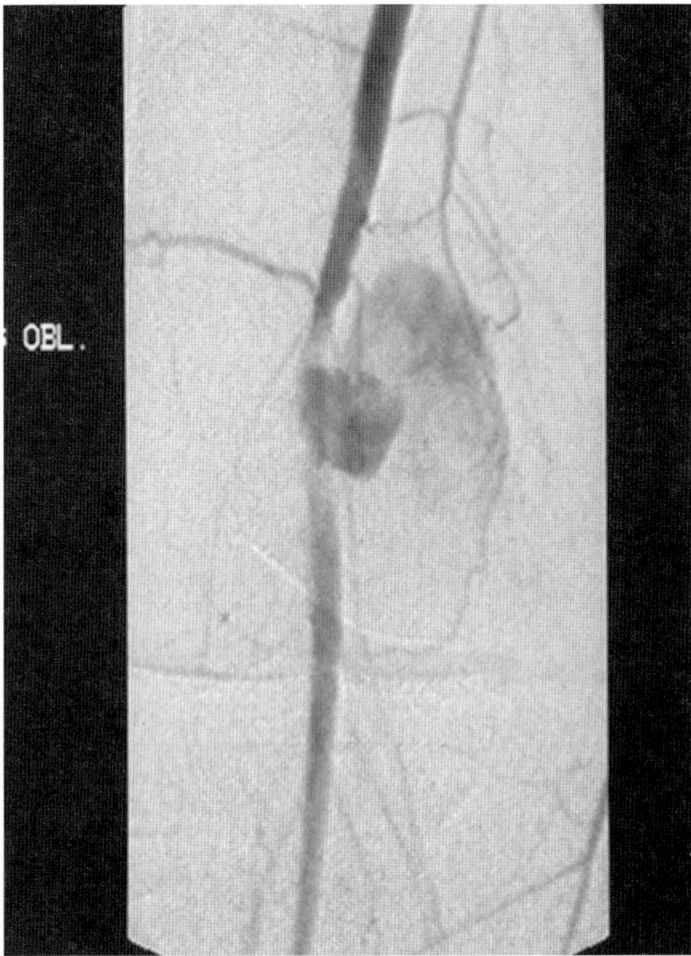

Figure 39-3. This pseudoaneurysm of the popliteal artery was detected by color-flow duplex scan. Arteriography was performed to delineate the distal arterial anatomy.

in only 23% of patients.[13] Other studies examining both upper and lower extremity have shown that routine angiography for proximity injury resulted in only a 5%–10% positive yield. However, some past studies were conditioned by the fact that angiography routinely required transfer of the patient to an interventional suite in a different location, delaying surgical treatment of other injuries, perhaps unnecessarily. Today's OR suite equipped with portable (or fixed) arteriographic imaging equipment allows prompt focused arteriographic examination of the injured extremity without delay. Since the risk of arteriography is low in the generally younger trauma population, consideration of the mechanism of injury (like suspected or obvious knee instability) can then be used to more liberally select patients for arteriography, even with relatively normal physical exams (Figure 39–4). Overall, in most cases, the decision to perform arteriography will be made based upon abnormalities found on physical exam and/or noninvasive testing. In these cases, arteriography can also help determine the reconstructive alternatives and precise surgical approach (Figures 39–5 and 39–6).

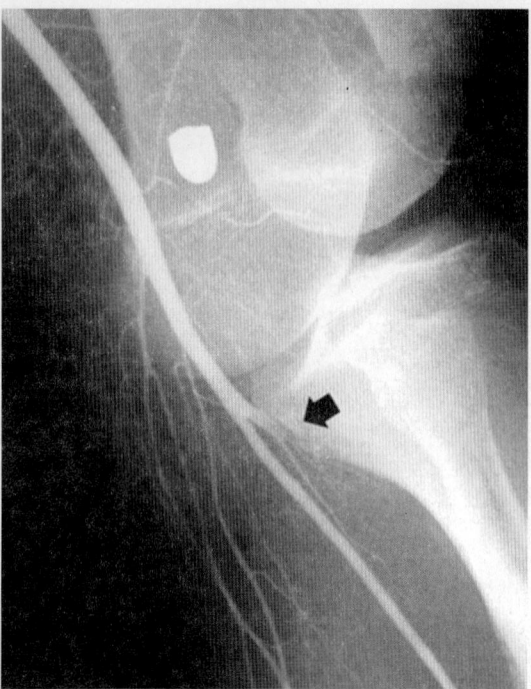

Figure 39-4. Arteriography following an obvious GSW reveals occlusion of a high take-off of the anterior tibial artery. The ABI was 1.0, but arteriography was performed due to proximity and the caliber of the bullet.

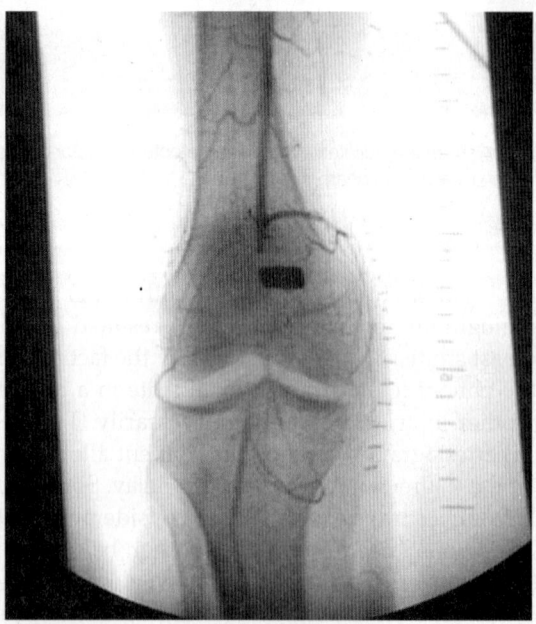

Figure 39-5. Following a GSW, this patient had an ABI = 0.4. Arteriography confirmed occlusion of the popliteal artery. The focal nature of the injury (with a normal distal popliteal artery and no major bony injury) allows consideration of the use of a posterior surgical approach.

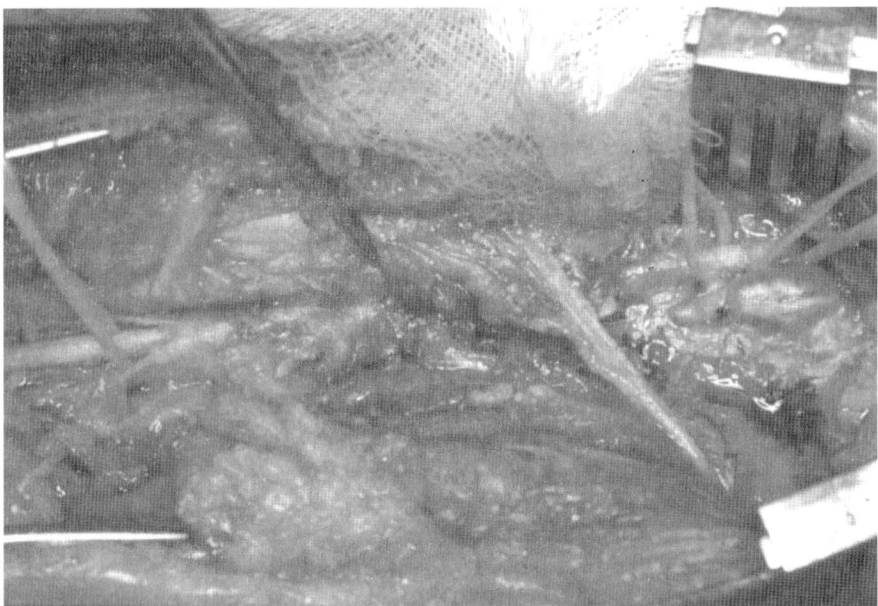

Figure 39-6A. Posterior approach to the popliteal fossa following GSW revealed focal significant arterial and venous injuries.

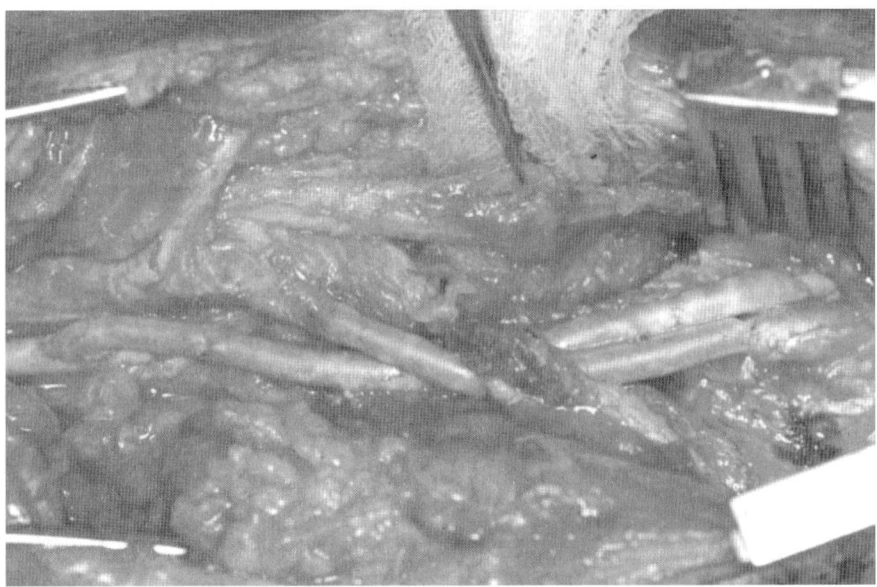

Figure 39-6B. Popliteal artery and vein reconstruction with saphenous vein grafts.

SURGICAL MANAGEMENT OF POPLITEAL INJURIES

The surgical management of popliteal vascular injuries is highly dependent on the mechanism of injury, the location of injury along the popliteal artery, and particularly, associated musculoskeletal injuries.

Both lower extremities should be prepared in the event that vein from the contralateral, noninjured extremity is required. Injuries to the popliteal artery are most often best approached initially through the standard medial thigh incision used for exposure in an above-knee femoropopliteal bypass. In most cases, this will allow proximal control of a normal vessel that can serve as inflow if bypass is required. A standard medial calf incision can then be used to expose the distal popliteal artery or extended to expose medial infragenicular vessels when required.

A very focal arterial injury may allow primary anastomosis, but the majority of popliteal artery injuries associated with significant limb ischemia will require bypass. Because of the significantly younger age of this population, vein bypass should be preferentially performed because of its superior durability. When there has been associated venous injury, saphenous vein from the contralateral leg may be preferred; otherwise, ipsilateral saphenous vein can be used successfully. The use of prosthetic grafts has been observed to be inferior to vein bypass when placed in this setting.[14] A prosthetic graft may be used in cases where vein is unavailable or unusable, or in the rare case of an older patient or one in whom instability has developed due to associated injuries or other medical conditions. Our experience suggests that vein bypass will be possible in over 90% of cases. In most cases, particularly when bypass is performed to crural vessels, intraoperative completion arteriography is recommended. Vasospasm (Figure 39–7) is often seen in these reactive small vessels and does not represent injury or technical error. The local infusion of papaverine (30–60 mg) may reverse this and enhance graft flow.

The direct posterior surgical approach to the popliteal fossa may be used in selected cases of popliteal vascular injury (Figure 39–6). The injury should not be above the adductor hiatus nor below the popliteal bifurcation. The patient cannot have musculoskeletal injury that requires associated surgical treatment since the patient will be

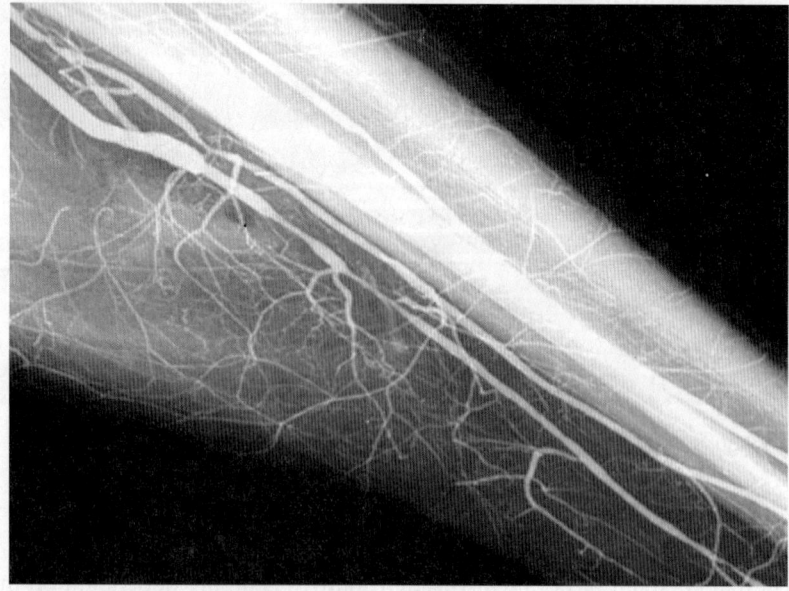

Figure 39-7. This completion arteriogram demonstrates typical areas of vasospasm in the native arteries beyond the distal anastomosis following popliteal-posterior tibial vein bypass.

prone on the table. This surgical approach has the advantage of providing easy access to the mid popliteal artery and vein that is impossible from a medial approach without extensive musculotendinous division and reconstruction. Young patients recover full mobility more quickly with the posterior approach and tend to have less leg edema.

The role of heparin in cases of popliteal vascular injury has been somewhat controversial.[15-16] Wagner et al[4] showed that the use of systemic heprinatization can improve limb salvage rates in the setting of popliteal injury with limb ischemia. However, in cases with extensive bony injury or associated visceral injuries, it may be prudent to use local heparin flushes during the revascularization procedure. In cases where there is no contraindication to systemic heparin therapy, complete anticoagulation should be initiated during the repair, and continued postoperatively.

UNIVERSITY OF MARYLAND EXPERIENCE

From 1995 through 2004, a total of 68 procedures were performed for popliteal artery injuries in 65 patients. This group included 58 men (89.2%) and seven women, and the average age of the patients treated was 35 years (range 16 to 87 years).

Procedures

Direct arterial repair by lateral suture, patch angioplasty, or direct anastomosis was performed in 12 patients. The remaining 53 patients had bypass of the area of arterial injury. In this population dominated by younger patients, the most proximate normal vessel (usually the superficial femoral or the proximal popliteal artery) was used as the origin for the bypass in most cases. The use of a more distal origin for the bypass also reduced the length of graft material required. The distal popliteal artery was the recipient vessel in 38 cases (68%) and bypass was performed to an infrapopliteal vessel in 18 cases.

Graft Materials

Autogenous vein was used for bypass in 45 cases (80%). An expanded polytetrafluoroethylene graft was used in six cases (10.7%), and the graft material could not be determined in five cases. Ipsilateral greater saphenous vein (GSV) was used for bypass in 32 cases (57%). Contralateral GSV was used in four cases, and lesser saphenous vein was used in one case; in another six cases, the precise origin of vein used could not be determined.

Outcome

No patient experienced failure of a direct arterial repair. Early bypass graft thrombosis (during the intitial hospitalization) occurred in four cases (15%). This group included one PTFE femoropopliteal graft and three vein bypasses (one femoropopliteal, two popliteal-tibial). Overall in this series, early graft occlusion occurred in 16.6% of PTFE grafts and 6.6% of vein bypasses (p = ???). Successful reoperation was performed in the three cases of vein bypass occlusion; two re-do vein bypasses, and one PTFE graft. The patient with thrombosis of the primary PTFE graft went on to AK amputation. Two other patients in this series required above-knee amputation with patent grafts (one PTFE, one vein) due to wound infection or infected orthopedic fixation hardware. The overall limb salvage rate for this series was 94.6%.

ASSOCIATED TOPICS

Popliteal Venous Injury

The majority of popliteal venous injuries occur with associated arterial trauma. Isolated venous injury was observed in only 5%–10% of cases.[17-18] Lower extremity postoperative edema occurs in significantly more patients that undergo popliteal vein ligation versus repair,[19] but the decision not to perform popliteal venous reconstruction does not impact on the success of arterial reconstruction or ultimate limb salvage as had once been thought. Popliteal vein injuries that were ligated versus repaired showed increased postoperative swelling and edema (45% versus 21%).[20] This may be somewhat disabling in the early postoperative period, but the majority of extremity edema resolves with time, leg elevation, and compression stockings. Patients with associated popliteal venous injury have typically suffered a more devastating injury, often with considerable surrounding soft tissue injury. Overall, the approach to repair of popliteal venous injuries with ligation, primary repair, or veno-venous bypass should be determined by the complexity of the procedure required in the setting of the stability of the patient and the extent of the patient's associated injuries.

Fasciotomy

Four compartment fasciotomies are recommended for all popliteal injuries associated with limb ischemia. Patients with known or suspected prolonged period of ischemia in the field, or those with obvious calf swelling due to direct crush injury or mass effect, may benefit from the fasciotomy prior to beginning a revascularization procedure. Delaying fasciotomies until compartmental hypertension has already developed results in increased amputation rates.

Concomitant Vascular and Skeletal Trauma

Debate is ongoing regarding management of patients suffering the most complex blunt trauma (usually vehicular) extremity injuries with multiple bone and joint injuries, and known or suspected vascular injury. One major issue is prioritization of vascular diagnosis and repair versus skeletal stabilization. In reality, this is often a fait accompli exercised by the first team on site in the OR. However, in an ideal world, particularly when the diagnosis of arterial trauma is in question or ischemia is moderate, arterial catheterization and arteriography can be performed while external skeletal stabilization is begun (as long as hardware does not obscure vessel visualization). In the presence of critical limb ischemia, primary revascularization is recommended because delayed revascularization in these cases results in reduced limb salvage rates. Another controversial issue in the severely injured extremity (or the multiply injured patient) is when reconstruction/revascularization should be abandoned and primary amputation performed. Intravascular shunts can provide rapid temporary arterial reperfusion and allow the orthopedic team to assess the extent of neurologic injury and/or the expectation for realistic skeletal salvage. These cases are rare and shunting remains relatively controversial. Hosseny[21] reporting on patients with blunt injury to the popliteal artery and demonstrating severe ischemia, related that amputation was required in 40% of those not-shunted versus 0% when a shunt was used. Vascular shunts have been used in the chest, neck, and abdomen routinely to provide time to further evaluate the surrounding structures and additional injuries. The data for popliteal artery shunting are limited, but do show an increased limb salvage rate when ischemia times are expected to be lengthy.[22] Overall, with injuries extensive enough to require these machinations, a serious consideration of primary amputation (with early mobilization and rehabilitation) is probably warranted, but this is a difficult decision in these very young individuals.

SUMMARY

The treatment of popliteal trauma has advanced considerably over the preceding 75 years and has seen amputation rates steeply decline. The combination of clinical examination, noninvasive vascular testing, and arteriography provides both accurate diagnosis and treatment planning. Modern operating facilities with state-of-the-art arteriographic imaging systems can allow vascular specialists to not only diagnose extremity vascular injuries, but also assess visceral perfusion, embolize pelvic bleeding, and even place an inferior vena cava filter when required as skeletal fixation of the extremity is performed. Standard limb revascularization procedures can be expected to restore normal distal arterial perfusion in over 90% of cases, and concommittant fasciotomy should be performed liberally in these cases. While long-term follow-up of trauma patients has been notoriously poor compared to other major vascular surgical procedures, late failure of limb revascularization procedures has not to date been recognized as a major health care problem. These observations continue to justify an aggressive approach to diagnosis and treatment of popliteal injuries with an expectation of excellent results. The most challenging cases remain those with severe associated neuromuscular and skeletal limb injuries where "limb salvage" can often result in a limb that may be attached but is functionless.

REFERENCES

1. DeBakey E, Simeone FA. Battle injuries of the arteries in World War II: An analysis of 2,471 cases. *Ann Surg*. 1946;123:534–579.
2. Hughes CW. Arterial repair during the Korean War. *Ann Surg*. 1958;147:155–561.
3. Rich NM, Baugh JH, Hughes CW. Acute arterial injuries in Vietnam: 1000 cases. *J Trauma*. 1970;10:359–369.
4. Wagner WH, Calkins ER, Weaver FA et al. Blunt popliteal artery trauma: One hundred consecutive injuries. *J Vasc Surg*. 19887: 5.
5. Hafez HM, Woolgar J, Robbs JV. Lower extremity arterial injury: Results of 550 casess and review of risk factors associated with limb loss. *J Vasc Surg*. 2001;33: 6.
6. Malan E, Tattoni G. Physio- and anatomo-pathology of acute ischemia of the extremities. *J Cardiovasc Surg*. 1996;4:214–221.
7. Pretre R, Bruschweiller I, Rossier J, et al. Lower limb trauma with injury to the popliteal popliteal vessels. *J Trauma*. 1996;40:595–601.
8. Majeski JA Gauto A. Management of perpherial arterial vascular injuries with a Javid shunt. *Am J Surg*. 1979;138:324–325.
9. Khalil IM, Livingston DH. Intravascualar shunts in complex lower limb trauma. *J Vasc Surg*. 19864:582–587.
10. Schwartz MR, Weaver FA, Yellin AE et al. Refining the indications for arteriography in penetrating extremity trauma: A prospective analysis. *J Vasc Surg*. 1993;17:166–170.
11. Klineberg EO, Crites BM, Flinn WR et al. The role of arteriography in assessing popliteal artery injury in knee dislocations. *J Trauma*. ?;56(4):786–790.
12. Byone RP, Miles WS, Bell RM, et al. Noninvasive diagnosis of vascular trauma by duplex ultrasonography. *J Vasc Surg*. 1991;123:534.

13. Dennis JW, Jagger C Dutcher JL, et al. Reassessing the role of arteriograms in the management of posterior knee dislocations. *J Trauma*. 1993;35:692.
14. Veterans Administration Cooperative Study Group 141. Comparative evaluation of prosthetic, reversed, an in situ vein bypass grafts in distal popliteal and tibial-peroneal revascularization. *Arch Surg*. 1988;123:434.
15. Yeager JA, Hobson RW, Lynch TG, et al. Popliteal and infrapopliteal arterial injuries: Differential management and amputation rates. *Am Surg*. 1984;50:155–158.
16. Melton SM, Croce MA, Patton JH, et al. Popliteal artery trauma: Systemic anticoagulation and intraoperative thrombolysis improves limb salvage. *Ann Surg*. 1997;225:518–529.
17. Borman KR, Jones GH, Snyder WH. A decade of lower extremity venous trauma. *Am J Surg*. 1987;154:608–612.
18. Edwards JM, Moneta GL. Peripheral venous injury. *Adv Tramua Crit Care*. 1993;8:217–228.
19. Rich NM, Hughes CW, Baugh JH, et al. Repair of lower extremity venous trauma: a more aggressive approach required. *J Trauma*. 1974;14:639–52.
20. Timberlake GA, Kerstein MD. Venous Injury: to repair or ligate, the dilemma revsited. *Am Surg*. 1995;61:139–145.
21. Hossney A. Blunt popliteal artery injury with complete lower limb ischemia: is routine use of temporary intraluminal arterial shunt justified? *J Vasc Surg*. 2004;40(1):?
22. Reber PU, Patel AG, Sapio NLD, et al. Selective use of temporary intravascular shunts in co-incident vascular and orthopedic upper and lower limb trauma. *J Trauma*. 1999;47:72–76.

40

The Management of Upper Extremity Arterial Trauma

David L. Gillespie, M.D., F.A.C.S.

Trauma is the fourth leading cause of all civilian deaths in the United States, and the leading cause of death among children and adults under age 45.[1] The development of endovascular therapies has been rapid over the last few years and has provided clinicians with more options for the treatment of life-threatening vascular injuries. A review of the literature on the endovascular management of upper extremity vascular trauma has shown it to be feasible.[2-4] This method of management in general is more rapid and less morbid than open repair of vascular injuries. It has the ability to accurately define the injury and treat it specifically. Most notably, endovascular management of vascular injuries results in extremely low blood loss in these already critically injured patients. As our comfort with endovascular techniques of managing traumatic injuries grows, however, there is still a great need to be immediately familiar with standard open methods of managing vascular injuries. This chapter will focus on several methods of managing upper extremity vascular trauma and show that there is still an important need for surgeons to be familiar with open surgery in the "endovascular era."

MECHANISM AND DISTRIBUTION OF UPPER EXTREMITY VASCULAR INJURIES

Trauma to the upper extremity in the civilian population is most often due to penetrating injuries (65–95%).[5-7] Blunt trauma accounts for roughly one-fourth of all injuries. Iatrogenic sources of trauma are reported to account for only 10% of vascular injuries in these same series. The majority of civilian firearm injuries is the result of low velocity handguns. Injuries from other causes occur much less frequently including stab wounds (1–28%), blunt trauma (1–23%), and shotguns (1–17%). The most common techniques of arterial repair in civilian injuries depends on mechanism of injury. High velocity gunshot wounds and shotguns tend to require more arterial resection and end-to-end anastomosis, or interposition saphenous vein grafting. Reports on the incidence of vascular injuries to the upper extremity report that injuries to the radial and ulnar arteries account for nearly 50%. Injuries to the brachial artery account for an additional 25% of upper extremity vascular trauma. Subclavian and axillary artery injuries are reported to be much less frequent, in the range of 10% each. Associated injuries in civilian trauma are generally low in comparison to military vascular injuries. Long bone fractures and soft tissue defects occur less common in association with civilian trauma than military trauma. Nerve and venous injuries, however, are nearly equally as frequent.[8-10] Injuries due to close range shotgun blasts are the exception to this as they have a very high incidence of associated bone, nerve, vein, and soft tissue defects approximating that of military trauma.[11]

Vascular injuries suffered during military conflicts are often more devastating, and associated with large soft tissue defects, fracture, and nerve injury. During the first three and a half years of the Afghanistan/Iraq war, known or suspected vascular injuries occurred in 304 (26%).[12] Twenty percent of these patients had injuries to an upper extremity artery. The majority of injuries (74%) was caused by fragments from explosive devices. High velocity gunshot wounds caused upper extremity vascular injuries in 17% patients. Blunt arterial injuries to the upper extremity have been reported very infrequently. Fully one-third of patients with vascular injury had associated bony fracture, and the majority had associated large soft tissue defect.[13] In this series, the subclavian artery was injured in three (5%) patients, axillary artery in eight (11%), brachial artery in 33 (50%), radial artery in 16 (24%), and ulnar in six (10%). To date, the majority of the early management of these injuries was performed by open surgical repair. Endovascular capabilities in the military field environment are still in evolution. Injury management was most often dictated by the arterial bed injured. All acute subclavian injuries in this series were managed by graft interposition. One subclavian artery pseudoaneurysm was diagnosed after evacuation to the United States, and was repaired endovascularly by insertion of stent graft. The majority of axillary artery injuries was repaired by lateral suture repair (37%). Interposition grafting was used in the minority (12%), usually by reversed saphenous vein. Endovascular stent grafting was performed in one patient with a late diagnosed pseudoaneurysm. Over half of the brachial artery injuries (19, 57%) were managed using interposition grafting. The majority of these was performed using reversed autologous saphenous vein. Lateral suture repair was used effectively in 10 (30%) and ligation in one patient. Half of the patients suffering radial artery injuries underwent successful ligation. Another third of patients with radial artery injuries underwent interposition grafting. Lateral suture repair was used in only one patient. Injuries to the ulnar artery were repaired more frequently than radial, most often by saphenous vein interposition graft. One-third of all ulnar artery injuries was successfully ligated while lateral suture repair was only used in a single case.

ENDOVASCULAR MANAGEMENT OF UPPER EXTREMITY VASCULAR INJURIES

A review of the literature finds an ever increasing number of reports on the use of endovascular techniques for the management of upper extremity trauma.[2-4,13-22] This is especially important for injuries to the subclavian artery where exposure is difficult, time-consuming, and potentially morbid. The first report of this application is attributed to Marin et. al.[2] In this article, the authors state that patency up to 14 months was achieved (mean follow-up 6.5 months) with these stented grafts. They found that the use of stented grafts appears to be associated with decreased blood loss, a less invasive insertion procedure, reduced requirements for anesthesia, and a limited need for an extensive dissection in the traumatized field. More recently, this method of management has been used to treat more devastating military injuries both for acute trauma[20] as well as for the management of pseudoaneurysms diagnosed late.[13] Interestingly, these stent grafts have also been reported to be used for the management of concomitant subclavian vein injuries in Iraq.[22]

Vascular access is obtained either at the common femoral or brachial artery in a standard fashion. After placement of a 5 Fr short sheath for access, a diagnostic arteriogram is obtained. A guidewire is placed into the aorta and followed by a 4 Fr pigtail catheter. The catheter is advanced to the root of the aorta to perform a diagnostic arch aortogram. Using a digital subtraction c-arm and a power injector with an injection protocol of 20/40 at 900 psi, the study is obtained. Either the innominate artery or left subclavian artery is selected. If unable to select using the pigtail catheter, the surgeon can choose another catheter such as 4 Fr angled glide catheter. Once selected, an injection protocol of 3/6 should demonstrate the site of the traumatic arteriotomy. Placement of a covered stent across this injury should provide adequate control and allow stabilization of the patient. Preplacement measurements are made in an attempt to preserve the vertebral artery, and not cross the sternoclavicular or acromioclavicular joints. We typically will use a 6–8 × 24 – 50 cm Viabahn™ (Gore) or Fluency™ (BARD) stent graft. The delivery catheter length on these stent grafts is often limiting (80–110 cm); therefore, brachial artery access is the preferred. Heparinization of the patient at 50–100 units/kg can be considered if the patient is stable and has a single injury. However, if the patient has multisystem injury, is coagulopathic, or has suffered large blood loss, no anticoagulation is given. The selected device is delivered to the zone of injury over the wire and a final positioning digital subtraction arteriogram is obtained. Once placement is confirmed, the device is delivered and a completion arteriogram is performed. On occasion, to ensure more accurate placement and collateral vessel preservation, one could consider using two shorter stent grafts and overlapping them (Figure 40–1).

OPERATIVE MANAGEMENT OF UPPER EXTREMITY VASCULAR TRAUMA

There is a robust body of knowledge on the operative management of upper extremity trauma in both civilian and military experience from around the world.[2,9-12,13,23-35] In today's environment, knowledge of how to perform surgical exposures that allow rapid control of vascular structures is extremely important. The decreasing volume of open vascular surgery makes it is even more important that the surgeon be familiar with surgical anatomy and various exposures of the vascular tree.

There are three main areas of exposure of vascular injuries to the upper extremity; the chest, the supraclavicular area, and the arm. The decision of which exposure to use will depend on the surgeon making some observations while examining the patient. In general, the incisions for exposure are placed just proximal to the site of injury in the arm. Through this incision, one can obtain proximal control of the injured vessel before exposing the arterial injury. Injuries to the chest, however, require the surgeon to use

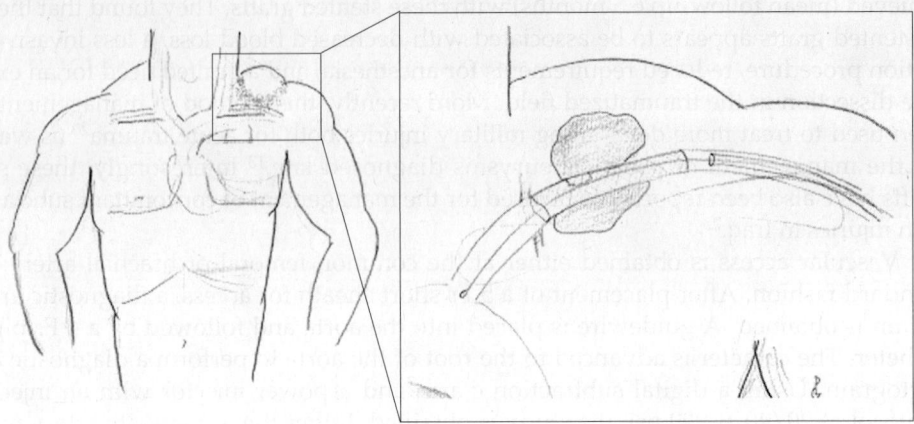

Figure 40-1. Endovascular approach using covered stent to exclude injury to left subclavian artery.

their judgment, and decide whether the injury involves the proximal left subclavian artery or not. This is usually evident, either by the trajectory of the missile or the presence of a hematoma in the left supraclavicular area. Anatomically, the left subclavian artery originates from the distal aortic arch and descends in the posterior mediastinum. This makes vascular control of the proximal left subclavian very difficult through a median sternotomy. Therefore, if the surgeon feels that proximal control of the left subclavian is necessary, a left anterior thoracotomy through the third intercostal space is needed. Injuries to all other major vessels in the chest, including the innominate artery and left and right common carotid artery, can usually be accomplished through a median sternotomy.

MEDIAN STERNOTOMY

Median sternotomy is the preferred method of exposure for suspected injuries to the innominate artery or vein, or right or left common carotid artery origins. An incision is made in the midline of the sternum (Figure 40–2). The sternum is exposed from the sternal notch to the xiphoid. At the ends of the sternum, the dissection is performed bluntly exposing the sternal notch and the subxiphoid area. The anesthesiologist is asked to hold ventilation and the sternum is divided using a sternal saw. Alternatively, the sternum may be divided using a Lipshke knife. The sternum is retracted using a Finochietto retractor. The surgeon should look for a hematoma obscuring the great vessels in the superior mediastinum. The hematoma should be explored in an attempt to identify the left innominate vein. This left innominate vein is a key landmark in the identification of the location of the great vessels. If visualization is obscured due to hematoma, the surgeon may open the pericardium in order to find the aortic root. By tracing the aorta as it ascends from the heart, one can identify the great vessels safely. The left innominate vein may be ligated and divided or retracted so as to give the surgeon greater visibility of the innominate and carotid arteries (Figure 40–3). Proximal control of injuries to these vessels can usually be achieved at their takeoff from the aortic arch using a vascular clamp. This incision may be combined with a left or right

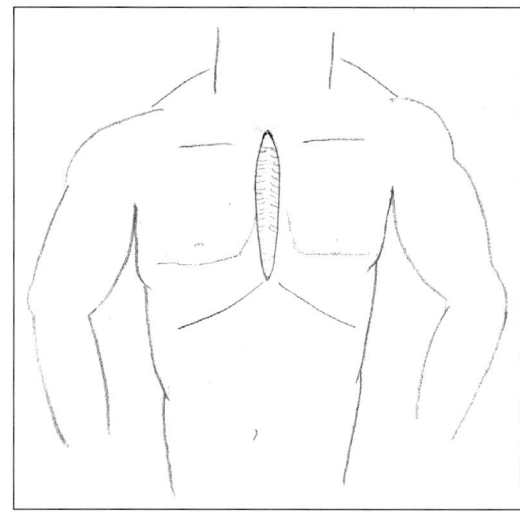

Figure 40-2. Median sternotomy.

supraclavicular incision for distal vascular control and facilitating arterial repair. After obtaining proximal and distal control of the vascular injury, a decision is made whether the injury can be repaired with lateral suture, patch angioplasty, or needs interposition grafting (Figures 40–4 and 40-5).

ANTERIOR THORACOTOMY

As stated previously, if the surgeon suspects injury to the left subclavian artery and there is a need to obtain proximal control at the aortic arch, an anterior thoracotomy is the incision of choice (Figure 40–6). With the patient in a supine position, an incision is made in the third interspace of the anterior surface of the left chest. The intercostal

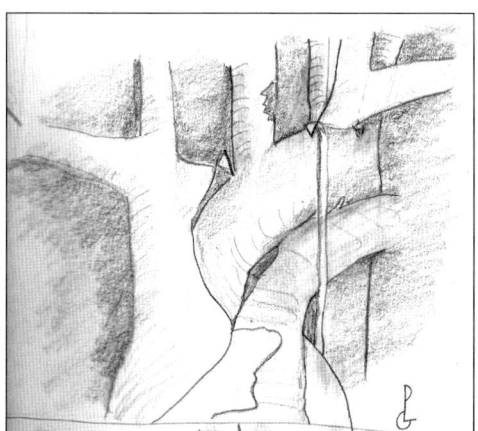
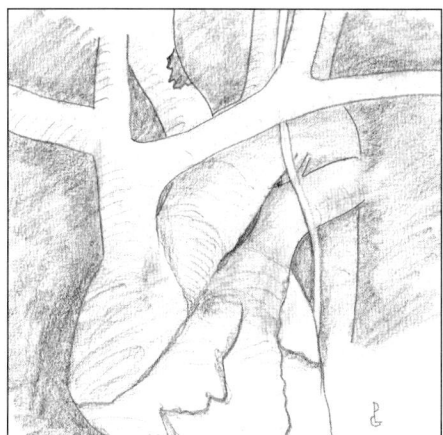

Figure 40-3. Division of the left innominate vein to improve exposure to proximal innominate artery injury through median sternotomy incision.

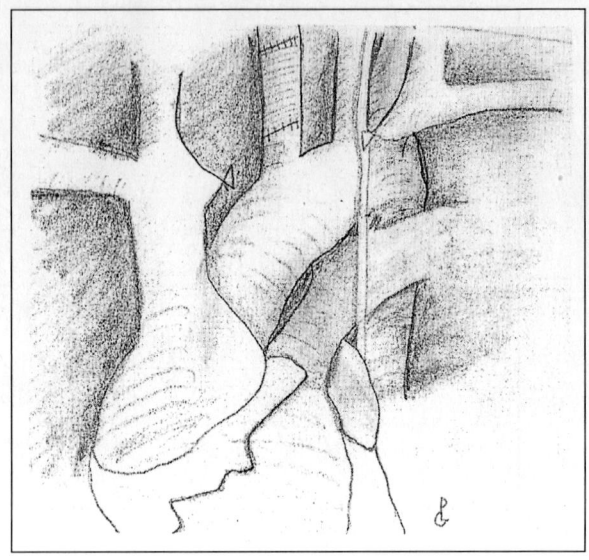

Figure 40-4. Repair of innominate artery injury using prosthetic interposition graft.

musculature is divided on the cephalad aspect of the rib to avoid injury to the intercostal neurovascular bundle. After entering the left chest, a Finochietto retractor is inserted between the ribs to improve exposure. The surgeon should ask the anesthesi-

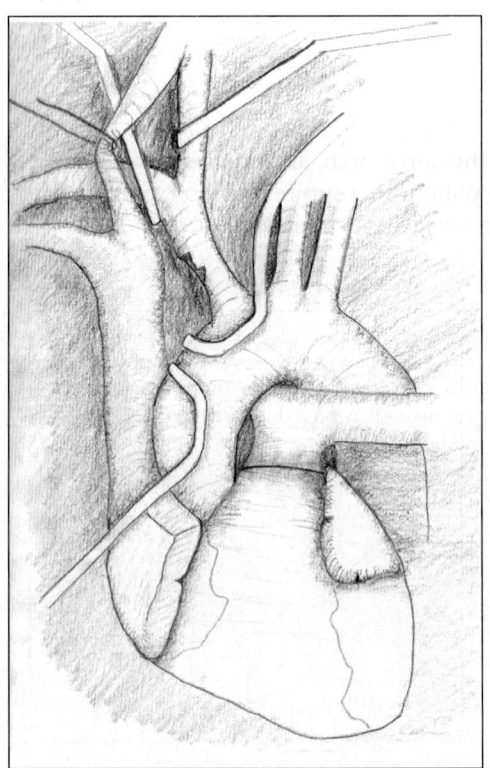 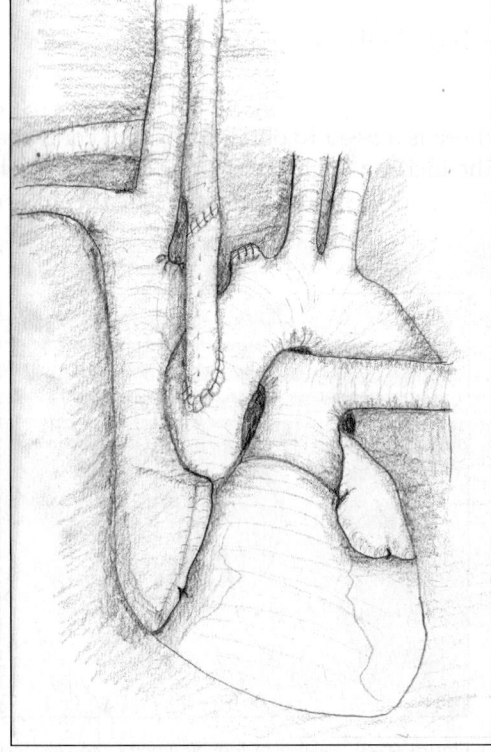

Figure 40-5. Repair of innominate artery injury using aorto-innominate bypass.

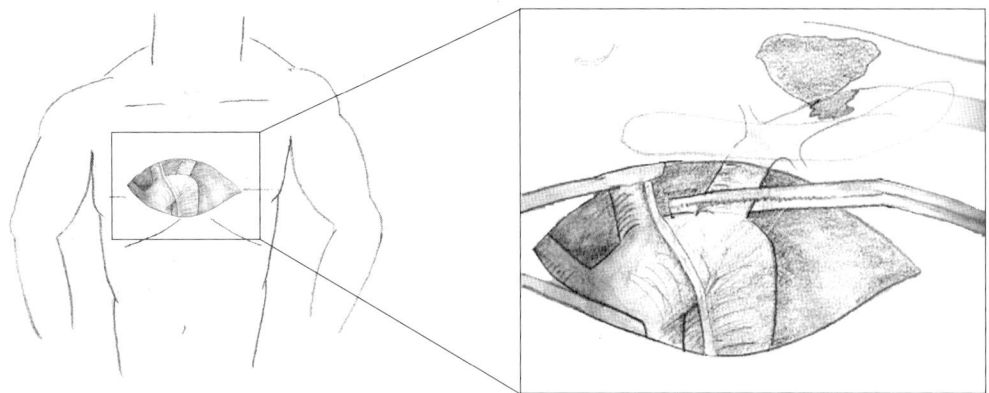

Figure 40-6. Left anterior thoracotomy to obtain proximal control of the left subclavian artery.

ologist to stop ventilating the left lung. The left lung is then retracted inferiorly, and the surgeon should focus his attention medially and cephalad to identify the aortic arch. With a combination of sharp and blunt dissection, the aortic arch and the left subclavian origin are exposed. Proximal control of the left subclavian is achieved using a straight vascular clamp. The surgeon should attempt to identify and protect the vagus nerve as it crosses the aortic arch proximal to the takeoff of the left subclavian. Once proximal control is obtained, attention is then turned to the supraclavicular region and the subclavian artery is exposed to obtain distal control.

SUPRACLAVICULAR APPROACH

The supraclavicular incision is very useful but requires a knowledgeable surgeon to avoid serious injury to important surrounding structures. It is not a surgical exposure to be taken lightly. The surgeon should also think twice about using this exposure if a large hematoma exists as exposure is the key to avoiding collateral injury. If there is significant hematoma in this area, obtaining distal control of the subclavian using an infraclavicular incision more laterally may be more appropriate.

To obtain supraclavicular control of the injured subclavian injury, an incision is made one finger breadth above the clavicle. The incision is carried down to the level of the platysma and it is divided using electrocautery. Exposure is maintained using self-retaining retractors. The scalene fat pad is identified and divided along its inferior and lateral margins. After retracting the scalene fat pad medially, the surgeon should attempt to identify the phrenic nerve as it crosses this region from lateral to medial on the anterior surface of the anterior scalene muscle. Once identified, it is retracted laterally by a vessel loop with the surgeon being cautious not to subject it to undo traction. The anterior scalene muscle is identified and divided from its insertion onto the first rib. The surgeon may need to remove a segment of this muscle to improve exposure of the underlying subclavian artery. Caution should also be used not to put undue traction on the brachial plexus: the roots exit the neck and run laterally to form the cords and innervate the arm. A segment of the subclavian artery should be able to be mobilized so as to allow vascular control. Most branches of the subclavian artery can be ligated with the exception of the vertebral artery. This artery should lie at the most

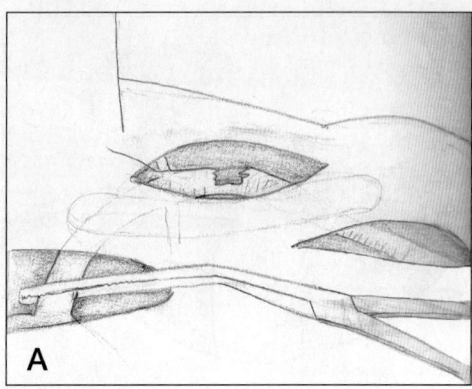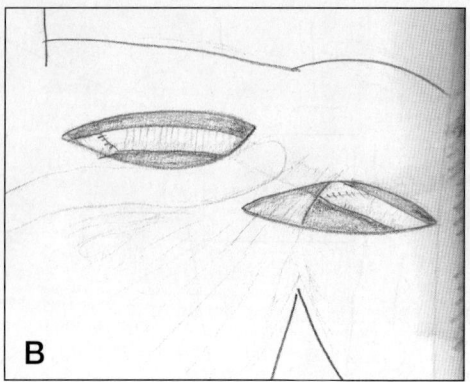

Figure 40-7. (A) Supraclavicular exposure of the subclavian injury after left anterior thoracotomy to obtain proximal control. **(B)** Prosthetic graft interposition repair of subclavian artery injury.

medial and cephalad portion of the subclavian artery adjacent from the internal mammary artery. Again, the surgeon should exercise caution along the medial aspect of this exposure where the thoracic duct on the left or large lymphatics on the right side reside (Figure 40–7A).

Once the subclavian artery is exposed, the surgeon can consider various methods of repair that include lateral suture, ligation and bypass, interposition graft, patch angioplasty, or subclavian transposition. The surgeon must consider the extent of injury, the overall status of the patient, and the need or availability of conduits to perform the operation. In general, there is no difference in long-term patency rate in the subclavian position whether vein or prosthetic is used. Prosthetic is usually larger than the patient's native vein and may be more resistant to infection in the short term. In this case, I usually prefer an 8 mm PTFE externally supported graft (Figure 40–7B). If no conduit is available, the surgeon can consider subclavian artery transposition to the proximal common carotid artery.

Subclavian-to-carotid transposition is performed by exposing the ipsilateral common carotid through the medial aspect of this same incision (Figure 40–8). The subclavian artery is divided proximal to the vertebral artery. The subclavian artery stump is oversewn, using a double suture technique both over and over as well as vertical mattress. Attention is turned to the exposed common carotid artery taking care to avoid injury to the vagus nerve. No cerebral protection is normally used when operating on the common carotid arteries. As long as the patient has no known carotid disease, the rich collateral network from the external to the internal carotid artery should suffice. After obtaining proximal and distal control, an incision is made in the lateral side of the common carotid and enlarged using a 3–4 mm arterial punch. The subclavian artery is then turned up and an end-to-side anastomosis is performed using a running 6–0 Proline suture.

Claviculectomy may be used as an alternate method of exposing distal subclavian artery injuries (Figure 40–9). This exposure has been reported to be associated with minimal blood loss, and permits direct repair of complex injuries of the subclavian artery and veins.[36-37] The procedure is relatively straightforward. An incision is made directly over the clavicle. The dissection is carried down to the level of the periostium using electrocautery. The periosteum is divided longitudinally along the axis of the clavicle. A Gigle saw or equivalent is used to transect the clavicle medially and laterally. This may be

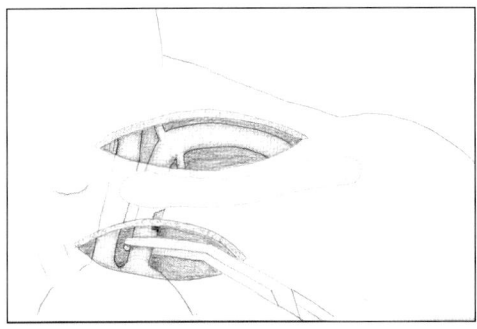
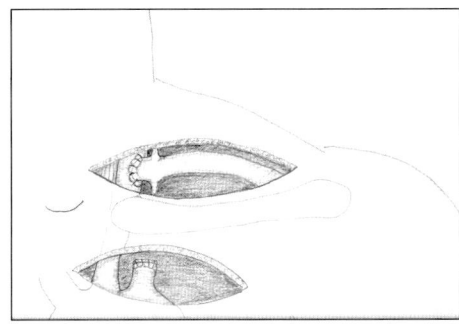

Figure 40-8. Subclavian carotid transposition repair of proximal subclavian injury.

more expedient and less morbid than attempting to remove the entire clavicle at the sternum. The underlying scalenus anticus muscle is identified and divided as it inserts on the first rib. The subclavian artery should then be easily exposed and controlled.

INFRACLAVICULAR INCISION

This exposure is normally used either to assist in repairing[38] distal subclavian artery injuries or to gain control of the proximal axillary artery as it exits the thoracic outlet (Figure 40–7B). An incision is made about 1 cm inferior to the clavicle over the lateral aspect of the deltopectoral groove. The fibers of the pectoralis major are split and the dissection is carried down to the level of the axillary artery. Arterial control can be obtained at this level to provide distal control of subclavian artery injuries or proximal control of vascular injuries more lateral in the arm. The insertion of the pectoralis major and minor can be preserved or divided to provide more exposure as needed. The surgeon should exercise caution to preserve the adjacent axillary nerve and vein.

BRACHIAL ARTERY INCISION

Exposure of vascular injuries of the upper arm and forearm are simpler than obtaining proximal control in the chest. Vascular control of the brachial artery should be

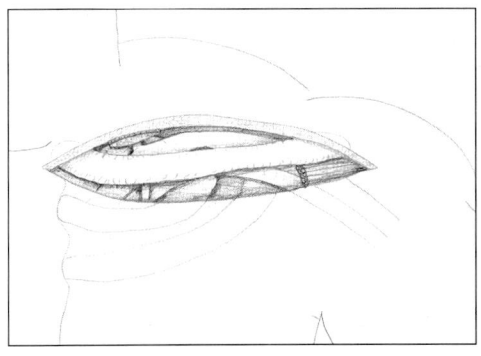
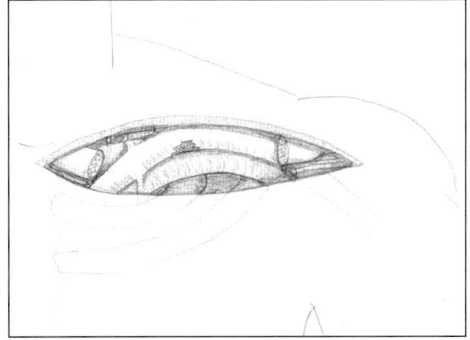

Figure 40-9. Claviculectomy for subclavian artery exposure.

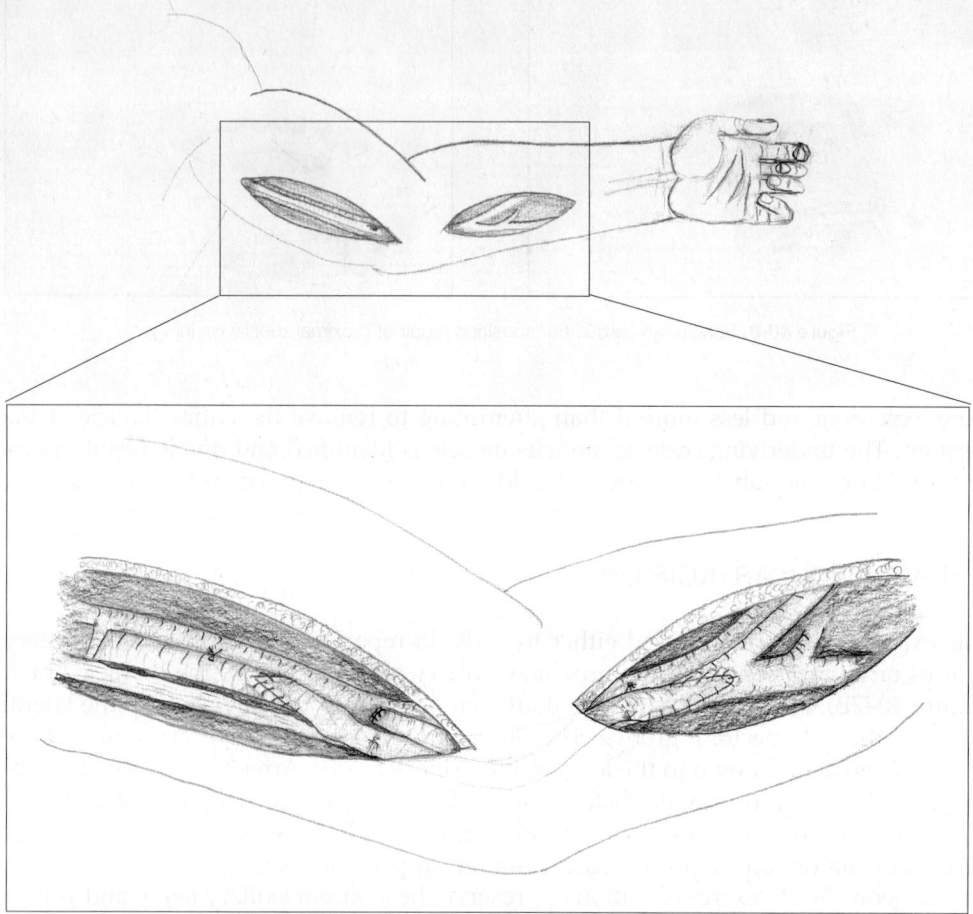

Figure 40-10. Brachial artery bypass using reversed saphenous vein.

obtained through clean tissue planes proximal to the zone of injury. An incision is made in the bicepital groove and the brachial artery is exposed, being careful not to injury the adjacent median nerve and paired brachial veins. Once exposed, vascular control can be achieved rapidly with a vascular clamp. Distal control of the brachial artery is obtained in a similar fashion through clean tissue planes away from the zone of injury. The artery is then exposed and the method of repair chosen. Interposition grafting, patch angioplasty, or lateral suture repair techniques are selected, depending on the extent of damage to the native artery (Figure 40–10).

FOREARM FASCIOTOMY

After revascularization of the upper extremity, assessment of the distal forearm and hand are essential to achieve successful limb salvage. It may be apparent at the time of revascularization that the extent of injury to the forearm requires a fasciotomy be per-

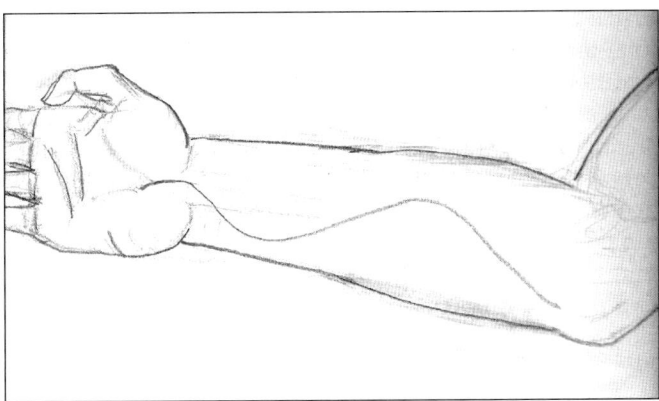

Figure 40-11. Forearm fasciotomy.

formed. More likely, the surgeon will have to make a decision based on the duration of ischemia. Although performed less frequently than in the lower extremity, the decision as to whether to perform forearm fasciotomies should not be taken lightly.[10,39-43] Monitoring of the patient may not be constant due to transportation issues, thereby leaving the patient at high risk for further muscle necrosis or nerve injury.

To perform forearm fasciotomies, an incision is made on the dorsal and volar aspects of the forearm. The volar incision is made in a curvilinear fashion in an attempt to provide adequate exposure and decompression of the flexor muscles and neurovasculature of the forearm (Figure 46–11). Using electrocautery, the dissection is carried down through the skin and subcutaneous tissue to the level of the fascia. The fascia is incised the length of the forearm from proximal to the elbow in a "lazy S" fashion, crossing from the ulnar side of the forearm to the radial side, and then back toward the ulnar side at the wrist. Finally, the incision is extended through the flexor retinaculum at the wrist to the middle of the palm so as to decompress the median nerve in the carpal tunnel. Caution should be used when extending this incision onto the palm of the hand not to injure the superficial palmar branch of the median nerve as it lies at the base of the third finger located in the palm. If the underlying muscle has been ischemic, it may immediately bulge out as the pressure in the compartment is released. Once the fasciotomies are complete, the surgeon should reconfirm good perfusion of the hand with palpable pulses. Examination of the epimysium of each of the underlying muscle bellies may reveal that they are also under tension. In the current conflict, this has been observed to be an additional source of late myonecrosis. In these cases, an epimysiotomy should be performed to ensure there is not a local unrecognized compartment syndrome. The use of vessel loops to place mild tension on the skin edges may assist in minimizing some of the morbidity of large gaping forearm fasciotomies, with the obvious caution not to cause a secondary compartment syndrome by using overzealous skin tension.[41] The incisions are then dressed with moist dressing or wound VAC™ prior to patient transport.[44-45]

CONCLUSION

The incidence trauma in the United States continues to increase. The development of catheter-based techniques for the treatment of vascular injuries has been revolutionary.

While current reports show these techniques to be successful, there are relatively little long-term data on the use of covered stents for the treatment of vascular injuries. In addition, widespread use of endovascular therapies for the treatment of innominate vein or artery injuries have not been reported. Finally, the widespread availability of stent grafts and radiographic equipment for use in emergency situations is still in the process of evolving. As such, even in the era of endovascular surgery, vascular surgeons must maintain their familiarity with open approaches to repairing vascular injuries. Our profession must remain vigilant and provide the best care for the vascularly injured patient that we can. This will only come about by recognizing vascular trauma as a priority for both training and maintenance of both open and endovascular surgical skill sets.

REFERENCES

1. Rice DP, MacKenzie EJ, et al. *Cost of Injury in the United States: A Report to Congress*. Institute for Health & Aging, University of California and Injury Prevention Center: The Johns Hopkins University; 1989. Ref Type: Generic
2. Marin ML, Veith FJ, Panetta TF et al. Transluminally placed endovascular stented graft repair for arterial trauma. *J Vasc Surg*. 1994;20(3):466–472.
3. Patel AV, Marin ML, Veith FJ, et al. Endovascular graft repair of penetrating subclavian artery injuries. *J Endovasc Surg*. 1996;3(4):382–388.
4. Ohki T, Veith FJ, Marin ML, et al. Endovascular approaches for traumatic arterial lesions. *Semin Vasc Surg*. 1997;10(4):272–285.
5. Hammond DC, Gould JS, Hanel DP. Management of acute and chronic vascular injuries to the arm and forearm. Indications and technique. *Hand Clin*. 1992;8(3):453–463.
6. Orcutt MB, Levine BA, Gaskill HV, Sirinek KR. Civilian vascular trauma of the upper extremity. *J Trauma*. 1986;26(1):63–67.
7. Borman KR, Snyder WH, III, Weigelt JA. Civilian arterial trauma of the upper extremity. An 11 year experience in 267 patients. *Am J Surg*. 1984;148(6):796–799.
8. Sitzmann JV, Ernst CB. Management of arm arterial injuries. *Surgery*. 1984;96(5):895–901.
9. Bongard F, Dubrow T, Klein S. Vascular injuries in the urban battleground: experience at a metropolitan trauma center. *Ann Vasc Surg*. 1990;4(5):415–418.
10. Myers SI, Harward TR, Maher DP, et al. Complex upper extremity vascular trauma in an urban population. *J Vasc Surg*. 1990;12(3):305–309.
11. Meyer JP, Lim LT, Schuler JJ et al. Peripheral vascular trauma from close-range shotgun injuries. *Arch Surg*. 1985;120(10):1126–1131.
12. Weber MA, Fox CJ, Adams E et al. Upper extremity arterial combat injury management. *Perspect Vasc Surg Endovasc Ther*. 2006;18(2):141–145.
13. Fox CJ, Gillespie DL, O'Donnell SD et al. Contemporary management of wartime vascular trauma. *J Vasc Surg*. 2005;41(4):638–644.
14. Ohki T, Veith FJ, Kraas C et al. Endovascular therapy for upper extremity injury. *Semin Vasc Surg*. 1998;11(2):106–115.
15. Dinkel HP, Eckstein FS, Triller J, Do DD. Emergent axillary artery stent-graft placement for massive hemorrhage from an avulsed subscapular artery. *J Endovasc Ther*. 2002;9(1):129–133.
16. Aerts NR, Poli de Figueiredo LF, Burihan E. Emergency room retrograde transbrachial arteriography for the management of axillosubclavian vascular injuries. *J Trauma*. 2003;55(1):69–73.
17. McArthur CS, Marin ML. Endovascular therapy for the treatment of arterial trauma. *Mt Sinai J Med*. 2004;71(1):4–11.
18. Valentin MD, Tulsyan N, James K. Endovascular management of traumatic axillary artery dissection—a case report and review of the literature. *Vasc Endovascular Surg*. 2004;38(5):473–475.

19. Danetz JS, Cassano AD, Stoner MC, et al. Feasibility of endovascular repair in penetrating axillosubclavian injuries: a retrospective review. *J Vasc Surg*. 2005;41(2):246–254.

20. Clouse WD, Rasmussen TE, Perlstein J et al. Upper extremity vascular injury: a current in-theater wartime report from Operation Iraqi Freedom. *Ann Vasc Surg*. 2006;20(4):429–434.

21. Starnes BW, Arthurs ZM. Endovascular management of vascular trauma. *Perspect Vasc Surg Endovasc Ther*. 2006;18(2):114–129.

22. Eliason JL, Rasmussen TE. *Stentgraft treatment of traumatic subclavian vein injury in Iraq*. 2007. Ref Type: Personal Communication

23. Diamond S, Gaspard D, Katz S. Vascular injuries to the extremities in a suburban trauma center. *Am Surg*. 2003;69(10):848–851.

24. Lin PH, Koffron AJ, Guske PJ et al. Penetrating injuries of the subclavian artery. *Am J Surg*. 2003;185(6):580–584.

25. Nanobashvili J, Kopadze T, Tvaladze M, et al. War injuries of major extremity arteries. *World J Surg*. 2003;27(2):134–139.

26. Katras T, Baltazar U, Rush DS et al. Subclavian arterial injury associated with blunt trauma. *Vasc Surg*. 2001;35(1):43–50.

27. Hyre CE, Cikrit DF, Lalka SG, et al. Aggressive management of vascular injuries of the thoracic outlet. *J Vasc Surg*. 1998;27(5):880–884.

28. Pillai L, Luchette FA, Romano KS, Ricotta JJ. Upper-extremity arterial injury. *Am Surg*. 1997;63(3):224–227.

29. Fitridge RA, Raptis S, Miller JH, Faris I. Upper extremity arterial injuries: experience at the Royal Adelaide Hospital, 1969 to 1991. *J Vasc Surg*. 1994;20(6):941–946.

30. Andreev A, Kavrakov T, Karakolev J, Penkov P. Management of acute arterial trauma of the upper extremity. *Eur J Vasc Surg*. 1992;6(6):593–598.

31. Sturm JT, Dorsey JS, Olson FR, Perry JF, Jr. The management of subclavian artery injuries following blunt thoracic trauma. *Ann Thorac Surg*. 1984;38(3):188–191.

32. Graham JM, Mattox KL, Feliciano DV, DeBakey ME. Vascular injuries of the axilla. *Ann Surg*. 1982;195(2):232–238.

33. Adar R, Schramek A, Khodadadi J, et al. Arterial combat injuries of the upper extremity. *J Trauma*. 1980;20(4):297–302.

34. Graham JM, Feliciano DV, Mattox KL, et al. Management of subclavian vascular injuries. *J Trauma*. 1980;20(7):537–544.

35. Rich NM, Hobson RW, Jarstfer BS, Geer TM. Subclavian artery trauma. *J Trauma*. 1973;13(6):485–496.

36. Buscaglia LC, Walsh JC, Wilson JD, Matolo NM. Surgical management of subclavian artery injury. *Am J Surg*. 1987;154(1):88–92.

37. George SM, Jr., Croce MA, Fabian TC et al. Cervicothoracic arterial injuries: recommendations for diagnosis and management. *World J Surg*. 1991;15(1):134–139.

38. Wall MJ, Jr., Granchi T, Liscum K, Mattox KL. Penetrating thoracic vascular injuries. *Surg Clin North Am*. 1996;76(4):749–761.

39. Dente CJ, Feliciano DV, Rozycki GS et al. A review of upper extremity fasciotomies in a level I trauma center. *Am Surg*. 2004;70(12):1088–1093.

40. Fields CE, Latifi R, Ivatury RR. Brachial and forearm vessel injuries. Surg Clin North Am. 2002;82(1):105–114.

41. Asgari MM, Spinelli HM. The vessel loop shoelace technique for closure of fasciotomy wounds. *Ann Plast Surg*. 2000;44(2):225–229.

42. Demirkilic U, Kuralay E, Yilmaz AT, et al. Surgical approach to military vascular injuries. *Cardiovasc Surg*. 1998;6(4):342–346.

43. Feliciano DV, Cruse PA, Spjut-Patrinely V, et al. Fasciotomy after trauma to the extremities. *Am J Surg*. 1988;156(6):533–536.

44. Fleck T, Gustafsson R, Harding K et al. The management of deep sternal wound infections using vacuum assisted closure (V.A.C.) therapy. *Int Wound J*. 2006;3(4):273–280.

45. Kneser U, Leffler M, Bach AD, et al. [Vacuum assisted closure (V.A.C.) therapy is an essential tool for treatment of complex defect injuries of the upper extremity]. *Zentralbl Chir*. 2006;131 Suppl 1:S7–12.

Upper Extremity
Ischemia

41

Quality Measures in Thoracic Outlet Syndrome

Julie Ann Freischlag, M.D.

The thoracic outlet syndrome (TOS) comprises a myriad of signs and symptoms related to compression of key anatomic structures that pass through a narrow space into the upper extremity. Three types of TOS are recognized: neurogenic, venous, and arterial. The neurogenic form is the most controversial as it has been difficult to diagnose by objective methods until recently. Additionally, no good tool or metric has previously been developed to assess improvement following surgical intervention in either the short or long term.

ANATOMY

The thoracic outlet is defined as the anatomic space that extends from the edge of the first rib to the upper mediastinum medially and the fifth cervical nerve superiorly. The roof of the space is the first rib and subclavius muscle, and the floor is determined by the superior surface of the first rib. Machleder was the first to describe this area as a triangle with its apex pointing toward the manubrium, which also lends to the understanding of how the dynamics in this area can lead to injury.[1] The clavicle and subclavius tendon overlap the first rib medially, and this relationship results in a fulcrum, similar to a pair of scissors opening and closing, causing the compression (Figure 41–1).

Most TOS symptoms are due to nerve compression. The brachial plexus lies lateral to the anterior scalene muscle which inserts onto the first rib. The C4–C6 nerve roots are superiorly oriented and the C7–T roots are inferiorly oriented. Posteriorly lateral to the brachial plexus is the middle scalene muscle, which broadly attaches to the first rib. The long thoracic nerve can be entwined in this muscle as it emerges to innervate the serratus anterior muscle.

Most patients with neurogenic TOS have some sort of soft tissue anomaly associated with an injury. Cervical ribs are only present in 10% of patients.[2] Multiple bands

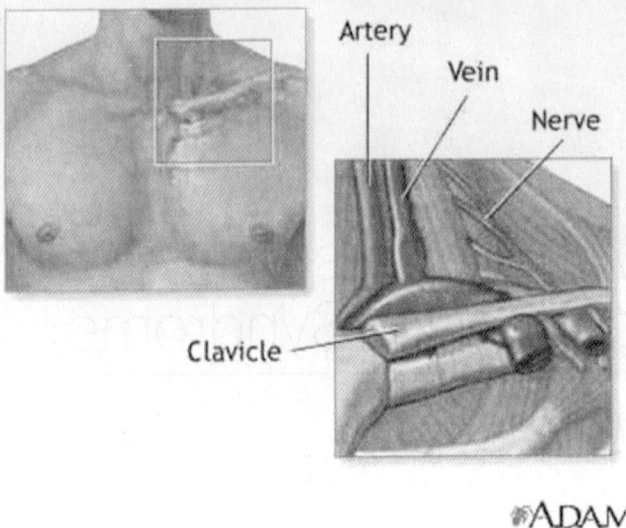

Figure 41-1. Diagram depicting the anatomy of the thoracic outlet space.

can be found that transverse the thoracic outlet and cause compression of the structures, especially the nerves as they can become trapped between the bands, muscles, and bony structures. The muscles themselves can cause compression by their presence between nerve roots and becoming attached to them. Hypertrophy of the muscle can cause compression as well, and this can be due to repetitive motion activity that involves athletics.

Trauma is implicated in many cases of neurogenic TOS, especially with injuries caused by hyperextension or whiplash. Additionally, repetitive motion type injuries due to occupational or recreational activities can play a significant role in those with neurogenic TOS.[3] In Machleder's series, no anatomic defect was found in 34% of patients, cervical ribs in 8.5%, scalene minimus in 10%, defect in the subclavius tendon or its insertion 19.5%, developmental defect or insertional defect in the scalene musculature in 43%, and unclear anatomic configurations in 7.5%.[4]

PRESENTATION

Patients can present with neurogenic TOS at any age although most patients are young to middle age with few other medical conditions. The symptoms can vary from intermittent discomfort to debilitating pain. Weakness can be present but nerve damage is rare. Pain originates in the back of the shoulder along the suprascapular portion of the trapezius muscle into the face, back of the head, and the arm. Headaches can be the most significant complaint. Lower plexus (C8–T1) symptoms in the arm tend to be more common than upper plexus (C5–C7), and are distributed in the ulnar nerve area of the fourth and fifth fingers with numbness and weakness. Stress due to overhead activity can exacerbate symptoms that may be present at rest. Some form of paresthesia is seen in over 90% of patients with similar numbers with complaints of upper limb pain. Suprascapular pain is reported by 80% of patients and headaches in 65%.[5]

DIAGNOSIS

An extensive history needs to be taken from the patient that includes any injuries that have occurred and the nature of the patient's occupation. Those activities that worsen the pain should be noted. The physical examination is important to confirm or deny the diagnosis of TOS and to identify any other possible etiology responsible for the symptoms the patient reports. The patient's general appearance should be noted with attention to the symmetry of the muscle groups of the shoulders and upper extremities. Serratus anterior atrophy can occasionally be present with TOS as noted by a winged scapula. Limited cervical range of motion and excessive tenderness over the cervical bodies is not characteristic of TOS and should be related to cervical spine disease as an alternative diagnosis. Grip strength, deep tendon reflexes, and pulses should be noted.

The region over the scalene muscle can be very tender. The most useful provocative test is the elevated arm stress test (EAST), which was originally described by Roos in 1966. Patients without TOS can do this maneuver for three minutes without pain or paresthesias. Those with TOS cannot, and within seconds may have weakness and paresthesias in the ulnar and median nerve distributions. The color of the hands is important, too, as pallor can indicate arterial compromise as well. The abduction and external rotation test—holding the arm in abduction and external rotation—can be helpful as well to elicit TOS symptoms. The Adson's sign is not as helpful as many patients without TOS symptoms will obliterate their pulse. One may hear a bruit with manipulation of the arm in the infraclavicular area that can better identify those with TOS.

Additionally, we administer a questionnaire that has been approved by the IRB to assess the patient's baseline functionality (Figures 41–2 through 41–5). These

TOS PATIENT FORM V3

LAST NAME	FIRST NAME

MRN	DOB	SEX
		(F) (M)

TODAY'S DATE	DATE OF SURGERY IF APPLICABLE

Please darken the one circle that best describes your/the patient's race.

American Indian or Alaskan Native	Asian	Black or African American	Hispanic	Native Hawaiian	White	More than one race	Prefer not to answer
①	②	③	④	⑤	⑥	⑦	⑧

Figures 41-2 through 41-5. SF 12 (short form 12) and DASH (Disability of the Arm, Shoulder and Hand).

TOS PATIENT FORM V3

1. In general, would you say your health is:

Excellent	Very Good	Good	Fair	Poor
①	②	③	④	⑤

2. The following questions are about activities you might do during a typical day. Does your health now limit you in these activities? If so, how much?

	Yes, limited a lot	Yes, limited a little	No, not limited at all
Moderate activities, such as moving a table, pushing a vacuum cleaner, bowling, or playing golf?	①	②	③
Climbing several flights of stairs.	①	②	③

3. During the past four weeks, have you had any of the following problems with your work or other regular daily activities as a result of your physical health?

	Yes	No
Accomplished less than you would like?	①	②
Were limited in the kind of work or other activities?	①	②

4. During the past four weeks, have you had any of the following problems with your work or other regular daily activities as a result of any emotional problems (such as feeling depressed or anxious)?

	Yes	No
Accomplished less than you would like?	①	②
Did work or other activities less carefully than usual?	①	②

5. During the past four weeks, how much did pain interfere with your normal work (including both work outside the home and housework)?

Not at all	A little bit	Moderately	Quite a bit	Extremely
①	②	③	④	⑤

6. These questions are about how you feel and how things have been with you during the past four weeks. For each question, please fill in the appropriate bubble to the one answer that comes closest to describing the way you have been feeling. How much of the time during the past four weeks...

	All of the time	Most of the time	A good bit of the time	Some of the time	None of the time
Have you felt calm and peaceful?	①	②	③	④	⑤
Did you have a lot of energy?	①	②	③	④	⑤
Have you felt downhearted and blue?	①	②	③	④	⑤

7. During the past four weeks, how much of the time has your physical health or emotional problems interfered with your social activities (e.g. visiting relatives, friends)?

All of the time	Most of the time	Some of the time	A little of the time	None of the time
①	②	③	④	⑤

TOS PATIENT FORM V3

Please indicate the importance of each of the following activities, and rate your ability to do them in the last week by circling the appropriate response.

Activities	Importance to me 1 = High importance 2 = Average importance 3 = Low importance	1 = No difficulty 2 = Mild difficulty 3 = Moderate difficulty 4 = Severe difficulty 5 = Unable
Open a tight or new jar	① ② ③	① ② ③ ④ ⑤
Write	① ② ③	① ② ③ ④ ⑤
Turn a key	① ② ③	① ② ③ ④ ⑤
Prepare a meal	① ② ③	① ② ③ ④ ⑤
Push open a heavy door	① ② ③	① ② ③ ④ ⑤
Place an object on a shelf above your head	① ② ③	① ② ③ ④ ⑤
Do heavy household chores (e.g., wash walls, wash floors)	① ② ③	① ② ③ ④ ⑤
Garden or do yard work	① ② ③	① ② ③ ④ ⑤
Make a bed	① ② ③	① ② ③ ④ ⑤
Carry a shopping bag or briefcase	① ② ③	① ② ③ ④ ⑤
Carry a heavy object (over 10 lbs)	① ② ③	① ② ③ ④ ⑤
Change a light bulb overhead	① ② ③	① ② ③ ④ ⑤
Wash or blow dry your hair	① ② ③	① ② ③ ④ ⑤
Wash your back	① ② ③	① ② ③ ④ ⑤
Put on a pullover sweater	① ② ③	① ② ③ ④ ⑤
Use a knife to cut food	① ② ③	① ② ③ ④ ⑤
Recreational activities which require little effort (e.g. card-playing, knitting, etc.)	① ② ③	① ② ③ ④ ⑤
Recreational activities in which you take some force or impact through your arm, shoulder, or hand (e.g. golf, hammering, tennis, etc.)	① ② ③	① ② ③ ④ ⑤
Recreational activities in which you move your arm freely	① ② ③	① ② ③ ④ ⑤
Manage transportation needs (able to get from one place to another)	① ② ③	① ② ③ ④ ⑤
Sexual activities	① ② ③	① ② ③ ④ ⑤
Driving a car	① ② ③	① ② ③ ④ ⑤
Typing on a computer keyboard	① ② ③	① ② ③ ④ ⑤
Hold a cup or a glass	① ② ③	① ② ③ ④ ⑤
Carrying a toddler	① ② ③	① ② ③ ④ ⑤

TOS PATIENT FORM V3

Please complete the following questions by darkening the appropriate bubble.

During the past week, to what extent has your arm, shoulder or hand problem interfered with your normal social activities with family, friends, neighbours or groups?	Not at all ①	Slightly ②	Moderately ③	Quite a bit ④	Extremely ⑤
During the past week, were you limited in your work or other regular daily activities as a result of your arm, shoulder or hand problem?	①	②	③	④	⑤

Please rate the severity of the following symptoms in the last week					
Arm, shoulder or hand pain	None ①	Mild ②	Moderate ③	Severe ④	Extreme ⑤
Arm, shoulder or hand pain when you performed any specific activity	①	②	③	④	⑤
Tingling (pins and needles) in your arm, shoulder or hand	①	②	③	④	⑤
Weakness in your arm, shoulder or hand	①	②	③	④	⑤
Stiffness in your arm, shoulder or hand	①	②	③	④	⑤

During the past week, how much difficulty have you had sleeping because of the pain in your arm, shoulder or hand?	No difficulty	Mild difficulty	Moderate difficulty	Severe difficulty	So much difficulty that I can't sleep
	①	②	③	④	⑤

I feel less capable, less confident or less useful because of my arm, shoulder or hand problem	Strongly disagree	Disagree	Neither agree nor disagree	Agree	Strongly agree
	①	②	③	④	⑤

questionnaires include the Short Form 12 (SF–12) and the Disability of the Arm, Shoulder, and Hand (DASH). A prospective observational study we did on 59 patients (44 women, 75%) revealed the physical component score (PCS) was 36.5 +/− 9.3, which is below 90% of the general population and is similar to patients with chronic heart failure. The mental component score (MCS) was 49.5 +/− 9.99, which was not different from the general population. ($p = 0.70$). The mean score for the DASH form was 41.1 +/−21.1, which is similar to those patients with chronic rotator cuff tears. The PCS was significantly associated with the DASH ($p<0.001$). These questionnaires will be administered to patients postoperatively to assess at three, six, 12, 18, and 24 months.

Other objective diagnostic testing should include a cervical spine film and a chest radiograph. MRI has not proven helpful except in a few unusual cases. Electrodiagnostic testing is mainly used to exclude other disease states as most patients with TOS will have normal electrodiagnostic studies. A recent study by Franklin and colleagues of 158 TOS patients found that only 7.6% had abnormalities in their electrodiagnostic tests.[5] Somatosensory evoked potentials (SSEPs) historically have played a role in the confirmation of a TOS diagnosis. Siivola was the first to demonstrate that multiple position recordings could be used to locate peripheral nerve deficits related to the brachial plexus.[6] Machleder and colleagues demonstrated that 74% of their patients who were thought to have TOS by history and physical examination had abnormal SSEPs. Additionally, when these patients were studied following transaxillary first rib resection and scalenectomy, over 90% had improvement in their symptoms that correlated with a change in their SSEPs to normal.[7] SSEPs can also be used in patients with signs and symptoms of recurrent TOS.

TREATMENT

Conservative treatment of patients with neurogenic TOS should always be initiated for at least six to eight weeks. This includes physical therapy that is specifically focused on relaxing muscle groups that tighten the thoracic outlet. Aligne and Barral described a program where the trapezius, levator scapulae, and sternocleidomastoid muscles are strengthened, and the middle scalene, subclavius, and pectoralis muscles are relaxed.[8] Anterior scalene blocks can be diagnostic with lidocaine and predictive of a good outcome following surgery. The use of botulinium toxin in the anterior scalene muscle has been shown to relieve symptoms in two-thirds of patients for a mean duration of 88 days.[9]

Successful surgical intervention requires a complete resection of the first rib, anterior scalene muscle, and any abnormal connective tissue and muscle bands. Using a special retractor (Figure 41–6), good visualization is obtained and injury to any of the vital structures is avoided.

We performed a retrospective analysis of the National Inpatient Sample Database between 1999–2003 from hospitals in 37 states with representative samples. TOS patients were selected by ICD 9 diagnosis of 353.0 or 353.3. Rib resection was also selected by ICD 9 code. Complications were identified by ICD 9 codes 953.4 or 997.09 for brachial plexus injury and 998.11 and 998.12 for vascular injury. A total of 2,016 TOS operations were identified ranging from 317 to 468 per year. Mean age was 37.3 with 1,409 (70.2%) women and 1,270 (63.0%) Caucasian. These patients were treated in 392 hospitals with an average volume of 1.03 cases per hospital per year (range 0–114 cases

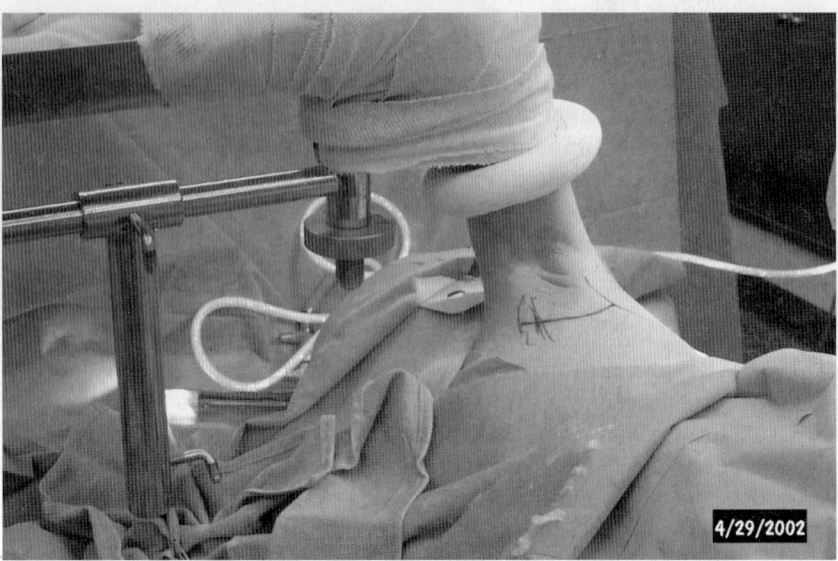

Figure 41-6. Thoracic outlet arm retractor.

per hospital per year). Their mean hospital stay was 2.51 days (median two days) with a mean total hospital charge of $16,160 in inflation, adjusted year 2005 dollars (median $11,824). The majority were treated at a teaching hospital (1,421 or 70.5%). There were two deaths (0.10%), 12 brachial plexus injuries (0.60%), and 35 vascular injuries (1.74%). The rate of vascular injuries was significantly lower among teaching hospitals (1.34% vs. 2.69% $p = 0.03$) and in women (1.35% vs. 2.67% $p = 0.03$). Vascular injuries had a significantly longer length of stay (7.7 days vs. 2.4 days $p<0.001$) and higher total hospital charges ($53,373 vs. $15,507, $p<0.001$) while no such difference was seen among those patients with brachial plexus injury.

RECURRENT TOS

Recurrent symptoms of TOS occur in approximately 10% of patients with a range of 2% to 20% that have been published.[10,11] The etiology of recurrence is not entirely clear; however, the main theory is that of scar tissue formation. Sometimes, the patient has suffered another injury similar to that previously, and the symptoms begin again. Conservative therapy with physical therapy and soft tissue massage should be initiatiated. Injections with botulinum toxin can aid in facilitating the ability of the patient to do the physical therapy. Reoperations by best reports result in improvement in symptoms in only 50% of patients and should be used only if conservative measures fail.

Prevention of recurrent TOS and scar tissue is, of course, the best treatment plan. Intense physical therapy following the initial operation with maintenance of the stretching and strengthening exercises is essential to prevent recurrent symptoms. No other topical agents that can be used at the time of operation have been shown to be efficacious.

PROGNOSIS

There are a few series reporting recurrence rates in TOS following surgical intervention. Sanders reported an immediate postoperative success rate of 84% decreased to 59% at two years, 69% at five years, and as low as 41% at the 10–15 year interval using life table analysis. Reoperations for these patients resulted in improvement in 86% of patients at five to 10 years. Patients with symptoms that were persistent rather than recurrent tended to do worse following reoperation.[11]

In a study by Sharp and colleagues, patients were able to return to work 80% of the time and 85% described their outcome as good to excellent.[12] In the study of Washington state workers, 40% of patients were still not working two years after the operation and 44% were not working at four years. Other studies have shown poorer results in patients with work-related or legal issues that complicate their TOS picture.[13,14] Roos reported his results in 1,844 patients and 90% were able to return to a level of activity that was markedly improved following surgical intervention. There was a 5% recurrence in this group of patients.[15]

SUMMARY

Outcomes in TOS surgery depend on making an accurate diagnosis, having a motivated patient, performing a complete and successful operation, and attention to extensive physical therapy in the postoperative period. Outcomes will only be specifically known as a tools such as our SF12 and DASH are used over time to confirm our results.

REFERENCES

1. Machleder HI. *Vascular Disorders of the Upper Extremity, 3rd Edition*. Future Press: Mt. Kiscon, New York; 1999.
2. Roos DB. Historical perspectives and anatomic considerations. Thoracic outlet syndrome. *Sem in Thor Cardiovasc Surg*. 1996;8:183–189.
3. Sanders RJ, Haug CE, Pearce WH, et al. Recurrent thoracic outlet syndrome. *J Vasc Surg*. 1990;12:390–400.
4. Machleder HI. Thoracic outlet syndrome's new concepts from a century of discovery. *Cardiovasc Surg*. 1994;2:137–145.
5. Franklin GM, Fulton-Kehoe D, Bradley C et al. Outcome of surgery for thoracic outlet syndrome in Washington State workers compensation. *Neurology*. 2000;54:1252–1257.
6. Siivola J, Myelyla VV, Sulg I et al. Brachial plexus and radicular neurography in relation to cortical evoked responses. *J Neurol Neurosurg Psychiatry*. 1979;42(12):1151–1158.
7. Machleder HI, Mill F, Nuwer M et al. Somatosensory evoked potentials in the potentials in the assessment of thoracic outlet compression syndrome. *J Vasc Surg*. 1987;6:177–184.
8. Aligne C, Barral. Rehabilitation of patients with Thoracic outlet syndrome. *Ann Vasc Surg*. 1992;6:381–389.
9. Jordan SE, Ahn SS, Freischlag JA et al. Selective botulinum chemodenervation of the scalene muscles for treatment of neurogenic thoracic outlet syndrome. *Ann Vas Surg*. 2000;14:365–369.
10. Lindgren KA, Leino E, Lepantalo M et al. Recurrent thoracic outlet syndrome after first rib resection. *Arch Phy Med Rehabil*. 1991;72:208–210.

11. Roos DB. Recurrent thoracic outlet syndrome after first rib resection. *Acta Chir Belg.* 1980;79:363–372.
12. Sanders RJ, Jackson CGR, Baushero N et al. Scalene muscle abnormalities in traumatic thoracic outlet syndrome. *Am J Surg.* 1990;159:231–236
13. Sharp WJ, Nowak LR, Zamani T et al. Long-term follow-up and patient satisfaction after surgery for thoracic outlet syndrome. *Ann Vasc Surg.* 2001;15:32–36.
14. Lepantalo M, Lindgren KA, Leino E et al. Long - term outcome after resection of the first rib for thoracic outlet syndrome. *Br J Surg.* 1989;76:1255–1256.
15. Roos DB, Edgar J. Poth. Lecture: Thoracic Outlet Syndrome: Update 1987. *Am J Surg.* 1987;154:568–573.

42

Arterial Injuries in Thoracic Outlet Compression

William H. Pearce, M.D., Jon S. Matsumura, M.D., and James S.T. Yao, M.D., Ph.D.

Upper extremity ischemia is an uncommon clinical problem. When it does occur, the etiology is rarely atherosclerosis and is more likely a manifestation of a systemic disease or a local mechanical problem. In general, it is easiest to identify the disease process based on the affected artery (Table 42–1). Large proximal arterial diseases include atherosclerosis, giant cell arteritis, and mechanical compression in the thoracic outlet. The arterial segments most commonly involved in the thoracic outlet include the second and third portion of the subclavian artery and the axillary artery. Figure 42–1 illustrates the compressive elements of the thoracic outlet and the affected arterial segments. The arterial pathology that may occur as a result of repetitive trauma in the thoracic outlet varies. Pathologic lesions vary from intimal ulceration, fibrointimal

TABLE 42-1. ARTERIAL RESPONSE TO TRAUMA IN THE THORACIC OUTLET

	Subclavian	Axillary	Brachial	Forearm	Hand
Atherosclerosis	—				
Giant Cell	—				
Takayasu's	—	—			
Arterial TOS	—	—		—	
FMD		—		—	
Embolic		—	—		—
Connective Tissue Disease				—	—
DM Repetitive Trauma				—	—
Hypercoagulation					—
Cryoglobulins					—
Pressors/PVC					—
Buerger's Disease					—

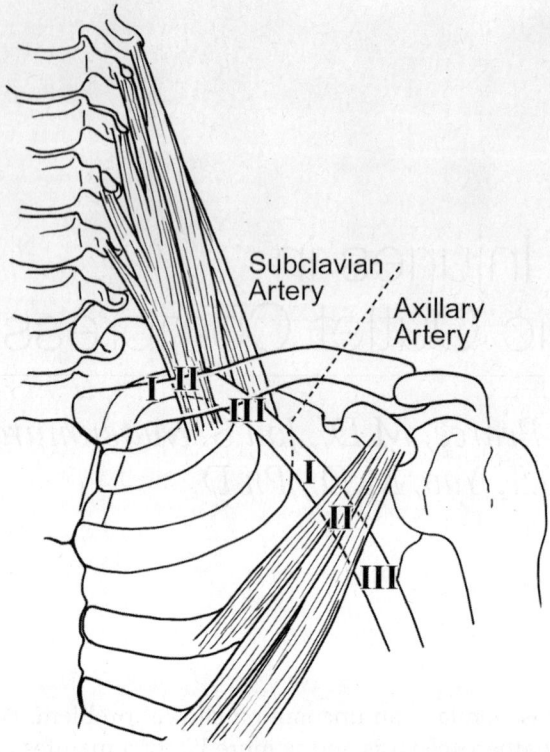

Figure 42-1. The compressive elements of the thoracic outlet and the affected arterial segments.

dysplasia, poststenotic aneurysms, and total occlusion (Table 42–2). In addition to the proximal arterial pathology, distal forearm and digital artery embolization is common. These distal lesions are the most common presenting symptoms of arterial injury in the thoracic outlet. This chapter will review the anatomy, presentation, diagnosis, and treatment of arterial injuries in the thoracic outlet.

PATHOPHYSIOLOGY AND ANATOMY

The clinical designation of the thoracic outlet as the area bounded by the cervical spine and first rib is actually anatomically incorrect. The true anatomic thoracic outlet is the diaphragm. However, the misidentification of the thoracic outlet is so ingrained in surgical history that correcting the designation would only confuse clinicians.

The thoracic outlet contains the subclavian and axillary artery and vein, brachial plexus, clavicle, first rib, humeral head, scalene muscles, subclavian, and pectoralis

TABLE 42-2. THE DISEASE PROCESS BASED ON THE ARTERIAL SEGMENT INVOLVED

Arterial Lesions
  Ulceration
  Stenosis
  Poststenotic aneurysm
  Occlusion

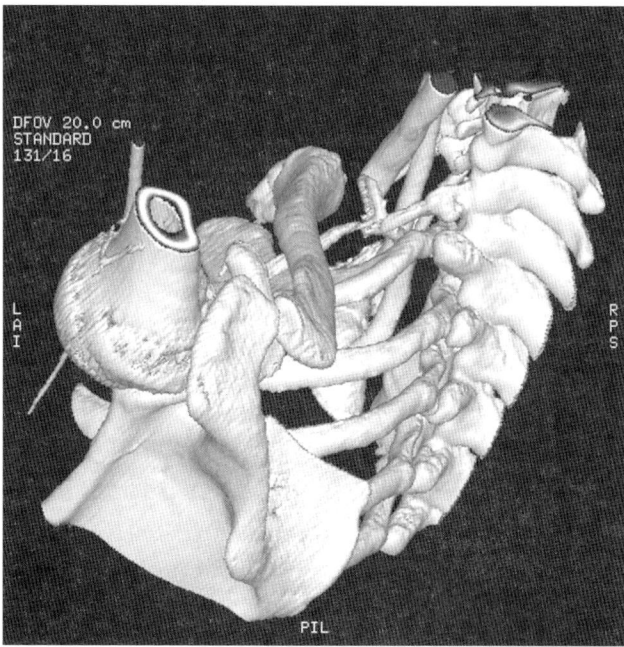

Figure 42-2. Hypertrophy of the scalenes in this 17-year-old swimmer.

muscles (major and minor). This anatomically compact area also contains the thoracic duct, and phrenic and long thoracic nerves. Because of the compact nature of the thoracic outlet, rigid boney, ligamentous structures, hypertrophy of muscles, or other abnormalities may compromise the arterial space leading to arterial damage. Hypertrophy of the scalenes is uncommon but has occurred in this 17-year-old swimmer (Figure 42–2). Further, hypertrophy of the pectoralis minor muscle is uncommon, occurring only in professional athletes.[1] In both instances, the hypertrophied muscles produce arterial compression only with stress positioning of the arm.

Boney abnormalities of the thoracic outlet are most frequently associated with arterial injury. Cervical ribs, anomalies of the first rib, and fracture calluses of the clavicle are the most common boney abnormalities. Cervical ribs occur in only 68 patients in 40,000 routine chest x-rays (0.17%).[2] Other radiographic studies have suggested a slightly higher incidence (0.27–0.74%).[3,4] Yet cervical ribs account for the majority of boney lesions associated with arterial injuries.[5-11] The length of the cervical rib may vary.[11] Shorter ribs (< 5.1cm) tend not to be associated with arterial injury but are more commonly associated with neurogenic symptoms A long cervical rib (> 5.5cm) will produce deviation of the subclavian artery and the rib (Figures 42–3A and 42–3B). Cervical ribs are bilateral in 33–47% of patients and are more common in females 3:1.

Cervical ribs are associated with abnormalities of the brachial plexus. During embryologic development, the limb bud develops at the interface between the cerivcal and thoracic vertebra. As the limb bud grows, it penetrates the scalene mass and competes with the evolving C7 rib. Thus, the lower plexus is less well-developed in patients with cervical ribs with greater contribution from higher nerve roots. As the neurovascular bundle penetrates the scalene mass, the mass is divided into the anterior and middle scalene muscles. If this process is slightly modified, a scalene minimus may occur. Furthermore, multiple abnormalities may occur with partial

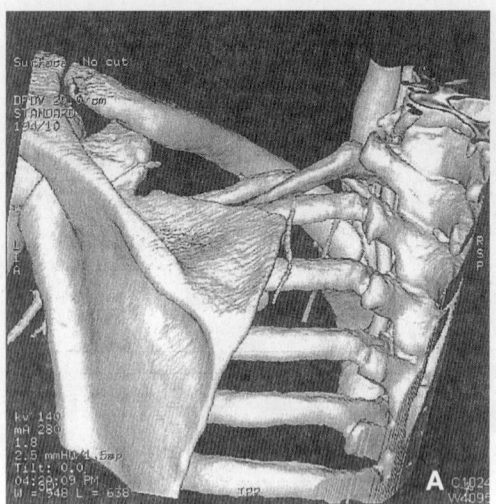 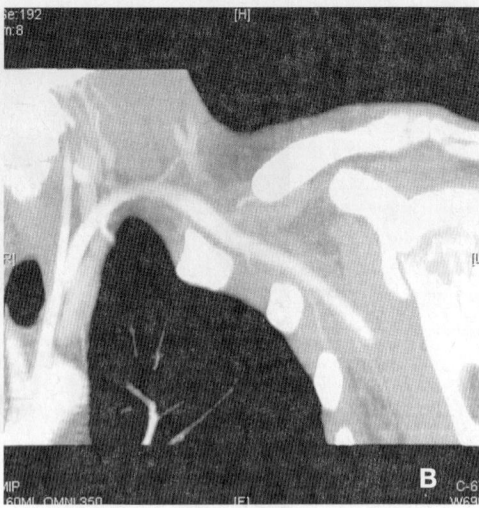

Figure 42-3. A long cervical rib (> 5.5 cm) will produce deviation of the (**A**) subclavian artery and (**B**) the rib.

ribs, bands, and muscle slips.[12, 13] Prefixation of the brachial plexus produces variability in both the trunks and cords of the brachial plexus and is important to remember when removing the anomolous rib. Anomalies of the first rib are less common than cervical ribs and are less likely to be associated with arterial injury.[14] These ribs usually have an exaggerated scalene insertion site or scalene slings.

PRESENTATION

Patients with arterial injury of the thoracic outlet may present with a spectrum of symptoms. Splinter hemorrhages and digital gangrene are the most obvious symptoms of distal embolization. A more subtle presentation is unilateral Raynaud's disease with or without a neurogenic component.[15] The unilateral Raynaud's may be attributed to vasospastic disease. Here, it is very important to obtain upper extremity blood flows and digital pressure. This test will demonstrate the underlying digital artery obstruction associated with the peripheral emboli.

Occlusive lesions produce arm discomfort with exercise. However, subclavian steal will not occur since the occlusion is distal to the vertebral artery origin. Patients with poststenotic aneurysms will feel the pulsatile artery and fullness of the supraclavicular space. Thirty percent of patients with arterial injuries will have co-existing neurogenic symptoms.[11, 16] These symptoms include numbness and/or pain in the ulnar nerve distribution. In addition, some patients will demonstrate motor weakness in the median nerve distribution.

EVALUATION

The history and physical examination provide important clues as to the pathology. Overuse and hypertrophy of muscles occurs primarily in high performance athletes. These athletes are usually involved in pitching motion or overhead strikes such as volleyball players, tennis, and kayaking.[1, 17-21] Arterial injuries in swimmers are less common but have been reported.

The physical exam involves a careful examination of the upper extremity pulses, hands, and nail beds. Splinter hemorrhages are subtle and often dismissed as an important sign by both the patient and the physician. The axillary, brachial, radial, and ulnar arteries are palpated. Monitoring the radial pulse, the patient's arm is abducted and externally rotated. The patient is then asked to look at the arm (Adson maneuver). In addition, the arm is exercised for symptoms in this position. Patients who are athletes are asked to reproduce the throwing or hitting motion to detect changes in the pulse. Pitchers have extreme external rotation and abduction. In this position, the shoulder is assessed for stability and subluxation of the humeral head. Similarly, the supraclavicular and infraclavicular spaces are auscultated as the arm changes position. Auscultated bruits signify arterial compression.

Noninvasive testing provides important information regarding the pathophysiology and the location of distal emboli. Segmented limb pressures, digital artery pressures, and waveforms will demonstrate fixed occlusions and their locations. The patency of the palmar arch is also determined. Using photoplethsymography, the arm is stressed (military, Adson, throwing motion). Obliteration of the signal is indicative of arterial compression. The duplex ultrasound is used to visualize the proximal subclavian and distal axillary arteries. Arterial aneurysms can be detected, but intimal ulcers beneath the clavicle are frequently missed. With the arm abducted and externally rotated, duplex ultrasound of the axillae may reveal humeral head compression.

Computed tomography (CT) is also useful in delineating boney and muscular compression. The thoracic outlet protocol used at Northwestern uses helical CT scan with bolus contrast infusion and three-dimensional reconstruction.[22, 23] The scan is repeated with the arm stressed. The value of the CT scan is that it can be reconstructed in three planes (transaxial, coroneal, and sagittal) and three dimensions. With this study, the dynamic nature of the thoracic outlet can be understood. Hypertrophied muscles, arterial pathology, and boney impingement can be readily demonstrated.

Arteriography is mandatory in patients requiring surgery. The questions to be answered are:

1. What is the location of the arterial compression?
2. What is the nature of the arterial injury?
3. What is the location and extent of the peripheral emboli?

The arteriogram is performed from the aortic arch to the hand and is repeated with the arm stressed. Visualization of the digital vessels is difficult with arterial vasospasm. Since Priscoline is no longer available, intra-arterial nitroglycerine as reactive hyperemia is used. However, neither technique is as effective as intra-arterial Priscoline.

Abnormalities of branch vessels are difficult to ascertain. Abrupt cutoffs imply thrombosis. On one occasion, we have seen a patient with a thrombosed thyrocervical branch with distal embolization. Aneurysm and thrombosis of the circumflex humeral artery have been reported. Damage to this artery occurs in the quadrilateral space.[24] This artery is difficult to visualize with both CT and arteriography. Occlusion of the artery with the arm abducted is an important finding since the artery often occludes with the arm abducted and externally rotated.

TREATMENT

The surgical treatment of arterial injuries of the thoracic outlet is tailored to the patient's pathologic anatomy. The principles are to remove the compressive elements, repair the damaged artery, and manage the peripheral emboli.

Muscular Decompression

Hypertrophied anterior scalene or pectoralis minor muscles may be identified as the source of compression. Anterior scalene muscle release is straightforward through a supraclavicular approach. Phrenic nerve injury is the most common complication and may be symptomatic. Pectoralis minor compression is rare and the muscle is resected via an infraclavicular approach. Resection of this muscle in the athlete must be weighed against potential difficulties with use of this muscle.

Osseous Decompression

Excision of a cervical or rudimentary first rib with arterial reconstruction is performed in our practice using supra- and infraclavicular approaches (Figure 42–4). Once the cervical rib is removed and the artery excised, the surgeon must decide whether the thoracic outlet is widely decompressed. With the arm prepped within the surgical field, the arm is placed in several positions with the surgeon's finger in the costoclavicular space. If the space remains compressive, additional resection of the first rib may be necessary. The artery is reconstructed with autogenous tissue (saphenous vein or arterial segment). Surgical treatment of clavicular abnormalities is more difficult. A fracture of the clavicle with malunion or callous formation narrows the costoclavicular space. In these instances, the clavicle should be removed. However, due to the trauma, scarring may be intense, making dissection of the proximal and distal arteries difficult. In addition, injury to the brachial plexus and subclavian vein is greater in these cases.

Humeral head compression is also difficult to manage. First, any laxity of the shoulder joint should be corrected by an orthopedic surgeon. If the shoulder joint is

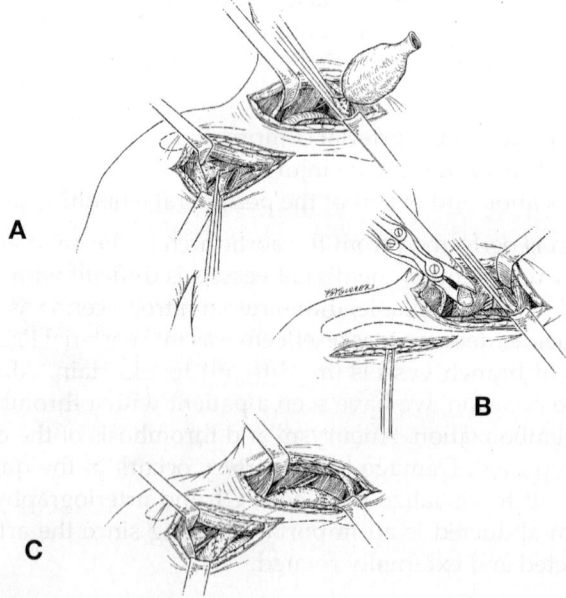

Figure 42-4. A. Resection of the subclavian aneurysm is needed to provide space for decompression. **B.** Removal of cervical rib by a bone rongeur. **C.** An interposed vein graft is placed underneath the clavicle. (Reprinted with permission from Saunders. Yao JST, Pearce Wh, Flinn WR, McCarthy WJ, Pearce WH. Upper Extremity Revascularization, In: *Techniques in Arterial Surgery,* Eds. Bergan JJ, Yao JST. WB Saunders, 1990, Philadelphia, page 335.)

stable, the artery is approached from a transaxillary incision.[1] Dissection of the neurovascular bundle is difficult in these patients (throwing athletes) due to multiple adhesions (personal observations). We have patched these arteries while others have used interposition grafts and bypasses to increase arterial length.[17]

Branch artery problems are generally treated with fresh ligation. In the few patients that present with these lesions, there appears to be an arterial stump, which is the nidus for clot formation.

Peripheral Emboli

Management of the peripheral emboli is variable. Thrombolysis of acute clot is possible and is usually performed with a direct brachial puncture. Like popliteal artery aneurysms, chronic embolization can occur that is asymptomatic. As a result, thrombolysis is generally ineffective. Similarly, Fogarty embolectomy can be performed at the time of arterial reconstruction. Occasionally, a distal bypass is needed to relieve hand symptoms.[1, 17]

COMMENT

Due to the infrequent occurrence of arterial injuries of the thoracic outlet due to compression and the variability of treatment options, large series are not available to provide long-term comprehensive studies. However, small series all provide a common theme of treatment: decompression followed by arterial reconstruction and management of distal emboli.

Controversy exists regarding the nature of the arterial conduit, open versus endovascular repair, and the treatment for humeral head compression. Prosthetic arterial replacement is rarely indicated unless all other autogenous sources have been used. We have generally used the greater saphenous. However, two have become aneurysmal in long-term follow up. Other surgeons have used external iliac or superficial femoral arteries with prosthetic replacement in the leg. Here, the feeling is that the arterial conduit will function better than a venous conduit in an area exposed to potentially repeated trauma. Humeral head compression presents a similar problem. Should the axillary artery be lengthened or simply patched?

Finally, the management of the athletic patient is complicated by economic and parental pressures. Professional, college, and high school athletes have made significant investments in their sports and hope to realize benefits (contracts, scholarships, endorsements). It is very important to be realistic with these patients about the operation, potential complications, and duration of rehabilitation.

REFERENCES

1. Durham JR, Yao JS, Pearce WH, et al. Arterial injuries in the thoracic outlet syndrome. *J Vasc Surg*. 1995;21(1):57–69.
2. Etter LE. Osseous abnormalities of the thoracic cage seen on forty thousand consecutive chest photoroentgenogram. *AJR*. 1944;51:359–363.
3. Adson AW. Cervical ribs: symptoms, differential diagnosis, and indication for section of the insertion of scalenous muscle. *J Int Coll Surg*. 1951;16:546–559.

4. Firsov GI. Cervical ribs and their distinction from underdeveloped first ribs. *Arkh Anat Gistol Embiol*. 1974;67:101–103.
5. Martin J, Gaspard DJ, Johnston PW, Kohl RD, Jr., Dietrick W. Vascular manifestations of the thoracic outlet syndrome. A surgical urgency. *Arch Surg*. 1976;111(7):779–782.
6. Matsumura JS. Thoracic outlet arterial compression: Clinical features and surgical management. In: Yao JST, editor. *Semin Vasc Surg*. 1996;9:125–133.
7. Scher LA, Veith FJ, Haimovici H, et al. Staging of arterial complications of cervical rib: guidelines for surgical management. *Surgery*. 1984;95(6):644–649.
8. Short DW. The subclavian artery in 16 patients with complete cervical ribs. *J Cardiovasc Surg (Torino)*. 1975;16(2):135–141.
9. Cormier JM, Amrane M, Ward A, et al. Arterial complications of the thoracic outlet syndrome: fifty-five operative cases. *J Vasc Surg*. 1989;9(6):778–787.
10. Hood DB, Kuehne J, Yellin AE, Weaver FA. Vascular complications of thoracic outlet syndrome. *Am Surg*. 1997;63(10):913–917.
11. Makhoul RG, Machleder HI. Developmental anomalies at the thoracic outlet: an analysis of 200 consecutive cases. *J Vasc Surg*. 1992;16(4):534–542.
12. Sanders RJ, Roos DB. Surgical anatomy of the scalene triangle. *Contemp Surg*. 1989;35:11–16.
13. Todd TW. Cervical rib: factors controlling its presence and its size, its bearing on the morphology of the shoulder, with four cases. *J Anat Physiol*. 1911-1912;45:293–304.
14. Baumgartner F, Nelson RJ, Robertson JM. The rudimentary first rib. A cause of thoracic outlet syndrome with arterial compromise. *Arch Surg*. 1989;124(9):1090–1092.
15. Bouhoutsos J, Morris T, Martin P. Unilateral Raynaud's phenomenon in the hand and its signficance. *Surgery*. 1977;82:547–551.
16. Sanders RJ, Hammond SL. Management of cervical ribs and anomalous first ribs causing neurogenic thoracic outlet syndrome. *J Vasc Surg*. 2002;36(1):51–56.
17. Arko FR, Harris EJ, Zarins CK, Olcott C. Vascular complications in high-performance athletes. *J Vasc Surg*. 2001;33(5):935–942.
18. Rohrer MJ, Cardullo PA, Pappas AM, et al. Axillary artery compression and thrombosis in throwing athletes. *J Vasc Surg*. 1990;11(6):761–768.
19. Jackson MR. Upper extremity arterial injuries in athletes. *Semin Vasc Surg*. 2003;16(3):232–239.
20. Kee ST, Dake MD, Wolfe-Johnson B, et al. Ischemia of the throwing hand in major league baseball pitchers: embolic occlusion from aneurysms of axillary artery branches. *J Vasc Interv Radiol*. 1995;6(6):979–982.
21. Mosley JG. Arterial problems in athletes. *Br J Surg*. 2003;90(12):1461–1469.
22. Matsumura JS, Rilling WS, Pearce WH, et al. Helical computed tomography of the normal thoracic outlet. *J Vasc Surg*. 1997;26(5):776–783.
23. Matsumura JS, Yao JS, Nemcek AA, Jr. Helical CT angiography of thoracic outlet syndrome. *AJR Am J Roentgenol*. 2001;177(3):714–715.
24. Cormier PJ, Matalon TA, Wolin PM. Quadrilateral space syndrome: a rare cause of shoulder pain. *Radiology*. 1988;167(3):797–798.

43

Supraclavicular (Paraclavicular) Approach for Thoracic Outlet Syndrome

Spencer J. Melby, M.D. Robert W. Thompson, M.D.

"All things being equal, the simplest solution tends to be the best one."
—William of Ockham

"Make everything as simple as possible, but not simpler."
—Albert Einstein

"If this was easy it wouldn't be so hard."
—Yogi Berra

Thoracic outlet syndrome (TOS) represents several different clinical conditions affecting the upper extremity, which most commonly occur in young, active, otherwise healthy individuals.[1] Each type of TOS is caused by extrinsic compression of neurovascular structures within the thoracic outlet, three forms of which are distinguished by the principal structure involved and the characteristic clinical manifestations produced: 1) *neurogenic TOS*, caused by compression of the brachial plexus nerve roots, which is characterized by arm, shoulder and/or neck pain, numbness and paresthesias, and functional disability; 2) *arterial TOS*, caused by compression of the subclavian artery, which typically leads to occlusive lesions or poststenotic aneurysm formation and the clinical sequelae of thromboembolism; and 3) *venous TOS*, caused by compression of the subclavian vein, which underlies the development of the effort thrombosis (Paget-Schroetter) syndrome.

Surgical treatment has an important role in the management of patients with all three forms of TOS.[2,3] However, there remains considerable controversy regarding optimal patient selection for operation, timing of surgical interventions, and the specific surgical techniques to be used. Current indications for surgery in TOS include the following: 1) patients with persistently disabling neurogenic TOS who have failed to achieve sufficient improvement with a conservative management program directed by a physical therapist with appropriate expertise in this condition; 2) patients with arterial TOS with any evidence of aneurysmal degeneration or a symptomatic occlusive lesion of the subclavian artery at the level of the first rib; and 3) patients with symptomatic venous TOS or recent effort thrombosis, preferably following initial treatment with catheter-directed thrombolysis (Figure 43–1).

Operations performed for TOS are designed to decompress the anatomic structures considered responsible for clinical symptoms. This may include removal of the first rib, anomalous cervical ribs, the anterior and middle scalene muscles, aberrant ligaments or fascial bands, and perineural or perivascular fibrosis, which all require an open operative procedure. In the treatment of vascular forms of TOS, these operative procedures also include arterial or venous reconstruction, either by direct open approaches or in combination with endovascular adjuncts (e.g., balloon angioplasty). The most commonly performed procedures for TOS are conducted through either the transaxillary or supraclavicular approach, with each approach having distinct advantages and disadvantages.[4-7] Over the past decade, our group has accumulated considerable experience with the surgical management of TOS, leading us to conclude that operative strategies based on supraclavicular exposure and its variations provide the most versatile, comprehensive, and safe approach to the treatment of all forms of TOS, with excellent surgical outcomes and low rates of symptomatic recurrence. In this chapter, we describe the specific operative techniques used for the treatment of patients with TOS using strategies based on supraclavicular/paraclavicular exposure.

SUPRACLAVICULAR EXPOSURE (ALL FORMS OF TOS)

Decompressive operations for all three forms of TOS begin with supraclavicular exposure. The patient is positioned supine under general anesthesia, with the head of the bed elevated 30 degrees, and the neck extended and turned to the opposite side. The neck, chest, and affected upper extremity are prepped into the field, with the arm wrapped in stockinette and held across the abdomen. This permits movement of the arm during the operation and provides access to the forearm and wrist when needed. The ipsilateral thigh is also included in the sterile field in order to provide access to the greater saphenous vein. We use an operating table compatible with C-arm portable fluoroscopy for the treatment of vascular forms of TOS, since intraoperative angiography with views of the shoulder and neck region is frequently utilized.

A transverse skin incision is made two finger breadths above and parallel to the clavicle, beginning at the lateral edge of the sternocleidomastoid muscle and following a skin crease for about 8 centimeters (Figure 43–2A). The incision is carried through the subcutaneous layer and subplatysmal flaps are developed to expose the scalene fat pad. Several small supraclavicular cutaneous nerves crossing the operative field are divided, if necessary, to ensure adequate exposure. The omohyoid muscle is identified and its central portion is excised, allowing each end to retract from the operative field.

One of the key elements in simplifying the supraclavicular exposure is proper elevation and lateral reflection of the scalene fat pad. The scalene fat pad is mobilized beginning at the lateral edge of the internal jugular vein. Then, using blunt dissection, it is progressively elevated from the medial to the lateral surface of the anterior scalene muscle (Figure 43–2B) Care is taken to identify and preserve the phrenic nerve, which

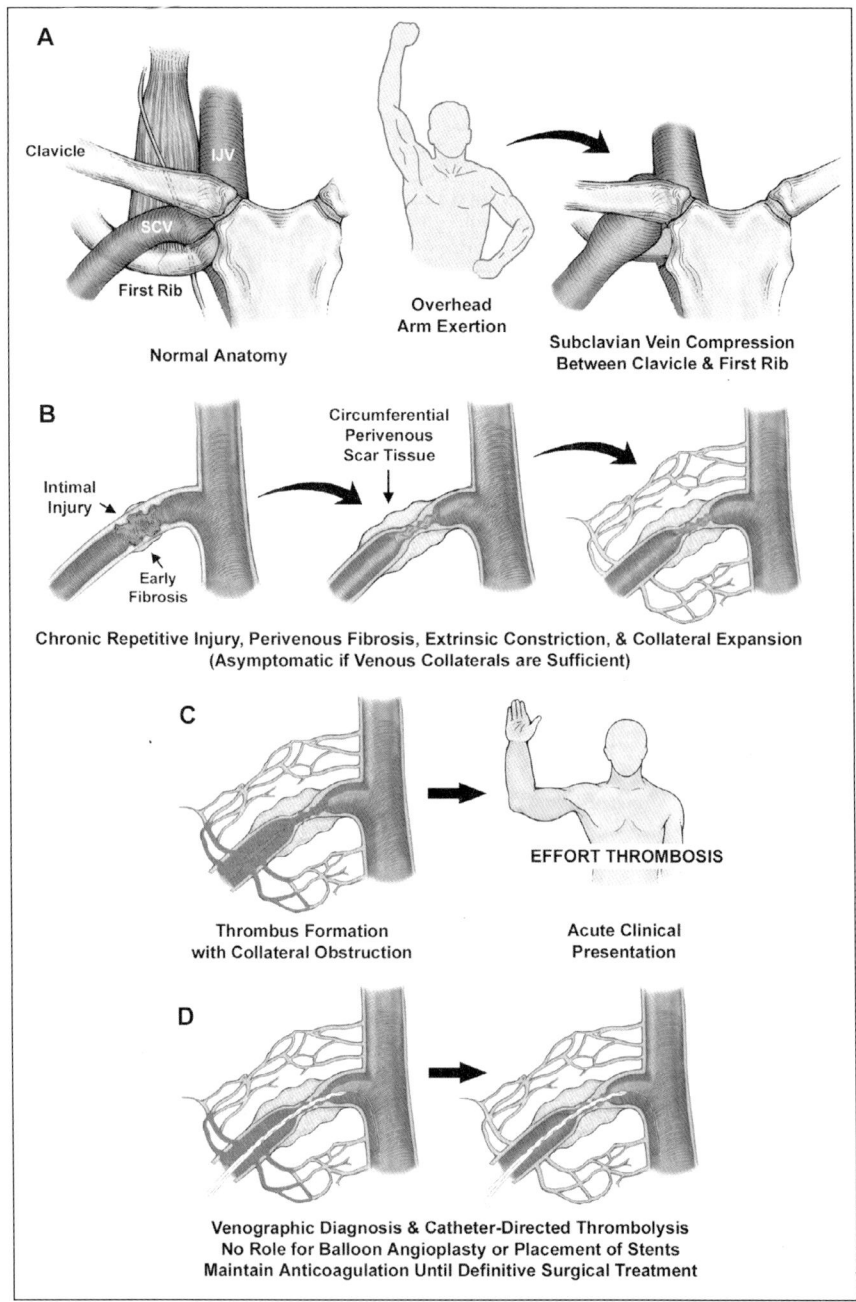

Figure 43-1. Pathophysiology of subclavian vein effort thrombosis. (**A**) Extrinsic compression of the subclavian vein between the clavicle and first rib, exacerbated by overhead arm activity. (**B**) Focal vein wall injury leading to a self-limited inflammatory response followed by perivenous and/or intramural fibrosis, with recurrent injury over a period of months to years causing progressive fibrosis and subclavian vein constriction. During this time, parallel expansion of venous collaterals may prevent symptomatic venous congestion. (**C**) Eventual formation of thrombus within the narrowed segment of the subclavian vein due to stagnant/turbulent flow distal to the obstruction. Distal propagation of clot obstructs the principal collateral veins, resulting in acute upper extremity swelling and cyanosis (the clinically evident "effort thrombosis" event). (**D**) Recommended treatment includes contrast venography for definitive diagnosis, and catheter-directed thrombolytic therapy followed by thoracic outlet decompression and subclavian vein reconstruction when necessary.

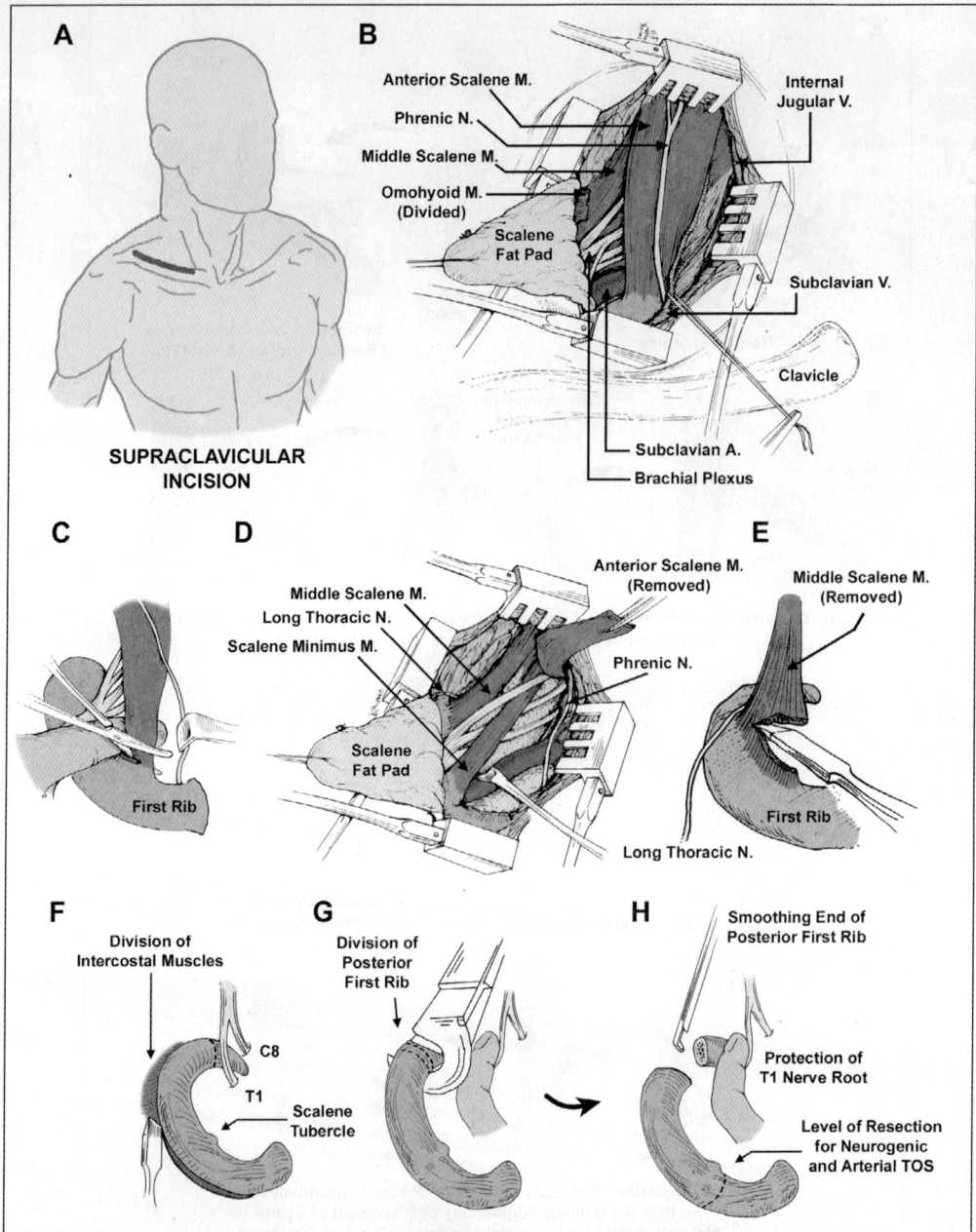

Figure 43-2. Supraclavicular exposure. (**A**) Incision. (**B**) Reflection of the scalene fat pad. (**C**) Division of the anterior scalene muscle from the first rib. (**D**) Anterior scalenectomy. (**E**) Middle scalenectomy. (**F-G**) Posterior division and resection of the first rib.

courses in a superolateral to inferomedial direction within the investing fascia of the anterior scalene muscle. The inferior and superior attachments of the scalene fat pad are divided between ligatures to secure small blood vessels and lymphatics. On the left side, the thoracic duct is usually observed at the medial edge of the scalene fat pad, coursing toward the junction of the internal jugular and subclavian veins where it is gently ligated and divided. Lateral mobilization of the scalene fat pad continues until there is sufficient exposure of the anterior scalene muscle and phrenic nerve, the brachial plexus, the middle scalene muscle and long thoracic nerve, as well as the lateral edge of the first rib. It is then held in position with several retraction sutures and kept moist during the remainder of the procedure (Figure 43–3A).

The anterior scalene muscle is next dissected circumferentially at the level of its insertion on the first rib. The subclavian artery and the brachial plexus nerve roots are visualized behind the anterior scalene muscle and protected from injury. Once exposure of

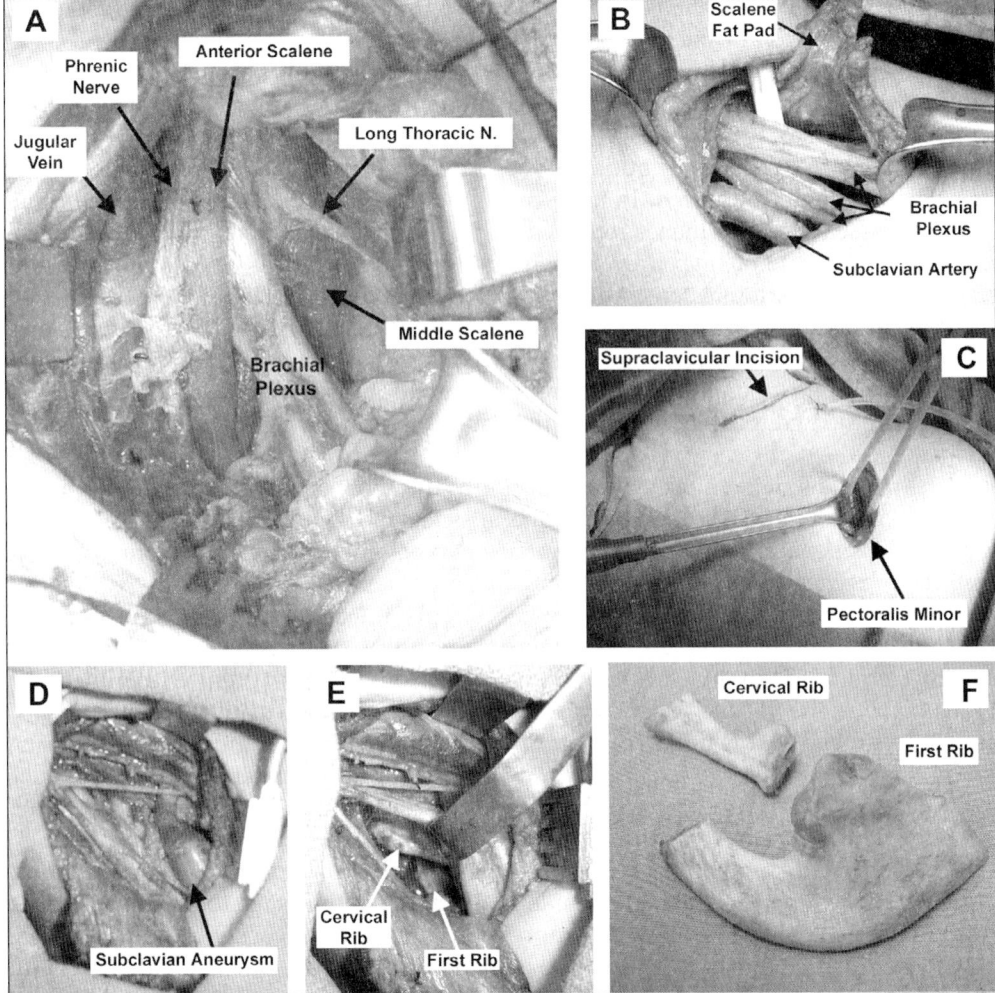

Figure 43-3. Operating room photographs. (**A**) Supraclavicular exposure of the left scalene triangle, following lateral reflection of the scalene fat pad. (**B**) Completion photograph after left-sided scalenectomy and brachial plexus neurolysis. (**C**) Infraclavicular isolation and division of the left pectoralis minor tendon near its insertion on the coracoid process, performed following left-sided supraclavicular decompression. (**D**) Cervical rib anomaly causing subclavian artery aneurysm. Exposure of the subclavian aneurysm following scalenectomy, with the phrenic nerve observed crossing the normal proximal subclavian artery. (**E**) Medial retraction of the brachial plexus with exposure of the cervical and first ribs. (**F**) Operative specimens of the resected cervical and first ribs.

the anterior scalene is sufficient to pass a finger behind the muscle at the level of the first rib, the muscle insertion is sharply divided under direct vision using curved Mayo scissors (Figure 43–2C). The anterior scalene muscle is then lifted superiorly and detached from the underlying subclavian artery, brachial plexus nerve roots, and extrapleural fascia (Sibson's fascia) (Figure 43–2D). It is also common at this stage to observe a scalene minimus muscle anomaly, which is characterized by fibers that originate in the plane of the middle scalene muscle and pass between the brachial plexus nerve roots to join the plane of the anterior scalene muscle. These fibers are divided, the remainder of which will be removed later with the middle scalene muscle. The superior dissection of the anterior scalene muscle is carried to the level of its origin on the transverse process of the sixth cervical vertebrae (which is easily palpated within the upper aspect of the operative field), where the muscle is then divided and removed. It is especially important to achieve full resection of the anterior scalene muscle for patients with neurogenic TOS, since incomplete scalenectomy is recognized as one of the principal causes for recurrent or persistent symptoms in patients undergoing either transaxillary or supraclavicular operations.[8-11]

The five nerve roots contributing to the brachial plexus (C5, C6, C7, C8, and T1) are then identified and mobilized. In most cases, these nerve roots are associated with inflammatory scar tissue, which is removed by performing a complete external neurolysis in order to alleviate or help prevent neurogenic symptoms. It is also common at this stage to identify various aberrant fibrous bands, ligaments, or fascial attachments that may contribute to nerve compression, as first described in detail by Roos.[12,13] Any such aberrant soft tissue structures are removed during dissection of the brachial plexus. This portion of the operation is not complete until all five nerve roots are dissected free throughout their course in the surgical field and fully mobilized without tension or fixation.

The middle scalene muscle lies posterior to the roots of the brachial plexus and it forms a broad oblique insertion on the lateral aspect of the first rib. The mid-portion of the muscle is penetrated by the long thoracic nerve, which is often represented by two or three branches at this level rather than a single nerve (Figure 43–3A). With gentle medial retraction of the brachial plexus nerve roots, the attachment of the middle scalene muscle is divided from the first rib using a cautery and periosteal elevator (Figure 43–2E). Cervical rib anomalies (or their soft tissue counterparts) occur within the same tissue plane as the middle scalene muscle, and if such structures are encountered, they are also removed at this time. The portion of the middle scalene muscle lying anterior to the long thoracic nerve is excised to its origin, and any remaining middle scalene muscle is detached from the posterior surface of the first rib.

Some authorities have described retention of the first rib following supraclavicular scalenectomy and brachial plexus neurolysis in selected patients with neurogenic TOS.[14,15] However, we have been unable to define any advantage to omitting first rib resection in achieving thorough decompression for neurogenic TOS, and there is general consensus that removal of the first rib is necessary in all patients with arterial or venous forms of TOS. To accomplish first rib resection at this stage in the supraclavicular dissection, gentle medial retraction of the brachial plexus nerve roots (particularly C8 and T1) is maintained and the intercostal muscle is divided from the lateral edge of the rib (Figure 43–2F). The tip of a right-angle clamp is then passed underneath the posterior neck of the first rib. The first intercostal nerve is pushed inferiorly away from the rib and the remaining intercostal muscle is separated. A modified Stille-Giertz rib cutter is applied to divide and excise a small segment of the first rib (Figure 43–2G). A

Kerrison bone rongeur is used to smooth the posterior end of the rib to a level immediately medial to the course of the T1 nerve root, and it is sealed with bone wax (Figure 43–2H). The free end of the first rib is elevated, and a fingertip is passed underneath the first rib to bluntly dissect away the extrapleural fascia. Additional intercostal muscles are detached underneath the lateral and anterior aspects of the rib in a similar manner to the level of the anterior scalene tubercle.

In operations for neurogenic and arterial TOS, the anterior portion of the first rib is next divided with the Stille-Giertz instrument just medial to the scalene tubercle, and the rib specimen is removed from the operative field (Figure 43–2H). The anterior edge of the rib is further debrided to a smooth flat surface with a bone rongeur, and then sealed with bone wax. This completes the operation for neurogenic TOS, and the wound is closed as described in a later section (Figure 43–3B). In operations for arterial TOS, this also completes the supraclavicular decompression phase of the procedure. In operations for venous TOS, the anterior portion of the first rib is not divided at this stage; rather, the procedure is continued by moving to the infraclavicular portion of the operation (see below).

INFRACLAVICULAR EXPOSURE FOR NEUROGENIC TOS

As part of the initial evaluation of patients with neurogenic TOS, the surgeon seeks to identify individuals that have distinct pain and tenderness localized to the area of the pectoralis minor muscle and tendon. Neurogenic symptoms in these patients may be attributable, at least in part, to compression of the brachial plexus nerves as they pass underneath the pectoralis minor tendon (also described as the "hyperabduction syndrome"). Such patients may thereby obtain significant improvement in symptoms following division of the pectoralis minor tendon, either as an isolated procedure or in combination with supraclavicular thoracic outlet decompression; individuals with distinct pectoralis minor symptoms following a previous operation for neurogenic TOS may also benefit from pectoralis minor tenotomy. When performed as an isolated procedure, pectoralis minor tenotomy is conducted as a short outpatient operation. In patients with evidence of hyperabduction syndrome in association with more typical neurogenic TOS (approximately 30% of patients in our experience), we prefer to include pectoralis minor tenotomy as part of the initial operative procedure immediately following supraclavicular decompression. To accomplish this, a 4-centimeter vertical incision is made inferior to the lateral clavicle and the coracoid process, along the border of the pectoralis major muscle. The pectoralis major muscle is identified, elevated, and retracted medially. The pectoralis minor muscle is identified and encircled near its attachment to the coracoid process, taking care to preserve the small pectoral nerves, and its tendon is then divided with the cautery under direct vision (Figure 43–3C).

INFRACLAVICULAR EXPOSURE FOR ARTERIAL TOS

In operations for arterial TOS (subclavian artery aneurysm or symptomatic occlusive lesions), the first rib is removed in the same manner as described above for neurogenic TOS. Attention is then turned to reconstruction of the subclavian artery, which typically exhibits fusiform dilatation immediately distal to the point of compression, often in association with a cervical rib anomaly (Figure 43–3, D through F). The thyrocervical trunk and other superior branches of the subclavian artery are ligated and divided, and the proximal subclavian artery is controlled circumferentially just distal to the origin of the internal thoracic and vertebral arteries. If the normal subclavian artery distal to the aneurysm can be mobilized sufficiently from the supraclavicular incision alone, the vessel is clamped and the aneurysmal segment is excised, followed by reconstruction with an interposition bypass graft. In most cases, however, further exposure is needed to control the distal subclavian artery, which is obtained using a second incision parallel and inferior to the lateral clavicle. After splitting the fibers of the pectoralis major muscle and opening the clavipectoral fascia, the axillary artery is exposed medial to the pectoralis minor muscle. The pectoralis minor tendon is divided if necessary, and the axillary artery is controlled just after it passes underneath the clavicle. Subclavian artery reconstruction is then performed with an interposition bypass graft. A number of different autologous conduits can be used for subclavian artery reconstruction, including the superficial femoral vein, reversed saphenous vein, construction of a saphenous vein panel graft, or an arterial autograft harvested from the external iliac artery (followed by iliac artery replacement with a prosthetic graft), and in some cases, a prosthetic bypass graft may be preferred. Regardless of the conduit selected, it is important to ensure the absence of positional graft tension, twisting, or kinking by observing the reconstruction with the arm placed through a full range of motion at the end of the procedure. Completion arteriography is also used for final assessment of the reconstruction. In situations complicated by distal arterial occlusion due to thromboembolism, further thrombectomy and reconstruction may be necessary at the brachial and/or radial/ulnar artery levels. When severe digital vasospasm is also present, cervical sympathectomy may be considered, which can be readily performed through the supraclavicular exposure already obtained.

INFRACLAVICULAR EXPOSURE FOR VENOUS TOS

In operations for venous TOS, the initial supraclavicular portion of the procedure is conducted as described above for neurogenic TOS, with the exception that the anterior portion of the first rib is not divided through the supraclavicular approach. Indeed, complete resection of the medial (cartilaginous) aspect of the first rib, which contributes most to subclavian vein compression in venous TOS, cannot be performed solely through the supraclavicular approach. To accomplish this component of the decompression for venous TOS, a transverse skin incision is made one finger breadth below the medial clavicle, extending laterally from the edge of the sternum for approximately 8 centimeters (Figure 43–4A). The incision is carried to the level of the fascia and then between the upper and middle portions of the pectoralis major muscle, and the cartilaginous portion of the first rib is identified by palpation. Using a finger placed within the supraclavicular incision, downward pressure is applied to the divided posterior segment of the first rib to place the attachments between the medial first rib and clavicle under tension, and the medial portion of the first rib is dissected from its soft tissue attachments through the infraclavicular incision. The subclavius muscle tendon, the costoclavicular ligament, and the muscles of the first intercostal space are all divided under direct vision extending to the lateral edge of the sternum (Figure 43–4B). The cartilaginous portion of the first rib is then divided adjacent to the sternum using the cutting cautery and/or curved Mayo scissors, and removed from the operative field as a single specimen. The remaining edge of the rib is remodeled with a Kerrison rongeur (Figure 43–4C).

The subclavian vein is then identified as it passes underneath the distal clavicle, as visualized through the lateral portion of the infraclavicular incision. It is carefully separated from the subclavius muscle moving toward the medial aspect of the surgical

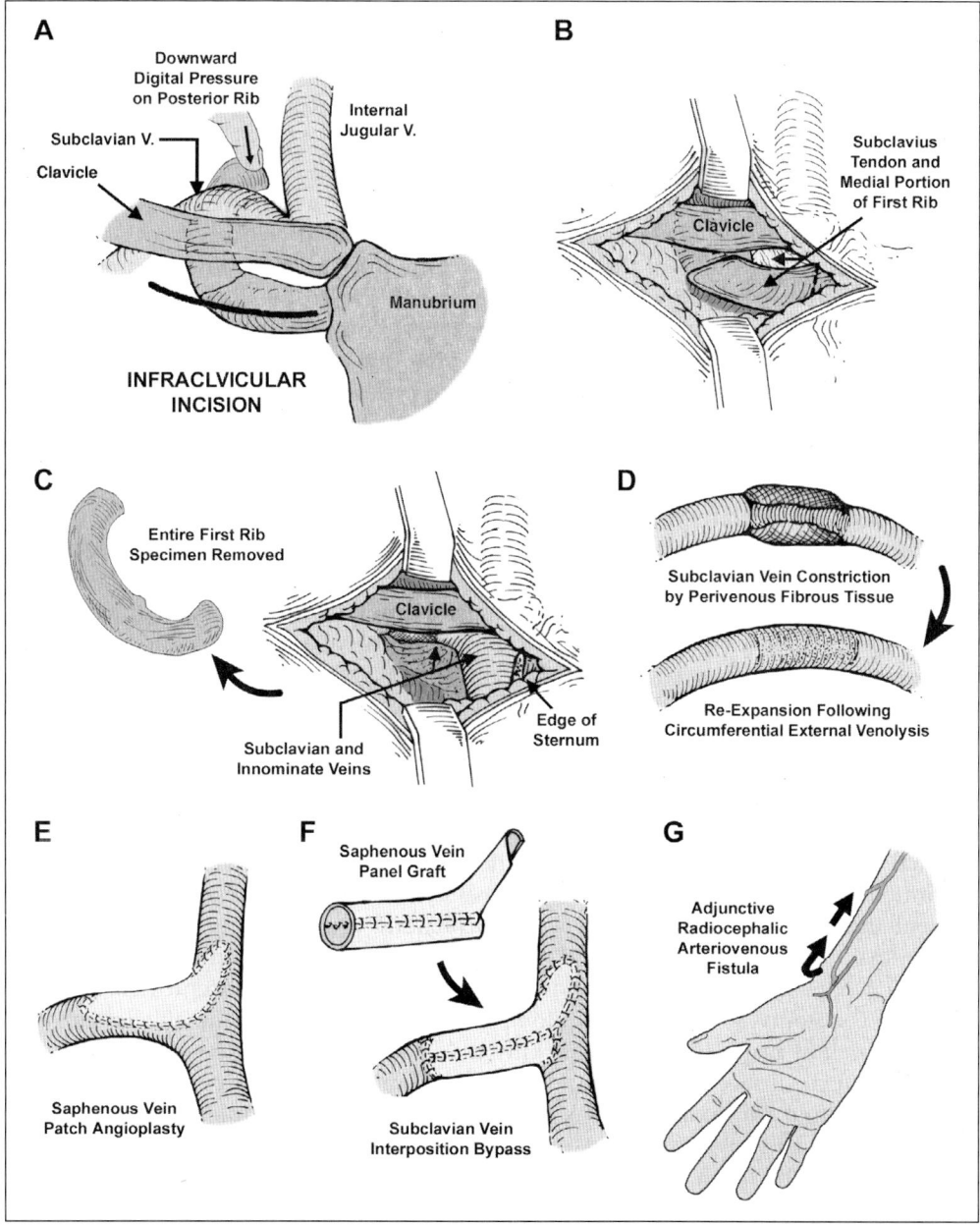

Figure 43-4. Infraclavicular exposure for venous TOS. (**A**) Infraclavicular incision overlying the medial first rib. (**B**) Exposure of medial first rib. (**C**) Excision of complete first rib specimen. (**D**) Circumferential external venolysis. (**E**) Patch angioplasty reconstruction of subclavian vein. (**F**) Panel graft bypass reconstruction of subclavian vein. (**G**) Radiocephalic arteriovenous fistula.

field, and any collateral vein branches that enter the subclavian vein are ligated and divided. Once the vein has been sufficiently separated from underneath the subclavius muscle, the muscle and its tendon are resected (Figure 43–4C). This completes the decompression portion of operations for venous TOS.

SUBCLAVIAN VEIN RECONSTRUCTION FOR VENOUS TOS

Further dissection of the subclavian vein is undertaken through the supraclavicular exposure. This is initiated along the lateral aspect of the subclavian vein and continued medially toward the junction of the subclavian and internal jugular veins to form the brachiocephalic (innominate) vein. Any residual scar tissue surrounding the proximal portion of the subclavian vein is completely excised ("circumferential external venolysis"), often resulting in reexpansion of the previously constricted segment of the vein (Figure 43–4D). The course of the phrenic nerve into the upper mediastinum is noted in order to identify situations where it passes anterior to the subclavian vein, and thereby contributes to venous obstruction (in this circumstance, the accessory phrenic nerve is mobilized away from the subclavian vein but not divided). The dissection is continued until the subclavian and internal jugular veins are fully mobilized to their junction, along with the first several centimeters of the innominate vein into the upper mediastinum. Complete dissection of the subclavian vein allows it to drop free of the clavicle, thereby facilitating the exposure required for further assessment and reconstruction as viewed from the supraclavicular incision.

The subclavian vein is next assessed by inspection and palpation. If there is no focal reduction in the diameter of the vein, if it is soft and easily compressible to palpation, and if it shows evidence of rapid filling and emptying, it is likely that no further venous reconstruction will be necessary. In this event, attention is turned to performance of an intraoperative venogram to confirm that the subclavian vein is widely patent. In our experience, this is the case in approximately 50% of patients with venous TOS, even in those with long-segment stenosis prior to operation (Figure 43–5).

Additional venous reconstruction is performed in situations where external venolysis alone has been insufficient to alleviate subclavian vein obstruction, or when intraoperative venography demonstrates a residual stenosis despite the apparent success of external venolysis. Following systemic anticoagulation with intravenous heparin and continuous infusion of Dextran, clamp control is obtained of the distal subclavian and internal jugular veins, as well as any smaller collateral veins entering this area. A pediatric Satinsky clamp is passed around the upper portion of the innominate vein, taking care not to damage posterior collateral veins and to exclude the phrenic nerve. A longitudinal venotomy is then created along the superior aspect of the subclavian vein and the lumen is inspected. If there is only mild focal stenosis of the subclavian vein, and the luminal surface is smooth and free of thrombus and/or irregularity following resection of any minimal intimal webs, a simple patch angioplasty is performed (Figure 43–4E). This is conducted using a short segment of the greater saphenous vein harvested from the thigh, or alternatively, with a segment of bovine pericardium. In each case, the patch angioplasty is constructed to span the entire affected area of the subclavian vein with extension onto the lateral aspect of the internal jugular vein to avoid obstructive kinking in the upright position (Figure 43–6, A through E).

When there is dense fibrosis within the wall of the vein despite external venolysis, or when another obvious abnormality is present on inspection of the opened vein, the

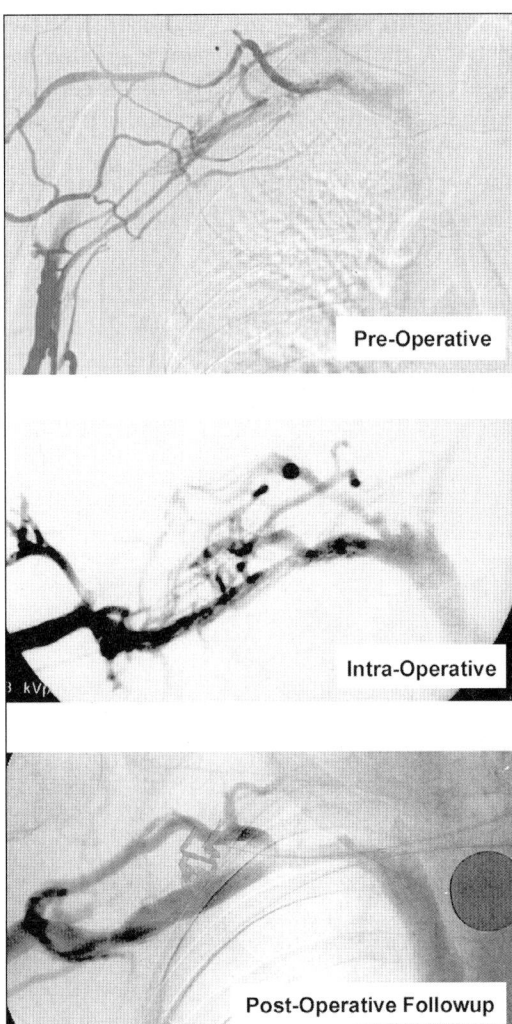

Figure 43-5. Venography in venous TOS. Patient with longstanding right-sided venous TOS with disabling congestive symptoms. **Upper panel:** Preoperative venogram demonstrating long-segment obstruction of axillary-subclavian vein with chronic collateral development. Middle panel: Intraoperative venogram following paraclavicular thoracic outlet decompression and external venolysis, demonstrating restoration of flow through the axillary-subclavian vein. No further reconstruction was performed. **Lower panel:** Followup venogram (six weeks), demonstrating sustained patency of axillary-subclavian vein with the patient experiencing complete relief of venous symptoms.

affected segment of the subclavian vein is replaced by interposition bypass. The intervening segment of the native subclavian vein is excised, and an interposition graft is constructed using an end-to-end anastomosis to the unaffected distal subclavian vein and an end-to-side anastomosis to the lateral aspect of the jugular-subclavian junction. As with patch angioplasty, the proximal portion is extended onto the jugular vein to avoid positional kinking of the graft. In some patients, subclavian vein reconstruction can be performed with reversed saphenous vein, but in most patients, the saphenous vein is too small to match the diameter of the subclavian vein. In this event, the saphenous vein is opened longitudinally and folded on itself after excising all valves; the closed end of the vein is then opened and the sides sutured together to create a panel graft with twice the diameter of the native saphenous vein (Figure 43–4F). In the event that the saphenous vein cannot be used, a conduit of similar size can be constructed from bovine pericardium. Intraoperative venography is used to confirm satisfactory subclavian vein reconstruction (Figure 43–6, F and G).

Creation of a temporary radiocephalic arteriovenous (AV) fistula is used with increasing frequency as an adjunct to the operative treatment of venous TOS in order to increase upper extremity venous blood flow during the first several months after operation. A short vertical incision is created at the wrist and the cephalic vein and radial artery are each exposed. The distal cephalic vein is divided and the proximal end is mobilized to the side of the radial artery, and a long end-to-side anastomosis is created (Figure 43–4G). If not performed at an earlier stage in the operation, the open end of the cephalic vein is also used at this point for contrast injection to perform intraoperative completion venography, immediately prior to the radiocephalic anastomosis.

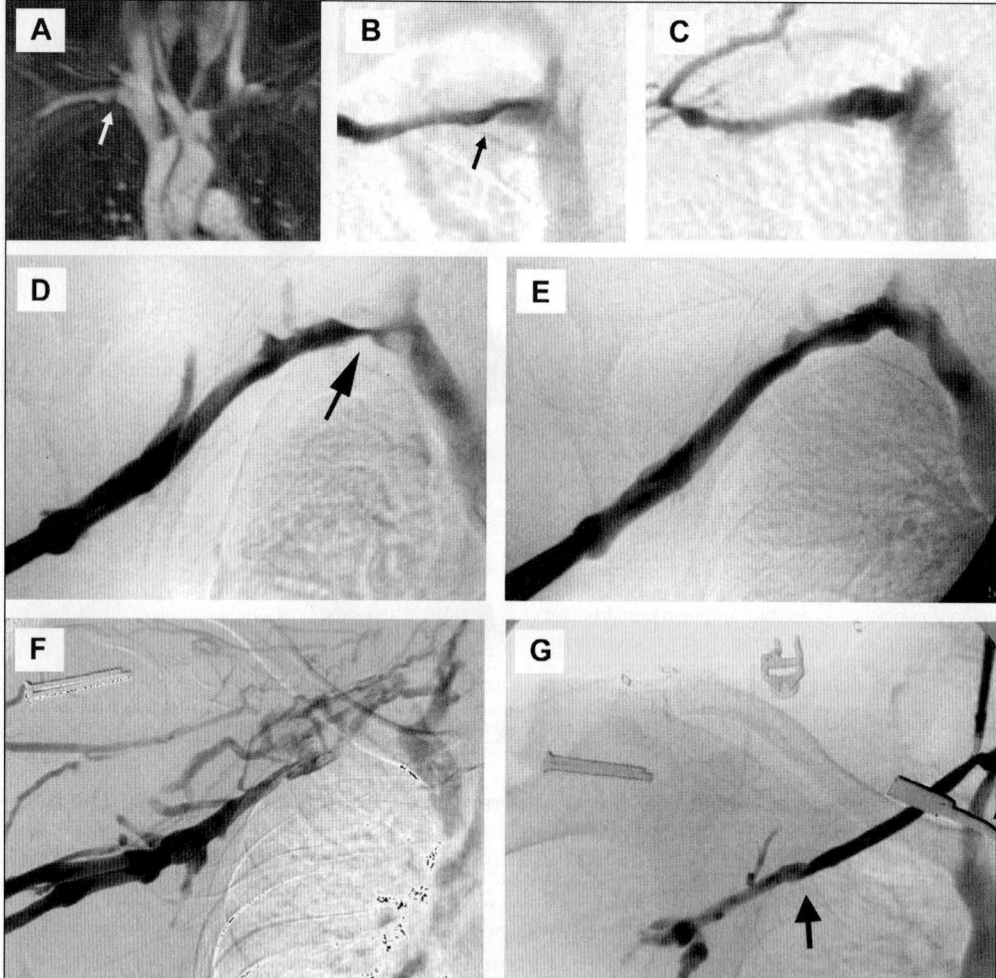

Figure 43-6. Venography in venous TOS. (**A**) Gadolinium-enhanced magnetic resonance venogram 8 weeks after right-sided effort thrombosis and thrombolytic therapy, demonstrating focal subclavian vein stenosis at the level of the first rib (arrow). (**B**) Intraoperative contrast venogram following paraclavicular thoracic outlet decompression and external venolysis, demonstrating residual subclavian vein lesion that was unresponsive to balloon angioplasty (arrow). (**C**) Completion intraoperative venogram following subclavian vein patch angioplasty. (**D**) Patient with right-sided effort thrombosis following paraclavicular decompression. Intraoperative venograms demonstrating residual subclavian vein stenosis after external venolysis, (**E**) with successful treatment by vein patch angioplasty. (**F**) Right-sided effort thrombosis. Preoperative venogram following thrombolysis, demonstrating persistent subclavian vein occlusion. (**G**) Intraoperative venogram following paraclavicular decompression, external venolysis, and subclavian vein reconstruction with a saphenous vein panel graft.

CLOSURE AND POSTOPERATIVE CARE

The supraclavicular and infraclavicular wounds are irrigated with saline. Hemostasis is achieved and any visible lymphatic leaks are controlled by suture ligature. If the pleura has been opened during the course of the operation, the chest cavity is evacuated of fluid; if not already entered, the pleural membrane is purposefully opened at the apex to facilitate postoperative drainage of fluid into the chest cavity. A #19 Blake closed-suction drain is passed through a stab wound adjacent to the supraclavicular incision and placed within the superior operative field lying posterior to the brachial plexus, with its tip extending into the pleura. The brachial plexus nerve roots are wrapped with a hyaluronidate-based gel membrane (Seprafilm, Genzyme Biosurgery, Cambridge, MA) to diminish postoperative adhesions, and the scalene fat pad is restored to its anatomic position and held in place with several tacking sutures. The platysma layer is closed with interrupted sutures and the skin is closed with a subcuticular stitch. Closure of the wrist wound is performed with a single layer of nylon skin sutures, with frequent palpation of the arteriovenous fistula to ensure the absence of compression.

Postoperative care includes ample use of pain medications, muscle relaxants, and anti-inflammatory agents. Chest radiographs are obtained for several days to monitor any collection of pleural fluid, which typically resolves over the course of the first week. The expected hospital stay is three to four days for patients undergoing operation for neurogenic TOS and five to six days for patients undergoing operation for arterial or venous TOS. The closed-suction drain is removed when daily output is less than 50 mL, which is typically in the office setting seven to 10 days after operation. In the presence of a substantial lymph leak (i.e., greater than 500 mL per day with chylous characteristics), the patient is maintained on a low-fat diet and treated with octreotide until the drainage diminishes. Inpatient physical therapy is started in all patients the day after operation to maintain range of motion. Postoperative rehabilitation is then overseen by a physical therapist from our institution with expertise in the management of TOS, in conjunction with a physical therapist located near the patient. No restrictions are placed on upper extremity activity beyond 12 weeks after operation.

In patients having operation for arterial or venous TOS, therapeutic anticoagulation is initiated several days after operation with intravenous heparin (with or without the addition of aspirin or clopidogrel), followed by low molecular weight heparin and conversion to warfarin. Anticoagulant and antiplatelet agents are maintained until 12 weeks after operation, then discontinued. For patients with venous TOS and a patent AV fistula, follow-up imaging studies are not performed in the absence of any symptoms of venous obstruction. These individuals undergo ligation of the AV fistula under local anesthesia 12 weeks after the primary operation, at which time follow-up contrast venography can be easily performed.

DISCUSSION

Supraclavicular exploration has become a widely utilized, versatile, and effective approach in the treatment of TOS. Although certain aspects of the surgical anatomy are quite familiar to most vascular surgeons, considerable attention must be given to procedural details in order to avoid inadequate decompression, serious injury to neurovascular structures, or predictable causes of recurrent compression. Compared to transaxillary first rib resection, supraclavicular exploration carries the advantage of wider exposure of all anatomic structures associated with thoracic outlet compression.[6,16,17] This allows complete resection of the anterior and middle scalene muscles to be achieved, as well as brachial plexus neurolysis with direct visualization of all five nerve roots. This approach also allows for resection of cervical ribs, anomalous first ribs, or the normal first rib. Another major advantage is that all forms of vascular reconstruction can also be accomplished through supraclavicular exposure and its variations without the need for repositioning the patient. Thus, thoracic outlet decompression through supraclavicular/ paraclavicular exploration is currently an ideal approach for all appropriately selected patients with all types of TOS, as well as for patients undergoing reoperations.

REFERENCES

1. Sanders RJ. *Thoracic Outlet Syndrome: A Common Sequelae of Neck Injuries*. Philadelphia: J. B. Lippincott Company; 1991.

2. Thompson RW, Petrinec D. Surgical treatment of thoracic outlet compression syndromes. I. Diagnostic considerations and transaxillary first rib resection. *Ann Vasc Surg*. 1997;11: 315–323.

3. Thompson RW, Petrinec D, Toursarkissian B. Surgical treatment of thoracic outlet compression syndromes. II. Supraclavicular exploration and vascular reconstruction. *Ann Vasc Surg*. 1997;11:442–451.

4. Roos DB. Transaxillary approach for first rib resection to relieve thoracic outlet syndrome. *Ann Surg*. 1966;163:354–358.

5. Qvarfordt PG, Ehrenfeld WK, Stoney RJ. Supraclavicular radical scalenectomy and transaxillary first rib resection for the thoracic outlet syndrome: a combined approach. *Am J Surg*. 1984;148:111–116.

6. Sanders RJ, Raymer S. The supraclavicular approach to scalenectomy and first rib resection: description of technique. *J Vasc Surg*. 1985;2:751–756.

7. Machleder HI. Transaxillary operative management of thoracic outlet syndrome. In: Ernst CB, Stanley JC, eds. *Current Therapy in Vascular Surgery, Second Edition*. Philadelphia: BC Decker; 1991:227–230.

8. Roos DB. Recurrent thoracic outlet syndrome after first rib resection. *Acta Chir Belg*. 1980; 79:363–372.

9. Cheng SW, Stoney RJ. Supraclavicular reoperation for neurogenic thoracic outlet syndrome. *J Vasc Surg*. 1994;19:565–572.

10. Ambrad-Chalela E, Thomas GI, Johansen KH. Recurrent neurogenic thoracic outlet syndrome. *Am J Surg*. 2004;187:505–510.

11. Altobelli GG, Kudo T, Haas BT, et al. Thoracic outlet syndrome: pattern of clinical success after operative decompression. *J Vasc Surg*. 2005;42:122–128.

12. Roos DB. Congenital anomalies associated with thoracic outlet syndrome. *Am J Surg*. 1976;132:771–778.

13. Thompson RW, Bartoli MA. Neurogenic thoracic outlet syndrome. In: Rutherford RB, ed. *Vascular Surgery, Sixth Edition*. Philadelphia: Elsevier Saunders; 2005:1347–1365.

14. Cheng SW, Reilly LM, Nelken NA, et al. Neurogenic thoracic outlet decompression: rationale for sparing the first rib. *Cardiovasc Surg*. 1995;3:617–623.

15. Fantini GA. Reserving supraclavicular first rib resection for vascular complications of thoracic outlet syndrome. *Am J Surg*. 1996;172:200–204.

16. Hempel GK, Shutze WP, Anderson JF, Bukhari HI. 770 consecutive supraclavicular first rib resections for thoracic outlet syndrome. *Ann Vasc Surg*. 1996;10:456–463.

17. Reilly LM, Stoney RJ. Supraclavicular approach for thoracic outlet decompression. *J Vasc Surg*. 1988; 8:329–334.

44

Axillary Approach for Thoracic Outlet Syndrome

Richard H. Pin, M.D. Ricardo Deleon, M.D.
Julie A. Freischlag, M.D.

Thoracic outlet syndrome (TOS) is a condition where the neurovascular structures leading to the arm are compressed in the space between the first rib and scalene muscles. There are three clinical types of TOS, depending on the primary structure involved. Neurogenic TOS is the most common type, comprising 95% of all cases. These patients often present with repetitive motion injury related to occupational stresses. Complaints of back and shoulder pain, or weakness and paresthesia in the hand, are common findings. These symptoms are usually caused by irritation of the C5-C7 and/or C8-T1 roots of the brachial plexus. The effects of C8-T1 root compression can be appreciated in ulnar nerve function that manifests as deficits in the fourth and fifth digits during physical examination. Oftentimes, a positive Tinel sign over the clavicle (Erb's point) will exacerbate symptoms down the affected arm. Tenderness may also be present over the anterior scalene muscle in the supraclavicular fossa.

Surgery for neurogenic TOS is reserved for patients who fail six to eight weeks of physical therapy targeted at increasing range of motion and reinforcing proper posture. Patients are encouraged to restructure their work environment to a more ergonomically appropriate setting. If physical therapy has already been attempted and unsuccessful, then a CT-guided anterior scalene block with lidocaine is usually performed. This block relaxes the anterior scalene muscle allowing the first rib to drop, which relieves tension on the brachial plexus. A successful anterior scalene block is an excellent indication that a first rib resection and anterior scalenectomy will benefit that patient.

The second most common type of thoracic outlet syndrome is the venous form that only constitutes 5% of all cases. This type of TOS is most often seen in athletes who have suffered an acute effort thrombosis of the axillosubclavian vein known as Paget-Schrotter Syndrome.[1] These patients are typically males in their late 20s to early 30s who have participated in some form of strenuous physical activity with the affected arm. They often present emergently with an acutely swollen upper extremity that has a bluish discoloration. A duplex scan is performed, indicating a partial or complete thrombosis of the subclavian and/or axillary vein. A venogram and catheter-directed lytic therapy may be used to recanalize the vein. These patients are then maintained on anticoagulation therapy. First rib resection is considered days to weeks later to prevent recurrent thrombosis of the vein. Following rib resection and scalenectomy, patients undergo repeat venogram, and any areas of venous stenosis can now be dilated in the absence of extrinsic compression. Even thrombosed veins will spontaneously open after rib resection while the patient is maintained on anticoagulation. Repeat duplex scans or venograms are essential studies for following a patient's progress.[2]

Arterial TOS is rare, constituting less than 1% of cases, and is often associated with a cervical rib. These patients present with complaints of intermittent arm or hand ischemia. These ischemic manifestations are due to stenosis caused by external compression or by embolization from an aneurysm. Patients can display numerous signs and symptoms including weakness, numbness, pain, pallor, and diminished pulses in the distal arm. An Adson's test helps in establishing the diagnosis. The patient is seated and the affected arm is elevated and flexed 90 degrees at the elbow. The patient is then asked to rotate his or her head toward the opposing side while the clinician feels for a radial pulse. Once the radial pulse is identified, the arm is maneuvered along a virtual horizontal plane while assessing if the pulse obliterates. A subclavian bruit can also be noted while performing the same maneuver. Patients have a duplex scan of the subclavian artery to assess the degree of stenosis or the presence of an aneurysm. In addition to first rib resection and scalenectomy, the artery frequently has to be replaced using the saphenous vein or prosthetic material to restore flow to the upper extremity.

Anatomically, the thoracic outlet is bounded by the first rib inferiorly and the clavicle medially, and spans the distance from the third portion of the subclavian artery to the axillary artery. Originating from the cervical spine, the anterior and middle scalene muscles insert onto the first rib, forming the scalene triangle within the thoracic outlet. These muscles have the potential to scar or hypertrophy, contributing to compression of neurovascular structures. The subclavius muscle, which occupies the angle between the clavicle and first rib, may also compress the subclavian vein contributing to venous TOS.

Patients that have been diagnosed with TOS and are considered to be surgical candidates can undergo either a transaxillary or supraclavicular approach to the thoracic outlet. The approach preferred for neurogenic and venous TOS is the transaxillary approach because of the anatomical visualization and effectiveness of decompression. The patient undergoes general anesthesia with a short acting neuromuscular blockade such as succinylcholine. The use of a short acting agent allows for safer dissection around the brachial plexus. After positioning in a lateral decubitus position, the patient is prepped from the neck to beyond the nipples, and an adjustable arm support (Machleder retractor) is attached to the OR bed (Figure 44–1). This device allows for elevation of the arm to facilitate exposure of the thoracic outlet. The arm is padded well prior to placement on the support to prevent injury to the median and ulnar nerves as they cross the elbow. The lateral edges of the lattisimus dorsi and pectoralis major muscles are palpated and marked. A skin incision is then made between these muscles on the lower border of the axillary hair line. The soft tissue of the axilla is divided with electrocautery to reach the flimsy areolar tissue superficial to the chest wall. Gentle finger dissection in an anterior and cephalad direction is used to reach the first rib as it approaches the clavicle. At this point, a self-retaining retractor is placed to separate the skin and superficial soft tissue, and the Machleder arm elevator is raised to gain exposure to the thoracic outlet.[3] The tissue overlying the brachial plexus, subclavian artery

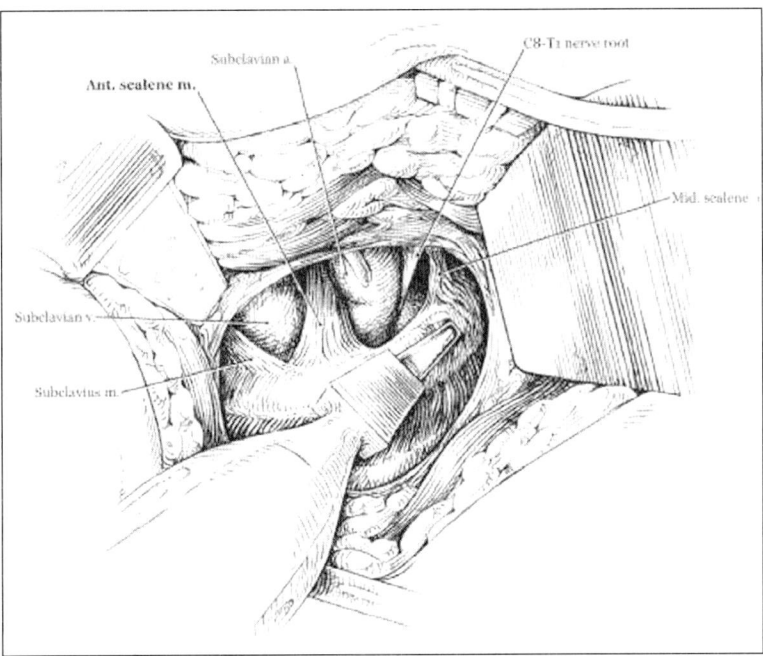

Figure 44-1. Machleder retractor used for positioning during transaxillary first rib resection. The patient is placed in a decubitus position with the nonoperative side down. Ample sterile towels are used for padding, and the arm is secured in the retractor with a combination of gauze and elastic wraps.

and vein, and scalene muscles are swept away with a Kitner dissector. Oftentimes, there is a branch of the subclavian artery that must be divided to fully expose and mobilize this vessel. The first rib is identified and the lower edge of the rib is bluntly cleared of its intercostal muscle attachments using a Kitner and a flat periosteal elevator (Figure 44–2). The first rib is lifted off the underlying pleura by gently sliding a small periosteal elevator between these structures. The pleura is pushed away from the rib; this mobilization should extend from behind the brachial plexus posteriorly to in front of the subclavian vein anteriorly. The subclavius muscle, which has a crescent-shaped ligamentous attachment on the first rib next to the subclavian vein, is sharply divided with a pair of scissors. Care is taken not to injure the vein. Division of the subclavius muscle provides greater anterior mobilization of first rib for resection, which is particularly important in situations of effort thrombosis. The scalene medius fibers that attach to the superior surface of the first rib are dissected off bluntly using a periosteal elevator. Sharp dissection of the scalene medius muscle is avoided because the long thoracic nerve courses adjacent to this muscle, and may be inadvertently divided. The anterior scalene muscle must be clearly visualized between the subclavian artery and vein. A right-angled clamp is then brought behind the anterior scalene muscle, lifting it away from the neighboring artery. The muscle is cut with scissors, leaving as much length attached to the rib as possible (Figure 44–3). This maneuver may need to be repeated in order to divide the entire muscle safely. A bone cutter is then placed anteriorly, and the first rib is divided adjacent to the subclavian vein. The posterior division of the rib occurs once the rest of the rib has been mobilized. This allows for optimal visualization of the brachial plexus to prevent injury when cutting the rib posteriorly. The rib cutter is gently applied to the rib just anterior to the brachial plexus (Figure 44–4). The rib is di-

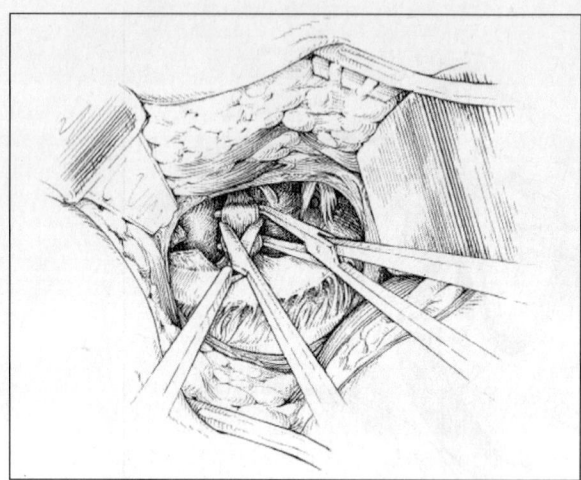

Figure 44-2. Gentle dissection of first rib with periosteal elevator.

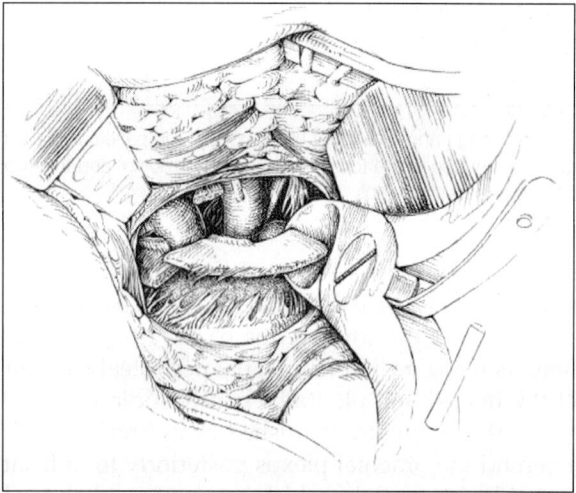

Figure 44-3. Anterior scalene muscle isolated by right-angle clamp prior to dissection.

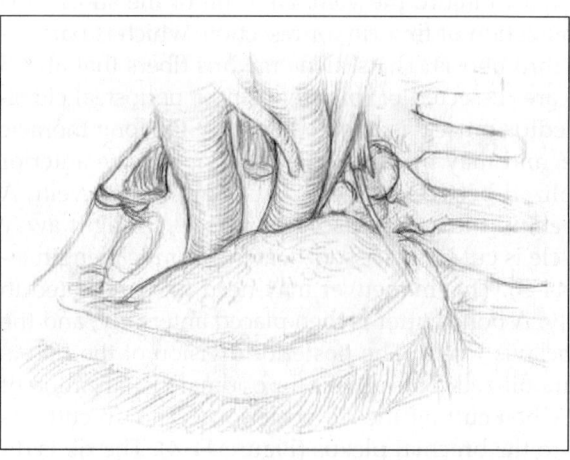

Figure 44-4. Bone cutter used to remove the first rib.

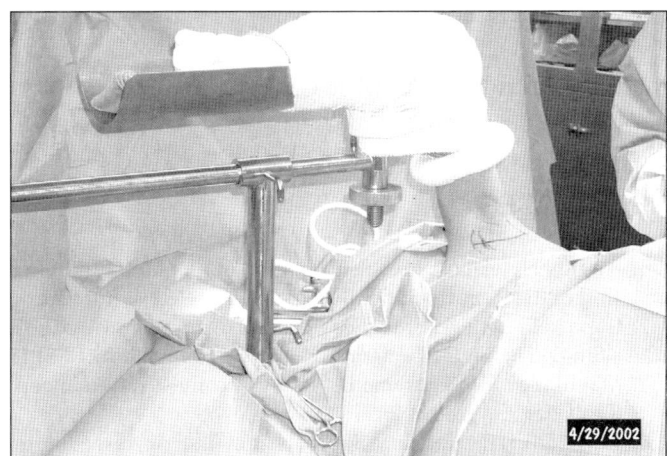

Figure 44-5. Anatomic space immediately prior to closure. The neurovascular structures are no longer restricted following rib resection.

vided and removed. The rib is always cut in front of the nerve so that posterior nerve roots are not unintentionally damaged. The remainder of the rib ends are then trimmed, using a bone rongeur. The nerve is pushed away from the bone and protected with a Roos retractor as the rib is rongeured posteriorly.[4] The bone edges should be fairly smooth and there should be no impingement on the neurovascular structures at this point (Figure 44–5) Saline is poured in the axillary cavity and the patient is given several positive pressure ventilations to check for tears in the parietal pleura. If a pneumothorax is present, a 12 Fr chest tube is inserted in the second intercostal space through a separate stab incision. The arm is then lowered and the axillary soft tissue is closed in two layers. If a chest tube has been placed, 20 cm of water suction is now applied.

Postoperatively, physical activity is restricted for two weeks and the patient's arm is supported in a sling. After two weeks, physical therapy is instituted, focusing on increased range of motion, stretching, and soft tissue massage. A patient's compliance with physical therapy plays a key role, not only for a successful recovery but also for minimizing the risk of recurrent injury. In cases of Paget-Schroetter Syndrome, patients should not resume anticoagulation until three days after surgery to lessen the chance of bleeding complications such as a chest wall hematoma or hemothorax. This cohort of occlusive venous patients undergoes a follow-up venogram two weeks postoperatively with additional venoplasty if necessary.[5] The patients are maintained on oral anticoagulation for three months at which time a follow-up duplex scan is performed. If no abnormalities are noted and the patient is asymptomatic, anticoagulation is stopped. Those who have undergone a vascular reconstruction of the subclavian artery, along with decompression, usually require antiplatelet therapy with aspirin alone for about three months, regardless of the conduit used (vein or prosthetic). Anticoagulation with warfarin is reserved for rare situations when repeat embolic events have compromised arterial flow and collateral circulation must be maintained. About 10% of all patients undergoing surgery for TOS will ultimately develop recurrent symptoms due to scar tissue formation. Scar tissue thickens and remodels for approximately two years following surgery, and its effects on the thoracic outlet can be minimized with physical therapy. For this reason, physical therapy and rehabilitation have become important for both functional recovery and avoiding recurring symptoms.

ACKNOWLEDGEMENT

Medical illustrations by Lydia Gregg.

REFERENCES

1. Angle N, Gelabert HA, Farooq MM, et al. Safety and efficacy of early surgical decompression of the thoracic outlet for Paget-Schoretter syndrome. *Ann Vasc Surg.* 2001;15:37–42.
2. Caparrelli DJ, Freischlag J. A Unified Approach to Axillosubclavian Venous Thrombosis in a Single Hospital Admission. *Semin Vasc Surg.* 2005;18(3):153–157.
3. Machleder HI. Thoracic outlet syndromes: new concepts from a century of discovery. *Cardiovasc Surg.* 1994;2:137–145.
4. Roos, DB. Transaxillary approach for first rib resection to relieve thoracic outlet compression syndrome. *Ann Surg.* 1966;163:354.
5. Perler BA, Mitchell SE. Percutaneous transluminal angioplasty and transaxillary first rib resection. A multidisciplinary approach to the thoracic outlet syndrome. *Am Surg.* 1986; 52:485–488.
6. Green RM, McNamara J, Ouriel K. Long-term follow-up after thoracic outlet decompression: An analysis of factors determining outcome. *J Vasc Surg.* 1991;14:739–746.

45

Palmar Ulnar Artery "Aneurysms"

Nicole M. Wheeler, M.D. Gregory L. Moneta, M.D.

Hand and finger ischemia may result from a variety of causes including autoimmune disorders, embolization from a cardiac or noncardiac proximal source, atherosclerotic occlusive disease, calciphylaxis, steal phenomenon from dialysis access procedures, or iatrogenic thrombosis of the brachial or forearm arteries. The initial clinical presentation is frequently Raynaud's syndrome and cold intolerance, but can also include ischemic digital pain, paresthesias, discoloration, ulceration or gangrene, and occasionally a palpable wrist or palmar mass. This chapter will focus on a specific cause of hand and finger ischemia: ulnar artery aneurysms in the palm. The etiology, diagnosis, and treatment of ulnar artery aneurysms will all be discussed.

The term ulnar artery aneurysm is a bit of a misnomer and somewhat misleading. Aneurysmal degeneration of the ulnar artery at the wrist is certainly observed; but in most cases of ulnar artery aneurysm, there is not a focal fusiform or sacular enlargement of the artery. Angiographically, the distal ulnar artery at the level of the wrist is not enlarged but rather has a somewhat "corkscrew" appearance, more consistent in appearance with fibromuscular disease than atherosclerotic aneurysmal degeneration (Figure 45–1). These lesions are associated with accumulation of what is presumed to be clot or platelet aggregates on an irregular luminal surface (Figure 45–2). Symptoms result from distal embolization of the accumulated material on the luminal surface of the ulnar artery to the digital arteries with resulting digital artery occlusion. Depending on the anatomy of the palmar arches, digital artery occlusions may occur in any finger and are not necessarily limited to the more medial fingers (Figure 45–1).

In adults, ulnar artery aneurysms are often associated with repetitive trauma to the hypothenar eminence. It is postulated the artery is damaged as it is crushed between some hard object and the hook of the hamate bone at the wrist. A typical patient is a blue collar worker who uses his hand, usually the dominant hand, as a hammer. Examples of so-called classic patients at risk for ulnar artery aneurysm include an auto mechanic who pounds hubcaps in place with his dominant hand, a carpenter aligning boards by striking them with the palm of his hand, or the machinists aligning metal parts. The lesions have also been associated with baseball players where presumably catching the hard baseball damages the artery. Other vocational situations involving repetitive hand trauma have also been implicated.

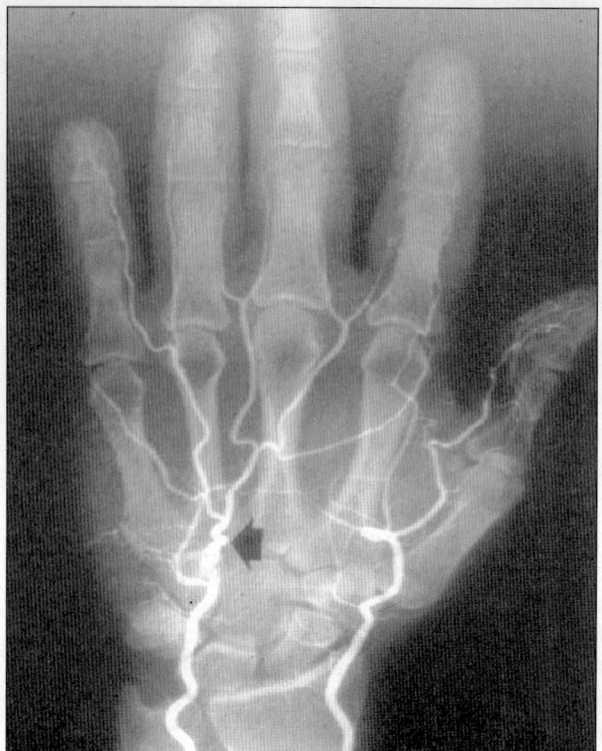

Figure 45-1. Arteriogram of a symptomatic hand demonstrating the typical "corkscrew" appearance of an abnormal ulnar artery. The palmar arch anatomy in this case permitted distal artery embolization to thesecond through fourth digits.

This clinical entity was first described in 1934 by Von Rosen[1] and later termed hypothenar hammer syndrome (HHS) by Conn et. al. in 1970.[2] A handful of pediatric cases of ulnar artery aneurysms have also been described. The existence of such cases raises the question of a congenital component to the etiology of this condition.[3-6] In addition, adults with ulnar artery aneurysms, when studied with bilateral hand angiography, can be found to have what appear to be changes in the ulnar artery of the nondominant hand, not subject to repetitive trauma, that mimic those of ulnar artery aneurysm. Given the presumed frequency of repetitive hand trauma in blue collar occupations, it seems logical that if repetitive trauma is the sole etiology of ulnar artery aneurysm, the condition ought to be more frequently encountered. Its rarity may re-

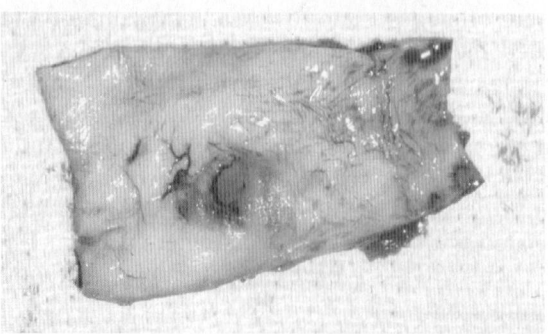

Figure 45-2. . Example of clot or platelet aggregate on the irregular luminal surface. Such material is the source of distal embolization to the digital arteries.

flect the fact that an infrequent underlying abnormality in association with repetitive trauma is required to produce a so-called ulnar artery aneurysm.

Evaluation of a patient for possible ulnar artery aneurysm begins with a history and physical examination, focusing on possible repetitive trauma to the hand and signs and symptoms of digital ischemia and Raynaud's syndrome. A palpable ulnar artery aneurysm or palmar mass is rarely present in patients embolizing from their distal ulnar artery.

Noninvasive upper extremity vascular laboratory testing should be performed. Upper extremity segmental pressures and Doppler derived waveforms should be obtained bilaterally from the axillary and brachial arteries, and from the radial and ulnar arteries at the level of the wrist. Finger photoplethysmographic waveforms and digital pressures should also be performed (Figure 45–3). Evaluation for autoimmune disease (complete blood count, erythrocyte sedimentation rate, multi-chem panel, antinuclear antibody, serum protein electrophoresis, rheumatoid factor, cold agglutinin assay, and hepatitis serology) can also be performed, but is not necessary if a large vessel source of embolization is discovered in a patient with unilateral symptoms of digital ischemia.

Duplex scanning may reveal occlusion or dilation of the distal ulnar artery. The absence of a duplex detected abnormality does not rule out ulnar artery pathology. The changes in the arterial lumen may be quite subtle; therefore, the gold standard for confirming or excluding "ulnar artery aneurysm" is contrast, catheter-based arteriography. The examination should include both upper extremities with visualization from the aortic arch to the fingertips, and magnification hand arteriography. Additional views using hand warming and intra-arterial vasodilators are used to visualize the digital arteries.

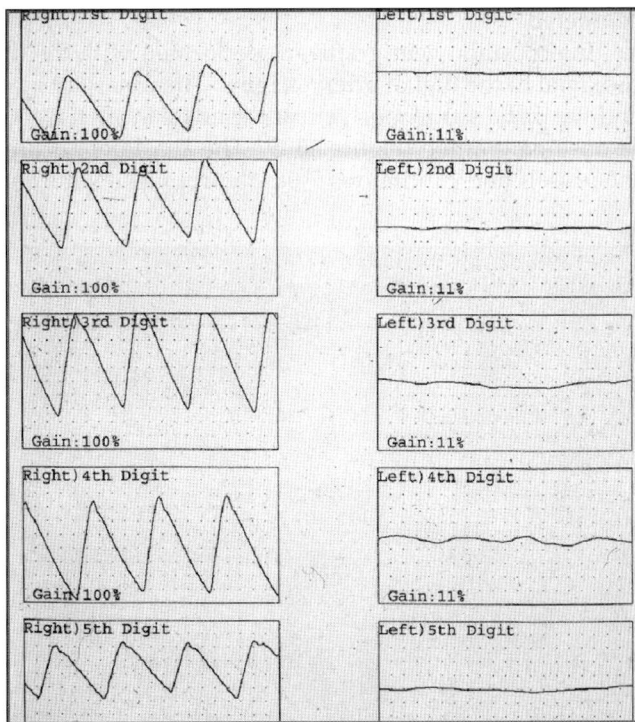

Figure 45-3. Finger plethysmography demonstrating unilateral dampened digital wave forms reflecting digital artery occlusions in a patient with a left-sided ulnar artery aneurysm.

The historical approach to treatment of symptomatic ulnar artery aneurysms in the palm has been observation with risk factor modification if symptoms were mild. Sympathectomy, with or without ligation/excision of the distal ulnar artery, was utilized for more severe symptoms. Currently, treatment is more commonly by excision and reconstruction, either by primary anastomosis or with autogenous vein interposition grafts.

It is tempting to consider thrombolytic therapy for digital artery occlusions secondary to embolization from an ulnar artery aneurysm. Such emboli are, however, likely to be chronic and, therefore, poorly responsive to thrombolytic therapy. The natural history of digital ischemic symptoms secondary to embolization from an ulnar artery aneurysm is to improve without tissue loss once the source of chronic embolization has been removed. The patients should be told to expect long-term cold intolerance of their affected digits, but that new or recurrent ulcers or a need for digital amputation is unusual.

Reconstruction of the ulnar artery is reserved for patent arteries at risk for persistent embolization. Collateralization in the hand is generally sufficient such that reconstruction of an occluded ulnar artery aneurysm is unlikely to provide a significant increase in digital blood flow. Exposure of the palmar ulnar artery is obtained through a longitudinal incision from the wrist crease to the superficial palmar arch. A sterile metal "hand" is used to hold the fingers extended (Figure 45–4). The artery is exposed where it lies just lateral to the hook of the hamate bone with the ulnar nerve lying immediately medial to the artery in the same plane. The deep branch of the ulnar artery generally courses medially between the pisiform bone and hook of the hamate bone, and then dives deep to join the deep palmar arch. There are no significant structures between the skin surface and the ulnar artery at this level, and exposure of the ulnar artery is quite straightforward, although periarterial inflammation is commonly encountered.

Interposition vein grafts are performed with the distal anastomosis generally just proximal to the digital artery origins. The ulnar artery is larger than one might expect; and the distal saphenous vein at the ankle is often a good size match for end-to-end interposition grafting (Figure 45–5). The anastomoses are performed with spatulation of the vessels and continuous 7-0 polypropylene suture under standard loop magnifica-

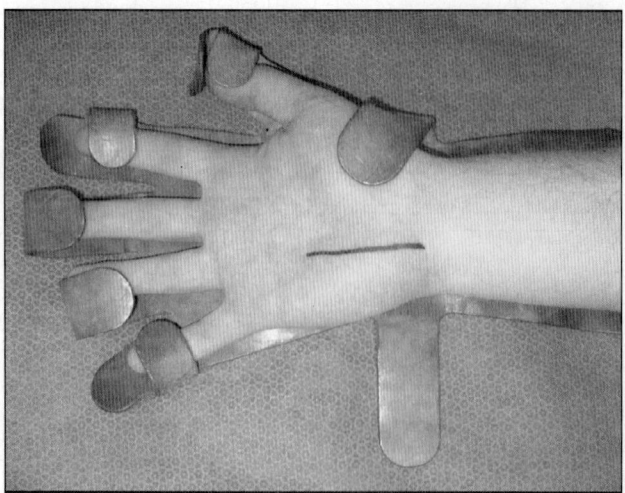

Figure 45-4. Lead-hand positioning device for repair of a palmar ulnar artery.

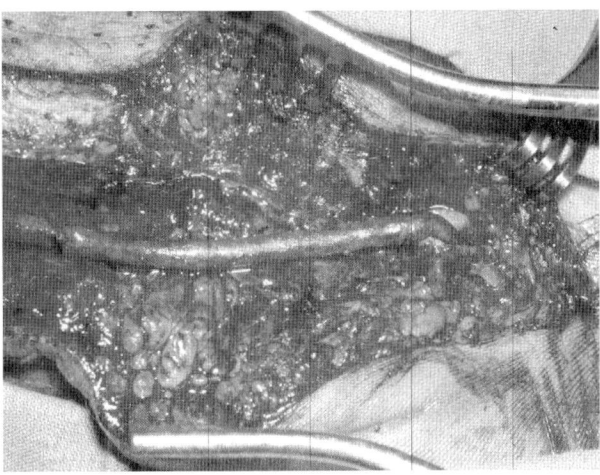

Figure 45-5. Palmar ulnar artery interposition vein graft.

tion. An operating microscope is not necessary in our opinion. Occasionally, the spatulation of the distal vein graft must be extended along with spatulation of the artery to include the origins of patent digital arteries into the distal anastomosis of the graft.

The largest series of abnormal palmar ulnar arteries treated by excision and reconstruction with reverse autogenous vein gafts was reported by Ferris et. al.[7] Twenty-one patients with occupational or avocational exposure to repetitive palmar trauma presented with symptoms of unilateral, and in one case bilateral, digital ischemia-digital pain, discoloration, and cold intolerance, with or without fingertip ulceration. Sixteen of the 21 patients were smokers, and none had a history of previous hand injury, Raynaud's syndrome, or connective tissue disorder. All patients underwent a preoperative work-up for hand ischemia as described above. Results of angiography proximal to the wrist were normal in all patients. Bilateral upper extremity angiography was completed in 13 patients, making a total of 34 ulnar arteries examined of which 33 were abnormal. Twelve of the abnormal ulnar arteries were found on an asymptomatic hand. The two most frequent angiographic findings were either occlusion of the palmar ulnar artery or the typical "corkscrew" appearance of the distal ulnar artery at the wrist.

Six patients with occluded palmar ulnar arteries had minimal symptoms that rapidly improved and, therefore, did not have an operation. The remaining 15 patients underwent a total of 21 operations consisting of one segmental excision and end-to-end anastomosis, one simple ligation, and 19 segmental excisions with interposition vein grafts. Minor ulcer debridement was required in one case; otherwise, all fingertip ulcers healed with conservative management. During the follow-up period, average 22 months, 16 grafts were clinically patent with palpable pulses. There were three graft occlusions, confirmed by imaging studies at 14, 15, and 35 months. Only one patient became symptomatic and required debridement of necrotic fingertips. These results are consistent with those published by Nehler et. al.[8] who had only one occluded graft out of 10 with an average of 15 months of follow-up. Other smaller case series of palmar ulnar artery "aneurysms" were treated by a variety of methods ranging from resection with reconstruction either by end-to-end anastomosis,[9-12] or via arterial[9] or venous interposition grafts,[9,11,13-16] ligation and resection alone,[12,17-22] or anticoagulation alone.[12] Two of the three largest series reported uniform improvement in vascular symptoms[11,12] with occasional persistent digital intolerance to cold.[11]

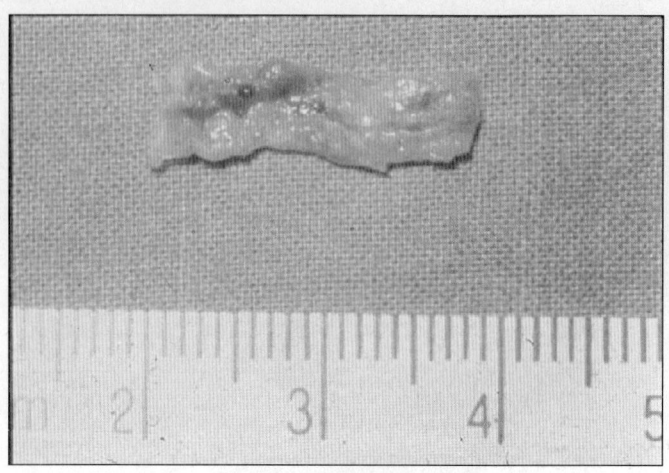

Figure 45-6. Operative specimen of an excised ulnar artery segment demonstrating luminal irregularity perhaps secondary to fibromuscular dysplasia.

As mentioned earlier, the histologic findings of ulnar artery specimens rarely show typical aneurysmal degeneration. Instead, histologic examination of 19 arterial specimens by Ferris et. al.[7] documented hyperplastic proliferation of the intima or media and disruption of the internal elastic lamina consistent with fibromuscular dysplasia supporting the hypothesis that development of HHS requires a preexisting abnormality of the ulnar artery (Figure 45–6). True palmar ulnar artery aneurysms[9-20,23-27] are an even rarer finding, as are pseudoaneurysms,[21-22,27] within the spectrum of HHS patients.

Hypothenar hammer syndrome is an infrequent condition when considering the large number of people who are exposed to repetitive palmar trauma. It should be thought of as a condition in which an abnormal ulnar artery, when subjected to repetitive trauma, forms a thrombus, resulting in symptomatic digital ischemia from distal embolization. Regardless of the pathology, surgical resection of the affected ulnar artery and vascular reconstruction has repeatedly shown generally good outcomes with minimal morbidity. The most experience has been with autogenous reverse interposition vein grafts or primary end-to-end anastomoses. This type of reconstruction should be the procedure of choice when there is a need to restore blood flow to affected digits, such as those cases of an incomplete palmar arch or poor collateral flow with impending digital necrosis.

REFERENCES

1. Von Rosen S. Ein Fall von Thrombose in der Arteria Ulnaris nach Einwirkung von Stumpfer Gewalt. *Acta Chir Scand*. 1934;73:500–506.
2. Conn J, Bergan JJ, Bell JL. Hypothenar hammer syndrome: posttraumatic digital ischemia. *Surgery*. 1970;68:1122–1128.
3. Al-Omran M. True ulnar artery aneurysm of the hand in an 18-month-old boy: a case report. *J Vasc Surg*. 2007;45(4):841–843.
4. Deune EG, McCarthy EF. Reconstruction of a true ulnar artery aneurysm in a 4-year-old patient with radial artery agenesis. *Orthopedics*. 2005;28(12):1459–1461.
5. Witt PD, Bowen KA, Johansen K. True ulnar artery aneurysm of the hand in an 8-year-old boy. *Plast Reconstr Surg*. 2003;111(7):2475–2476.

6. Offer GJ, Sully L. Congenital aneurysm of the ulnar artery in the palm. *J Hand Surg [Br]*. 1999;24(6):735–737.

7. Ferris BL, et al. Hypothenar hammer syndrome: proposed etiology. *J Vasc Surg*. 2000; 31:104–113.

8. Nehler MR, et al. Upper extremity arterial bypass distal to the wrist. *J Vasc Surg*. 1992;16(4): 633–640.

9. Dethmers RS, Houpt P. Surgical management of hypothenar and thenar hammer syndromes: a retrospective study of 31 instances in 28 patients. *J Hand Surg [Br]*. 2005;30(4): 419–423.

10. Unlu Y, Ceviz M, Polat P. False aneurysm in the palmar segment of the ulnar artery: report of a case. *Surg Today*. 2003;33(2):148–150.

11. De Monaco D, et al. Hypothenar hammer syndrome: retrospective study of nine cases. *J Hand Surg [Br]*. 1999;4(6):731–734.

12. Rothkopf DM et al. Surgical management of ulnar artery aneurysms. *J Hand Surg*. 1990; 15(6):891–897.

13. Troum SJ, Floyd WE, Sapp J. Ulnar artery thrombosis: a 6-year experience. *J South Orthop Assoc*. 2001;10(3):147–154.

14. Brodmann M, et al. Hypothenar hammer syndrome caused by posttraumatic aneurysm of the ulnar artery. *Wien Klin Wochenschr*. 2001;113(17–18):698–700.

15. Bakhach J, Chahidi N, Conde A. Hypothenar hammer syndrome: management of distal embolization by intra-arterial fibrinolytics. *Chir Main*. 1998;17(30):215–220.

16. Taylor LM. Hypothenar hammer syndrome. *J Vasc Surg*. 2003;37(3):697.

17. Galati G, et al. True aneurysm of the ulnar artery in a soccer goalkeeper: a case report and surgical considerations. *Am J Sports Med*. 2003;31(3):457–458.

18. Rainer C, et al. Compression of the ulnar nerve caused by an aneurysm of the ulnar artery in an HIV-positive patient. *Plast Reconstr Surg*. 2002;110(2):533–536.

19. Yoshii S, Ikeda K, Murakami H. Ulnar nerve compression secondary to ulnar artery true aneurysm at Guyon's canal. *J Neurosurg Sci*. 1999;43(4):295–297.

20. Balakrishnan C, et al. Mycotic aneurysm of the ulnar artery distal to the wrist. *Clin Infect Dis*. 1998;26(6):1470–1471.

21. Erdoes LS, Brown WC. Ruptured ulnar artery pseudoaneurysm. *Ann Vasc Surg*. 1995;9(4): 394–396.

22. Birrer M, Baumgartner I. Images in clinical medicine: work-related vascular injuries of the hand-hypothenar hammer syndrome. *N Engl J Med*. 2002;347(5):339.

23. Coulier B, et al. Colour duplex sonographic and multislice spiral CT angiographic diagnosis of ulnar artery aneurysm in hypothenar hammer syndrome. *JBR-BTR*. 2003;86(4):211–214.

24. Lorelli DR, Shepard AD. Hypothenar hammer syndrome: an uncommon and correctable cause of digital ischemia. *J Cardiovasc Surg*. 2002;43(1):83–85.

25. Velling TE, et al. Sonographic diagnosis of ulnar artery aneurysm in hypothenar hammer syndrome: report of 2 cases. *J Ultrasound Med*. 2001;20(8):921–924.

26. Torre J. Ulnar artery aneurysm with digital ischemia. *Vasc Med*. 1999;4(3):143–145.

27. Filis K, et al. Expanding ulnar artery aneurysm presenting with signs of threatened rupture. *Acta Chir Belg*. 2006;106(1):101–103.

46

Hand Ischemia in End-Stage Renal Disease

Paul B. Kreienberg, M.D., Benjamin B. Chang, M.D.,
Sean P. Roddy, M.D., R. Clement Darling III, M.D.,
Philip S.K. Paty, M.D., Kathleen J. Ozsvath, M.D.,
Manish Mehta, M.D., M.P.H., and Dhiraj M. Shah, M.D.

Unlike the lower extremity, the upper extremity is less likely to be involved with critical ischemia. Even in those few patients presenting with symptomatic occlusive disease, involvement of the axillary, subclavian, and brachial arteries are more commonly seen. In fact, the arteries of the forearm are so infrequently encountered that a standard text encompassing upper extremity vascular disorders does no more than briefly mention this topic.[1] While it seems to be virtually nonexistent in the majority of patients, even in those with diabetes, occlusive disease of the infrabrachial arteries combined with critical limb ischemia is encountered in patients with end-stage renal failure. Hand and finger ischemia has been reported with increasing frequency in patients with end-stage renal disease (ESRD). The etiologic backgrounds of this disease process are multiple and include thrombosis, accelerated atherosclerosis, and diffuse arterial calcification. The origin of this condition may well involve atherosclerosis, but the association with calciphylaxis does exist.[2] Presentations range from digital rest pain and ulceration to gangrene. These conditions occasionally require digital amputation, and in severe cases, hand amputation. It is difficult to accurately determine the prevalence of this problem. Management of these patients may require vascular reconstructive techniques that are more commonly applied to the lower extremity to prevent or delay amputation.

Another clinical situation of hand ischemia encountered in the patient with ESRD is that associated with ipsilateral upper extremity arteriovenous fistula. The onset of hand ischemia is a devastating complication of upper extremity hemodialysis access. Arteriovenous shunts are almost always associated with some degree of reduced arterial flow to the distal circulation.[3] Untreated, this may produce pain, ulceration, and gangrene in a previously viable extremity. While prevention of this complication remains paramount, several techniques are available to manage this problem once diagnosed. This chapter describes the diagnosis and management of steal associated ischemia as well as our experience with critical upper extremity ischemia caused by infrabrachial disease in renal failure patients.

ISCHEMIC STEAL IN PATIENTS WITH ARTERIOVENOUS FISTULAE

Arterial insufficiency usually manifests itself as a steal syndrome. This syndrome can occur at any time after creation of the vascular access formation with signs and symptoms of ischemia, and in some situations, may be worse while the patient is on dialysis. In its severe form, patients may have the classic signs of pain, paresthesia and paralysis, and pallor and coolness. Ischemic steal can be found in 2–9% of access operations and are more commonly found the higher one places the fistula in the arm.[4]

It is important to make the diagnosis early in order to maximize limb salvage. Helpful tests in the diagnosis of ischemic steal include pulse volume recordings of the extremity with and without compression. Angiography of the extremity with and without compression of the fistula is then also performed to confirm the diagnosis as well as to plan operative therapy. Angiographic evaluation should also include the inflow vessels as a significant percentage of patients with steal will have it secondary to an inflow stenosis.

A number of steps can be taken to reduce the incidence of this problem. These include making the fistula as distal as possible in the extremity with the wrist being preferred to the elbow. Additionally, there is benefit in reducing steal complications by making end-to-side rather than side-to-side anastomosis and limiting the size of the arteriotomies to 5–7 mm.

Patients with mild symptoms can be managed conservatively as long as they are closely monitored. Patients with more severe presentations should be evaluated expeditiously and promptly treated.

A number of treatment options exist for management of this problem. Obviously, ligation of the fistula is the most rapid solution of the ischemic problem; however, this leaves the patient without a conduit for dialysis. This option should be reserved for situations where the ischemia manifests early and with severe symptoms. Ligation of the fistula is a quick, simple, and effective way to reverse steal.

Other techniques available are designed to maintain patency of this fistula while reducing or limiting the symptoms of vascular steal. Banding of the venous conduit has been described to decrease the blood flow through the conduit and, therefore, reduce the symptoms.[5] The main drawback to the banding of the outflow tract is that a fine line is walked between reducing steal and maintaining adequate flow through the conduit to prevent thrombosis. Use of intraoperative pulse volume recordings may be of benefit to determine how much plication should be performed.

Presently, the technique receiving the most attention is that of distal arterial ligation and bypass (DRIL). This procedure combines correction of the vascular steal with continuing use of the access site.[6] The technique involves ligating the artery just distal to the anastomosis and placing a bypass graft of vein from above the access anastomosis to just below the site of the ligation. This procedure offers benefits overbanding because the plication technique increases the resistance in the fistula, and in the face of fixed inflow pressure, a smaller amount is shunted through the fistula.[7] Although this will improve distal perfusion, it creates a lowered flow state in the fistula that may produce thrombosis. Unlike banding, the DRIL procedure functions as a low resistance parallel circuit. By reducing the ratios between the systemic circulation and the fistula, the shunt fraction is decreased and distal perfusion is increased. The net result is increased distal perfusion while maintaining shunt flow. Results show access patency of 94% at 18 months with resolution of ischemic symptoms in almost all patients.[6]

HAND ISCHEMIA IN PATIENTS WITH ESRD

Patients with ESRD and upper extremity occlusive disease occasionally present with limb threatening upper extremity ischemia. This may be in the absence of functioning shunts as described above. These are often patients with advanced arteriosclerosis and calciphylaxsis. The following is our experience in the management of this subset of patients who required bypass for limb salvage.

MATERIALS AND METHODS

All patients with end-stage renal disease presenting with ulceration or gangrene of the upper extremities were reviewed from 1992 to 2002. Patients with documented arteritis, myeloproliferative disorders, immunoglobulin abnormalities, disseminated intravascular coagulation, acute ischemia, embolization, or iatrogenic causes of upper extremity ischemia were excluded. Patients with previous radial artery fistulas or patent upper arm fistulas were also removed from analysis.

Patients were evaluated initially via clinical exam coupled with pulse volume recordings and segmental arterial pressures down to the finger level. Blood samples were obtained and tested for evidence of connective tissue disorders, immunoglobulin abnormalities, and coagulation disorders.

Patients found to have significant occlusive disease by noninvasive testing underwent further arterial imaging. Patients who were determined to have nonreconstructible disease by angiography were excluded. Patients were deemed nonreconstructible if there were no bypassable segmental stenosis or occlusions seen on arteriography (true small-vessel.disease). The remainder underwent vein mapping by ultrasound to locate a suitable venous conduit. After successful reconstruction, patients with digital gangrene had debridement and/or amputation of the affected digits as necessary.

Data were retrieved through our computerized vascular registry and medical records. Bypass patency was monitored at office visits at least every three months during the first postoperative year followed by six-month intervals thereafter. Follow-up noninvasive studies also included Duplex evaluation of the forearm graft. Patency, salvage, and survival rates were determined using life table methods.

RESULTS

Over this 10-year period, fifteen patients and eighteen upper extremities with chronic critical ischemia were found to be reconstructible and underwent autogenous vein bypass using the brachial artery as the inflow site. The mean age of this patient group was 52 (range: 32–74). Eight (53%) patients were diabetic; nine (60%) patients were male. Fifteen (83%) limbs had digital and hand gangrene while the remaining three (17%) had ischemic digital ulcers. Five patients (seven limbs) had lower extremity necrotic lesions that had been previously diagnosed as calciphylaxis. Four patients (five limbs) presented with nonhealing, gangrenous digital amputation sites. All had evidence of cellulitis and wet gangrene in the face of intravenous antibiotics and aggressive wound care. In addition, pain was a marked symptom in all cases. Six other patients underwent arteriography only to be deemed nonreconstructible. Palmar arch patency was not used as a criterion for selection and was completely intact in none of these cases in this series.

All 15 patients had chronic renal failure; six patients had functioning renal transplants and three had previous nonfunctioning renal transplants. Those patients lacking functional transplants were maintained on hemodialysis in six cases and peritoneal dialysis in three cases. Two patients had had previous brachial arteriovenous loop PTFE fistulas that were occluded in the affected limb. Neither of these limbs showed evidence of stenosis at the arterial anastomotic site.

Arteriography employed standard contrast agents in 12 patients. In those patients who had renal transplants but elevated serum creatinine levels, carbon dioxide and gadolinium were used to image the arteries. No limbs had significant axillosubclavian lesions. One limb had a 50% stenosis of the brachial artery related to an old nonfunctioning arteriovenous fistula (treated with a PTFE patch angioplasty).

Distal bypasses were attempted in all 18 limbs using autogenous vein grafts (upper arm vein in eight and greater saphenous vein in 10). The inflow site for every bypass was the distal brachial artery at or below the elbow crease. The outflow vessel was the radial artery in the anatomic snuffbox in 15 (83%) cases and the distal ulnar artery in three (17%) cases. Veins were reversed in nine cases and orthograde in nine.

There was no perioperative mortality in this series. Several patients required prolonged hospitalizations for the management of associated medical problems. The average length of stay postoperatively was seven days.

Two (11%) bypasses occluded in the early postoperative period. One bypass to the ulnar artery occluded within a few hours of completion and thrombosis was felt to be secondary to poor outflow. No revision was attempted because there was no reasonable alternative to salvage the bypass. The other bypass occlusion occurred one week after surgery and the patient declined reoperation. In the remaining 16 bypasses in 13 patients, patency was maintained during a follow-up ranging from 3–40 months, (mean 18 months, no bypass was revised). One bypass was found on routine Duplex scan to have a layer of nonocclusive thrombus but is patent 23 months postoperatively.

All patent bypasses produced improved hand perfusion as assessed by clinical and vascular laboratory testing. The pulsatility of digital plethysmography, which was uniformly flat (Class 4 or 5) preoperatively, returned in all cases postoperatively (Class 2 or 3). Digital pressure measurements were not useful due to the heavy arterial calcification in this group.

Pain relief was the most notable benefit of successful bypass. All patients reported significant reduction in pain and the need for narcotic analgesia. Several of the patients were able to leave the hospital where they had been kept for up to several weeks simply for pain relief.

Limbs presenting with gangrene underwent numerous digital amputations and debridements. There were 28 finger amputations in this group, all for preexisting gangrene. Twelve involved the distal phalanx. Twelve involved the proximal phalanx. Four involved the entire finger and metacarpal head. While healing of these amputations was slow, none had to be revised. The goals of revascularization, pain reduction, and limb/tissue salvage were achieved in all patients (16/18) with patent bypass grafts.

Postoperative survival was poor, as one would expect in this group of patients. One of the two patients with occluded bypasses died eight months postoperatively. Of the 13 patients with 16 patent bypasses, six patients with seven bypasses died 18, 20, 23, 24, 27, and 30 months postoperatively. The cause of death was cardiac arrest in five patients (four during or immediately after dialysis) and multisystem organ failure with refusal to continue dialysis in one patient (two bypasses).

DISCUSSION

Access induced ischemia is an infrequently occurring problem that carries significant consequences. Ideal management of this mandates resolving the ischemia while maintaining functioning access for dialysis. Experience with banding as treatment has been mixed but generally poor, and often long-term relief of steal is not realized. As mentioned previously, the inherent problem with banding is the increased resistance in the outflow conduit. At present, the DRIL procedure represents the most sound, physiologic solution to the problem of angio-access induced steal. By functioning as a large, low resistance arterial collateral, it improves perfusion in the distal arteries beyond the access while the ligation eliminates steal. In this matter, it improves distal perfusion and maintains access patency. The DRIL procedure provides the method that most reliably achieves the goals of eliminating steal and maintaining access patency in a durable manner.

Although the occurrence of symptomatic distal upper extremity chronic occlusive disease is decreasingly small in most large series, it may present more frequently in patients with chronic renal failure. Though grossly resembling occlusions seen in atherosclerotic lower extremity disease, there are clearly other factors that make some patients more prone to tissue loss than others. The presentation of occlusive lesions in the relatively young (as compared to the general population with symptomatic atherosclerosis) may in some way be related to their renal failure. Since several of these patients were known to have calciphylaxis, it seems likely that this was also a principal contributor to the development of ischemic lesions. Whether the entire group of patients had some degree of calciphylaxis is difficult to determine, as tissue samples were not available for retrospective review in most cases. However, calciphylaxis usually involves medial calcification of cutaneous arteries in the range of 0.1 mm in diameter, not the larger ulnar and radial arteries seen to be occluded in this series.[8] Calciphylaxis is relatively poorly understood at this time and its relationship to the arterial calcification seen in many patients with and without renal failure is not clear. What is clear is that calciphylaxis is associated with a high mortality rate, estimated at 60–90%, and many patients survive only a few months, even with aggressive management and parathyroidectomy.[2, 8, 9] Patient mortality appears to be related to sepsis from wound infections. Foot gangrene in these patients has a high association with death from sepsis.[10] More proximal leg lesions may not carry quite as dismal a prognosis.[11]

Given the atypical nature and location of their occlusive disease, the patients in this series presented with the familiar hallmarks of chronic critical ischemia, ischemic pain, ulceration, and gangrene, and lent themselves to conventional bypass techniques. Patient evaluation utilized conventional arteriography augmented with the use of non-nephrotoxic contrast materials when indicated. Bypasses, utilizing reversed or nonreversed excised vein grafts, were performed from the distal brachial artery, which was only mildly or moderately calcified. The distal bypass sites, the radial and ulnar arteries were, however, very densely calcified and difficult to manipulate. Performing the distal arteriotomy was the most difficult part of the procedure and the two failures in this series may have been related to disruption of the plaque during this step. Arterial control was achieved utilizing Yasargil clips; however, continued bleeding during the performance of the anastomosis was common and managed with the combined use of irrigation and continuous aspiration.

The results of the arterial bypasses in this series have been gratifying. Reported experiences with distal lower extremity bypass in renal failure patients have not generally carried a good outcome, with significantly lower bypass patency and higher limb loss compared to patients without renal failure.[12-14] Calciphylaxis, present in many of our cases, has been reported to be a poor prognostic indicator for limb salvage after lower leg bypass.[15] We attribute the satisfactory patency in this group of forearm bypasses to the use of short autogenous vein bypass grafts, careful anastomotic technique, and the selection of patients with favorable arterial anatomy, i.e., segmental forearm artery occlusions with preservation of enough of the palmar arteries to provide adequate outflow.

In addition, we feel that limb salvage was aided by the upper extremity location in that the absence of the stress of weight-bearing allowed patients to better protect their fingers and hands from trauma. Furthermore, the principal indication in this group of patients was not so much the tissue loss but rather the attendant pain and infection, which deterred the use of the limb and hand. A patent bypass uniformly reduced pain to much more manageable levels, which we regard as the most important benefit of these reconstructions.

Patient survival in this group was, not surprisingly, relatively poor given the limited survival of renal failure patients in general and of patients with calciphylaxis in particular.[2,8,9] Remarkably, no patient with a functioning transplant died during the study period, while half the patients maintained on dialysis died during follow-up.

These bypasses have only been performed at our institution for the past decade, and principally during the past five years. This does not infer that such patients did not exist previously; rather, they were managed with cervical sympathectomy, amputation, and pain medications. However, the increased success achieved with lower extremity bypass procedures convinced us that some of these cases might also benefit from revascularization. A successful bypass produced a significant and gratifying improvement in the quality of life of these chronically ill individuals with admittedly limited longevity. The relative roles and benefits of bypass surgery versus parathyroidectomy in renal failure patients with upper extremity occlusive disease and calciphylaxis remains to be elucidated.

REFERENCES

1. Williamson K, Edwards JM, Taylor LM, et al. Small Artery Disease of the Upper Extremity. In: Machleder HI, ed. *Vascular Disorders of the Upper Extremity, 3rd edition.* New York: Futura; 1998:289–314.

2. Coates T, Kirkland GS, Dymock RB, et al. Cutaneous necrosis from calcific uremic arteriopathy. *Am J Kidney Dis.* 1995; 32(3):384–391.
3. Goff CD, Sato DT, Bloch PH, et al. Steal syndrome complicating hemodialysis access procedures: can it be predicted? *Ann Vasc Surg.* 2000;14:138–144.
4. Morsy AH, Kulbaski M, Chen C, et al. Incidence and characteristics of patients with hand ischemia after a hemodialysis access procedure *J Surg Res.* 1998;74:8–10.
5. Rivers SP, Scher LA, Veith FJ. Correction of steal syndrome secondary to hemodialysis access fistula: A simplified quantitative technique. *Surgery.* 1992;112(3):593–597.
6. Berman, SS, Gentile AT, Glickman MH, et al. Distal revascularization-interval ligation for limb salvage and maintenance of dialysis access in ischemic steal syndrome *J Vasc Surg.* 1997;26(3):393–402.
7. Wixon CL, Hughes JD, Mills JL. Understanding strategies for the treatment of ischemic steal syndrome after hemodialysis access. *J Am Coll Surg* 2000;191(3):301–310.
8. Fischer AH, Morris DJ. Pathogenesis of calciphylaxis: Study of three cases with literature review. *Hum Pathol.* 1995;26:1055–1064.
9. Hafner J, Keusch G, Wahl K, et al. Uremic small-artery disease with medial calcification and intimal hyperplasia (so-called calciphylaxis): A complication of chronic renal failure and benefit of parathyroidectomy. *J Am Acad Dermatol.* 1995;33(6):954–962.
10. Davis CA, Valentine, RJ. Wet gangrene in hemodialysis patients with calciphylaxis is associated with a poor prognosis. *Cardiovasc Surg.* 2001; 9:565–570.
11. Howe SC, Murray JD, Reeves RT, et al. Calciphylaxis, a poorly understood clinical syndrome: Three case reports and a review of the literature. *Ann Vasc Surg.* 2001;15(4):470–473.
12. Mills JL, Gahtan V, Fujitani RM, et al. The Utility and Durability of Vein Bypass Grafts Originating from the Popliteal Artery for Limb Salvage. *Am J of Surg* 1994;168: 646–651.
13. Edwards JM, Taylor LM, Porter JM. Limb Salvage in End-Stage Renal Disease. *Arch Surg.* 1998;123:1164–1168.
14. Chang BB, Paty PSK, Shah DM, Kaufman JL, Leather RP. Results of infrainguinal bypass for limb salvage in patients with end-stage renal disease. *Surgery.* 1990;108:742–747.
15. Mureebe L, Moy M, Balfour E, et al. Calciphylaxis: A poor prognostic indicator for limb salvage. *J Vasc Surg.* 2001;33(6):1275–1279.

Index